CLINICAL NEUROSURGERY

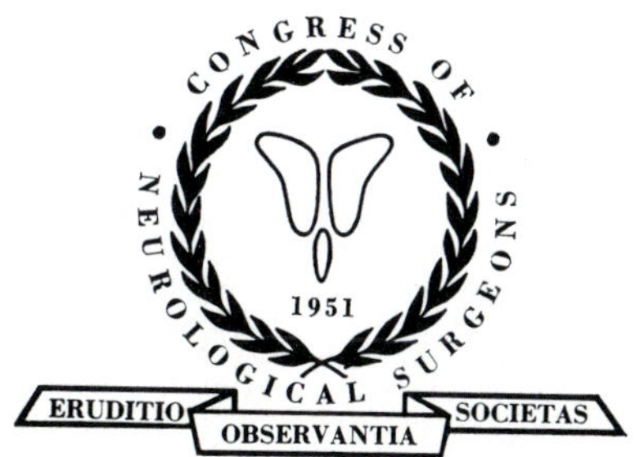

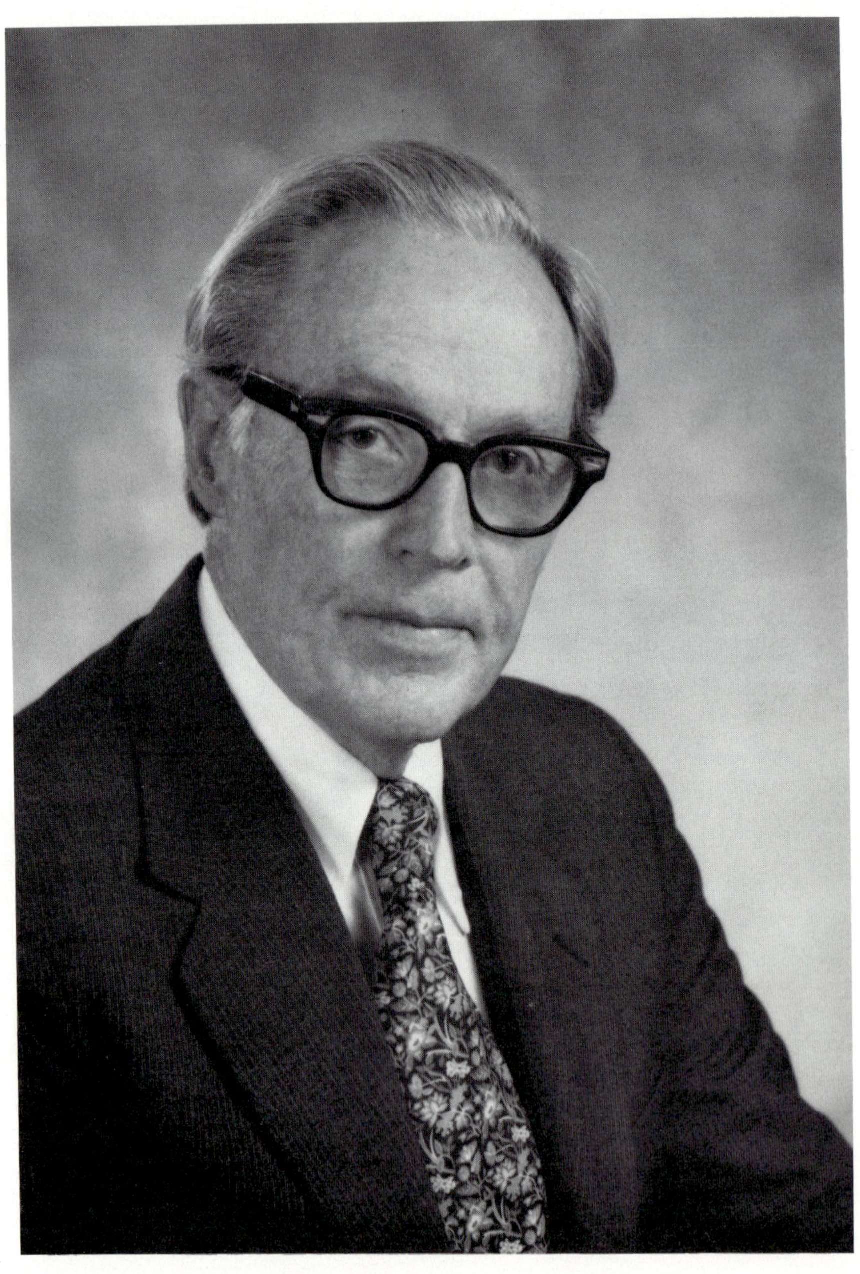

Eben Alexander, Jr., M.D.

CLINICAL NEUROSURGERY

Proceedings

OF THE

CONGRESS OF NEUROLOGICAL SURGEONS

Houston, Texas

1980

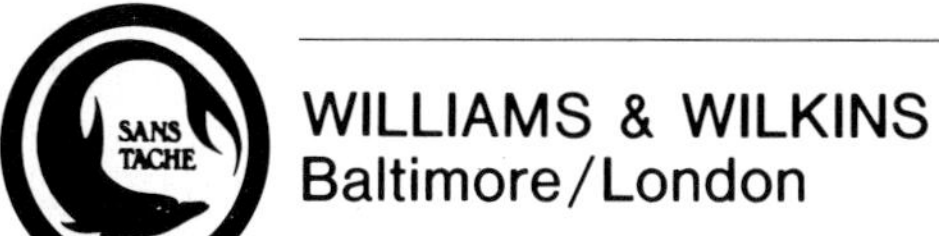

WILLIAMS & WILKINS
Baltimore/London

1981

Made in the United States of America

Library of Congress Cataloging in Publication Data

Clinical neurosurgery. The Library of Congress cataloged the first printing as follows:

Congress of Neurological Surgeons.
Clinical neurosurgery. Proceedings. v.1-1953-
Baltimore, Williams & Wilkins
v. illus. 24 cm. annual.

1. Nervous system—Surgery. I. Title.

RD593.A1C63 617.48 54-12666 rev

Library of Congress [r57fl]

ISBN 0-683--02023-4

COMPOSED AND PRINTED AT
WAVERLY PRESS, INC.
Mt. Royal and Guilford Aves.
BALTIMORE, MD. 21202, U.S.A.

Honored Guests

1952—Professor Herbert Olivecrona, Stockholm, Sweden
1953—Sir Geoffrey Jefferson, Manchester, England
1954—Dr. Kenneth G. McKenzie, Toronto, Canada
1955—Dr. Carl W. Rand, Los Angeles, California
1956—Dr. Wilder G. Penfield, Montreal, Canada
1957—Dr. Francis C. Grant, Philadelphia, Pennsylvania
1958—Dr. A. Earl Walker, Baltimore, Maryland
1959—Dr. William J. German, New Haven, Connecticut
1960—Dr. Paul C. Bucy, Chicago, Illinois
1961—Professor Eduard A. V. Busch, Copenhagen, Denmark
1962—Dr. Bronson S. Ray, New York, New York
1963—Dr. James L. Poppen, Boston, Massachusetts
1964—Dr. Edgar A. Kahn, Ann Arbor, Michigan
1965—Dr. James C. White, Boston, Massachusetts
1966—Dr. Hugo A. Krayenbuhl, Zurich, Switzerland
1967—Dr. W. James Gardner, Cleveland, Ohio
1968—Professor Norman M. Dott, Edinburgh, Scotland
1969—Dr. Wallace B. Hamby, Cleveland, Ohio
1970—Dr. Barnes Woodhall, Durham, North Carolina
1971—Dr. Elisha S. Gurdjian, Detroit, Michigan
1972—Dr. Francis Murphey, Memphis, Tennessee
1973—Dr. Henry G. Schwartz, St. Louis, Missouri
1974—Dr. Guy L. Odom, Durham, North Carolina
1975—Dr. William H. Sweet, Boston, Massachusetts
1976—Dr. Lyle A. French, Minneapolis, Minnesota
1977—Dr. Richard C. Schneider, Ann Arbor, Michigan
1978—Dr. Charles G. Drake, London, Ontario, Canada
1979—Dr. Frank H. Mayfield, Cincinnati, Ohio
1980—Dr. Eben Alexander, Jr., Winston-Salem, North Carolina

Officers of the Congress of Neurological Surgeons 1980

ROBERT H. WILKINS, M.D.
President

J. FLETCHER LEE, M.D.
President-Elect

JULIAN T. HOFF, M.D.
Vice-President

EDWARD R. LAWS, JR., M.D.
Secretary

EDWARD F. DOWNING, M.D.
Treasurer

EXECUTIVE COMMITTEE
David L. Kelly, Jr., M.D.

PETER W. CARMEL, M.D.
E. FLETCHER EYSTER, M.D.
JOSEPH C. MAROON, M.D.
GEORGE OJEMANN, M.D.
J. CHARLES RICH, M.D.

CHRISTOPHER B. SHIELDS, M.D.
DONALD O. QUEST, M.D.
BRUCE F. SORENSEN, M.D.
DONALD H. STEWART, JR., M.D.
JOHN M. TEW, JR., M.D.

J. CHARLES RICH, JR., *Chairman, Annual Meeting Committee*
CLARK WATTS, *Chairman, Scientific Program Committee*

Contributors

Charles F. Abboud, M.D., Department of Neurological Surgery, Mayo Medical School and Mayo Clinic, Rochester, Minnesota (*Chapter 6*)

Eben Alexander, Jr., M.D., Professor, Section of Neurosurgery, Bowman Gray School of Medicine, Winston-Salem, North Carolina (*Chapters 17, 18, 19*)

A. Allen, M.D., Department of Neurology, University of California, California College of Medicine, Irvine, California (*Chapter 26*)

Ronald I. Apfelbaum, M.D., Department of Neurological Surgery, Albert Einstein College of Medicine and Montefiore Hospital and Medical Center, Bronx, New York (*Chapter 15*)

James I. Ausman, M.D., Ph.D., Chairman, Department of Neurosurgery, Henry Ford Hospital, Detroit, Michigan (*Chapter 5*)

Stephen C. Boone, M.D., Division of Neurosurgery, University of North Carolina, Chapel Hill, North Carolina (*Chapter 21*)

John A. Byer, M.D., Associate Professor, Department of Neurology, University of Missouri School of Medicine, Columbia, Missouri (*Chapter 3*)

Larry V. Carson, M.D., Section of Neurosurgery, Medical College of Georgia, Augusta, Georgia (*Chapter 30*)

R. A. de Los Reyes, M.D., Department of Neurosurgery, Henry Ford Hospital, Detroit, Michigan (*Chapter 5*)

F. G. Diaz, M.D., Ph.D., Staff Associate, Department of Neurosurgery, Henry Ford Hospital, Detroit, Michigan (*Chapter 5*)

Gernot S. Doetsch, Ph.D., Dept. of Surgery, Section of Neurosurgery, Dept. of Physiology, Medical College of Georgia, Augusta, Georgia (*Chapter 30*)

J. Donald Easton, M.D., Professor and Chairman, Department of Neurology, University of Missouri School of Medicine, Columbia, Missouri (*Chapter 3*)

Marc A. Flitter, M.D., Chairman, Department of Neurosurgery, St. Francis Hospital, Miami Beach, Florida (*Chapter 31*)

Stanley F. Handel, M.D., Professor and Chief, Diagnostic Radiology and Neuroradiology, The University of Texas Medical School at Houston, Houston, Texas (*Chapter 28*)

Alvin B. Hayles, M.D., 200 First Street SW, Rochester, Minnesota (*Chapter 6*)

Richard M. Hodosh, M.D., 10 Parrott Mill Road, Chatham, New Jersey (*Chapter 21*)

Peter Jannetta, M.D., Professor and Chairman, Department of Neurological Surgery, University of Pittsburgh School of Medicine, Pittsburgh, Pennsylvania (*Chapter 25*)

Mark M. Kartchner, M.D., Medical Director, Ocular Pulse and Vascular Laboratory, Tucson Medical Center, Tucson, Arizona (*Chapter 23*)

Andrew M. Kelahan, B.S., Medical College of Georgia, Augusta, Georgia (*Chapter 30*)

Robert B. King, M.D., Professor and Chairman, Department of Neurosurgery, State University of New York, College of Medicine, Syracuse, New York (*Chapter 7*)

Edward R. Laws, Jr., M.D., Professor, Department of Neurological Surgery, Mayo Medical School and Mayo Clinic, Rochester, Minnesota (*Chapter 6*)

Carla J. Lenkey, Associate in Medical Illustration, Neurological Surgery, University of Florida, Gainesville, Florida (*Chapter 16*)

James P. Luby, M.D., Associate Professor of Medicine, University of Texas Health Science Center, Dallas, Texas (*Chapter 4*)

Leonard I. Malis, M.D., Professor and Chairman, Department of Neurosurgery, Mt. Sinai School of Medicine, New York, New York (*Chapter 14*)

Kenneth R. Maravilla, M.D., Associate Professor, Department of Radiology, University of Texas Health Science Center, Dallas, Texas (*Chapter 27*)

John Martin, M.D., Professor, Department of Anesthesiology, Medical College of Ohio, Toledo, Ohio (*Chapter 1*)

Clinton E. Massey, M.D., Medical College of Georgia, Augusta, Georgia (*Chapter 30*)

Lorin P. McRae, Ph.D., Tucson Medical Center, Tucson, Arizona (*Chapter 23*)

Bruce E. Mickey, M.D., Division of Neurological Surgery, University of Texas Health Science Center, Dallas, Texas (*Chapter 24*)

Robert C. Murry, Jr., Ph.D., Department of Radiology, University of Texas Health Science Center, Dallas, Texas (*Chapter 27*)

Frank H. Netter, M.D., Point Manalapan, Florida (*Chapter 13*)

Edward A. Neuwelt, M.D., Associate Professor of Surgery (Division of Neurosurgery), Assistant Professor of Biochemistry, University of Oregon Medical School, 3181 Southwest Sam Jackson Park Road, Portland, Oregon, 97201 (*Chapter 30*)

K. Nudleman, M.D., Department of Neurology, California College of Medicine, Irvine, California (*Chapter 26*)

C. Warren Olanow, M.D., Director of Clinical Neurology, Duke University Medical Center, Durham, North Carolina (*Chapter 8*)

Donald J. Prolo, M.D., Practice of Neurosurgery, San Jose, California (*Chapter 22*)

Morris Pulliam, M.D., Assistant Clinical Professor of Neurosurgery, Department of Neuroscience, School of Medicine, University of North Dakota, Fargo, North Dakota (*Chapter 2*)

Charles D. Ray, M.D., Senior Consulting Neurosurgeon, Department of Neuroaugmentive Surgery, Sister Kenny Institute, Minneapolis, Minnesota (*Chapter 31*)

Richard H. Ray, Ph.D., Medical College of Georgia, Augusta, Georgia (*Chapter 30*)

Robert Reeder, M.D., The Plastic Surgery Group of Memphis, Memphis, Tennessee (*Chapter 11*)

Albert L. Rhoton, Jr., M.D., Professor and Chief, Neurological Surgery, J. Hillis Miller Health Center College of Medicine, University of Florida, Gainesville, Florida (*Chapter 16*)

Duke Samson, M.D., Associate Professor of Neurosurgery, University of Texas Health Science Center, Dallas, Texas (*Chapter 24*)

Paul C. Sharkey, M.D., Clinical Associate Professor of Neurological Surgery and Rehabilitation, Baylor College of Medicine, Houston, Texas (*Chapter 33*)

David G. Sherman, M.D., Associate Professor, Department of Neurology, University of Missouri School of Medicine, Columbia, Missouri (*Chapter 3*)

Arnold Starr, M.D., Professor of Neurology, University of California College of Medicine, Irvine, California (*Chapter 26*)

William H. Sweet, M.D., Professor of Surgery, Harvard Medical School, Boston, Massachusetts (*Chapter 10*)

Bryce K.A. Weir, M.D., Clinical Professor of Neurological Surgery, University of Alberta, Edmonton, Alberta, Canada (*Chapter 12*)

Martin H. Weiss, M.D., Professor and Chairman, Division of Neurological Surgery, University of Southern California Medical School, Los Angeles, California (*Chapter 20*)

Robert H. Wilkins, M.D., Professor and Chief, Division of Neurosurgery, Duke University Medical Center, Durham, North Carolina (*Chapter 19*)

Eben Alexander, Jr., M.D.: A Biographical Sketch

DAVID L. KELLY, JR., M.D.

Dr. Eben Alexander, Jr., was born on September 14, 1913, to Dr. and Mrs. Eben Alexander, Sr., of Knoxville, Tennessee, where Dr. Alexander was a prominent general surgeon. Eben, Jr., attended the University of North Carolina and received his A.B. degree at Chapel Hill, where his grandfather was a professor of Greek. He then went on to Harvard Medical School, receiving his M.D. degree Cum Laude in 1939. Among his classmates were Drs. John Adams, Kenneth Livingston, Francis Moore, and the late and beloved Dr. Donald Matson. Dr. Alexander is the permanent President of the Class of 1939 and is now serving as the President of the Harvard Medical Alumni Association for 1980 and 1981.

Dr. Alexander was attracted into neurological surgery by Dr. Franc Ingraham, who was his teacher and great friend. Dr. Ingraham, one of the finest and most respected gentlemen in neurological surgery, had a great influence upon Dr. Alexander's career.

Dr. Alexander's internship and residency at Peter Bent Brigham and Children's Hospital in Boston spanned a 9-year period from 1939 to 1948, being interrupted by World War II. He returned from the war with a rank of Major, the Bronze Star, and a great appreciation for the comforts of home. His home fires had been lit when he married Elizabeth West in 1942. Betty has been a source of strength for him. Her graciousness and charm are appreciated by members of many neurosurgical organizations, by civic groups, and by their many friends.

Dr. Alexander was fortunate enough to serve a year of neurosurgical residency from 1948 to 1949 under Dr. Kenneth McKenzie in Toronto, Canada. That year was rewarding to Dr. Alexander, not only because he was exposed to Dr. McKenzie's outstanding skills but also because he had the opportunity to review Dr. McKenzie's series of patients with eighth nerve tumors. That published review represented the state of the art at that time.

In 1949, Dr. Alexander was appointed Assistant Professor of Surgery in charge of Neurological Surgery and in 1954 became Professor and Head of the Section on Neurological Surgery, Bowman Gray School of Medicine of Wake Forest University. He held this position until October 1978. As director of the neurosurgical program, he was responsible for the training of 31 residents. His emphasis on the clinical practice of neurosurgery caused his program to be recognized as one of the best in the nation.

From 1953 through 1973, Dr. Alexander served as Chief of Professional Services of North Carolina Baptist Hospital. During that period the Medical Center in Winston-Salem grew, and much of the present prominence of both the Bowman Gray School of Medicine and North Carolina Baptist Hospital is the result of his efforts and leadership.

Dr. Alexander's contribution to neurological surgery, both at the laboratory and clinical levels, is documented in over 100 publications. His research projects have focused on hydrocephalus, peripheral nerve injuries, craniosynostosis, spinal cord injuries, and brain tumor chemotherapy. He was one of the first neurosurgeons to recognize the value of plastics in neurosurgery. His clinical interests cover a wide range of subjects, but most often have related to cranial and spinal injuries, brain tumors, and intracranial aneurysms. He has maintained his interest and enthusiasm for pediatric neurosurgery by continuing to contribute to the surgical treatment of many congenital lesions.

His influence on organized neurosurgery at the national level has been truly remarkable. He has made contributions to the National Institutes of Health and the American Association of Medical Colleges. He has served as president of the Society of Neurological Surgeons, the American Academy of Neurological Surgeons, and the American Association of Neurological Surgeons. He served on the Executive Committee of the American Association of Neurological Surgeons and was an officer from 1959 to 1967 when he became president of that association. He also served on the editorial board of the *Journal of Neurosurgery* from 1961 to 1970.

For the past few years, Dr. Alexander has made a great effort on our behalf in the AMA. He has participated in the development of the AMA Section Council for Neurosurgery. He has also served on the Interspecialty Advisory Board, the Council of Medical Specialty Societies, and the Council on Medical Education. He has recently been appointed to the National Board of Medical Examiners and the Liaison Committee for Graduate Medical Education.

Dr. Alexander has earned the respect of all neurosurgeons. For those who have had the privilege of knowing him well for many years, he is appreciated for his attention to detail, demand for excellence, compassion and dedication to his patients, positive and optimistic attitudes, honesty and fairness in all endeavors, and for his perseverance and commitment to organization and progress.

He has earned the privilege to be recognized as the Honored Guest of the Congress for 1980.

BIBLIOGRAPHY OF EBEN ALEXANDER, JR., M.D.

1. Ingraham, F. D., and Alexander, E. Jr. Experimental application of sulfonamide drugs to the cerebral cortex. N. Engl. J. Med., *227:* 374–378, 1942.
2. Alexander, E. Jr. Adaptation of government issue spectacles as holder for nasal tube. Milit. Surg., *94:* 166, 1944.
3. Campbell, J. B., and Alexander, E. Jr. Eosinophilic granuloma of the skull. Report of a case. J. Neurosurg., *1:* 365–370, 1944.
4. Lamon, J. D. Jr., and Alexander, E. Jr. Secondary closure of decubitus ulcers with the aid of penicillin. J.A.M.A., *127:* 396, 1945.
5. Alexander, E. Jr., Morris, D. P., and Eslick, R. L. Atropine poisoning. N. Engl. J. Med., *234:* 258, 1946.
6. Ingraham, F. D., Alexander, E. Jr., and Matson, D. D. Synthetic plastic materials in surgery. N. Engl. J. Med., *236:* 362–368, 402–407, 1947.
7. Ingraham, F. D., Alexander, E. Jr., and Matson, D. D. Polyethylene: a new synthetic plastic for use in surgery. Experimental applications in neurosurgery. J.A.M.A., *135:* 82–87, 1947.
8. Ingraham, F. D., Alexander, E. Jr., and Matson, D. D. Experimental hydrocephalus. J. Neurosurg., *4:* 164–176, 1947.
9. Ingraham, F. D., Matson, D. D., Alexander, E. Jr., and Woods, R. P. Studies in the treatment of experimental hydrocephalus. J. Neuropathol. Exp. Neurol., *7:* 123–143, 1948.
10. Alexander, E. Jr., Small, W., and Campbell, J. B. A dependable method for constant intravenous therapy in infants using polyethylene tubing. Ann. Surg., *127:* 1212–1216, 1948.
11. Matson, D. D., Alexander, E. Jr., and Weiss, P. Experiments on the bridging of gaps in severed peripheral nerves of monkeys. J. Neurosurg., *5:* 230–248, 1948.
12. Alexander, E. Jr., Woods, R. P., and Weiss, P. Further experiments on bridging of long nerve gaps in monkeys. Proc. Soc. Exp. Biol. Med., *68:* 380–382, 1948.
13. Ingraham, F. D., Matson, D. D., and Alexander, E. Jr. Experimental observations in the treatment of craniosynostosis. Surgery, *23:* 252–268, 1948.
14. Ingraham, F. D., Alexander, E. Jr., and Matson, D. D. Clinical studies in craniosynostosis. Analysis of fifty cases and description of a method of surgical treatment. Surgery, *24:* 518–541, 1949.
15. Ingraham, F. D., Alexander, E. Jr., and Matson, D. D. Current therapeutics. XIV. The use of synthetic plastic materials in surgery. Practitioner, *162:* 152–159, 1949.
16. Alexander, E. Jr., and Janes, R. M. Neurofibroma: benign intraspinal-intrathoracic "hour-glass" tumor with paraplegia. Ann. Surg., *129:* 267–273, 1949.
17. Alexander, E. Jr., and Botterell, E. H. Unilateral hydrocephalus resulting from occlusion of foramen of Monro: complication of radical removal of brain abscess. J. Neurosurg., *6:* 197–206, 1949.
18. Alexander, E. Jr., and Dillard, P. H. Cerebral angiography. N.C. Med. J., *11:* 116–122, 1950.
19. Alexander, E. Jr., and Dillard, P. H. The use of pure polyethylene plate for cranioplasty. J. Neurosurg., *7:* 492–498, 1950.
20. McKenzie, K. G., and Alexander, E. Jr. Restoration of facial function by nerve anastomosis. Ann. Surg., *132:* 411–415, 1950.
21. Alexander, E. Jr., Beamer, P. R., and Williams, J. O. Tumor of the glomus jugulare with extension into the middle ear. J. Neurosurg., *8:* 515–523, 1950.
22. Alexander, E. Jr., Masland, R., and Harris, C. Anterior dislocation of first cervical vertebra simulating cerebral birth injury in infancy. Am. J. Dis. Child., *85:* 173–181, 1953.
23. Alexander, E. Jr., and Davis, C. H. Jr. Trigeminal neuralgia. Conservative management with massive vitamin B_{12} therapy. N.C. Med. J., *14:* 206–207, 1953.

24. Alexander, E. Jr. Treatment of traumatic paraplegia. N.C. Med. J., *14:* 32–34, 1953.
25. Alexander, E. Jr. Benign subtentorial supracollicular cyst as a cause of obstructive hydrocephalus. Report of a case. J. Neurosurg., *10:* 317–323, 1953.
26. Davis, C. H. Jr., Stoll, J. Jr., and Alexander, E. Jr. The use of concentrated human serum albumin in the management of increased intracranial pressure. A preliminary report. N.C. Med. J., *14:* 569–574, 1953.
27. Alexander, E. Jr., and Adams, S. Tumor of the glomus jugulare. Follow-up study two years after roentgen therapy. J. Neurosurg., *10:* 672–674, 1953.
28. Alexander, E. Jr., Garvey, F. K., and Boyce, W. Congenital lumbosacral myelomeningocele with incontinence. A contribution to the understanding of bladder physiology. J. Neurosurg., *11:* 183–192, 1954.
29. Alexander, E. Jr., and Davis, C. H. Jr. Recent advances in the treatment of infantile hydrocephalus. N.C. Med. J., *14:* 610–613, 1953.
30. McKenzie, K. G., and Alexander, E. Jr. Acoustic neuroma. Clin. Neurosurg., *2:* 21–36, 1955.
31. Kitahata, L. M., Alexander, E. Jr., and Davis, C. H. Jr. Head injuries in children: falls from moving automobiles. N.C. Med. J., *16:* 180–183, 1955.
32. Alexander, E. Jr., and Davis, C. H. Jr. Correction of peripheral paralysis of the facial nerve by hypoglossal-facial anastomosis. South. Med. J., *47:* 299–303, 1954.
33. Fowler, F. D., Alexander, E. Jr., and Davis, C. H. Jr. Pinealoma with metastases in the central nervous system. A rationale of treatment. J. Neurosurg., *13:* 271–288, 1956.
34. Alexander, E. Jr., Davis, C. H. Jr., and Field, C. H. Metastatic lesions of the vertebral column causing cord compression. Neurology, *6:* 103–107, 1956.
35. Norris, F. G., Alexander, E. Jr., and Davis, C. H. Jr. The analysis of the carotid artery syndrome. N.C. Med. J., *17:* 8–14, 1956.
36. Taylor, L., Dent, J., Lynch, G., and Alexander, E. Jr. An apparatus for photography of transillumination of the head. J. Neurosurg., *13:* 219–220, 1956.
37. Fowler, F. D., and Alexander, E. Jr. Atresia of the foramina of Luschka and Magendie. A cause of obstructive internal hydrocephalus. Am. J. Dis. Child., *92:* 131–137, 1956.
38. Alexander, E. Jr., and Nashold, B. S. Jr. Agenesis of the sacrococcygeal region. J. Neurosurg., *13:* 507–513, 1956.
39. Alexander, E. Jr., Davis, C. H. Jr., and Kitahata, L. M. Hydranencephaly: observations on transillumination of the head of infants. Arch. Neurol. Psychiatry, *76:* 578–584, 1956.
40. Alexander, E. Jr., Davis, C. H. Jr., and Field, C. H. Hyperextension injuries of the cervical spine. Arch. Neurol. Psychiatry, *79:* 146–150, 1958.
41. Alexander, E. Jr. Head injuries in children. *In* Current Therapy, edited by H. F. Conn, W. B. Saunders, Philadelphia, 1958, pp. 613–618.
42. Alexander, E. Jr., Forsyth, H. F., Davis, C. H. Jr., and Nashold, B. S. Jr. Dislocation of the atlas on the axis. The value of early fusion of C1, C2, and C3. J. Neurosurg., *15:* 353–371, 1958.
43. Morgan, Z. V. Jr., Headley, R. N., Alexander, E. Jr., and Sawyer, C. G. Atrial fibrillation and epidural hematoma associated with lightning stroke. Report of a case. N. Engl. J. Med., *259:* 956–959, 1958.
44. Strobos, R. J., Alexander, E. Jr., and Masland, R. L. Brain tumor presenting as convulsive disorder. Dis. Nerv. Syst., *19:* 518–522, 1958.
45. Forsyth, H. F., Alexander, E. Jr., Davis, C. H. Jr., and Underdal, R. The advantages of early spine fusion in the treatment of fracture-dislocation of the cervical spine. J. Bone Joint Surg., *41A:* 17–36, 1959.
46. Davis, C. H. Jr., and Alexander, E. Jr. Intracranial aneurysms: an evaluation of methods of treatment. Southern Med. J., *52:* 357–360, 1959.
47. Alexander, E. Jr., Davis, C. H. Jr., and Kester, N. C. Intracranial aneurysms: methods

of treatment; the value of hypothermia in the surgical approach. Arch. Neurol. Psychiatry, *81:* 684–692, 1959.

48. Davis, C. H. Jr., and Alexander, E. Jr. Congenital nasofrontal encephalomeningoceles and teratomas. Review of seven cases. J. Neurosurg., *16:* 365–377, 1959.
49. Strobos, R. R. J., and Alexander, E. Jr. The electroencephalogram in cerebellar or tonic fits. Electroencephalogr. Clin. Neurophysiol., *12:* 491–494, 1960.
50. Alexander, E. Jr., Myers, R. T., and Davis, C. H. Jr. Run-over (überfahren) accidents. N.C. Med. J., *22:* 47–54, 1961.
51. Suwanwela, C., Alexander, E. Jr., and Davis, C. H. Jr. Prognosis in spinal cord injury, with special reference to patients with motor paralysis and sensory preservation. J. Neurosurg., *19:* 220–227, 1962.
52. Suwanwela, C., Alexander, E. Jr., and Davis, C. H. Jr. Extradural aerocele. J. Neurosurg., *19:* 401–404, 1962.
53. Mitchell, O. C., de la Torre, E., Alexander, E. Jr., and Davis, C. H. Jr. The nonfilling phenomenon during angiography in acute intracranial hypertension. Report of 5 cases and experimental study. J. Neurosurg., *19:* 766–774, 1962.
54. Spudis, E. V., Scharyj, M., Alexander, E. Jr., and Martin, J. F. Dissecting aneurysms in the neck and head. Neurology, *12:* 867–875, 1962.
55. de la Torre, E., Alexander, E. Jr., Davis, C. H. Jr., and Crandell, D. L. Tumors of the lateral ventricles of the brain. Report of eight cases, with suggestions for clinical management. J. Neurosurg., *20:* 461–470, 1963.
56. Alexander, E. Jr., Adams, J. E., and Davis, C. H. Jr. Complications in the use of temporary intracranial arterial clip. J. Neurosurg., *20:* 810–811, 1963.
57. Yarborough, W. L., Harrill, J. A., and Alexander, E. Jr. Traumatic internal carotid aneurysm. Rupture in sphenoid sinus with angiographic demonstration. Laryngoscope, *73:* 1313–1324, 1963.
58. Alexander, E. Jr., and Davis, C. H. Jr. The radiographic demonstration of cysts and abscesses of the brain. Use of micropaque barium in suspension. J. Neurosurg., *21:* 288–291, 1964.
59. Alexander, E. Jr., Mitchell, O. C., Ferguson, K. G. S., and Leinbach, L. B. Excretory urography; by-product of cerebral angiography. J. South Carolina Med. Assoc., *60:* 237–239, 1964.
60. Alexander, E. Jr. Questions and answers: acute and chronic disk disease. J.A.M.A., *190:* 404–405, 1964.
61. Alexander, E. Jr., Harrill, J. A., and Satterwhite, W. M. Jr. Skeletal traction for facial fractures. Surg. Gynecol. Obstet., *119:* 1326–1327, 1964.
62. Alexander, E. Jr., Davis, C. H. Jr., and Mitchell, O. C.: Treatment of craniosynostosis. Clin. Neurosurg., *11:* 32–45, 1964.
63. Toglia, J. U., Netsky, M. G., and Alexander, E. Jr. Epithelial (epidermoid) tumors of the cranium. Their common nature and pathogenesis. J. Neurosurg., *23:* 384–393, 1965.
64. Alexander, E. Jr., Davis, C. H. Jr., and Pikula, L. Aneurysm of the posterior inferior cerebellar artery filling the fourth ventricle. J. Neurosurg., *24:* 99–101, 1966.
65. Alexander, E. Jr. Neurosurgical techniques: introduction. J. Neurosurg., *24:* 817–819, 1966.
66. Davis, C. H. Jr., Alexander, E. Jr., Witcofski, R. L., and Maynard, C. D. Brain scanning with ^{99m}technetium. J. Neurosurg., *24:* 987–992, 1966.
67. Alexander, E. Jr., Wigser, S. M., and Davis, C. H. Jr. Bilateral extracranial aneurysms of the internal carotid artery. Case report. J. Neurosurg., *25:* 437–442, 1966.
68. Kelly, D. L. Jr., and Alexander, E. Jr. Radiofrequency cordotomy for intractable pain. N.C. Med. J., *27:* 457–462, 1966.
69. Alexander, E. Jr. Questions and answers: facial paralysis. J.A.M.A., *199:* 681, 1967.

70. Alexander, E. Jr. Preliminary report of the national conference on education in the neurological sciences. J. Neurosurg., *26:* 297–298, 1967.
71. Alexander, E. Jr. Editorial: neurosurgery and the health services. J. Neurosurg., *26:* 377, 1967.
72. Alexander, E. Jr. Presidential address: perspective on neurosurgery. J. Neurosurg., *27:* 189–206, 1967.
73. Alexander, E. Jr., Davis, C. H. Jr., and Forsyth, H. F. Neurosurgical technique: reduction and fusion of fracture dislocation of the cervical spine. J. Neurosurg., *27:* 587–591, 1967.
74. Alexander, E. Jr. Lumbar puncture. J.A.M.A., *201:* 316–317, 1967.
75. Alexander, E. Jr., Farrell, F. W. Jr., and Davis, C. H. Jr. The *in vitro* evaluation of the PSP and indigo carmine tests for obstruction in hydrocephalus. Am. Surg., *33:* 936–942, 1967.
76. Kelly, D. L. Jr., and Alexander, E. Jr. Lateral cervical puncture for myelography. Technical note. J. Neurosurg., *29:* 106–110, 1968.
77. Kelly, D. L. Jr., and Alexander, E. Jr. Expanding intraspinal lesions. *In* Current Diagnosis, edited by H. F. Conn and R. B. Conn Jr., pp. 730–732. Philadelphia, W. B. Saunders, 1968.
78. Alexander, E. Jr., and Davis, C. H. Jr. Intra-uterine fracture of the infant's skull. J. Neurosurg., *30:* 446–454, 1969.
79. Davis, C. H. Jr., Alexander, E. Jr., and Kelly, D. L. Jr. Treatment of craniosynostosis. Neurosurgical technique. J. Neurosurg., *30:* 630–636, 1969.
80. Alexander, E. Jr. Donald Darrow Matson. November 28, 1913 to May 10, 1969. J. Neurosurg., *31:* 249–252, 1969.
81. Kelly, D. L. Jr., Alexander, E. Jr., Davis, C. H. Jr., and Maynard, C. D. Intracranial arteriovenous malformations. Clinical review and evaluation of brain scans. J. Neurosurg., *31:* 422–428, 1969.
82. Alexander, E. Jr. Donald Darrow Matson. N. Engl. J. Med., *281:* 327–328, 1969.
83. Alexander, E. Jr., and Anderson, P. C. How should graduate medical education be financed? J. Med. Educ., *44:* 847–849, 1969.
84. Alexander, E. Jr. Significance of the small lumbar spinal canal: cauda equina compression syndromes due to spondylosis. Part 5. Achondroplasia. J. Neurosurg., *31:* 513–519, 1969.
85. Alexander, E. Jr., and Davis, C. H. Jr. Neurosurgical technique: reduction and fusion of fracture of the odontoid process. J. Neurosurg., *31:* 580–582, 1969.
86. Alexander, E. Jr. Book review: *Neurosurgery of Infancy and Childhood.* J.A.M.A., *211:* 832, 1970.
87. Kushner, J., and Alexander, E. Jr. Partial spontaneous regressive arteriovenous malformation. Case report with angiographic evidence. J. Neurosurg., *32:* 360–366, 1970.
88. Kelly, D. L. Jr., Lassiter, K. R. L., Calogero, J. A., and Alexander, E. Jr. Effects of local hypothermia and tissue oxygen studies in experimental paraplegia. J. Neurosurg., *33:* 554–563, 1970.
89. Calogero, J. A., and Alexander, E. Jr. Unilateral amaurosis in hydrocephalic child with an obstructed shunt. Case report. J. Neurosurg., *34:* 236–240, 1971.
90. Lassiter, K. R. L., Alexander, E. Jr., Davis, C. H. Jr., and Kelly, D. L. Jr. Surgical treatment of brain stem gliomas. J. Neurosurg., *34:* 719–725, 1971.
91. Kushner, J., Alexander, E. Jr., Davis, C. H. Jr., and Kelly, D. L. Jr. Kyphoscoliosis following lumbar subarachnoid shunts. J. Neurosurg., *34:* 783–791, 1971.
92. Kelly, D. L. Jr., Alexander, E. Jr., Davis, C. H. Jr., and Smith, J. M. Acrylic fixation of atlanto-axial dislocations. Technical note. J. Neurosurg., *36:* 366–367, 1973.

93. Alexander, E. Jr. Medical management of closed head injuries. Clin. Neurosurg., *19:* 240–250, 1972.
94. Alexander, E. Jr. Surgical management of head injuries in children in the acute phase. Clin. Neurosurg., *19:* 251–262, 1972.
95. Kushner, J., Alexander, E. Jr., Davis, C. H. Jr., Kelly, D. L. Jr., and Kushner, A. H. Crouzon's disease (craniofacial dysostosis). Modern diagnosis and treatment. J. Neurosurg., *37:* 434–441, 1972.
96. Alexander, E. Jr. Fractures of the odontoid process. J. Neurosurg. Nurs., *4:* 141–153, 1972.
97. Alexander, E. Jr. Spinal cord injuries. Method of Eben Alexander, Jr., M.D. In: *Current Therapy*, pp. 720–733. W. B. Saunders, Philadelphia, 1972.
98. Alexander, E. Jr. Cancer in the central nervous system: current status and a look to the future. In: *Seventh National Cancer Conference Proceedings*, pp. 839–842. American Cancer Society, Inc., 1973.
99. Kushner, J., Meschan, I., and Alexander, E. Jr. Cerebrospinal fluid rhinorrhea, aqueductal stenosis, and the empty sella. Md. Med. J., *22:* 51–54, 1973.
100. Norwood, C. W., Kelly, D. L. Jr., Davis, C. H. Jr., and Alexander, E. Jr. Irradiation-induced mesodermal tumors of the central nervous system: report of two meningiomas following x-ray treatment for gliomas. Surg. Neurol., *2:* 161–164, 1974.
101. Alexander, E. Jr. Kenneth George McKenzie, Canada's first neurosurgeon. J. Neurosurg., *41:* 1–9, 1974.
102. Alexander, E. Jr. Harvey Cushing operating. Surg. Neurol., *2:* 228–229, 1974.
103. Norwood, C. W., Alexander, E. Jr., Davis, C. H. Jr., and Kelly, D. L. Jr. Recurrent and multiple suture closures after craniotomy for craniosynostosis. J. Neurosurg., *41:* 715–719, 1974.
104. Pollock, M. L., Miller, H. S., Linnerud, A. C., Laughridge, E., Coleman, E., and Alexander, E. Jr. Arm pedaling as an endurance training regimen for the disabled. Arch. Phys. Med., *55:* 418–424, 1974.
105. Alexander, E. Jr. Henry L. Heyl, 1906–1975. Surg. Neurol., *4:* 205–207, 1975.
106. Alexander, E. Jr., and Kushner, J. Intrauterine head injuries. In: *Handbook of Clinical Neurology*, Vol. 23, Chap. 23, pp. 471–476. American Elsevier, New York, 1975.
107. McWhorter, J. M., Alexander, E. Jr., Davis, C. H. Jr., and Kelly, D. L. Jr. Posterior cervical fusion in children. J. Neurosurg., *45:* 211–215, 1976.
108. Alexander, E. Jr. Lumbar subarachnoid-peritoneal shunt and the development of scoliosis: Is there a place for it now? In: *Current Controversies in Neurosurgery*, edited by T. P. Morley, pp. 686–690. Philadelphia, W. B. Saunders, 1976.
109. Alexander, E. Jr. Franc Douglas Ingraham (1898–1965). Surg. Neurol., *7:* 107–108, 1977.
110. McGraw, C. P., and Alexander, E. Jr. Durometer for measurement of intracranial pressure. Surg. Neurol., *7:* 293–295, 1977.
111. Alexander, E. Jr. Editorial: the role of the neurosurgeon in the medical school curriculum. Surg. Neurol., *7:* 357–358, 1977.
112. Ghatak, N. R., Kasoff, I., and Alexander, E. Jr. Further observation on the fine structure of a colloid cyst of the third ventricle. Acta Neuropathol., *39:* 101–107, 1977.
113. Alexander, E. Jr. Classics in neurosurgery: fractures of the odontoid. Surg. Neurol., *8:* 239–242, 1977.
114. Alexander, E. Jr. Special article: a surgeon's belated look at the past. Surg. Neurol., *9:* 61–67, 1978.
115. Alexander, E. Jr. Tumors of the brain. In *Practice of Medicine*, edited by P. G. H. Wolber, Vol. 10, Chap. 28, pp. 1–27. Harper & Row, Hagerstown, Md., 1978.

116. McGraw, C. P., Alexander, E. Jr., and Howard, G. Effect of dose schedule on the response of intracranial pressure to mannitol. Surg. Neurol., *10:* 127–130, 1978.
117. Walker, M. D., Alexander, E. Jr., Hunt, W. E., MacCarty, C. S., Mahaley, M. S. Jr., Mealey, J. Jr., Norell, H. A., Owens, G., Ransohoff, J., Wilson, C. B., Behan, E. A., and Strike, T. A. Evaluation of BCNU and/or radiotherapy in the treatment of anaplastic gliomas. J. Neurosurg., *49:* 333–343, 1978.
118. Smith, H. P., Russell, J. M., Boyce, W. H., and Alexander, E. Jr. Results of urinary diversion in patients with myelomeningocele. J. Neurosurg., *50:* 773–778, 1979.
119. Six, E., Alexander, E. Jr., Kelly, D. L. Jr., Davis, C. H. Jr., and McWhorter, J. M. Gunshot wounds to the spinal cord. Southern Med. J., *72:* 699–702, 1979.
120. Smith, H., Moody, D., Ball, M., Laster, W., Kelly, D. L. Jr., and Alexander, E. Jr. The trapped temporal horn: a trap in neuroradiological diagnosis. Neurosurgery, *5:* 245–249, 1979.
121. Cowley, A. R., Moody, D. M., Alexander, E. Jr., Ball, M. R., and Laster, D. W. Distinctive CT appearance of cyst of the cavum septi pellucidi. Am. J. Roentgenol., *133:* 548–550, 1979.
122. Kline, D. G., Alexander, E. Jr., Carey, M. E., and Clark, W. K. The battered brain (from meeting reports). In: *Back to Basics. Common Emergencies in Daily Practice*, pp. 309–322. New York, EM Books, 1979.
123. Shuping, J. R., Toole, J. F., and Alexander, E. Jr. Transient global amnesia due to glioma in the dominant hemisphere. Neurology, *30:* 88–90, 1980.
124. Alexander, E. Jr. A "truth in mending" act. J.A.M.A., *243:* 1239–1240, 1980.
125. Alexander, E. Jr. Fractures of the cervical spine: indications for and techniques of decompression and fixation. Surg. Rounds, *3:* 50–56, 1980.
126. Smith, H. P., Challa, V. R., and Alexander, E. Jr. Odontoid compression of the brain stem in a patient with rheumatoid arthritis. J. Neurosurg., *53:* 841–845, 1980.

Contents

II
SCIENTIFIC COMMUNICATION

III
REVIEW OF CURRENT ADJUNCTS OF NEUROSURGERY

I

Practical Pharmacology for the Neurosurgeon

CHAPTER

1

Selected Aspects of Neuroanesthesia

JOHN T. MARTIN, M.D.

A brief resume of recent controversies and innovations in neuroanesthesiology can seek perspective but cannot do justice to every development in the field. What seem to be important issues will be considered in several categories: namely, management of airway pressure, premedication, carbon dioxide effects, actions of anesthetic agents, controlled hypotension, and the effects of diuretics.

AIRWAY PRESSURE MANAGEMENT

Spontaneous ventilation is depressed by anesthetic drugs and may lead to CO_2 retention, cerebral vasodilaton, and increased intracranial pressure (ICP). Intermittent positive pressure ventilation is usually substituted for spontaneous ventilation in order to control $PaCO_2$ at about 30 torr, reduce cerebral blood flow by approximately 25 to 30%, lower ICP, and decongest the cerebral surgical field. Proper management of airway pressure during intermittent positive pressure ventilation is, therefore, a significant issue in neuroanesthesia.

Excessive mean airway pressure can occur accidentally if the patient is allowed to cough or strain, and it easily results in congestion of the superior vena cava, obstruction to venous drainage of the brain, and an acute increase in brain mass. At the operative site this may extrude brain into the field. In two situations, however, the Valsalva maneuver can be made to work for us during neuroanesthesia. A briefly sustained elevation of intrathoracic pressure, gently administered and carefully monitored, can be used to evaluate hemostasis in a craniotomy just prior to dural closure. When an air embolus is suspected, continuously sustained positive airway pressure will increase venous pressure in the superior cava and head, stop entrainment of air, and allow the site of air entry to be identified as it bleeds.

The peak of each positive pressure inflation of the lung is of short duration and is usually inoffensive to the cranial contents if expiratory pressure returns to atmospheric and mean airway pressure remains low. Positive end expiratory pressure (PEEP) is a common device employed to improve gas exchange in emphysematous and injured lungs. When autoregulation of cerebral vasculature is intact, PEEP may have little effect on cranial contents. When autoregulation is impaired by anesthetics, injury, acidosis, or hypoxia, the brain becomes regionally or globally susceptible to fluctuations in flood pressure, and the effect of PEEP is unpredictable. An additional variable factor is the tendency of the noncompliant abnormal lung to absorb the airway pressure increases and thereby buffer their transmission to the CNS.

Investigators from the University of Pennsylvania (1) studied cerebral perfusion in cats that were subjected to the application and removal of graded levels of PEEP with and without the presence of an intracranial balloon, which served as a variable mass lesion. They found that the majority of PEEP applications had no effect on ICP. In some instances of previously elevated ICP, abrupt further rises in ICP followed additions of PEEP. When oleic acid was used to produce fulminant pulmonary edema, the PEEP effect was attenuated. In hypovolemic cats PEEP was capable of reducing systemic blood pressure and impairing cerebral perfusion. Shapiro and Marshall (28) in 1978 measured ICP in 12 head-injured patients who required 4 to 8 cm H_2O PEEP, found increased ICP in 6 patients, decreased mean arterial pressure in 10 patients, and cerebral perfusion pressure (CPP) less than 50 mm Hg in 6 patients. Two had neurologic deterioration associated with the PEEP. They concluded that ICP monitoring should be used to titrate the effect of PEEP in a head-injured patient.

A new ventilatory modality has appeared in the last 2 years, utilizing positive pressure ventilation at high rates and low tidal volumes (HFPPV). Todd and coworkers (32) have just presented evidence that the exposed cat brain is quieter with HFPPV and that ventilation-related changes in ICP were minimized compared to those accompanying usual ventilation methods. Both modes can be arranged to produce similar pulmonary gas exchange. This new work looks most promising, but its evaluation awaits a broader experience.

We should digress briefly to touch on an issue that should have been settled long ago but which still seems to stir discussion. It involves spontaneous vs. controlled ventilation of patients during surgical procedures in the posterior fossa. Folklore demands preservation of spontaneous respiratory activity as an index of intact brain stem function. However, experience in major centers, now quite extensive, plus the careful study of Millar (23), validates careful ECG monitoring as the most sensitive index of brain stem function and permits controlled ventillation and proper CO_2 management even in these patients.

Schettini and coworkers (27) examined dogs with hypoxic hypercarbia sufficient to produce brain swelling. Subsequent hyperventilation with oxygen for 60 minutes produced a rapid drop in cisternal CSF pressure but did not decrease brain bulk, and in some instances a continued increase in swelling occurred. Suggested mechanisms for this included a direct action of hypercarbia to increase the permeability of the cerebral capillary walls and thereby aid edema formation.

The effects of hypocarbia and hypotension were recently studied by Levin's group (17) using dogs hyperventilated to $PaCO_2$ 25 while receiving sodium nitroprusside-induced hypotension to 50mm Hg mean arterial pressure (MAP). They examined CSF lactate levels and noted that the most significant rises occurred in the hypocarbic dogs made hypotensive. Their conclusion was that the combination of low CO_2 and low BP yielded poor cerebral oxygenation. Since this combination is a familiar and useful neuroanesthetic maneuver, the duration of hypotension should be carefully limited to the period of maximum surgical need.

PREMEDICATION

While quietude is the goal in preoperative neurosurgical patients, undue drug depression of the central nervous system is to be feared and avoided. Premedication-induced ventilatory depression, CO_2 accumulation, and dangerous cerebral vasodilation can imperil a patient whose ICP is already elevated. On the other hand, a restless straining patient is equally at risk from increased vena cava pressure reflected to an injured head. Adequate oxygenation, mild sedation with an ataraxic such as phenergan, and a belladonna derivative for its antisecretory effect usually provide sufficient premedication for the conscious and responsive patient. As obtundation increases, premedication becomes less necessary, and atropine or scopolamine alone may suffice.

The relatively new benzodiazapine drug, lorazepam, has been examined by Gagnon and coworkers (11) as a potential premedicant for neuroanesthesia. Using cats with epidural balloons serving as controllable mass lesions, they found that lorazepam did not cause significant respiratory depression and did lower elevated ICP, presumably by decreasing CBF. They suggested lorazepam as a useful premedicant for neurosurgical patients.

CARBON DIOXIDE

What role does CO_2 play in neuroanesthesia? Ventilation directly affects $PaCO_2$. That is, as minute ventilation increases, more CO_2 is eliminated, and $PaCO_2$ falls if the lung is properly perfused; reduced ventilation causes CO_2 accumulation and $PaCO_2$ rises. In normal lungs only a very slight gradient exists for CO_2 from capillary to alveolus, so arterial blood gases, end tidal CO_2 and probably transcutaneous CO_2

values are all good measurements of systemic carbon dioxide tensions. Cerebral blood flow has been shown (12) to be roughly linear with $PaCO_2$ changes between 20 and 80 torr. If normal $PaCO_2$ 40 is halved by hyperventilation, normal CBF of 44 to 50 ml/100 g brain/minute falls to about 25 ml/100 g/minute, presumably by vasoconstriction. $PaCO_2$ doubled to 80 torr implies that CBF becomes 90 to 100 ml/100 g/minute. I believe that most neuroanesthesiologists strive to keep $PaCO_2$ about 30 torr during a craniotomy to aid in reducing the volume of vault contents. $PaCO_2$ levels lower than about 25 torr often reduce PaO_2, presumably by pulmonary vasoconstriction, and progressively lower values for $PaCO_2$ threaten cerebral ischemia from reduced CBF. $PaCO_2$ levels above 40 torr lead to various degrees of cerebral vascular engorgement. How long the cerebral circulation maintains these acute responses to alteration of the $PaCO_2$ steady state is uncertain, but the presumed prompt advantage during neuroanesthesia seems a firm part of our folklore. Careful $PaCO_2$ monitoring by some method, therefore, seems necessary to establish the required degree of mechanical ventilation during anesthesia.

INHALATION AGENTS

Shapiro (29) has displayed the degree to which volatile anesthetics alter intracranial pressure and cerebral metabolism (Fig. 1.1). They increase cerebral blood flow despite minor depression of cerebral metabolism and do so in a dose-related pattern. Nitrous oxide is somewhat unique in that it increases both CBF and CMR simultaneously and to a considerable degree. Enflurane, and the new drug isoflurane just now being introduced into limited clinical use, seem by these data to be better suited to neuroanesthesia than does our familiar workhorse, halothane.

AGENT	CMR	CBF
NITROUS OXIDE 0.6-0.7MAC	↑↑	↑↑↑
HALOTHANE 1.0MAC	↓	↑↑↑
ENFLURANE 1.0MAC	↓	↑
ISOFLURANE 1.0MAC	↓	↑
METHOXYFLURANE 1.0MAC	↓	↑

↓=SLIGHT ↓↓=MODERATE ↓↓↓=MARKED

FIG. 1.1. Inhalation agents. (After Shapiro (29).)

Enflurane has been shown to produce epileptiform cortical and motor activity which is accentuated by the low levels of $PaCO_2$ achieved by hyperventilation. Many consider this to be a detriment to its use in neuroanesthesia. A recent report by Flemming and associates (9) demonstrates that this trait of enflurane can be used to deliberately activate silent epileptogenic foci during electrocorticography and thereby guide proper location and depth of cortical resections.

Nitrous oxide diffuses readily into nitrogen-filled body cavities and is known to threaten intracranial pressure if used following a pneumoencephalogram. Artru and associates (2) have emphasized that resorption of air in the ventricles may not be complete for as long as 5 days and that nitrous oxide may be hazardous to use during that period unless a preanesthetic skull film has confirmed the absence of air.

INTRAVENOUS AGENTS

Barbiturates, and thiopental in particular, decrease both cerebral blood flow and cerebral metabolism to about the same extent (29) (Fig. 1.2). Innovar, and each of its components, droperidol and fentanyl, used separately, also reduce CBF and CMR but with flow being more markedly affected than is metabolism. Morphine reduces CMR by about 50% but its CBF depression is not that great, and these effects are reversed by the administration of naloxone, a narcotic antagonist which by itself has no CNS affect (3). Ketamine (34) has been shown to severely increase cerebral blood flow while increasing metabolism to a lesser degree. Since other properties of ketamine initially seemed to make it a good choice for

AGENT	CMR	CBF
THIOPENTAL TO SLOW EEG	↓↓	↓↓
MORPHINE 1MG/KG	↓↓	↓
DROPERIDOL 0.3MG/KG	↓	↓↓
FENTANYL 0.06MG/KG	↓	↓↓
INNOVAR (D+F)	↓	↓↓
DIAZEPAM 0.25MG/KG	↓	↓
KETAMINE 3MG/KG	↑	↑↑↑

↓=SLIGHT ↓↓=MODERATE ↓↓↓=MARKED

FIG. 1.2. Intravenous agents. (After Shapiro (29).)

$PaCO_2$ and PaO_2 levels and concluded that when ICP is increased, slow onset of induced hypotension during hypocarbic hyperoxia did not increase ICP. In man, sodium nitroprusside-induced hypotension has been shown (15) to increase plasma renin levels and to produce a reactive hypertension when the drug was stopped. Khambatta and associates (16) found that previous administration of propranolol blunted the renin release, reduced the amount of nitroprusside needed to effect hypotension, and prevented the hypertensive rebound. Frost *et al.* (10) found sodium nitroprusside to be much less likely than was trimethaphan to produce tachycardia, tachyphylaxis, or a failed response, and used it to relieve postoperative cerebral vasospasm following vascular surgery.

Recognition and treatment of cyanide intoxication from prolonged administration of sodium nitroprusside by infusion is a significant issue, and useful antidotes plus oxygen therapy should be available. Michenfelder and Tinker (25) noted that progressive metabolic acidosis and increasing oxygen levels in mixed venous blood were the most reliable indicators of the development of cyanide intoxication. They found that doses of more than 0.75 mg/kg/hour produced cyanide toxicity. Simultaneous administration of sodium thiosulfate (6 mg/kg/hour) permitted much higher nitroprusside doses without evidence of cyanide toxicity, presumably by supplying a source of sulfur for conversion of cyanide to thiocyanate by the enzyme rhodanase. Because thiocyanate formation apparently results in diuresis, careful attention must be directed toward fluid balance management. Ivankovich's group (14) infused potassium cyanide into dogs and compared the effectiveness of sodium nitrate, sodium thiosulfate, hydroxycobalamine, and cysteine as antidotes. Hydroxycobalamine and cysteine did not prevent KCN-induced circulatory failure; nitrate infusion produced high levels of methemoglobin; and thiosulfate appeared safe and effective as an antidote when given as a 30 mg/kg bolus IV followed by an infusion of 60 mg/kg/hour.

Nitroglycerine has been shown (13) to diminish autoregulation of CBF and allow any increases in MAP to significantly increase ICP. Stevenson *et al.* (30) induced hypoxemia in dogs and demonstrated increased CBF and ICP; addition of nitroglycerine reduced CBF but further increased ICP and caused the authors to urge caution in its use.

We must conclude, then, that induced hypotension is a technique widely used to promote safer surgical manipulation of cerebral vasculature. However, it carries a significant risk of increasing intracranial pressure, reducing cerebral perfusion, and removing the autoregulative protection of the cerebral vasculature against sudden increases in mean arterial pressure. Careful monitoring of blood pressure levels and restriction of the hypotension technique to the period of definite surgical need should be standard intraoperative precautions.

during deliberate hypotension. Anesthesiology, *53:* S91, 1980.

20. Marsh, M. L., Shapiro, H. M., Smith, R. W., and Marshall, L. F. Changes in neurologic status and intracranial pressure associated with sodium nitroprusside administration. Anesthesiology, *51:* 336–338, 1979.
21. Marsh, M. L., Aidinis, S. J., Naughton, K. V. H., Marshall, L. F., and Shapiro, H. M. The technique of nitroprusside administration modifies the intracranial pressure response. Anesthesiology, *51:* 538–541, 1979.
22. Marx, G. F., Andrews, I. C., and Orkin, L. R. Cerebrospinal fluid pressures during halothane anesthesia. Can. Anaesth. Soc. J., *9:* 239–245, 1962.
23. Millar, R. A. Neurosurgical anesthesia in the sitting position. Br. J. Anaesth., *44:* 495–505, 1972.
24. Michenfelder, J. D., and Theye, R. A. Canine systemic and cerebral effects of hypotension induced by hemorrhage, trimethaphan, halothane or nitroprusside. Anesthesiology, *46:* 188–195, 1977.
25. Michenfelder, J. D., and Tinker, J. H. Cyanide toxicity and thiosulfate protection during chronic administration of sodium nitroprusside in the dog. Anesthesiology, *47:* 441–448, 1977.
26. Sakabe, T., Maekawa, T., Ishikawa T., and Takeshita, H. The effects of lidocaine on canine cerebral metabolism and circulation related to the EEG. Anesthesiology, *40:* 433–441, 1974.
27. Schettini, A., McKay, L., Mahig, J., Modell, J. H. The response of brain surface pressure to hypercapnic hypoxia and hyperventilation. Anesthesiology, *36:* 4–12, 1972.
28. Shapiro, H. M., and Marshall, L. F. Intracranial responses to PEEP in head-injured patients. J. Trauma, *18:* 254–256, 1978.
29. Shapiro, H. M. Neuroanesthesia: physiologic and pharmacologic principles, American Society of Anesthesiologists Refresher Course Lectures, 1980. p. 205.
30. Stevenson, R. L., Traystman, R. J., and Rogers, M. C. Cerebral responses to nitroglycerin with hypoxia. Anesthesiology, *53:* S76, 1980.
31. Stullken, E. H., and Sokoll, M. D. Anesthesia and subarachnoid intracranial pressure. Anaesth. Analg., *54:* 494–500, 1975.
32. Todd, M. M., Toutant, S. M., Shapiro, H. M., and Smith, N. T. Intracranial effects of low and high frequency ventilation. Anesthesiology, *53:* S196, 1980.
33. Wang, H. W., Liu, L. M. P., and Katz, R. L. A comparison of the cardiovascular effects of sodium nitroprusside and trimethaphan. Anesthesiology, *46:* 40–48, 1977.
34. Wyte, S. R., Shapiro, H. M., Turner, P., and Harris, A. B. Ketamine-induced intracranial hypertension. Anesthesiology, *36:* 174–176, 1972.

CHAPTER

2

Use of Blood and Its Components

MORRIS W. PULLIAM, M.D.

INTRODUCTION

Use of blood transfusion dates back over 300 years to 1667 when Jean Baptiste Denis and a surgeon, Emmerez, transfused blood of a sheep into a 15-year-old boy who had been bled repeatedly for treatment of a fever (19). Two subsequent patients of Denis succumbed, due at least in part to a transfusion, resulting in his prosecution. The "FDA" of his day and country, the Faculty of Medicine in Paris, immediately placed severe restrictions on further transfusions. About 200 years later, *human* blood was recognized to be the only appropriate source for use in replacement.

A major step toward safe transfusion occurred in 1900 with the discovery by Landsteiner of blood grouping, and the A, B, and O groups. With discovery of the Rh and other blood groups, development of sensitive cross-matching procedures, and the impetus of World War II, blood transfusion became commonplace (49). Improved preservatives such as acid-citrate dextrose (ACD) and citrate-phosphate-dextrose (CPD) allowed development of large-scale blood banking.

Rapid advances in blood component therapy have fostered new concepts of transfusion. Blood or its components may be indicated for correction of blood volume, inadequacies of oxygen transport, bleeding disorders, and decreased capability to combat infection. It is or should be realized that routine use of *whole blood* is not only inappropriate and unnecessary, but also wasteful and hazardous. In most cases today, correction of a hematologic deficiency is possible with one specific component. This selectivity in transfusion allows a single, sometimes scarce unit of blood to serve many patients (43). Table 2.1 presents a list of components available for use today (10).

WHOLE BLOOD

Whole blood is commonly considered in two forms—fresh and stored(banked). It can be obtained from donors or, in the case of autologous transfusions, from the recipient himself. In either case, it is collected into a citrate-containing medium to prevent clotting; kept at reduced temperature (4°C), unless it is to be used within four hours for transfusion

*Summary Chart of Blood Components**

Component	Contents	Indications for use	Approximate volume	Amount of active substance per transfused unit	Risk of hepatitis†	Shelf life of product
Red cells	Red cells, some plasma, some WBC and platelets or their degradation products	Increase patient red cell mass	250–350 ml	200-ml packed red cell mass	2	21 days
Leukocyte-poor blood	Red cells, some plasma, few WBCs	Prevent febrile reactions from leukoagglutinins	200–250 ml	185 ml red cells	2	21 days closed 24 hr open
Frozen red cells	Red cells—no plasma minimal WBCs and platelets	Increase red cell mass, prevent tissue antigen sensitization, prevent febrile or anaphylactic IgA reaction, provide rare bloods	200 ml	169–190 ml red cells	3	3 yr frozen 24 hr thawed
Concentrated leukocytes	WBCs, few platelets	Agranulocytosis	Variable 50–100 ml	Variable no. granulocytes	2	12 hr
Platelets	Platelets, few WBCs, some plasma	Bleeding due to thrombocytopenia	30–50 ml	5.5×10^{10} platelets or more	2	6–72 hr depending on storage
Single donor plasma	Plasma—no labile coagulation factors	Blood volume expansion	220–250 ml	NA	2	5 yr
Fresh frozen plasma	Plasma—all coagulation factors, no platelets	Treatment of coagulation disorders	220–250 ml	220–250 units factor VIII	2	2 hr thawed 12 mo frozen
Cryoprecipitate	Coagulation factors I and VIII	Hemophilia and von Willebrand's disease, fibrinogen deficiency	10–25 ml	80–100 units factor VIII	2	4–6 hr thawed 12 mo frozen
AHG concentrate	Factor VIII	Hemophilia	Lyophilized	Unit concentrates labeled on vial	1	Dated period
II-X complex	Factors II, VII, IX, X	Christmas disease	Lyophilized	See text	1	Dated period
Albumin	Albumin	Blood volume expansion-replacement of protein	250 or 50 ml	12.5 gm albumin	3	3–5 yr
Plasma protein fraction (PPF)	PFF-albumin α- and β-globulin	Blood volume expansion	250 ml	12.5 gm protein 39% ; ga- and β globulin	3	3–5 yr α
Immune serum globulins	Globulin	Disease prophylaxis or attenuation, agammaglobulinemia	Varies with patient's weight	NA	3	3 yr

* Adapted from ref. 10, with permission of American Association of Blood Banks.
† 1, greater than whole blood (W.B.); 2, same as W.B.; 3, less than W.B.

or separation into its components; and transfused through a blood filter to remove microaggregates.

Fresh Whole Blood

Ideal replacement for acute blood loss is an autologous transfusion of *fresh whole blood.* However, in the acute situation, except in the case of use of blood collected from a patient's hemothorax (autotransfusion), this is not of much practical importance. Fresh whole blood, obtained from donors (homologous) and transfused within 24 hours of collection, provides all of the components of normal blood except platelets with little loss of function. Platelet function is improved if blood is less than 6 hours old (45, 59). A relative indication proposed for use of fresh whole blood is in replacement of massive blood loss (10 to 14 units) within a 24-hour period in a patient who is continuing to bleed (10,45,49,59,61). Even here, however, blood components almost always play a major role due to frequent geographic and/or temporal unavailability of sufficient emergency donors. A few blood banks consider fresh whole blood a "component" and charge extra for it. No real justification exists for use of fresh whole blood. Most patients will benefit from components (especially platelets and clotting factors) infused in a much higher concentration and less volume than is possible with fresh whole blood.

Stored Whole Blood

The usefulness of *stored or banked whole blood* is even more limited. The red blood cells (RBC) in whole blood, collected in the anticoagulant-preservative ACD or CPD and stored at 4°C (1 to 6°), have a 70% *in vivo* survival of 21 and 28 days, respectively. For this reason ACD is no longer used. Addition of adenine to CPD as the preservative increases RBC survival rate to 35 days and, as a result, is becoming a common additive (23,45,49). Federal regulations allow use of CPD and CPD-adenine-preserved blood to be stored up to 21 and 35 days respectively (23). Albumin, immunoglobulin, and some coagulant factors (Table 2.9) are relatively well preserved. However, platelets and leukocytes lose their viability rapidly. Therefore stored whole blood may be useful for replacement of volume and oxygen-carrying capacity. However, other than finding some use in replacement of major surgical or traumatic blood loss, stored whole blood finds itself being increasingly supplanted with selective component therapy, even though such selectivity may require more complete diagnostic evaluation before transfusion is performed.

Transfusion of whole blood, whether stored or fresh, is associated with numerous untoward side effects of varying frequency. Unfortunately, most blood components have, to greater or lesser extent, the same drawback. One of the chief adverse effects of using whole blood as the only form of replacement is production of circulatory overload before adequate *in vivo* blood or plasma concentration of some components (*e.g.*, RBC, platelets, several coagulation factors) is reached. This concern is epitomized in transfusion of the anemic neonate or geriatric patient with cardiac failure and the young hemophiliac, low in factor VIII. In an attempt to decrease complications and obtain maximal use of each precious unit of donated blood, the virtues of component therapy have been increasingly extolled (9–11,13,14,43,45,49,57,59,70).

BLOOD COMPONENTS

Red Cells

A primary indication for blood transfusion is to restore and maintain blood's oxygen-transport capability. Oxygen content of blood may be calculated as follows:

$$(O_2) = (\text{Hgb} \times 1.3584 \times Sat) + (pO_2 \times 0.0031)$$

Where (O_2) = O_2 concentration in 1 dl of blood in ml
Hgb = hemoglobin concentration in g/d
Sat = measured percent O_2 saturation of Hgb
pO_2 = measured partial pressure of O_2
0.0031 = ml O_2 *dissolved* in plasma per mm Hg pO_2

Therefore, given an average hemoglobin concentration of 14 g/dl, oxygen percent saturation = 95, and pO_2 = 90 mm Hg, it can be calculated that, of a total (O_2) of 18.346 ml, 98% is carried by hemoglobin and, thus, the RBC.

This vividly demonstrates the importance of maintaining an "adequate" hematocrit (Hct). What constitutes an adequate hematocrit remains the subject of controversy, but for surgical patients, especially trauma patients, a lower limit of 30% is still used (67). Whereas a healthy adult can tolerate a loss of up to 50 to 60% of his red cell mass (Hct = 20%), a patient with coronary artery disease may experience organ ischemia and failure with as little as a 30% fall (Hct = 30%) in circulating RBC numbers (35).

RED CELL CONCENTRATES

Red cell concentrates are prepared by removal of most of the plasma from whole blood. Separation can be accomplished either by centrifugation ("packed" red cells) or gravity sedimentation ("sedimented" red cells) with resultant Hct ranges of 60 to 90% and an average of 70 to 80% (11,45,49). A simple comparison of some properties of typical red cell concentrates whole blood is given in Table 2.2.

The important parameters of posttransfusion viability and oxygen-transport ability of red cells, whether in the form of whole blood or *liquid*

TABLE 2.2

Properties of Red Cell Concentrates vs. Whole Blood

Property	Whole blood	Red cell concentrates
Volume (ml)	500 ± 25	300 ± 25
Hematocrit (%)	40 ± 5	70 ± 5
Red cell volume (ml)	200 ± 25	200 ± 25
Plasma volume (ml)	300 ± 25	100 ± 25
Albumin content (g)	10–12	4–5
Hepatitis risk, per 1000 transfusions	2.1	2.1

concentrates, are influenced by methods of storage (49). Viability is influenced by several aspects of red cell metabolism, but one of the most important factors is maintenance of adequate levels of adenosine triphosphate (ATP). At a red cell ATP level of one-third normal, only 50% remain viable. Reduction in ATP levels also produces several other changes in red cells, among which are change in shape from a disc to a sphere, and striking increase in cellular rigidity. It is fortunate, from the standpoint of circulation through capillary beds, that these latter alterations are reversed within a reasonably short time after transfusion.

Oxygen-transport characteristics of red cells are influenced significantly by cellular levels of 2,3-diphosphoglycerate (DPG). With depletion of DPG during storage, affinity of oxygen for hemoglobin increases (*i.e.*, shift of oxyhemoglobin dissociation curve to the left). Thus, peripheral (capillary) release of O_2 and the resultant amount of O_2 available for tissue metabolism is reduced. This RBC storage defect appears of questionable clinical significance (4,6,49,54). Its importance is greater in massive transfusions in infants, older patients, and those with cardiovascular or pulmonary disease. Even here no problem exists if blood no older than 7 days is used (23). Optimal posttransfusion viability and function for liquid storage is best maintained by refrigeration at 4°C (range = 1° to 6°C) (49). While acid-citrate-dextrose (ACD) was a standard early storage medium, it has been entirely supplanted by citrate-phosphate-dextrose (CPD). The latter medium has been found to improve both viability and oxygen affinity of stored red cells. This results in maintenance of higher pH with resultant reduction in depletion of ATP and DPG. A recent modification has been addition of adenine which further improves viability, but appears to decrease maintenance of DPG (49). On balance, the benefit of increased viability outweighs the drawbacks, so that adenine is now a routine additive to CPD (23). With ACD posttransfusion red cell survival after 21 days of storage was about 70%. With CPD-adenine, survival at 28 and 35 days is 80 and 76%, respectively (49).

Indications for use of red cell concentrates include **chronic anemia, slow blood loss**, and **rapid blood loss**. In the last case concentrates are combined with volume expanders and, if necessary, coagulation factors. Perusal of Table 2.3 allows recognition of several conditions that afflict neurosurgical patients, in which RBC concentrates are specifically indicated. In these conditions, as is the case with over 80% of all blood transfusions, restoration or maintenance of oxygen transport is the primary goal. Most of these conditions would be adversely affected by excessive volume—occasionally in a dramatic manner in patients with severe **chronic anemia** (Hgb below 4 g/dl) with high output failure (49). Infusion of unneeded potassium present in plasma of stored whole blood is reduced approximately two-thirds by use of RBC concentrates. This is of particular importance in many burn patients and those with renal failure. Potassium reduction can be maximized by removing the plasma near time of transfusion.

Some leukocytes and platelets are removed during concentration which reduces frequency and severity of immunologic reactions to antigens on these cells (54). However, if this is of great concern, special leukocyte-poor preparations or frozen red cells are necessary. Reduction of plasma volume may reduce chance of side effects associated with immunologic and nonimmunologic reactions to plasma proteins and peptides. Removal of plasma decreases the quantity of anti-A and/or anti-B blood group antibodies normally found in individuals lacking the corresponding antigen (see Table 2.4). This is of particular value when faced with the rare

TABLE 2.3

Specific Indications for Use of Packed Cells

1. Cirrhosis of the liver
2. Uremia
3. Burns with hyperkalemia
4. Anemia secondary to marrow failure
5. Cachectic patients
6. Debilitated patients
7. Elderly patients
8. Patients of small stature
9. Severe chronic anemia (Hgb <4 g/dl)
10. Pre- and postoperative transfusions

TABLE 2.4

*Compatibility of Red Cells and Plasma**

Recipient's blood group	Donor's red cells		Donor's plasma
	Elective	Emergency†	
O	O	O	O, A, B, AB
A	A	O	A, AB
B	B	O	B, AB
AB	A, AB	A, O	AB

* Table shows which donor phenotype is compatible with a potential recipient's ABO blood group for transfusion of red cells or plasma.

† Risk of *serious* hemolytic reactions when emergency substitutions are made can be significantly decreased with use of packed cells.

need to use group O blood for recipients that are other than group O. Unfortunately, risk of hepatitis is not reduced by the decrease in plasma administered in red cell concentrates.

For those that argue, as many surgeons do, that, "my patient needs the protein" found in plasma of whole blood, it should be recognized that more efficacious means exist for providing it. If the patient is on a regular diet, one to two eggs or an average serving of meat provide more assimilable protein than plasma from one unit of whole blood. Similar reasoning applies to use of nasogastric feedings in preference to plasma for protein administration.

Slow blood loss should be treated with RBC concentrates to avoid increased venous pressure that might aggravate capillary and venous oozing. **Total blood volume expansion** advocated in perioperative management of patients with subarachnoid hemorrhage and vasospasm can use RBC concentrates (52). Infusion of a unit of packed cells plus 250 ml of 5% albumin or 50 ml of 25% albumin plus 200 ml D5S provides the same amount of RBC, protein, and volume expansion as one unit of whole blood.

Small to moderate intraoperative blood loss can be successfully managed with packed cells. In two studies of general surgery patients, no difference could be found between patients receiving operative transfusion of packed RBC and those receiving whole blood with respect to biochemical changes, complications, or mortality (54,56). No patient required fresh frozen plasma for bleeding problems, and no differences were demonstrated in cardiac output between groups. The authors concluded that blood replacement of less than 1 blood volume (about 10 units) can be accomplished safely with RBC concentrates, without requirement for whole blood.

Massive, acute blood loss can be replaced with packed red cells, saline or Ringer's lactate, plasma (especially fresh frozen plasma), cryoprecipitate, platelet concentrates, and albumin.

The **method of infusion** of packed red cells is seldom a problem, except when very rapid rates are needed. For rapid infusion, a 17 gauge (18 gauge, thin-walled) needle, or larger, is recommended, with application of pressure to the bag, if necessary. Addition of 50 ml of saline to each packed unit gives it flow properties similar to whole blood. Use of glucose solutions, which can produce red cell agglomerations, and Ringer's lactate or other calcium-containing solutions, which may partially reverse the anticoagulant action of citrate, is discouraged.

Hematocrit increment achieved with infusion of each unit of packed RBCs is usually 2 to 3% (1 to 2% for whole blood) for a 70-kg man. This takes into account blood volume readjustment which may not be stabilized for as long as 24 hours after a 500-ml transfusion (49). For those who may wish to make a more precise estimate, the increment can be evaluated as follows:

$$\frac{(\text{Blood volume} \times \text{Hct}_i) + (\text{Transfused red cell volume} \times \text{Hct}_r)}{(\text{Blood volume} + \text{transfused red cell volume})} \times 100 = \text{Hct}_f$$

where Hct_i = Hct before transfusion
Hct_r = Hct of transfused unit
Hct_f = patient's new Hct.

LEUKOCYTE-POOR BLOOD (RED CELLS)

Leukocyte-poor blood is the component remaining after removal of most leukocytes and platelets from whole blood. Sedimentation of fresh blood through dextran or hydroxyethyl starch or filtration through nylon mesh removes about 95% of leukocytes at the expense of 10 to 20% red cell loss. Reconstituted **frozen red cells** are also about 95% depleted of leukocytes and provide a more convenient source (49).

Need for this somewhat expensive component is infrequent. The two most common *indications* are: (a) to avoid transfusion-associated, febrile reactions caused by recipient antibodies to white cells and platelets, which developed in response to previous transfusions or pregnancies, and (b) to avoid alloimmunization to histocompatibility antigens on these cells in potential transplant recipients (10,45,49).

FROZEN AND/OR WASHED RED CELLS

Washed red cells are prepared by batch or continuous-flow centrifugation using normal saline. Because of high risk of bacterial contamination, the preparations must be used promptly. While containing significantly reduced numbers of leukocytes and platelets, this infrequently used preparation is **indicated** in the rare patient who is hypersensitive to plasma. Such patients develop allergic or febrile reactions to very small amounts of plasma, frequently on the basis of antibodies to IgA formed after a previous transfusion or pregnancy (45). A second indication is in patients with paroxysmal hemoglobinuria. Washing also reduces the amount of anti-A and anti-B blood group antibodies present in plasma, permitting safer transfusion of group O red cells into non-O recipients (11). However, this process does not reduce the risk of transfusion-induced hepatitis (32).

Frozen red cells became a feasible component when it was discovered that addition of glycerol before freezing prevented postthaw damage, especially hemolysis (10,45,49). Depending on the method used storage is at −20 to −150°C (2,5,11). After thawing, a laborious washing process is required to reduce the 20 to 50% glycerol concentrations present. Fortunately, this process is now automated. Frozen red cells are several times more expensive than those stored in liquid state.

Storage for 3 months at −20°C gives a posttransfusion survival only slightly less than fresh cells; cells stored at −80 to 120°C for up to 3.7 years have a 95% posttransfusion survival. The freeze-thaw-wash process does produce small losses of red cells, so that the overall therapeutic efficiency of cells stored at −80°C is about 78% that of fresh red cells (49). DPG levels and oxygen affinity are maintained near normal (70). Because of the freeze-thaw-repeated washing process, this component is 95% or more leukocyte- and platelet-free, and markedly reduced in blood group antibodies, microaggregates, plasma proteins, plasma electrolytes and other potentially toxic products (10). However, as with saline-washed red cells, risk of hepatitis remains the same as whole blood (20).

Indications for frozen red cells include: maintenance of an inventory of rare blood types, autologous transfusion for patients with rare blood types or unidentifiable blood group antibodies, decrease in incidence of nonhemolytic transfusion reactions, supplying metabolically superior cells and reduced sensitization to tissue antigens in potential transplant recipients (10,45,49). Should improved technology reduce the cost of this component, more liberal indications may become applicable.

AUTOLOGOUS BLOOD

A patient's own blood has several advantages over blood from another source. Blood group incompatibility is not a problem, immunogenicity is nil, and hepatitis transmission is obviated. In many situations it is possible for the patient to predeposit up to 4 units of blood within 15 days before elective surgery without significant reduction in hematocrit or plasma volume by time of surgery (22,23,25). **Frozen autologous blood** is ideal for patients with rare blood types or with multiple antibodies, such that compatible units of homologous blood are virtually impossible to acquire.

Two basic problems exist with this component. First, advanced planning is mandatory, precluding availability to trauma victims or patients presenting with rapidly progressing neurosurgical conditions. Second, patients with chronic illnesses or with impaired nutritional status may not be able to replenish the lost red cells with sufficient speed, if at all. In the latter category use of infrequently drawn, frozen red cells is an option.

SINGLE-UNIT TRANSFUSIONS

Although single-unit transfusions cannot be condemned outright, they often do represent an unwarranted use of blood. It has been suggested that the patient who needs only one unit of blood is no more in need of transfusion than its donor. This is certainly the case in "elective" transfusions, such as administration of a unit of blood to correct a preoperative hemoglobin or blood volume deficit which could be corrected by other means or to hasten recovery of convalescing patients. Single-unit transfusion is justifiable in the elderly surgical patient with coronary disease, the patient who has sustained an acute blood loss of 2 or 3 units who achieves circulatory stability with 1 unit, and patients whose bleeding during surgery or from the gastrointestinal tract is controlled after transfusion of the first unit. Such transfusions represent good judgment and therapeutic skill. It has been suggested that an empirical guide for evaluating appropriateness of single-unit transfusions is that they should represent not more than 10% of the total hospital blood usage (45).

COMPATIBILITY

More than 400 different antigens have been detected in human red cells (23,25,49). Their corresponding alleles vary greatly, but several million possible phenotypes exist. When a recipient is transfused with serologically compatible blood based only on ABO and Rh(D) phenotype, it probably contains one or more antigens foreign to the patient. Fortunately, most red cell antigens are not very immunogenic. About 12 antigens are clinically significant from the standpoint of stimulating nonnaturally occurring antibody production. Among naturally occurring antibodies, anti-A and anti-B present a very serious transfusion hazard, whereas most others have little capacity for destroying red cells.

TYPE AND CROSS-MATCHING

Type and cross-matching usually involve determination of the recipient's ABO and Rh(D) phenotypes. In addition a "major" cross-match (donor's cells and recipient's serum) is performed before release of blood by the blood bank except in life-threatening emergencies. The "minor" cross-match has become obsolescent with development of other antibody screening techniques for the donor's serum.

Screen of the recipient's serum, for presence of alloantibodies to red cell antigens, has become mandatory. These can occur as result of receipt of previous transfusions or delivery of an Rh-positive infant by an Rh-negative mother. The advantage of this method is that it can be performed well in advance of transfusion, so that when alloantibodies are detected, sufficient time for antibody identification and compatible donor selection exists. Further, highly sensitive red cells can be used for the test, allowing detection of much weaker antibodies than commonly possible in cross-matching. This has led to the **"type and screen"** commonly suggested as a cost-effective means of preparing patients for elective surgery where some blood use is possible but not probable. This allows determination of presence in the blood bank of units that are type-specific (ABO and Rh) and a determination that these units do not have antigens to which the surgical patient has antibodies. If the latter exist, a consultation between surgeon and blood bank director may lead to preoperative cross-matching even in patients undergoing procedures seldom requiring blood (23,49). On the other hand, if there is a high likelihood of need for intraoperative transfusion, especially of several units, then a preoperative cross-match in addition to antibody screen usually becomes routine.

SUBSTITUTION

Substitution of non-type-specific (ABO and Rh) blood, while never ideal, does have some relative indications and reasonable risk based on the ABO compatibility listed in Table 2.4. In the elective group AB patient it is commonly necessary to substitute blood from group A donors because of a lack of available AB donors.

In case of Rh incompatibility, it is not uncommon to electively transfuse Rh-negative recipients with Rh-positive blood (85% of donor population), particularly if the recipient is an elderly male or a postmenopausal female. In women of child-bearing age this Rh substitution is permissible only in serious emergencies. In this case the recipient should be given an Rh-immune globulin injection to prevent the likelihood of sensitization (25, 49). However, this is impractical except in the case of small transfusions. It requires one vial (2 ml each) of Rh-immune globulin to neutralize each 15 ml packed RBC. Therefore, for 1 unit of packed RBC (about 300 ml) injection of 40 ml of Rh immunoglobulin would be required. The difficulty of complete neutralization of, for example, a 4-unit emergency transfusion is obvious. It is for this reason that most good blood banks always keep 4 to 6 units of group O-negative RBC on hand, even if this requires cancellation of elective surgery. In those **very rare** situations where an emergency dictates use of Rh-positive RBC in an Rh-negative young woman, it is suggested to give sufficient Rh immunoglobulin (20 vials) to neutralize 1 unit of packed cells (23).

In **serious emergencies** blood group O-packed RBC can be substituted for all other groups. Once again, risk of severe hemolytic transfusion reaction can be reduced by use of packed cells rather than whole blood. However, use of **"universal donor," O-negative** blood, without at least determining the recipient's blood type, and preferably also performing a "major" cross-match, must be reserved for life-threatening situations. In most cases type-specific blood can be made available within 30 to 45 minutes (23, 59).

Platelets

Platelet transfusion is used for patients with platelet disorders of quantity (thrombocytopenia) or quality (dysfunction) sufficiently severe to produce actual or highly probable spontaneous posttraumatic or surgical bleeding. Although this blood component was first used 60 years ago, it has been in real clinical usage for 10 to 15 years (22, 23). Platelets can be obtained by transfusion of fresh whole blood or platelet concentrates. Since use of the former generally entails infusion of unacceptable large volumes to obtain desired platelet levels, the latter is the usual source.

Platelet concentrates are prepared by one of two centrifugation techniques (22, 49, 64). Using one of the techniques, involving intermittent- or continuous-flow centrifugation (cell separation), large quantities of platelets from a single donor may be collected. This technique is frequently termed **plateletphereis.** The second method is separation by centrifugation of platelet-rich plasma from single units of blood and is called random unit platelets.

Storage of random unit platelets is usually in **liquid state** in approximately 50 ml of plasma (with CPD) per unit of platelets. Packs prepared by plateletpheresis are the equivalent of 6 units of random-donor platelets and have volume of about 400 ml. While virtues of liquid storage at 4°C versus 22°C (room temperature) continue to arouse some discussion, most agree that the best balance of viability and posttransfusion function is achieved at the latter temperature (9, 22, 23, 49, 64). Platelets stored in this manner are acceptable for clinical use for up to 72 hours. Each random unit contains an average of 6×10^{10} viable platelets, although with some collection methods, each unit can obtain about 1.0×10^{11} platelets (41). A plateletpheresis pack contains about 3.6×10^{11} platelets. Platelets should be transfused promptly after receipt from the blood bank to prevent further storage losses. With application of strict **precautions** of collection, processing, and storage, bacterial contamination and proliferation is unusual, even at 22°C. Nevertheless, such contamination must be considered and investigated in any patient exhibiting fever or chills during or after infusion (9, 49). Techniques have been developed for storage of platelets in the **frozen state** using either glycerol or dimethylsulfoxide (DMSO) (22, 49). While moderate increases in loss of functioning platelets occur as a result of freeze-thawing, clinically useful units have been maintained for up to 400 days (58).

The **role of platelets in the hemostatic process** can be appreciated from Fig. 2.1. They contribute to primary clot formation by adhering to damaged endothelium and subendothelial substances such as collagen. Their intracellular granules which contain adenosine diphosphate (ADP) are released. ADP recruits other platelets into the aggregate. Platelet factor 3, a phospholipid found on the inner surface of platelet cell membranes, helps form a matrix upon which factors VIII, V, and X aid in clot formation (8, 50, 80).

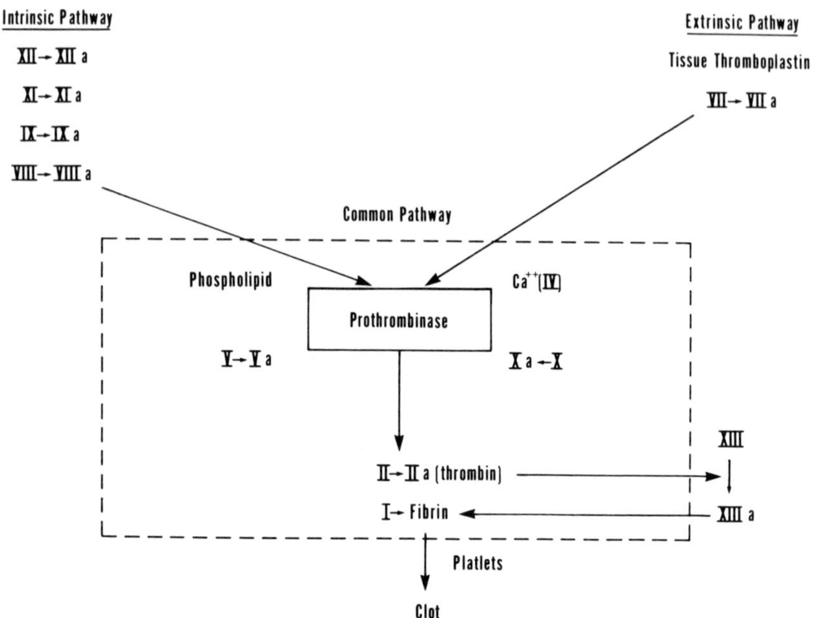

FIG. 2.1. Simplified scheme of hemostatic mechanism demonstrating interaction of the clotting factors (Roman numerals; *a*, activated form) in the intrinsic, extrinsic, and common pathways to form fibrin which provides a meshwork to stabilize platelets in the clot.

Indications for platelet transfusion include thrombocytopenia and disorders of platelet function sufficient to prevent fulfillment of the above role. A list of some of the more common clinical conditions associated with these two general abnormalities is presented in Table 2.5. It is important to recognize that disorders of platelets account for a significant proportion of bleeding problems enountered in surgical patients.

A key part of averting surgical disasters secondary to platelet abnormalities is a good history. **Manifestations** consist of complaints of epistaxis, gum bleeds, ecchymoses, hemoptysis, hematuria, and uterine and gastrointestinal bleeds. However, the classic symptom and sign is diffuse petechial hemorrhage on the dependent extremities. At operation, the hemorrhage of thrombocytopenia is a continuously bloody field from the time of the opening incision.

Conditions commonly confronting neurosurgeons, such as leukemia, malignant lymphoma, and carcinomas, are important to establish, since marrow involvement in these can produce decreased numbers and function of platelets. Patients who have been on cytotoxic agents frequently manifest thrombocytopenia. A host of other drugs, some of which are used by neurosurgical patients (*e.g.*, dilantin, aspirin, diuretics), can produce immunologically mediated thrombocytopenia (4). Of course,

TABLE 2.5
Disorders of Platelets

Thrombocytopenia: acquired	
drug-induced	Cyclic thrombocytopenia
(marrow poisons)	Paroxysmal nocturnal hemglobinuria
immune	Merritt Kassack
dilutional	Hypersplenism
posttransfusion purpura	Hypothermia
aplastic marrow	DIC
malignant invasion of marrow	
tTrombocytopenia: congenital (several types, all rare)	
Platelet dysfunction of cellular origin	
thrombosthenia	Leukemia
thrombopathia	Myelofibrosis
Platelet dysfunction of metabolic origin	
drugs (esp. aspirin)	Hyperbilirubinemia
uremia	Hyperglobulinemia
fibrin degradation products	

aspirin, currently in high use on neurosurgical and neurological services, is a prime offender in producing qualitative platelet function disorders. However, other antiinflammatory drugs, phenothiazines, and some penicillins (*e.g.*, carbenicillin) must be suspected and/or inquired about. Finally, thrombocytopenia, due to dilution with massive transfusions or to consumption with disseminated intravascular coagulation (DIC) is not unusual in neurosurgical patients.

Examination of a **peripheral smear** by a hematologist or pathologist for **platelet morphology** may detect rare platelet disorders that could predispose to bleeding. For a quantitative knowledge of platelet numbers present in the circulation a **platelet count** is necessary. Assuming **normal function** of all platelets present and counted, spontaneous bleeding is uncommon with counts above 20,000 to 30,000/μl. Counts of 30,000 to 50,000/μl are usually sufficient for most minor surgical procedures, while 50,000 to 70,000/μl are adequate for hemostasis in major surgery or trauma. With platelet counts below 10,000/μl, risk of spontaneous hemorrhage rises significantly (49).

Simple presence of adequate numbers may not provide sufficient hemostasis if qualitative dysfunctions afflict some or all of the platelets. For instance, aspirin uniformly affects all circulating platelets by producing an irreversible inhibition of prostaglandins and thromboxane A_2. This compromises platelet aggregation and clot formation. Until aspirin is stopped, cleared from the blood, and sufficient new unaffected platelets appear in the blood, platelet function and clot formation will be disturbed.

This may require at least 5 to 7 days and may require 14 days after chronic aspirin usage (23, 49).

The simplest and **pathognomonic test** for clinically significant platelet disorders is the **bleeding time.** A frequently used version of this test is the modified Ivy bleeding time (Miekle template method) which is performed, as follows (38, 47): (a) a blood pressure cuff is placed on the arm and inflated to 40 mm Hg; (b) an incision 9 mm long and 1 mm deep is made using a standardized template; and (c) filter paper is gently applied to the wound every 30 seconds until bleeding stops. Average bleeding time is 5 minutes, while a time greater than 10 minutes strongly suggests platelet problems. The possible role of platelets in unexpected intraoperative bleeding can be evaluated by the lancet version of the Ivy bleeding time on an exposed extremity (8, 38). While von Willebrands's disease prolongs the bleeding time and produces poor platelet adhesiveness, factor VIII is the substance needed to stop bleeding in this condition. More sophisticated tests of platelet function can be performed as necessary after consultation with a coagulation expert. Some of these include: platelet aggregation, platelet retention in glass bead columns (adhesion), clot retraction, and platelet factor 3 activity (80).

Once it is established that a bleeding problem exists on the basis of platelets, **appropriate therapy** can be commenced (Table 2.6). Of course, if active bleeding is not occurring and an anticipated surgical procedure is elective, time will allow consideration of all therapeutic options. When possible it is best to delay surgery until the safest form of treatment has corrected the platelet abnormality.

In more urgent situations, it is frequently necessary to transfuse the necessary numbers of functioning platelets, either to stop active hemorrhage or to decrease risk of serious bleeding during nonelective surgery. It also is appropriate to electively transfuse patients with platelet counts of less than 10,000/μl to decrease the high risk of spontaneous hemorrhage under these circumstances, although exceptions exist (22, 49).

Fresh whole blood could be used to increase platelet number. Use of fresh whole blood has one other serious drawback in addition to the problem of lack of available emergency donors. This is the volume required. A 70-lb child with a platelet count of 10,000/μl would need 1,000 ml of fresh whole blood to increase the count to 30,000/μl and a full blood volume replacement to achieve a count of 70,000/μl. Similar calculations and their results in adults show that it is not only impractical, but nearly always dangerous, to use fresh whole blood in treatment of thrombocytopenia. Therefore, use of platelet concentrates is a must.

The anticipated number of random units of platelets to be given is calculated and pooled. These are then infused rapidly through an administration set with filter. The expected increment in platelet count is approximately 6,000 to 12,000/μl/m^2/unit (22). As a general rule the increment in the average-sized adult is 5,000/μl per unit transfused, measured 1 hour after the infusion (9). The average adult will require about 4 to 5 units as an initial infusion to give the increment of 25,000/μl for 24 to 48 hours (9, 10). Another rule of thumb that can be used is to initially give 0.1 unit/kg body weight.

Effectiveness should be monitored by platelet counts taken 1 to 2 hours after an infusion and by repeated checks of the bleeding time. Depending on the underlying condition producing the platelet disorder, as well as the bleeding problem (*e.g.*, surgery, trauma), repeated transfusions may be necessary at intervals of 3 times per week (8, 22).

In some situations transfusion requirements may be much greater than those suggested above. These conditions include: fever, sepsis, splenomegaly, antiplatelet antibodies, and DIC (9, 10, 22). In the case of fever and sepsis, increasing the initial calculated infusion by three-fold has been suggested (22).

A special case worth noting is idiopathic thrombocytopenic purpura (ITP). Here platelet counts of 20,000/μl and below are common but are seldom associated with bleeding. Platelet transfusions in these patients give short-lived increments and should not be used. Steroid therapy is the initial treatment of choice. Should serious central nervous system bleeding intervene, emergency splenectomy has been recommended (59).

Presence of antibodies to histocompatibility antigens (HLA) may be responsible for posttransfusion platelet increments smaller than expected. These antigens usually appear as a result of previous platelet or leukocyte transfusions or pregnancy with resultant alloimmunization (9, 10, 49). Some patients are immunized by a single transfusion. Even whole blood can produce this state because of the presence of nonviable platelets. Infusion of histocompatible platelets into such patients is frequently effective (9, 22).

ABO-incompatibility can produce low increments after platelet administration and, thus, should be taken into account when possible (9, 10, 22). However, use of ABO-incompatible platelets is certainly permissible if they are the only ones available and need is urgent (9). In this case, a larger dose may be needed to achieve the desired increment. Practically speaking, ABO-incompatibility is not important unless the patient is smaller than $1.0\ m^2$ body surface area (23). Rh factor incompatibility does not influence platelet increment since they do not contain Rh (D) antigens (13).

Risks involved in platelet transfusions include some that are similar to those encountered with whole blood and red cell administration. The risk of transfusion-induced hepatitis is similar to that of red cells or whole blood (10). While Rh(D) incompatibility does not alter expected platelet

TABLE 2.6

*Partial List of Coagulopathies Encountered in Surgery and the Available Therapy**

Effective level for hemostasis		Emergency therapy		Dosage†	
Coagulopathy	Major trauma or surgery (% normal)	1st Choice	2nd Choice	Initial	Maintenance per day
Factor XIII deficiency	5	Plasma, 1, 2, 3‡	Cryoprecipitate§	2–3 U	None needed
Factor XII deficiency	NA	None needed			
Factor XI deficiency	15–25	Plasma 1, 2, 3		10–20 U	5 U
Factor IX	40–50‖	Plasma 1, 2	Prothrombin complex	40–60 U	5–10 U q 12 hr
Von Willebrand's disease (factor VIII assayed)	40–50	Plasma 1, 2		10 U (factor VIII)	1 of U (factor VIII)
			Cryoprecipitate	1 bag/10 kg 1 bag/2 kg	1 bag/10 kg/1–2 days 1 bag/4 kg q 12 hr
Factor VIII deficiency	40–50‖	Cryoprecipitate	Lyophilized factor VIII plasma 1, 2 (0.8 U/ml)	40 U 30 U	20 U q 12 hr 15 U q 12 hr
				(Dose limited by vol. of plasma given)	
Factor VII deficiency	10–20	Plasma 1, 2	Prothrombin complex	5–10 U	5 U q.i.d.
Factor X deficiency	15–20	Plasma 1, 2	Prothrombin complex	10–15 U	10 U
Factor V deficiency	25	Plasma 1, 2	Plasma 1, 2	15–25 U	15–20 U
Factor II deficiency	20–40	Plasma 1, 2		20 U	15–20 U b.i.d.
			Prothrombin complex	40 U	15–20 U b.i.d.
Factor I deficiency	100 mg/100 ml	Cryoprecipitate	Plasma 1,2	2 bags/10 kg	1 bag/15 kg
Vitamin K deficiency (Factors II, VII, IX, X deficient)	30–50	Vitamin K replacement#		25–50 mg IV (See text) 15–20 U	10 mg q.i.d. IM or PO 10–20 U b.i.d.-q.i.d.

Liver disease chronic	Same as vitamin K deficiency				
DIC	See text	Remove precipitating cause	Heparin	7,000 IU	1,000 IU/hr¶
			Plasma 1, 2	7–15 U	See text
			Cryoprecipitate	12 bags**	See text
			Platelets	8–10 packs**	See text
Thrombocytopenia: acquired	50,000 to 60,000/μl	Platelet transfusion	See text	See text	See text
Platelet dysfunction of cell origin	Same	Same	Same	Same	Same
Platelet dysfunction of metabolic origin	Same	Same	Delay procedures and correct metabolic defect	Same	Same

* Modified from refs. 8 and 39, with permission of *Surgical Rounds* and McGraw-Hill Book Company.

† Dosage is per kilogram of body weight unless specified otherwise. Units of activity (expressed above as U) is in terms of plasma equivalents: 1 unit is the amount present in 1.0 ml fresh normal male plasma. The range of values encountered under normal clinical conditions is likely to be much wider than depicted here (effective level for hemostasis, above). The disparities are due primarily to differences in patients, in particular clinical state being treated, and in assay employed. When therapy is initiated in a particular patient, dosage employed should maintain plasma levels above the recommended minimum to allow for those variables.

‡ 1, fresh plasma; 2, fresh-frozen plasma; 3, outdated plasma, approximately 21 days old.

§ One bag cryoprecipitate contains 70 to 100 units factor VIII_{ahf}.

‖ Level suggested is specifically for CNS bleeding or surgery.

¶ Must be in form of vitamin K_1.

≡ Dosage is in terms of International Units (IU) and is dose for average-sized adult. Initial dose given IV bolus; subsequent dose given by continuous infusion.

** Dosage is that suggested for average-sized adult.

increments, platelet concentrates do contain a small quantity of red cells (about 0.4 ml/unit of platelets) (13). As with red cell or whole blood transfusions in which Rh(D) incompatibility exists, Rh-immunization of an Rh-negative recipient could occur with infusion of platelets from an Rh-positive donor. This is of particular significance in women of child-bearing age or younger. In such patients, if urgency dictates the use of platelets containing Rh-incompatible RBC, administration of Rh(D) immune globulin within 72 hours of transfusion is strongly recommended (9, 10). The small quantity of RBC infused here makes use of Rh(D) immune globulin much more practical than is the case when the latter is used for protection in large volume emergency RBC transfusions. Platelet transfusions carry the risk of immunization to HLA histocompatibility antigens. This possibility is of larger concern in those patients expected to require repeated platelet transfusions (*e.g.*, leukemia). In such patients consideration should be given to use of donor platelets with the best possible histocompatibility or perhaps, more ideally, to use autologous frozen platelets (58).

Leukocytes

Transfusion of **leukocytes** for treatment of bone marrow failure dates back to 1934; early success was minimal (51). Refinement of techniques and indications has improved usefulness of this form of component therapy, although it is still frequently considered investigational (10–12, 49, 51, 57). Transfusion of *lymphocytes* remains even less well established and carries the major hazard of initiating graft *vs.* host (GVH) disease in the immunosuppressed patients commonly considered for such transfusions (49).

Collection of leukocytes, with return of the rest of the blood to the donor, is done by plasmapheresis (leukapheresis) using either a nylon filtration technique or a cell separator (19, 43, 49). Using filtration techniques, an average of 3.7×10^{10} leukocytes can be collected from a single donor. Storage for 24 hours at 4 to 6°C maintains function and immediate posttransfusion survival adequately; however, the subsequent rate of disappearance from the bloodstream is increased, and it is doubtful whether 24-hour stored leukocytes are as effective as fresh ones (49). Frequently, they are kept at room temperature after collection and transfused within 12 hours (23).

Indication for leukocyte transfusion is generally considered to be for treatment of fever or sepsis with granulocytopenia (less than 500/μl) following cancer chemotherapy in patients who have culture results known or pending (11, 12, 49, 51). Its use as a prophylatic measure to prevent infection in patients receiving bone-marrow transplants has been suggested (17).

To date no reports of use of this component in patients with typical neurosurgical problems are known (44). However, it may be possible that leukocyte transfusions may play a role in some future chemotherapy protocols used for treatment of malignant central nervous system tumors. This may be even more likely in patients subjected to high-dose BCNU with subsequent bone marrow rescue (45, 48).

Risks of use of this component include hepatitis (same as whole blood) and alloimmunization to histocompatibility antigens as well as leukocyte-specific antigens (10, 49, 57). As with platelet transfusions, risk of histocompatibility antigen sensitization can probably be reduced by use of closely HLA-matched donors (57).

Plasma

Plasma is commonly available in two forms: stored plasma and fresh frozen plasma (FFP). **Pooled plasma** carries an unacceptably high hepatitis risk and is no longer used clinically (10). It still finds use as a starting material for blood fractionation, such as production of albumin and prothrombin complex. While stored plasma (single donor) occasionally finds use as a volume expander, it and FFP find their major role in replacement of clotting factors. For this reason it is appropriate to briefly review the role of these clotting factors in hemostasis. This will also be germane to subsequent discussions of factor VIII and prothrombin complexes and DIC.

THE HEMOSTATIC MECHANISM

Hemostasis and problems related to its defects are too complex for a complete presentation and only some points relevant to use of blood components will be presented. Activation of clotting begins with factor XII, and the Fletcher factor, kininogens, kinins, bradykinins, and complement. The activation phase initiates changes in vessel tone, immune system, fibrinolytic system, and coagulant system. Since clinical use of blood components usually plays a role only in management of disorders of the latter two systems, only they will be considered further.

A simplified version of the clotting pathway (*i.e.*, cascade) is presented in Figure 2.1. A list of clotting factors are given in Table 2.7 along with their **synonyms.** Table 2.6 details the levels of each factor (in terms of percent of normal level) required for adequate surgical hemostasis. The **intrinsic** (intravascular) **pathway** involves factors XII, XI, IX, and VIII, including factor VIII_{vwf} or "von Willebrand factor" which contribute activated VIII (VIII_a) toward activation of factor X to X_a in the **common pathway.** As noted earlier, platelet factor 3 is important in the intrinsic pathway. In addition, calcium (factor IV) is needed. In the **extrinsic** (extravascular) **pathway**, tissue thromboplastin activates factor VII

TABLE 2.7

*Coagulation Factor Nomenclature**

Factor	Synonyms
I	Fibrinogen
II	Prothrombin, prethrombin
III	Tissue factor, tissue thromboplastin
IV	Calcium
V	Proaccelerin, labile factor, Ac globulin
(VI)	Not assigned
VII	Proconvertin, SPCA, stable actor, autoprothrombin I
VIII	Antihemophilic factor (AHF), antihemophilic globulin, antihemophilic factor A, platelet cofactor I
IX	Plasma thromboplastin component (PTC), Christmas factor, antihemophilic factor B, autoprothrombin II, platelet cofactor II
X	Stuart-Prower factor, Stuart factor, autoprothrombin III
XI	Plasma thromboplastin antecedent (PTA), antihemophilic factor C
XII	Hageman factor
XIII	Fibrin-stabilizing factor, fibrinase, Laki-Lorand factor

* Activated factors are designated by an "a" after the Roman numeral.

which contributes to activation of factor X to X_a in the **common pathway.** In the **common pathway** factors X_a and V_a form a complex together with calcium and platelet phospholipid which can be termed prothrombinase. This complex activates II to II_a (thrombin), an esterase which cleaves fibrinopeptides A and B from fibrinogen (factor I) to form fibrin monomers (factor I_a) which polymerize. Factor XIII is also activated by II_a to XIII_a which serves to stabilize polymerized fibrin monomers. Without XIII_a the fibrin gel is soft and fragile and it disintegrates rapidly *in vivo*. Patients lacking factor XIII bleed severely. The fibrin meshwork serves to seal the platelet plug.

INHERITED DEFECTS OF CLOTTING FACTORS

While genetic defects can be responsible for deficiency of every one of the coagulation proteins, most are extremely rare. Hemophilia-A and -B are X-linked, hemophilia-C is autosomal recessive, and von Willebrand's disease is autosomal dominant. All share the variable expressivity characteristic of many genetic disease (37, 75).

The first four factors in the intrinsic pathway have been called "hemophilioid factors" because deficiency of three of them is responsible for the three types of hemophilia: classic hemophilia or hemophilia-A (factor VIII), Christmas's disease or hemophilia-B (factor IX), and hemophilia-C (factor XI). Deficiency of the fourth hemophilioid factor, factor XII, while important to normal laboratory tests of clotting, does not produce abnormal bleeding.

In von Willebrand's disease there is a defect in factor VIII activity, with a resultant defect in platelet function (adhesion and ristocetin aggregation), producing prolongation of the bleeding time. That a portion of the active fragment of factor VIII plays a role in this disease can be demonstrated by the correction of platelet aggregation (ristocetin induced), bleeding time, and patient hemorrhage by administration of factor VIII. This apparent dual, yet separable activity of factor VIII has led to a suggestion of the following nomenclature to prevent some of the confusion that might otherwise arise: (a) Factor VIII_{ahf} is the procoagulant activity of factor VIII, *i.e.*, antihemophilic factor activity. (b) Factor VIII_{vwf} is the activity which supports platelet aggregation with ristocetin, *i.e.*, von Willebrand factor activity. (c) factor VIII_{agn} is the protein which reacts in an immunoassay with rabbit antibodies to factor VIII, *i.e.*, factor VIII antigen (39). Thus, in hemophilia-A factor VIII_{ahf} is reduced, while both factor VIII_{vwf} and VIII_{agn} are normal or elevated; whereas, in von Willebrand's disease factor VIII_{vwf} is reduced along with factor VIII_{agn}. Some patients with von Willebrand's will also have somewhat low factor VIII_{ahf} (75).

ACQUIRED DEFECTS OF CLOTTING FACTORS

The classical example of acquired factor deficiencies is that associated with **vitamin K deficiency**, including its iatrogenic relative, oral anticoagulation. Four hepatically produced factors—factors II, VII, IX, and X—are defective and poorly functioning. Note that the intrinsic (factor IX), extrinsic (factor VII), and common (factor X and II) pathways are all affected, in a dramatic "shot-gunning" of the entire clotting mechanism. **Severe liver disease** in any form can produce deficiencies of these factors as well as others, since most coagulation factors are produced by the liver (60).

FIBRINOLYSIS

The last step in the hemostatic process is not designed to stop bleeding. On the contrary, fibrinolysis dissolves fibrin so as to scavenge fibrin from the vessel wall undergoing repair. Further, it prevents indefinite accumulation of fibrin which could seriously compromise blood flow.

The key elements of this process are depicted in Figure 2.2. As a result of appearance of as yet structurally uncharacterized activator substances, produced in the liver and vessel walls, plasminogen is converted to plasmin. This latter trypsin-like enzyme hydrolyzes susceptible bonds in fibrin, forming several degradation products. The same enzymatic action against fibrinogen is possible, so that fibrinolysis always involves some fibrinogenolysis (62). When this mechanism goes awry, not only will fibrin be dissolved before the vessel wall is repaired, resulting in bleeding, but fibinogen also may be consumed so that clotting cannot occur. Further,

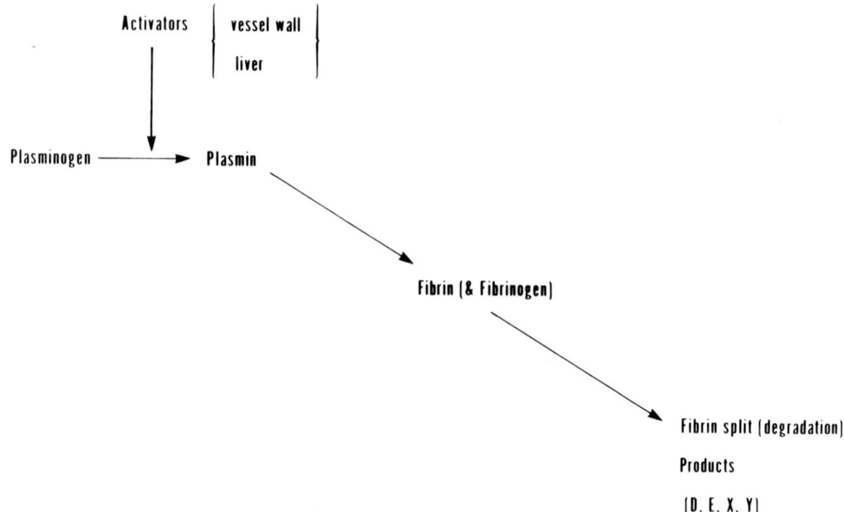

FIG. 2.2. Simplified scheme of fibrinolysis (fibrinogenolysis). Basic process is the same under normal condition (clot formation and resorption) and abnormal conditions (DIC).

fibrin degradation products may act as anticoagulants. Epsilon-aminocaproic acid (EACA) blocks the activation of plasminogen to plasmin, preventing fibrinolysis.

SCREENING TESTS OF COAGULATION

Full laboratory evaluation of the entire coagulation mechanism involves a host of tests ranging from gross (clotting time and bleeding time) to quite refined (specific factor assay) (8, 50, 79). The single most useful **"screening test"** is a good **bleeding history** which will uncover most coagulopathies (8, 50, 79). It is paramount to inquire about **previous surgery** with emphasis on bleeding during the operation or delayed bleeding after surgery, and excessive gum bleeding after dental extractions or bleeding after tonsillectomies. In females excessive menstrual bleeding may be significant. History of excessive bleeding from the umbilical stump should be a concern.

The details of the bleeding history can often point in the direction of a specific factor deficiency. Epistaxsis in childhood which improves after puberty is suggestive of von Willebrand's disease. With this disease bleeding usually occurs only after a challenge to the system, while in moderate to severe hemophilia spontaneous bleeding occurs. Excessive bleeding from the umbilical stump and/or a history of poor wound healing should prompt a closer look for factor XIII deficiency. Clotting factor deficiencies may produce a history of bleeding that stops and later starts.

A history of delayed bleeding after extraction or surgery is significant. History of solid or hematologic malignancy, liver disease, or drug intake (*e.g.*, aspirin, anticoagulants) is important.

A good history can be supplemented by appropriate laboratory tests. The tests ordered may be so insensitive as to miss all but the most florid deficiencies. An example of this is the whole blood clotting time, which becomes prolonged only when a factor VIII deficit reaches 1% of normal. By contrast, the more sensitive activated partial thromboplastin time (PTT) will be abnormal with factor VIII and IX levels of 30 to 40%. Even use of a battery, including bleeding time, platelet count, prothrombin time, and partial thromboplastin time, preoperatively, tends to expose the wrong patients. Those with moderate to severe hemophilia and severe liver disease usually should already be known on the basis of history and more sensitive laboratory tests of liver function. The patient with mild clotting factor abnormalities and negative bleeding history will not always be detected by screening tests,, and mild defects may produce major hemostatic problems under stress of surgery. Intraoperative blood loss and replacement with crystalloids and banked blood can further dilute borderline levels of factors in such patients. It must be realized that the above screening tests do not become abnormal until concentration of any single clotting factor falls below about one-fourth of its normal level (50).

A second problem is the matter of cost-effectiveness. A commonly suggested coagulation screen which consists of platelet count, bleeding time, prothrombin time (PT), partial thromboplastin time (PTT), and thrombin time (TT) can add $40.00 or more to the hospital bill. All those with a positive or questionable bleeding history should have these tests performed, supplemented with even more sophisticated tests as needed.

For the present, general use of the above screening tests in patients undergoing major CNS surgery cannot be strongly condemned and, in fact, is recommended. For those patients manifesting unexpected intraoperative, postoperative, or posttraumatic bleeding, these tests provide a key starting point in diagnostic evaluation and therapeutic decision-making. Table 2.8 outlines this five-test screening battery with some possible interpretations of abnormalities and other tests to use as supplements. Relationship of these tests to the clotting cascade and three pathways described above can be appreciated from Fig. 2.3. Armed with this basic knowledge of hemostasis, an examination of use of plasma and some of its components in treatment of hemostatic and other disorders is possible.

FRESH FROZEN PLASMA (FFP)

Preparation of this component is from single donor, CPD-preserved, fresh whole blood separated within 4 to 6 hours of collection. Following

TABLE 2.8
Five-Test Coagulation Battery

Test pattern*					Character of disorder	Possible causes	Supplementary tests
PC	BT	PT	PTT	TT			
D	I	N	N	N	Thrombocytopenia	See Table 2.5	Peripheral smear for platelet morphology, platelet antibodies
N	I	N	N	N	Platelet dysfunction vessel wall	See Table 2.5 esp. aspirin and uremia	Platelet aggregation and adhesion
N	I	N	I(±)	N	Hybrid disorder	Von Willebrand's	Factor VIII activity, platelet adhesion
N	N	N	I	N	Intrinsic pathway	Hemophilia incl XI & XII, heparin	Specific factor activity; correction with normal plasma, not with old plasma
N	N	I	N	N	Extrinsic pathway	Factor VII deficiency (rare)	Specific factor assay
N	N	I	I	N	Common pathway or extrinsic and intrinsic	Multiple factor: vitamin K defect liver disease coumarin	*In vitro* correction with normal plasma
N	N	I	I	I	Common pathway	Factor I defect DIC Circulating anticoagulant (heparin) primary fibrinolysis	Fibrinogen assay FDP*, poor *in vitro* correction with normal plasma
D	I	I	I	I	Hybrid disorder	DIC†	FDP, fibrinogen level, antithrombin III, paracoagulation tests
N	N(I)‡	I	I	N	Intrinsic and extrinsic pathways	Multiple transfusion (banked blood)	*In vitro* correction of PT, PTT, with normal plasma

* PC, platelet count; BT, bleeding time; PT, prothrombin time; PTT, partial thromboplastin time; TT, thrombin time; N, normal; D, decreased; I, increased; FDP, Fibrin degradation products.
† Abnormalities may vary widely with severity.
‡ PC usually = 50 to 100,000/μl.

centrifugation at 4°C, 200 to 250 ml of plasma is harvested and frozen in a −60°C bath or a −80°C freezer. **Storage** at −30°C or colder maintains stability of all coagulation factors (see Table 2.9), including labile factor V and 75% of factor VIII, for at least 1 year (9, 10, 23, 49). Immediately before use, FFP is thawed in the blood bank in a 37°C water bath for about 20 minutes. Once thawed it should be infused promptly (within 6 hours, preferably less) to provide maximal levels of factors V and VIII. It should be infused through a blood administration filter at the highest possible rate for maximal clotting factor recovery.

While plasma does not have to be blood group-specific, it should be ABO-compatible as indicated in Table 2.4. Analysis of the table should

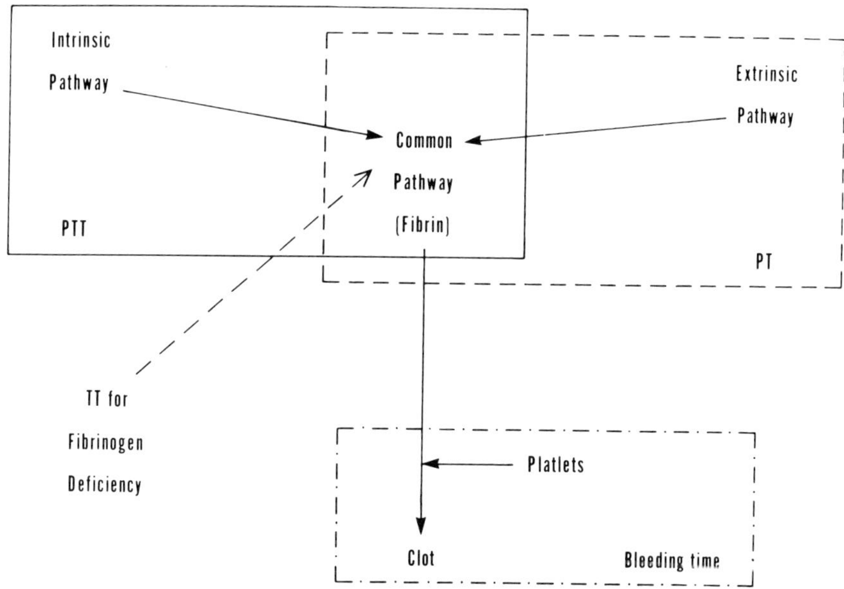

FIG. 2.3. Demonstration of portion of hemostatic mechanism assayed by each of the tests in the five-test coagulation battery (Table 2.8). PTT, partial thromboplastin time; PT, prothrombin time; TT, thrombin time. Platelet count assays platelet numbers; bleeding time assays platelet numbers and/or function.

TABLE 2.9
Clotting Factor Content of Blood Components

Component	Clotting factor*								
	I	II	V	VII	VIII	IX	X	XI	XIII
Stored plasma and whole blood	+	+	−	+	−	+	+	+	+
FFP	+	+	+	+	+	+	+	+	+
Cryoprecipitate	+	−	−	−	+	−	−	−	+
Factor VIII concentrate (lyophilized)	−	−	−	−	+	−	−	−	−
Prothrombin complex (factor II-X complex)	−	+	−	+	−	+	+	+	−

* +, therapeutic quantities present; −, therapeutic quantities not present.

make it obvious why many blood banks attempt to stockpile group AB plasma. Rh-specific plasma is not usually given because sentitization or other complications related to Rh have rarely been noted. However, if large volumes of plasma are used, Rh-negative individuals may become sensitized by small amounts of red cells always present in plasma (9). In

Stored plasma as a volume expander has **limited** use in conditions where considerable colloid may be lost rather acutely. These might include burns, peritoneal injuries, acute pancreatitis, mesenteric thrombosis, and initial treatment of hemorrhagic shock (10). No attempt will be made here to address the crystalloid *vs.* colloid debate or its relation to treatment of any of the above conditions (67). It can be stated that albumin along with appropriate amounts of crystalloid can achieve the same purpose as plasma with a risk of hepatitis near zero. Those choosing to use plasma for the "nutrition" provided should again be reminded that one and two-thirds eggs, a thin slice of meat, or a glass of milk provide the same amount of protein as 200 ml of plasma.

FACTOR VIII PREPARATIONS

Factor VIII_{ahf} or antihemophilia factor (AHF) is a clotting factor involved in the intrinsic pathway for hemostasis. Classic hemophilia (hemophilia-A) is a disease in which this factor is deficient. In addition to its relationship to this disease, factor VIII_{ahf} and factor VIII_{vwf} is important in treatment of von Willebrand's disease and plays an uncommon role in management of DIC and unexplained intraoperative blood loss.

Before 1964 FFP was the primary source of factor VIII_{ahf}. Since 1964, major advances in producing concentrated forms of factor VIII_{ahf} have made available two preparations, cryoprecipitate and factor VIII concentrate, for therapy in hemophilia and other appropriate disorders.

CRYOPRECIPITATE

Cryoprecipitate is prepared from single donor plasma by thawing a unit of FFP at 4°C and recovering th cold-precipitated factor VIII by centrifugation and decantation. The resultant bag contains 30 to 50% (70 to 100 units) of factor VIII_{ahf} and 10 to 60% of factor VIII_{vwf} in a volume of 10 to 25 ml representing a 2- to 12-fold concentration (9, 39, 49). Also present is factor I (200 to 250 mg/bag) and factor XIII (10 to 35% of plasma content). Yield in each case depends on the original activity in donor plasma and amount of plasma retained. By definition, a unit of any clotting factor is that amount of activity present in 1 ml of normal, fresh pooled plasma. Stored at −30°C or colder, stability of the three factors is maintained for 1 year.

Simple reconstitution is performed by thawing for 10 minutes at 37°C followed by prompt (within 4 to 6 hours) administration through a blood filter. It may be infused as single units or pooled into several units. If slight dilution is necessary, normal saline should be used. Whenever possible ABO-compatibility should be observed since hemolytic reactions have occurred when this was not done (9). The use of cryoprecipitate in hemophilia-A and von Willebrand's disease, as well as DIC and other intraoperative bleeding will be discussed below. It should also be recognized that cryoprecipitate serves as the best source of fibrinogen (factor I) in the clinical situations in which fibrinogen is indicated. This is because purified fibrinogen preparations carry an exceptionally high hepatitis risk and have been removed from the market. Cryoprecipitate has a hepatitis risk which is similar to that of whole blood or FFP, but a lower risk of febrile and allergic reactions.

FACTOR VIII CONCENTRATE

Factor VIII concentrates are commercial preparations made by polyethelene glycol fractionation of FFP (2, 3, 13, 57). The resultant material is lyophilized (freeze-dried). When stored at 4°C or room temperature it is usable for several months or several days, respectively. This latter feature makes it useful for severe hemophiliacs, since it allows some freedom of travel with outpatient administration.

Factor VIII_{ahf} activity (shown on the label of each vial) ranges from 100 to 1000 units per 25- to 30-ml vial (11). However, the factor VIII_{vwf} activity is quite variable and often low. Therefore, while these concentrates prove useful in management of hemophilia-A (see below), they are not recommended for therapy of von Willebrand's disease unless combined with cryoprecipitate. In this case factor VIII concentrates serve to boost levels of factor VIII_{ahf}, while cryoprecipitate boosts both factors VIII_{ahf} and VIII_{vwf} (9, 39). No significant amount of fibrinogen (factor I) is present. Administration after reconstitution can be intravenously or intramuscularly (10, 57).

Risk of hepatitis with factor VIII concentrates, as with other *commercially* provided blood components, is definitely greater than that of single donor whole blood, FFP, or cryoprecipitate. This is due, in large part, to the preparation of this material from large pools of plasma. Allergic reactions can also occur with this material (11). Since home use of factor VIII concentrate is common, some physicians routinely provide antihistamines, steroids, and isoproterenol for use by outpatient hemophiliacs.

HEMOPHILIA-A (FACTOR VIII_{AHF} DEFICIENCY)

Hemophilia-A is a genetic disease transmitted as a sex-lined recessive trait with an incidence of 1 per 10,000 to 100,000 population. Patients with this disease fail to synthesize normal amounts of factor VIII_{ahf}. However, degree of deficit is variable amount patients, producing varying severity of clinical manifestations (37, 50, 80).

Severe cases have less than 1% of normal factor VIII_{ahf} levels and suffer from repeated episodes of spontaneous hemorrhages, especially hemarthroses. They commonly bleed excessively at circumcision. Factor VIII_{ahf}

levels in moderate cases range from 1 to 5% of normal. These patients have infrequent spontaneous bleeding attacks and may reach adulthood without crippling deformities. Mild cases have levels in the 6 to 30% range and rarely have spontaneous bleeding. This latter group may first come to recognition when excessive bleeding occurs after dental extraction or other relatively minor surgery.

Another serious problem that occurs in 6 to 21% of patients is the development of circulating inhibiting antibodies (usually after previous treatment with factor VIII preparations) to factor VIII_{ahf} (*i.e.*, directed at the procoagulant portion of the molecule). When these appear, severity of the bleeding problem may increase, but management always becomes more difficult (21, 37, 49).

A recent study found 56 cases of central nervous system (CNS) bleeding among 2,100 patients (27%) with hemophilia-A (21). Fifty-four patients had intracranial bleeding. In nearly one-half, there was no history of trauma. **No** etiology was apparent in 38%. Of those with trauma one-half had a long (4 ± 2.2 days) symptom-free interval. Combined mortality was 34%. Of 27 survivors, six had recurrent CNS bleeding in absence of trauma. Twenty-one percent developed factor VIII_{ahf}-inhibiting antibodies.

The PTT is prolonged in all patients with factor VIII_{ahf} levels of less than 20% normal and is borderline in patients with levels in the range of 20 to 30% normal. While this test is helpful in uncovering mild cases with no past history of bleeding, modern management of these patients requires ability to perform factor VIII assays.

Level of factor VIII_{ahf} required in most patients with hemophilia changes based on the clinical situation: (a) minor hemorrhage and prophylaxis, about 15% of normal; (b) minor surgery about 30% normal, and (c) major surgery (the majority of neurosurgical procedures) 40 to 50% normal (9). However, for major surgery (especially intracranial) other-shave recommended factor VIII_{ahf} levels of 80 to 100% normal (measured immediately after transfusion) with a continuation of these levels until healing is well under way (23, 55).

The recommendations of the study on CNS bleeding in hemophiliacs (21) were: (a) **Severe hemophiliacs** need immediate treatment for head and spine injury. With **minor trauma** a single dose of factor VIII sufficient to raise the plasma level to **40 to 50% normal is** proposed (Table 2.6). With **more significant injury**, including that associated with signs and symptoms, treatment should be repeated one or more times on a 12- to 24-hour basis. Because of the long symptom-free interval observed, untreated cases seen within 5 days of previous significant head trauma should receive at least one dose of replacement therapy. **Back injuries** should also receive prompt treatment. (b) If intracranial or intraspinal bleeding is documented, minimal levels of 30 to 50% should be maintained for at least 10 to 14 days. (c) If bleeding is not documented but symptoms are present, treatment during a few days of observation is recommended. (d) Mild hemophiliacs need treatment only for significant trauma; however, poor history reliability in children under 8 to 10 years makes treatment of trivial injuries in this group wise. (e) **Rapid infusion** of factor VIII_{ahf} for any known hemophiliac suspected of CNS bleeding **before** institution of definitive investigation is emphasized. (f) Activated prothrombin complex (see below) should be considered for CNS bleeding in those with high-titer factor VIII_{ahf}-inhibiting antibodies.

In planning dosage schedules it must be recalled that the metabolic half-life of factor VIII_{ahf} is about 12 hours. Table 2.6 provides some rough guidelines regarding initial and maintenance dosage for cryoprecipitate and lyophilized factor VIII_{ahf} concentrate. A rough calculation of dosage can be made as follows:

$$\text{Dose (units)} = (\text{desired factor VIII concentration} - \text{initial factor VIII concentration}) \times \text{plasma volume}$$

where factor concentrations are in units per ml.

Approximate adult plasma volume is 41 ml/kg of body weight. Nomograms are available for more accurate estimates of plasma volume. To predict the eventual factor VIII_{ahf} concentration (in terms of percent normal), half-life and volume of distribution need to be considered. When this is done, it is discovered that **one unit of factor VIII_{ahf} per kilogram of body weight produces a 2% rise in plasma levels in adults (about 1.5% in children)**. The amount of lyophilized Factor VIII_{ahf} concentrate required can be determined from these calculations plus information provided on each vial regarding number of units in the vial. When using **cryoprecipitate** which has a variable number of units per bag, a good approximation is that **each bag** (average number of units = 80) will produce a **2% rise** in plasma factor VIII_{ahf} levels in an average adult (70 kg) (9, 39).

The difficulty of attempting to use **FFP** in total management of hemophiliacs can be demonstrated as follows:

1. A severe hemophiliac (less than 1% activity) sustains a head injury with acute subdural hematoma, intracerebral hematoma, and cerebral swelling. The patient weighs 70 kg.
2. At least 50% of normal factor VIII_{ahf} level would be desired.
3. From the above information about 1750 units of factor VIII_{ahf} would be needed as an initial dose, followed (because of the 12-hour half-life) by an equivalent dose every 8 hours for, perhaps, 24 hours, then every 12 hours for 10 to 14 days.
4. FFP contains about 0.8 units factor VIII_{ahf} per milliliter.

5. Therefore, roughly 2200 ml of FFP would be needed for each dose per the schedule immediately above. It should be obvious that such volumes would not only adversely affect the course of cerebral swelling, but also would almost certainly compromise cardiac function. By contrast, the volume of each dose of cryoprecipitate required to achieve equivalent levels of factor VIII_{ahf} would be about 350 ml (even lower with better cryoprecipitate preparations). Therefore, use of FFP in most hemophiliacs needing factor VIII_{ahf} replacement is an emergency, stop-gap measure to be reserved for the rare situation in which sufficient concentrated forms of factor VIII are not readily available.

Prophylactic treatment of severe hemophiliacs with factor VIII_{ahf} concentrates can reduce overall frequency of bleeding by 15% but necessitate administration of 73% more factor VIII to these patients than required for intermittent bleeds (49). A 66% reduction in bleeding incidence would require 160% more factor VIII administration. It has been estimated that, to prophylactically convert all severe hemophiliacs to moderate hemophiliacs with factor VIII concentrates would require fractionation of over 20 million units of plasma (donations) per year for the U. S. alone (39). In 1976 only 6 million units of plasma were fractionated into factor VIII. A potentially serious side effect of such a course would be an increase in cases of hepatitis in these patients, since practical outpatient therapy favors use of the hepatitis-prone, lyophilized concentrates. Therefore selection of patients for prophylactic therapy should be left to those with wide experience in its use.

Optimal management of hemophiliacs mandates the ready availability of factor VIII_{ahf} assays. In those situations in which the assay is not readily available, Table 2.10 can be used for guidelines for therapy until the patient can be transferred to an adequate facility. **Management** of hemophiliacs **requires** constant assistance of a **competent hematologist** in addition to excellent laboratory and blood bank facilities.

VON WILLEBRAND'S DISEASE

This genetic disorder is transmitted as an autosomal dominant with variable expression (resulting in variable clinical severity). **Clinical manifestations** tend to be of the **"platelet type"** with epistaxis, gum bleeds, ecchymoses, and gastrointestinal and uterine bleeds (27). These may improve somewhat at puberty only to reappear as a serious bleeding problem during surgery. Laboratory diagnosis rests in part on prolongation of the bleeding time and decreased **ristocetin-induced platelet aggregation**. Factor VIII_{ahf} levels are usually higher than in hemophilia-

TABLE 2.10

Factor VIII_{ahf} Dosage in Severe Hemophiliacs Where Factor VIII Assays Not Available

Clinical condition	Initial dose	Maintenance dose
Intracranial or intraspinal surgery	1 PV* 1 to 2 hr preoperatively	1 PV q 8 hr for 24 hr, then 1 PV q 12 hr for 10 to 14 days, then ¼ PV q 12 hr for 14–28 days
Other surgical procedures (*e.g.*, ulnar nerve transposition)	1 PV 1 to 2 hr preoperatively	½ PV q 8 hr for 24 hr, then 1/2 PV q 12 hr for 7–10 days; then 1/4 PV q 12 hr for 3–7 days
Major hemorrhage† (incl. all intracranial and intraspinal)	1 PV	1/2 PV 1 8 hr for 24 hr, then 1/2 PV q 12 hr until 3–5 days after bleeding stops (10–14 days for intracranial or intraspinal bleeding)

* PV, plasma volume (about 41 ml/kg body weight); the number of ml in the PV corresponds to the number of units of factor VIII to be given.

†, Give initial dose prophylactically in head injuries even if minor; consider maintenance dosage in more serious injuries even if bleeding not apparent.

A, but values of 1 to 5% may be found (75). Factor VIII_{vwf} assayed by the ristocetin method gives levels of 25% or less in patients with severe clinical symptoms, but may be normal in less severely affected patients. A more recent study suggests that ratio of factor VIII_{ahf} level to factor VIII_{agn} level and factor VIII_{agn} level are more sensitive and specific in diagnosis than the other tests mentioned (42).

Therapy is directed toward increasing factor VIII_{vwf} level and VIII_{ahf} and reducing the bleeding time, although the latter effect is variable. Infusion of FFP or cryoprecipitate may raise the level of factor VIII_{ahf} for 12 to 24 hours. Patients with mild disease usually respond more readily than severe cases (39). However, precise knowledge is not available on the specific factors required to correct hemostatic defects in this disease, nor the metabolic half-life of the plasma component(s) effective in therapy. At present diagnosis and monitoring of therapy combines factor VIII_{ahf} assay, ristocetin-induced platelet aggregation, factor VIII_{agn} levels, and bleeding time.

FFP in doses of 10 to 15 ml plasma/kg body weight per day (Table 2.6) have been recommended and may suffice in milder cases (39). However, in more severe cases volumes required frequently become prohibitive. Therefore, except under the most unusual circumstances, cryoprecipitate serves as the component for treatment of von Willebrand's disease. Initial doses of 1 to 1.5 bags of cryoprecipitate/ 10kg/day may suffice for a 70-kg man; however, larger doses may be required. Patients scheduled for surgery should have therapy instituted 48 hours preoperatively. Postoperative maintenance should continue for periods similar to those in hemophilia-A. As already noted, lyophilized factor VIII concentrates do not seem to be as effective as cryoprecipitate in this disease.

PROTHROMBIN COMPLEX CONCENTRATE

Prothrombin complex concentrate (also called factor II-X complex or factor IX complex) is prepared by fractionation of pooled, stored plasma, since all of the contained factors (II, VII, IX, X) are stable for up to 26 days at 4°C. It is then lyophilized and stored in vials for periods indicated on the label. Each vial contains 500 units of factor IX and variable amounts of factors II, VII, and X (usually about 250 units each) (9). The reconstitution volume is on the label of the vial and is small. Administration is by the intravenous route.

HEMOPHILIA-B (FACTOR IX DEFICIENCY)

Hemophilia-B (factor IX deficiency or Christmas disease) serves as the primary indication for use of this concentrate. Hemophilia-B is one-fourth to one-tenth as common as hemophilia-A; it also is inherited as a sex-linked recessive. As with hemophilia-A it is variable in severity and usually produces prolongation of the PTT. It also requires capacity to perform specific factor assays (here, factor IX) for precise diagnosis and management. Its involvement of the central nervous system is quite similar in frequency and character to that discussed above with hemophilia-A (21). Likewise, therapeutic recommendations regarding management of head trauma and CNS bleeding are similar (21).

Dosage calculations for use of prothrombin complex in hemophilia-B must take into account an *in vivo* recovery of factor IX of only 30 to 60% of that infused. Therefore, a dose arrived at using calculations described under hemophilia-A should be doubled. Half-life shows an initial rapid phase (5 hours) followed by a slower phase (24 hours), giving a functional half-life of 15 to 20 hours (9, 39). This allows maintenance of adequate levels, in most cases, with infusion once every 24 hours.

For most major surgery and CNS bleeding or bleeding after major trauma, a factor IX level of 40 to 50% of normal is usually adequate. As with classic hemophilia, immediate postinfusion levels of 80 to 100% are desirable in intracranial surgery (23). An initial dose of 40 to 60 units/kg of body weight, followed by 10 to 20 units/kg/day is suggested (Table 2.6). The caveat regarding appropriate consultation and laboratory facilities pertains.

Use of prothrombin complex to treat deficiencies of other factors available in this complex will not be detailed here, as they are very rare. Some guidelines regarding adequate levels and suggested doses of these factors are contained in Table 2.6.

Prothrombin complex (partially "activated") can bypass the function of factor VIII_{ahf} and, therefore, may be useful in managing hemophilia-A patients who have circulating inhibiting antibodies to factor VIII_{ahf} (see above) (9, 21, 39, 49). "Nonactivated" complex concentrates also seem to work, perhaps because some preformed coagulant activity is present in most concentrates.

Use of this complex in treatment of patients with severe liver disease and in neonates is contraindicated because thrombosis or DIC may occur after infusion (9). Other risks include a significant risk of hepatitis since it is prepared from pooled plasma (39). Therefore, prothrombin complex should not be used in patients without compelling reasons, the primary of which is management of hemophilia.

DISSEMINATED INTRAVASCULAR COAGULATION AND UNEXPECTED SURGICAL BLEEDING

It is appropriate to discuss DIC and unexpected surgical bleeding under the same heading since the former may be a cause of the latter. In either case blood component therapy often plays a significant role. **DIC** is a syndrome with many synonyms, including consumption coagulopathy, defibrination syndrome, and intravascular coagulation with fibrinolysis (24, 50). Over the past 15 years numerous papers have addressed this problem (for 388 such papers see reference 53).

The syndrome reflects presence in the circulation of the enzyme and clotting factor, thrombin (53). Thrombin, in turn, activates platelets and other clotting factors with the result being their consumption and the formation of fibrin thrombi. The latter two events can lead to production of hemostatic defects and tissue ischemia from thrombi in the microcirculation. Finally, fibrinolysis is activated which also may compound hemostatic problems.

Many different disorders can predispose to DIC (24, 50, 53). In a consideration of all cases (acute and chronic) the most common underlying conditions are infection and neoplasm (53). Infection, especially with gram-negative bacteria and liberation of endotoxin, can play a role. Coagulant proteins from a number of sources can be important. Chief among these is tissue juice or thromboplastin, of which damaged brain is a rich source. Shock and hypoxia are other important predisposing factors in surgical patients. A more unusual inciting factor in surgical patients is transfusion reactions.

In neurosurgical populations head trauma is a common cause (72). One study found 9 of 13 patients with head trauma and brain destruction to have laboratory evidence of DIC; whereas 13 patients with head trauma but without brain damage showed no evidence of DIC (27). Platelet counts and plasma fibrinogen fall after injury, and acute DIC may occur (7, 20). In one group of 150 head-injured patients clinical evidence of DIC was observed in 12 and laboratory evidence of it in another 48 patients (71). A recent study discovered 12 **delayed** or **recurrent** intracranial hematomas in 340 patients with head injuries (40). Eleven had some laboratory evidence of DIC, while seven of the eight with delayed traumatic intracerebral hematomas (31) had associated clotting abnormalities. DIC may present in acute and chronic forms; the former being most common in neurosurgical patients. In the former onset is rapid, the patient is critically ill, and the predominant event is bleeding; mortality can be high. In the latter, onset is slow, thrombosis predominates, and mortality relates to the underlying disease process.

Numerous **changes** occur **in** the **coagulation mechanism** (24, 50, 53). If tissue thromboplastin is present, as it frequently is in DIC in neurosurgical patients, factor X will be depleted. The inevitable presence of thrombin in DIC activates and, thereby, variably depletes fibrinogen (converted to fibrin monomers); factors V, VIII, and XIII; and platelets. Prothrombin (factor II) levels are only partially reduced.

In predictable response to intravascular coagulation, secondary fibrinolysis is activated (Fig. 2.2, above). The resultant fibrin degradation products (FDP) inhibit polymerization of fibrin monomers into a clot, impair the action of thrombin on fibrinogen, and inhibit platelet function (24, 53). Further, the enzyme plasmin, which attacks fibrin, also may attack fibrinogen, leading to further depletion of this already reduced clotting factor.

Laboratory abnormalities in the "screening" tests of the hemostatic mechanism can be seen in Table 2.8. However, the four most useful tests for the diagnosis and monitoring of therapy are the PT, fibrinogen assay, platelet count, and FDP determination (24). A modern coagulation lab should be able to complete this battery in slightly more than 1 hour from receipt of a blood sample. All but the quantitative FDP should be done in about 30 minutes. A qualitative FDP can be done in about 15 minutes, but a final answer takes about 1 hour. Table 2.11 demonstrates the changes in these tests in DIC (61). Trends in the above tests (especially platelet count, fibrinogen level, and FDP) are often of more value than a single test (24).

While many consider the FDP test to be confirmatory, it should be recognized that elevated FDP levels can occur in conditions other than DIC, such as the postoperative state (1 to 7 days postop), trauma, and

TABLE 2.11

Four Useful Tests in DIC

Test	Level in DIC*	Comment
PT	E	Abnormal in 90%
Fibrinogen	R	Abnormal in 70%
Platelet count	R	Abnormal in 90%
FDP	E	Abnormal in 95% Consider paracoagulation tests

* E, elevated; R, reduced.

venous thrombosis (61, 68). For this reason some recommend addition of paracoagulation tests for fibrin monomers (protamine sulfate tests, ethanol gelation test), which identify a fibrinolytic state as being secondary to DIC (24, 53, 71). Unfortunately, they are frequently negative in patients who apparently have DIC (23, 24).

Before proceeding with a discussion of therapy for DIC some attention to the topic of **unexplained surgical bleeding** is appropriate since it may be due to DIC, especially in brain surgery. The commonest cause of unexplained surgical bleeding is "factor XIV or XV deficiency." "Factor XIV," depending on the surgical specialty, can be defined as a catgut, silk, or electrocoagulation. "Factor XV," common to all specialties, is an inadequate preoperative coagulation evaluation including, most importantly, a good bleeding history and the laboratory screening battery described earlier. Neglecting to note that a patient is on aspirin, has liver disease, or has a history of epistaxis or postdental surgery bleeding can provide for many unnecessary anxious moments during a craniotomy.

The nature of operative bleeding may provide some clues. Preexisting platelet disorders, as well as some severe clotting factor deficiencies (whether congenital or acquired), will present as a bloody field from the beginning of the operation. This is especially true of thrombocytopenia. On the other hand, some mild disorders of clotting factors and platelets will present only later in the operation, as clotting factors and platelets become further depleted through use in the normal clotting process or through dilution by fluid administration or transfusion of stored blood.

Somewhat delayed intraoperative bleeding is common with DIC. The first warning is oozing from the incision, first a trickle, then progressively more severe bleeding from the entire surgical field. If mismatched blood is the cause, clumping of red cells may be noted on surgical instruments. As DIC progresses the anesthesiologist may notice appearance of ecchymoses and bleeding from recent venipuncture sites. Unexplained bleeding that is delayed until the early postoperative period may be due to a rare factor XIII deficiency (50).

When confronted with unexplained intraoperative bleeding, several steps should be taken. First, inspect the area to rule out a "factor XIV deficiency" (uncoagulated bleeders). Next, have the anesthesiologist draw blood for appropriate laboratory studies including: peripheral smear, platelet count, PT, PTT, fibrogen assay, and FDP assay; as well as, factor VIII, IX, and XI assays if the first group does not provide a satisfactory answer. As already mentioned, a good coagulation lab should be able to complete all of the above, including specific factor assays, in slightly over 1 hour, if needed. The anesthesiologist or a nurse or technician can usually perform a bleeding time on an exposed extremity. Next, or simultaneous with the above, any obviously damaged brain (a predisposing agent for DIC) that can be removed should be; the anesthesiologist should recheck blood bags for possible mismatch; and hypotension and hypoxia should be searched for and corrected, if found. Finally, an urgent call to the local coagulation expert is not only appropriate, but necessary, if the above simple therapeutic measures have failed and bleeding is becoming progressively more severe.

The therapy of DIC during surgery or in neurosurgical patients not needing surgery remains controversial (24, 27, 53, 71). It is generally agreed that whenever possible the most important first step in neurosurgical treatment of DIC is to remove the predisposing factor—damaged brain tissue. Of course, this is not always safe from the standpoint of neurological morbidity. Also all would agree that hypoxia and hypotension must be corrected. Opinion is divided over the role of heparin for DIC in patients in general, and neurosurgical patients, in particular (24, 27, 53). While it is beneficial in selected patients, problems of monitoring and safely dealing with continued bleeding, which sometimes can occur with heparin therapy for DIC, can be particularly difficult and dangerous in the CNS (27). When the neurosurgeon and his coagulation consultant feel **heparin** is indicated, the usual **dosage** is an initial bolus of 5,000 to 10,000 units IV, then 700 to 1,500 units IV per hour by continuous infusion (24, 53). It is generally agreed that the antifibrinolytic drug, **epsilon-aminocaproic acid is rarely indicated** in DIC and should never be given without concurrent heparin therapy (24, 27).

Use of **blood component therapy in DIC** also finds opinions divided (24). The theoretical role is for replacement therapy of the recognized clotting factor and platelet deficiencies in DIC. Cryoprecipitate (for factor VIII and fibrinogen), FFP (for factors V, X, and also VIII and fibrinogen), and platelet concentrates (for the thrombocytopenia) are components to consider (Table 2.12).

Because DIC in patients with severe head trauma and brain destruction has been associated with increased morbidity and mortality (27, 71), prophylactic administration of cryoprecipitate (12 bags), FFP (2 to 4

TABLE 2.12

Component Therapy in DIC

Clotting material	Hemostatic level required	Source	Amount (approx)
Fibrinogen	100–125 mg/dl	Cryoprecipitate FFP	250 mg/bag 600 mg unit
Factor VIII	40–50% normal activity	Cryoprecipitate FFP	80 units/bag 300 units/bag
Factor V	25% normal activity	FFP	250 units/bag
Factor X (seldom needed)	15–20% normal activity	FFP	250 units/bag
Platelets	30,000–50,000/μl	Platelets	5.5×10^{10} /bag

units), and platelet concentrates (calculated to increase platelet count to at least 75,000/ml) has been suggested (27). This recommendation was made in spite of a 5 to 20% risk of hepatitis with such therapy (23).

When confronted with possible DIC at surgery, it is reasonable to consider component therapy while awaiting laboratory results. In this case the initial dose is 10 to 15 bags of cryoprecipitate and 4 units of FFP (24). Since an estimation of platelet numbers can be obtained so rapidly from a peripheral smear, platelet transfusion might be reserved until this result, if not the platelet count (15 minutes), is available. When thrombocytopenia is confirmed, platelet units (commonly called "packs") should be given to raise the platelet count to 30,000 to 50,000/ml. However, prophylactic administration of 8 to 10 units of platelets in severe situations, along with FFP and cryoprecipitate, could not be strongly criticized. Maintenance dosages of these same materials should be given to keep platelet counts in the range of 30,00 to 50,000/ml and fibrinogen level at 100 to 125 mg/dl. Although commercial preparations of fibrinogen were used for replacing the latter in the past, they are no longer available. Factor VIII levels should be kept in the range of 80 to 100% of normal (measured 1 hour postinfusion) using cryoprecipitate primarily. Factor V has an adequate hemostatic effect when present in the range of 25% of normal. FFP, which contains 200 to 300 units of factor V per bag, can be used to maintain this coagulant protein. Factor X is seldom a replacement consideration in DIC, but, if necessary, it can be given as FFP which contains 200 to 300 units per bag. Effective hemostatic levels of Factor X are 15 to 20% for major surgical and CNS bleeding problems (24). Component therapy using cryoprecipitate, FFP, and platelet concentrates to maintain the levels suggested above usually is a supplement to heparin therapy for those favoring use of the latter drug (24).

Whereas rough calculation of maintenance dosage of clotting factors in most congenital deficiency states is a possibility, since rates of production, half-life, and distribution volumes are somewhat established, it is not possible in DIC, where half-lives and volumes of distribution are greatly affected by the "consumptive" process. This consumption is a dynamic process, but the rates and volume involved are constantly changing. Production may also be perturbed in a varying manner. Therefore no formulae presently exist to provide guidelines for estimation of maintanence requirements of clotting factors or platelets in DIC. The best guidance is frequent use of the coagulation lab with particular attention to platelet and fibrinogen levels as well as FDP and PT.

THERAPY OF UNEXPLAINED INTRAOPERATIVE BLEEDING

Reflection on the above recommendations for initial component management of DIC (cryoprecipitate, 10 to 12 units; FFP, 4 units; and, perhaps, platelets, 4 to 6 units) demonstrates that adequate initial treatment for DIC covers **unexplained intraoperative bleeding** as well. This would include such conditions as: the mild, previously unrecognized hemophilia-A and -B or von Willebrand's disease, vitamin K deficiency or coumarin anticoagulant drugs, most of the rare congenital clotting factor deficiencies, and most platelet disorders (if platelet units are part of the prophylaxis). Further treatment can usually wait for the 1 to 2 hours required for a good coagulation lab to do a major clotting evaluation, including specific factor assays.

ALBUMIN

It is now appropriate to discuss the last three commonly available blood components—albumin, plasma protein fraction, and immunoglobulin. **Albumin** (human) is a serum protein with a molecular weight of about 68,000 (9, 68, 69). It is prepared by the Cohn cold-ethanol precipitation technique from pooled plasma. In the resultant product not less than 96% of the protein is albumin. In the U. S. each unit of plasma used in preparation is nonreactive for hepatitis B surface antigen and the product is pasturized at 60°C for 10 hours. This renders the final material nearly **free of risk of hepatitis** induction. Albumin solutions contain no clinically significant isoagglutinins or other antibodies and may be given without concern over the recipient's blood group or Rh type. None of the recognized components of the clotting mechanism is present.

Solutions are available in two concentrations. The **5% solution** is supplied in 250 or 500 ml quantities and the **25% solution** in 50 or 100 ml. The sodium concentration of each ranges from 130 to 150 mEq/liter. This has produced the **misnomer, "salt-poor" albumin,** which is occasionally applied to the 25% solution. The sodium present in this solution has been concentrated several times less than the albumin; however, it remains relatively equivalent to solutions such as normal saline or Ringer's solution. The 5% albumin is iso-oncotic with human plasma; 25% solutions are oncotically equivalent to 5 times their volume of human plasma. Solutions may be stored at 37°C or less for up to 3 years or 2 to 10°C for up to 5 years, depending on instructions on the label. The solutions are compatible for infusion in conjunction or combined with whole blood, plasma, sterile water for injection, and dextrose, sodium lactate, or sodium chloride solutions.

A great deal of information is available on the pharmacology of albumin (68). Briefly, it is a factor of some importance in regulating plasma volume and tissue fluid balance because of its colloidal oncotic effects. Normally, it constitutes 50 to 60% of plasma protein and exerts 80 to 85% of the colloid oncotic pressure of the blood. Intravenous infusion of concentrated (25%) albumin produces a shift of fluid from interstitial spaces into the circulation and a slight increase in plasma protein concentration. When given to a well-hydrated patient, each volume of 25% albumin solution draws about 3.5 volumes of additional fluid into the circulation within 15 minutes, reducing hemoconcentration and blood viscosity. In those with reduced blood volume (from hemorrhages, exudates, edema), hemodilution persists for many hours; however, in patients with normal blood volume excess fluid and protein are lost from the circulation within a few hours. In dehydrated patients, albumin usually produces little or no clinical improvement unless other additional fluids are administered. While albumin contains some amino acids, it provides only **minimal to modest** nutritional effect. However, it binds and acts as a carrier of intermediate metabolites (such as bilirubin), trace metals, some drugs, dyes, fatty acids, hormones, and enzymes, so that it affects the transport, inactivation, and/or exchange of many tissue products.

Uses of albumin still remain controversial (9, 10, 23, 39, 49, 59, 69). Table 2.13 provides a list for consideration (69). In the table the terms "appropriate," "unjustified use," etc. are those of Tullis and are based on a consideration of potential usefulness of albumin in a given clinical situation compared with costs of the material and probable lack of sufficient supplies, if it were used in an unbridled manner (69).

It is sufficient to say that no indication listed meets with universal agreement among surgeons or fluid physiologists. For many years it has

TABLE 2.13
Possible Uses of Human Albumin

1. Appropriate use:
   a. Shock, hypovolemic
   b. Burns
   c. Adult respiratory distress syndrome
   d. Cardiopulmonary bypass
   e. Induction of hypervolemia*
2. Occasional use:
   a. Acute liver failure
   b. RBC resuspension media
   c. Ascites
   d. Postoperatively
   e. Acute nephrosis
   f. Renal dialysis
3. Uses requiring more data:
   a. Detoxification
4. Unjustified use:
   a. Undernutrition
   b. Chronic nephrosis
   c. Chronic cirrhosis

* Special neurosurgical use

been suggested that albumin can be of value in fluid resuscitation in hypovolemic (including hemorrhagic) shock. However, no conclusive data can be mustered to show it to be clinically or experimentally better than crystalloids and packed cells, or whole blood (26, 59, 63, 67). A possible exception, on which many agree is that colloid therapy including albumin, plays a role in burn management in the period after the first 24 hours (9, 18, 59, 69). In such situations the 5% solution is preferred. Occasionally, in hypoalbuminemia of acute liver failure and rarely in ascites albumin may play a role in drawing fluid back into the circulation. Here, the 25% solution is suggested. However, its use in treating the hypoalbuminemia of undernutrition and chronic renal or liver failure is strongly discouraged as a waste of a costly and scarce commodity (69).

Albumin, especially 25% solutions, might have some theoretical advantage in severe head trauma with cerebral edema; however, there is no known clinical or experimental evidence to support this. The one recent indication is induction and maintenance of elevated blood volumes in patients with vasospasm following subarachnoid hemorrhage in ruptured intracranial aneurysms (52). From the considerations presented above it is probably advisable to use repeated doses of 25% albumin solutions. In addition, should the patient have initial evidence of dehydration, some additional fluid over normal maintenance needs should be given to correct this problem. Techniques are available to monitor the increase in blood volume and its cardiovascular side effects, if any (52). Production of circulatory overload is the only significant risk associated with use of albumin.

PLASMA PROTEIN FRACTION

This material is prepared in 5% solutions (50 mg/ml) from pooled human plasma. It is subjected to the same precautions applied to albumin, including pasteurization, to prevent hepatitis (10). The proteins present consist of 83 to 90% albumin, 17% or less α and β-globulins, and 1% or less γ-globulin. Depending on method of storage it has a 3 to 5 year shelf life. Its indications are similar to those for 5% albumin solutions, and, therefore, are quite limited. Unfortunately, this component has been noted to produce episodes of serious hypotension secondary to presence of Hageman factor fragments (2), and its use is strongly discouraged.

IMMUNE SERUM GLOBULIN (ISG) AND SPECIFIC IMMUNOGLOBULINS

Immune serum globulin (ISG) is a blood component prepared from large batches of pooled plasma (usually 1000 donors) by an alcohol fractionation technique. It is supplied as a 16% solution of ISG in 2-, 5-, or 10-ml vials. It may be stored at 2 to 8°C for up to 3 years. It contains antibodies to which the general population has been exposed and must have specified titers of neutralizing antibodies to diptheria antitoxin, poliovirus, and measles. Administration of ISG (and other, specific immunoglobulins) serves to provide passive immunity by increasing the patient's antibody titer and his antigen-antibody reaction potential. **Indications** for ISG, may include congenital immunodeficiency disorders, acquired hypogammaglobulinemia, and prevention or modification of hepatitis-A (9, 11). It has limited effectiveness in preventing hepatitis-B and does not seem to be effective in preventing posttransfusion (non-A, non-B) hepatitis (11).

It may contain the IgG blood group isohemagglutinins anti-A and anti-B. It should be given intramuscularly to prevent complications including sensitization to ISG and possible anaphylaxis. Its use entails a very small risk of hepatitis (11).

Specific immunoglobulins are prepared by the same techniques as ISG, from pooled donor plasma which is known to have a high titer to a specific antigen. Table 2.14 lists the currently available types and suggested uses (9, 11). A few are of sufficient interest to neurosurgeons to merit further discussion.

Rh_o(D) immune globulin is prepared from plasma from RH-negative volunteers who have produced high titers of anti-D following immunization. It suppresses antibody response of Rh_o(D) negative individuals to foreign Rh_o(D) positive antigen, which may be in the form of fetal cells introduced at birth, abortion, amniocentesis, or antepartum hemorrhage. Its prime use in relation to surgery is to prevent Rh (D) sensitization in

TABLE 2.14

Immune Serum Globulins (Human)

Generic name	Therapeutic uses
Immune serum globulin (ISG)	Congenital immunodeficiency, acquired hypogammaglobulinemia, hepatitis-A, measles (rubeola and rubella), chicken pox, herpes zoster, bacterial infections
RH_o (D) immune globulin	To reduce frequency of sensitization *of Rh-negative women:* after birth of Rh-positive child, after abortion, after serious antepartum hemorrhage, and *when Rh-positive RBC must be infused during childbearing age*
Tetanus immune globulin	Used vice horse antitetanus serum for prevention and treatment of tetanus in previously unimmunized
Rabies immune globulin	To provide passive immunity to those exposed to rabies infection
Hepatitis B immune globulin	Prevention or modification of hepatitis
Zoster immune globulin	Prevention of varicella and disseminated zoster in exposed patients with immunodeficiencies

women of child-bearing age when, in emergency situations, it is necessary to transfuse them with blood components containing Rh-positive cells (RBC, platelets, and, rarely, leukocytes). To be effective it must be administered within 72 hours of exposure. Dosage is 1 vial, IM. A cross-match against the patient's RBC must be performed before administration. If a vial is incompatible by cross-match, a vial from another lot should be tested.

Tetanus immune globulin is prepared from plasma donors previously immunized and having high titers of antibody to tetanus toxoid. Each vial contains 250 units of hyperimmune γ-globulin. Injections with this material can provide protective levels of antibody for 24 to 32 days. It does not seem to cross the blood-brain barrier except when the meninges are inflamed. It is used for passive immunization of patients with tetanus-prone injuries who have not been actively immunized and boosted in the past 5 years. It is no substitute for active (elective) immunization, good surgical debridement, or antibiotics for active infection. It has also been used in attempts to modify active infections. It is given by intramuscular injection. The prophylactic dose, if given soon after injury, is 250 units for the adult and 4 units per kg of body weight for thc child. Doses of 400 to 500 units are recommended with extremely tetanus-prone wounds or when more than 24 hours have elapsed since injury. Single doses of 3,000 to 6,000 units have been suggested for active tetanus infections, but optimal dosage schedules are not available for this condition.

Rabies-immune globulin is prepared with plasma from donors who have been hyperimmunized with rabies vaccine. The resultant product contains 150 IU per ml. It is used to afford passive immunity to rabies in the initial prophylactic treatment of individuals exposed to rabies infection. Current best treatment is felt to entail use of this material, in addition to rabies vaccine and thorough local wound care. Usual dose is 20 IU per kg of body weight at the time of the first dose of rabies vaccine. Up to one-half of the dose should be used to infiltrate the wound and the rest given IM.

TREATMENT OF MASSIVE HEMORRHAGE

Massive transfusion is usually defined as a single transfusion of 2,500 ml in 1 hour or transfusion of 5,000 ml or more over a 24-hour period. These volumes represent one-half and one blood volume, respectively, for the average adult. However, evidence suggests that after a 5,000-ml transfusion only 27% (at best) and 18% (at worst) of the recipient's original blood volume remains (59).

The purpose of massive transfusion is to maintain sufficient intravascular volume to prevent shock and ensure tissue perfusion. Along with this must come replacement of sufficient functioning RBC to provide adequate oxygen transport. Platelets and soluble clotting factors must be replaced in sufficient quantities to ensure adequate hemostasis. Finally, the potential side effects of massive transfusion must be appreciated and treated if they appear.

When rapid bleeding is encountered, the blood bank and its director should be informed so that early thought can be given to need for special components, such as **FFP, platelets, cryoprecipitate,** or, perhaps, **whole blood,** including **fresh whole blood**. The potential need for special coagulation tests also can be anticipated.

Few situations occur where type-specific **RBC concentrates** cannot be waited for, even if time does not allow for a complete cross-match. The limitation to restoration of blood loss with balanced salt solutions (BSS) alone is 20% of blood volume, or 1,000 ml. However, quantities of up to 3 to 4 liters of BSS can be used in iniitial resuscitation, if type-specific blood or components are being prepared (26, 67). In those rare instances in which type-specific blood is not readily available, group O negative packed RBC can be used. In even more unusual situations, where Rh-negative blood is not available, Rh-positive can be used in an Rh-negative person. Because of the future hazard this entails in a woman of child-bearing age she should be given **Rh_o(D) immune globulin**, sufficient to neutralize about one unit packed RBC within 72 hours of transfusion.

Once transfusion of **RBC concentrates** is started they can be used as the only red cell replacement, indefinitely if needed. However, after replacement of 2 liters of blood loss with red cell concentrates some would recommend adding whole blood to the transfusion regimen, but a preponderance of **red cell concentrates** plus BSS can still prevail (49).

For those who prefer colloid, 250 ml of 5% **albumin** could be added to, or infused along with, each unit of **red cell concentrate**. A somewhat more risky (*i.e.,* hepatitis) source would be **stored plasma** used for the same purpose, although this would have the possible advantage of providing some stable clotting factors (all except factors V and VIII). However, in my opinion neither albumin nor stored plasma is needed, or appropriate, in the problem under discussion, since substitution of BSS and RBC concentrates is preferable.

After rapid transfusion of the equivalent of about 5 to 6 units of blood (2,500 ml), 1 to 2 units of **FFP** are appropriate for replacement of all clotting factors, including the labile ones. Certainly by the time a 10-unit replacement is approached 2 units of **FFP** are indicated (26, 61). When bleeding has reached this magnitude it is also time to become concerned about DIC and other coagulopathies and to institute the intraoperative coagulation work-up previously suggested, and to seriously consider administration of **platelet concentrates**. At this point platelet numbers are decreasing and platelet function is below normal. Therefore administration of at least 2 units of **platelet concentrates** has been suggested (71). However, if bleeding at this point is still quite brisk, 4 to 6 units of **platelet concentrates** would be appropriate if a platelet count found less than 50,000/ml (61). By the time replacement of 14 to 15 units of blood in less than 24 hours has occurred, bleeding secondary to thrombocytopenia is virtually certain, and is a more likely cause for continued bleeding than clotting factor deficiencies. Here, transfusion of 4 to 6 units of platelet concentrates is necessary, but 8 to 10 units are recommended.

Although not endorsed by all, administration of **fresh whole blood** for part of replacement after transfusion of over 10 units of blood in a 12-hour period has been suggested (18). Administration of 44.8 mEq calcium chloride for each 5 units of blood given has been suggested (61). However, with use of good EKG monitoring this is usually not necessary. Should the EKG suggest the rare case of hypocalcemia or hyperkalemia associated with massive transfusion (even more rare when **red cell concentrates** are used) calcium chloride can be given or hyperkalemia treated.

Should the coagulation lab suggest the presence of DIC, finding low fibrinogen and platelets as well as increased FDP, **cryoprecipitate** (10 to 15 bags) should be added to the regimen already described.

It is only through use of components as described above, or as an individual surgeon's experience or his coagulation consultant's advice dictates, that patients with massive hemorrhage have a remarkable chance for survival.

RISKS OF TRANSFUSION

Transfusion of blood and its components is associated with a relatively high incidence of side effects. Some of these are minor (febrile and minor allergic reactions), causing little morbidity and virtually no mortality; while others (hepatitis and hemolytic reactions) can lead to significant morbidity and mortality. A list of some unfavorable effects of transfusion is presented in Table 2.15 (49). A few of the more common and/or more serious will be reviewed in a bit more detail.

HEMOLYTIC TRANSFUSION REACTIONS

Most side effects of transfusion are not the result of serologic incompatibilities. It has been estimated that only 5% of reactions resulting from serologic incompatibility are due to factors that can be detected. Hemolytic transfusion reaction occurs in about 1 to 40,000 units of blood transfused. Even today, the majority of transfusion reactions due to serologic incompatibilities are the result of clerical error—the wrong unit of blood is given to the patient (10).

Hemolytic reactions are characterized by intravascular destruction of

TABLE 2.15

Some Unfavorable Effects of Transfusion

1. Hemolytic transfusion reactions
2. Immunological reactions involving:
   a. Leukocytes
   b. Platelets
   c. Proteins
3. Nonimmunological reactions
   a. Vasoactive substances
   b. Ice-cold blood
   c. Citrate toxicity
   d. Potassium toxicity
4. Infusion of extraneous matter
   a. Air embolism
   b. Particulate matter
   c. Toxic substances in plastic
5. Thrombophlebitis
6. Infusion of blood contaminated with bacteria or pyrogens
7. Transmission of disease
   a. Hepatitis
   b. Malaria
   c. Syphilis
   d. Cytomegalovirus
8. Hemosiderosis

red blood cells and consequent hemoglobinemia and hemoglobinuria. Clinical manifestations observed depend on whether the patient is awake or under anesthesia. If the patient is awake, common symptoms include a sensation of heat or pain along the vein in which the blood is being infused, flushing of the face, pain in the lumbar region, and constricting pain in the chest. Chills, fever, and respiratory distress may be seen early and hypotension and tachycardia can occur from amounts as small as 50 ml (59). In patients who are anesthetized and undergoing surgery, two signs which commonly call attention to a possible hemolytic reaction are abnormal bleeding and continued hypotension, despite adequate volume replacement. The abnormal bleeding is frequently secondary to DIC. In some series acute hemorrhagic diathases occurred in 8 to 30% of patients with hemolytic reactions (59).

Laboratory criteria for diagnosis of hemolytic transfusion reaction include: hemoglobinemia with a concentration of free hemoglobin over 5 mg/100 ml, a serum haptoglobin level below 50 mg/100 ml and serologic criteria (positive Direct Coomb's test) to show antigen incompatibility of the donor and recipient's blood.

If a hemolytic transfusion reaction is suspected, the following measures should be instituted without delay: (a) stop the transfusion immediately, but keep the vein open with intravenous fluids infused through a new administration set; (b) send a sample of the recipient's blood, drawn without anticoagulants, in a clot tube and EDTA tube along with the suspected unit of blood (administration tubing tied in a knot to prevent bacterial contamination) to the blood bank for comparison with pretransfusion samples; (c) monitor the patient's blood pressure and urine output carefully and institute appropriate therapy immediately if shock supervenes; (d) culture residual blood from the transfusion and determine a serum bilirubin in the recipient; (e) if not already present insert a Foley catheter and record hourly urine output (color and volume of excreted urine are evaluated since hemoglobinuria and oliguria are the most characteristic signs); (f) submit the first posttransfusion urine to the laboratory, with the transfusion reaction notice attached for analysis for free hemoglobin; (g) to minimize renal toxicity from precipitation of hemoglobin within the renal tubules, initiate a diuresis along with alkalinization of the urine by administering 100 ml of 20% mannitol plus 45 mEq of bicarbonate; (h) if marked oliguria or anuria occurs, restrict fluid and potassium intake, and treat the patient as a case of renal shutdown; and (i) dialysis may eventually be required. Administration of 5,000 IU heparin IV bolus is generally recommended to reduce likelihood of DIC; however, in intracranial or intraspinal surgery this course may carry excessive risk of hematoma formation (23).

Mortality and morbidity resulting from hemolytic reactions is high, particularly if the patient receives a full unit of incompatible blood. This mortality may approach 40 to 60%.

IMMUNOLOGICAL REACTIONS

Transfusion reactions secondary to immunologic events are usually related to transfusion of leukocytes, platelets, or certain proteins (49). Reactions occurring in association with transfusion of platelets and leukocytes are secondary to antibodies in the recipient to surface antigens on the transfused cells. The commonest effect noted is a febrile reaction appearing 30 to 80 minutes after beginning transfusion. Occasionally the reaction may appear within 5 minutes. In general these reactions are self-limited if the transfusion is stopped immediately; however, fibrinolysis has been observed in rare cases (49). Aspirin may be effective in ameliorating some febrile reactions secondary to these antigens.

Reactions due to transfused protein can be the "immediate type" hypersensitivity reaction. Severe anaphylactic-type reactions, characterized by flushing of skin, dyspnea, and hypotension are rare. Mild reactions, sometimes described as "anaphylactoid," characterized by urticaria are much commoner. Probably the commonest cause for severe anaphylactic reactions following transfusions is an interaction between transfused IgA and a class-specific anti-IgA in the recipient's plasma. At present little is known about the relative importance of antigens and antibodies known to be associated with the mild reaction described as anaphylactoid (49). With exception of severe anaphylactic reactions, these side effects of transfusion are usually self-limited and disappear soon after stopping transfusion. Therapy with antihistamines has been successful in reducing the incidence of these allergic reactions and is also frequently beneficial in treatment of reactions once they have occurred.

SOME NONIMMUNOLOGIC REACTIONS

Reactions to **vasoactive substances** have occasionally been observed after transfusion of blood or its components. Severe hypotension after infusion of a unit of plasma protein fraction was recently reported. It was found that the reaction was secondary to Hageman factor fragments in the transfused material (2).

With transfusion of massive quantities of blood the cold temperature resulting from refrigerator storage of blood can become a factor. Massive transfusion of ice-cold blood has been proven very dangerous (49). For this reason use of blood warmers with transfusions involving more than 2 units in a short period of time is strongly recommended.

Possible **toxicity of citrate** in CPD has been a concern for years (49). At least part of the toxicity is secondary to binding of ionized calcium by infused citrate. However, some toxicity seems to be due to citrate itself. Review of considerable data suggests that signs of citrate toxicity are likely to develop when several units of blood are transfused at the rate of 1 liter in 10 minutes and that toxic effects can be minimized by giving calcium (*e.g.,* 10 ml. of 10% calcium gluconate for every liter of citrated blood) (49). With higher rates of transfusion, larger amounts of calcium may be advisable. Dosage of calcium chloride is one fourth of that of calcium gluconate.

Toxicity from infused **potassium** can occur in the form of hyperkalemia. This problem can be minimized by use of red cell concentrates whenever possible. Apart from circumstances in which large amounts of blood are rapidly transfused, potassium toxicity need be considered only when transfusing patients whose plasma potassium is already raised (*e.g.,* anuric patients with extensive wounds involving muscle). One guideline worth considering is that severely injured patients should not be transfused with more than 10 units of 10-day-old whole blood in less than 10 hours (49). Use of RBC packed immediately before transfusion obviates this risk.

TRANSFUSION OF EXTRANEOUS MATERIAL

Air embolism was a significant problem in the past when transfused blood was contained in glass bottles. When this was used in combination with an air pump to increase pressure within the bottle and, therefore, the rate of transfusion, the incidence of air embolism was significant. Today it is an unusual problem if care is taken to keep the air in the transfusion line at the beginning of transfusion and with each bag change to a minimum. **Particulate matter** has already been discussed in some detail in the section on RBC. The potential importance of use of filters to remove these microaggregates is increased when massive transfusions become necessary. In this case it is highly advisable to include a 20 to 40 μm pore size filter in the transfusion system (2, 49). While this will slow the rate of transfusion slightly the decreased risks afforded by its use are probably worth the effort.

TRANSFUSION OF BLOOD CONTAMINATED WITH BACTERIA OR BACTERIAL PRODUCTS

In most American blood banks bacterial contamination of blood and its components at the time of transfusion is an extremely rare problem (10). The same statement holds true for transfusions of significant quantities of bacterial pyrogens. When this does happen and the pyrogens are from gram-negative organisms (endotoxins), a medical emergency comparable to that associated with hemolytic transfusion results. Profound gram-negative shock is well known to be difficult to manage, and is associated with a mortality approaching 50%. Less dangerous bacterial pyrogens may be present and produce febrile reactions. These can be minimized by using scrupulous care in preparing anticoagulant solutions, as well as all transfusion equipment. When they do occur, stopping the transfusion and administration of aspirin usually limit the reaction to a minor inconvenience.

POSTTRANSFUSION VIRAL HEPATITIS

Viral hepatitis acquired from the donor remains the commonest lethal complication of blood transfusion. Discovery in 1968 of the **hepatitis B virus** and the "Australia antigen" associated with it allowed development of a radioimmunoassay for screening of donors for the virus. Use of such screening has markedly reduced the incidence of posttransfusion hepatitis secondary to this virus. **Hepatitis A virus** seems to be a very rare cause of posttransfusion hepatitis (49). Likewise, it can be recognized in donors and avoided. Unfortunately, the commonest form of posttransfusion hepatitis today is non-A, non-B posttransfusion hepatitis. The most effective way of preventing posttransfusion hepatitis is careful screening of donors by history along with appropriate antigen-screening techniques, and limiting use of poorly screened, paid volunteers. Use of blood components prepared from large pools of plasma or serum should be limited to those cases in which it is absolutely necessary. If careful use of volunteer donors is made, incidence of clinically evident transfusion-induced hepatitis can be kept in the range of 2 per 1,000 transfusions (32). If subclinical cases diagnosed via liver function tests and/or biopsy are included, incidence approaches 10%. This incidence is even higher with use of **fresh whole blood** since performance of hepatitis antigen screening is usually not possible.

Transmission of other diseases such as malaria, syphilis, cytomegalovirus, infectious mononucleosis, brucellosis, toxoplasmosis, and other bacterial and parasitic infections are extremely rare in modern American blood banks.

FUTURE PROSPECTS IN COMPONENT THERAPY

Blood Substitutes

Since acquisition of adequate supplies of blood and its components is frequently difficult under the best of circumstances, and extremely difficult under some (*e.g.*, wartime), interest in artificial replacements for blood components, including the cellular components, has existed for a long time. To this end, an interest and considerable research in the use of perfluorochemicals has developed. These substances can dissolve as much as 60% oxygen by volume; whole blood, in contrast can dissolve only 20% oxygen by volume (46). However, pure perfluorochemicals are immiscible with blood. In 1968 a major advance was made when techniques for emulsification of these chemicals were developed, allowing suspension in solution with albumin and surfactants. Considerable work in this country and Japan has continued to the present. In April of 1979 a 65-year-old Japanese patient was bleeding heavily after a prostate operation. Sufficient blood of his particular rare type could not be found. Faced with this critical problem, his surgeon gave him an infusion of 1 liter of an oxygenated perfluorocarbon emulsion. This material was able to carry sufficient oxygen to keep the patient alive until his blood type could be found. Subsequently eight additional patients have been transfused with this artificial oxygen-carrying material. All nine patients are well today (46).

While it is widely agreed that significant problems still exist with use of such materials, their potential availability has caused a great deal of interest. It should be obvious that use of such materials could reduce the number of the unfavorable effects of transfusion toward zero. Not the least of these would be the commonest complication of transfusion—hepatitis. In addition, those patients who have religious objections to standard blood transfusions may now have a satisfactory alternate approach.

Bone Marrow Transplantation

Marrow transplantation between genotypically HLA identical siblings has an established and expanding place in management of leukemia and aplastic anemia (65, 66). Recently, techniques have been developed to allow use of this therapy in leukemic patients utilizing unrelated donors (33). In many of these cases the patients developed a normal hematopoetic system of donor origin which remained functional for many months.

While modern techniques make actual harvesting of marrow and its transfer to the recipient relatively simple, some potential side effects of such transfusions can be devastating. One of the leading side effects is known as graft-versus-host (GVH) disease or reaction (49). When there is successful engraftment of tissue which includes immunologically competent cells (*i.e.,* lymphocytes or their precursors), the foreign cells may mount an attack against host cells and produce the syndrome known as GVH disease. Features of this disease are: diarrhea, dermatitis, lymphadenopathy, hepatosplenomegaly, hemolytic anemia, pancytopenia, and a high mortality rate. This disease has been the commonest fatal complication of bone-marrow grafting (49). Such grafts are successful and GVH disease does not appear only when there is complete identity of histocompatibility antigens between donor and recipient or when the recipient's immunological responses are virtually nonexistent. The latter may occur either because of a rare disease of the immune system or as a result of treatment with immunosuppressive agents. Of course, the problem could be averted if the donor and patient are one-and-the-same. With most of the indications for bone-marrow transplantation however, the patient cannot serve as his own donor, since the underlying disease has precluded use of his own marrow. Complete identity of histocompatibility antigens is assured only when donor and recipient are identical twins or donor and recipient are one-and-the-same. Nevertheless, siblings who are HLA identical at the A, B, and D loci can be expected to have relatively minor differences in their histocompatibility antigens so that when the recipient's immune responses are suppressed by an otherwise lethal dose of radiation or some other means, a very high rate of engraftment of donor tissue has been observed.

Use of this technique has recently appeared in neurosurgical circles for the purpose of allowing high dose chemotherapy in the management of malignant brain tumors (36). This technique makes it possible to administer to the patient massive doses of cytotoxic agents which not only kill large numbers of tumor cells but also effectively wipe out the patient's bone marrow. By harvesting the patient's marrow prior to institution of the high dose chemotherapy, and then infusing it back into the patient after the chemotherapy has been completed, it is possible to safely use such high dose chemotherapy and still have a patient with a reasonably normally functioning hematopoietic system.

Further experience with this technique, and the high dose chemotherapy it allows, may prove the regimen to be another useful platoon in the slowly growing army directed at increasing the survival of patients with malignant gliomas.

ACKNOWLEDGMENTS

The author is indebted to Dr. L. W. Gaston, Professor of Pathology and Director of Blood Bank and Coagulation Laboratory, University of Missouri Health Sciences Center, Columbia, Missouri and Dr. C. Watts, Professor and Chief, Division of Neurological Surgery, University of Missouri Health Sciences Center, Columbia, Missouri for their knowledgable assistance in preparation and review of the manuscript. Drs. H.H. Kaufman, J.L. Moake, J.D. Olson, M.E. Miner, R.T. duCret, J.L. Pruessner, and P.L. Gildenberg are thanked for allowing use of material from their paper (reference 40) before publication. The author is also deeply indebted to Ms. D. Peterson for her diligence in typing and revising the manuscript and Ms. Cathy Ferris for assistance in proofreading.

REFERENCES

1. Alavi, J. B., Root, R. K., Djerassi, I., Evans, A. E., Gluckman, S. J., MacGregor, R. R., Guerry, D., Schreiber, A. D., Shaw, J. M., Koch, P., and Cooper, R. A. A randomized clinical trial of granulocyte transfusions for infection in acute leukemia. N. Engl. J. Med., *296:* 706–711, 1977.
2. Alving, B. M., Hojima, Y., Pisano, J. J., Mason, B. L., Buckingham, R. E., Mozen, M. M., and Finlayson, J. S. Hypotension associated with prekallikrein activator (Hageman-factor fragments) in plasma protein fraction. N. Engl. J. Med., *299:* 66–70, 1978.
3. Aster, R. H. Thrombocytopenia due to diminished or defective platelet production. *In* Hematology, edited by W. J. Williams, Ed. 2, pp. 1317–1325. McGraw-Hill, New York, 1977.
4. Aster, R. H. Thrombocytopenia due to enhanced platelet destruction. *In* Hematology, edited by W. J. Williams, Ed. 2, pp. 1326–1360. McGraw-Hill, New York, 1977.
5. Aster, R. H. Thrombocytopenia due to sequestration of platelets. *In* Hematology, edited by W. J. Williams, Ed. 2, pp. 1360–1362. McGraw-Hill, New York, 1977.
6. Aster, R. H. Thrombocytopenia due to platelet loss. *In* Hematology, edited by W. J. Williams, Ed. 2, pp. 1362–1364. McGraw-Hill, New York, 1977.
7. Auer, L. Disturbances of the coagulatory system in patients with severe cerebral trauma. Acta Neurochir. (Wien), *43:* 51–59, 1978.
8. Bern, M. M. Management of hemorrhage during surgery. Surg. Rounds, *3:* 36–46, 1980.
9. Blajchman, M. A., Shepherd, F. A., and Perrault, R. A. Clinical use of blood components and blood products. Can. Med. Assoc. J., *121:* 33–42, 1979.
10. Blood Component Therapy. A Physician's Handbook. Am. Assoc. Blood Banks, Washington, D.C., 1975.
11. Blood Products. Med. Lett. Drugs Ther., *21:* 93–96, 1979.
12. Boggs, D. R. Neutrophils in the blood bank. N. Engl. J. Med., *296:* 748–750, 1977.
13. Buchholz, D. H. Blood transfusion: merits of component therapy. I. The clinical use of red cells, platelets, and granulocytes. J. Pediatr., *84:* 1–15, 1974.
14. Buchholz, D. H. Blood transfusion: merits of component therapy. I. The clinical use of plasma and plasma components. J. Pediatr., *84:* 165–172, 1974.

15. Buchholz, D. H., Blumberg, N., and Bove, J. R. Long-term granulocyte transfusion in patients with malignant neoplasmas. Arch. Intern. Med., *139:* 317–320, 1979.
16. Chaplin, H., Jr. Frozen blood. N. Engl. J. Med., *298:* 679–681, 1978.
17. Clift, R. A., Sanders, J. E., Thomas, E. D., Williams, B., and Buckner, C.D. Granulocyte transfusions for the prevention of infection in patients receiving bone-marrow transplants. N. Engl. J. Med., *298:* 1052–1057, 1978.
18. Curreri, P. W. Burns. *In* Care of the Trauma Patient, Ed. 2, pp. 139–161. McGraw-Hill, New York, 1979.
19. Denis, J. Letter to the publisher. Philos. Trans. R. Soc. Lond. [Biol. Sci.], No. 32:617, 1667–1668.
20. Drayer, B. P., and Poser, C. M. Disseminated intravascular coagulation and head trauma. Two case studies. J.A.M.A., *231:* 174–175, 1975.
21. Eyster, M. E., Gill, F. M., Blatt, P. M., Hilgartner, M. W., Ballard, J. O., Kinney, T. R., and the Hemophilia Study Group. Central nervous system bleeding in hemophiliacs. Blood, *51:* 1179–1188, 1978.
22. Gardner, F. H. Preservation and clinical use of platelets. *In* Hematology, edited by W. J. Williams, Ed. 2, pp. 1553–1561. McGraw-Hill, New York, 1977.
23. Gaston, L. W. Personal communication, 1980.
24. Gaston, L. W. Component use in the treatment of disseminated intravascular coagulation. *In* Blood, Blood Components, and Derivatives in Transfusion Therapy. Am. Assoc. Blood Banks, Washington, D.C., in press, 1981.
25. Giblett, E. R. Erythrocyte antigens and antibodies. *In* Hematology, edited by W. J. Williams, Ed. 2, pp. 1497–1512. McGraw-Hill, New York, 1977.
26. Giesecke, A. H., and Jenkins, M. T. Anesthesia considerations. *In* Care of the Trauma Patient, Ed. 2, pp. 83–106. McGraw-Hill, New York, 1979.
27. Goodnight, S. H., Kenoyer, G., Rapaport, S. I., Patch, M. J., Lee, J. A., and Kurze, T. Defibrination after brain-tissue destruction. N. Engl. J. Med., *290:* 1043–1047, 1974.
28. Gottlieb, A. J. Nonallergic purpura. *In* Hematology, edited by W. J. Williams, Ed. 2, pp. 1385–1391. McGraw-Hill, New York, 1977.
29. Gottlieb, A. J. Allergic purpura. *In* Hematology, edited by W. J. Williams, Ed. 2, pp. 1393–1399. McGraw-Hill, New York, 1977.
30. Gottlieb, A. J. Hereditary hemorrhagic telangiectasia. *In* Hematology, edited by W. J. Williams, Ed. 2, pp. 1400–1403. McGraw-Hill, New York, 1977.
31. Gudeman, S. K., Kishore, P. R. S., Miller, J. D., Girevendulis, A. K., Lipper, M. H., and Becker, D. P. The genesis and significance of delayed traumatic intracerebral hematomas. Neurosurgery, *5:* 309–313, 1979.
32. Haugen, R. K. Hepatitis after the transfusion of frozen red cells and washed red cells. N. Engl. J. Med., *301:* 393–395, 1979.
33. Hansen, J. A., Clift, R. A., Thomas, E. D., Buckner, C. D., Storb, R., and Giblett, E. R. Transplantation of marrow from an unrelated donor to a patient with acute leukemia. N. Engl. J. Med., *303:* 565–567, 1980.
34. Herzig, R. H., Herzig, G. P., Graw, R. G., Jr., Bull, M. I., and Ray, K. K. Successful granulocyte transfusion therapy for gram-negative septicemia. N. Engl. J. Med., *296:* 701–705, 1977.
35. Hillman, R. S. Acute blood loss anemia. *In* Hematology, edited by W. J. Williams, Ed. 2, pp. 618–623. McGraw-Hill, New York, 1977.
36. Hochberg, F. H., Parker, L. M., Takvorian, T., Canellos, G., and Zervas, N. High-dose BCNU with autologous bone marrow rescue for recurrent glioblastoma multiforme. Presented at the Annual Meeting of the American Association of Neurological Surgeons, New York, 1980.
37. Hougie, C. Hemophilia and related conditions—congenital deficiencies of prothrombin

(factor II), factor V, and factors VII to XII. *In* Hematology, edited by W. J. Williams, Ed. 2, pp. 1404–1422. McGraw-Hill, New York, 1977.
38. Hougie, C. Bleeding time. *In* Hematology, edited by W. J. Williams, Ed. 2, p. 1655. McGraw-Hill, New York, 1977.
39. Johnson, A. J., Aronson, D. L., and Williams, W. J. Preparation and clinical use of plasma and plasma factors. *In* Hematology, edited by W. J. Williams, Ed. 2, pp. 1561–1583. McGraw-Hill, New York, 1977.
40. Kaufman, H. H., Moake, J. L., Olson, J. D., Miner, M. E., duCret, R. P., Pruessner, J. L., and Gildenberg, P. L. Delayed and recurrent intracranial hematomas related to DICF in head injury. Neurosurgery, in press, 1981.
41. Koepke, J. A., Wu, K. K., Hoak, J. C., and Thompson, J. S. A comparison of platelet production methods suitable for a service-oriented blood donor center. Transfusion, *15:* 39–42, 1975.
42. Lian, E. C., and Deykin, D. Diagnosis of von Willebrand's disease. Am. J. Med., *60:* 344–356, 1976.
43. Lundsgaard-Hansen, P., Bucher, U., Tschirren, B., Haase, S., Kuske, B., Ludi, A., Stankiewicz, L. A., and Hassig, A. Red cells and gelatin as the core of a unified program for the national procurement of blood components and derivatives. Vox Sang., *34:* 261–275, 1978.
44. Mahaley, S. Personal communication, 1980.
45. Masouredis, S. P. Preservation and clinical use of erythrocytes and whole blood. *In* Hematology, edited by W. J. Williams, Ed. 2, pp. 1530–1561. McGraw-Hill, New York, 1977.
46. Maugh, T. H., II. Blood substitute passes its first test. Science, *206:* 205, 1979.
47. Mielke, C. H., Jr., Kaneshiro, M. M., Maher, I. A., Weiner, J. M., and Rapaport, S. I. The standardized normal Ivy bleeding time and its prolongation by aspirin. Blood, *34:* 204–215, 1969.
48. Miller, R. D., Robbins, T. O., Tong, M. J., and Barton S. L. Ann. Surg., *174:* 794-801, 1971.
49. Mollison, P. L. Blood Transfusion in Clinical Medicine. Blackwell Scientific Publications, Oxford, 1979.
50. Owen, C. A., Jr., and Bowie, E. J. W. Surgical hemostasis. J. Neurosurg., *51:* 137–142, 1979.
51. Perry, S. Preservation and clinical use of leukocytes. *In* Hematology, edited by W. J. Williams, Ed. 2, pp. 1547–1553. McGraw-Hill, New York, 1977.
52. Pritz, M. B., Giannotta, S. L., Kindt, G. W., McGillicuddy, J. E., and Prager, R. L. Treatment of patients with neurological deficits associated with cerebral vasospasm by intravascular volume expansion. Neurosurgery *3:* 364–368, 1978.
53. Rapaport, S. I. Defibrination syndromes. *In* Hematology, edited by W. J. Williams, Ed. 2, pp. 1454–1480. McGraw-Hill, New York, 1977.
54. Rice, C. L., and Moss, G. S. Blood and blood substitutes: current practice. Adv. Surg., *13:* 93–114, 1979.
55. Rizza, C. R. Coagulation factor therapy. Clin. Haematol., *5:* 113–133, 1976.
56. Robertson, H. D., and Polk, H. C., Jr. Blood transfusions in elective operations: comparison of whole blood versus packed red cells. Ann. Surg., *181:* 778–783, 1975.
57. Schiffer, C. A. Annotation. Some aspects of recent advances in the use of blood cell components. Br. J. Haematol., *39:* 289–294, 1978.
58. Schiffer, C. A., Aisner, J., and Wiernik, P. H. Frozen autologous platelet transfusion for patients with leukemia. N. Engl. J. Med., *299:* 7–12, 1978.
59. Schwartz, S. I. Hemostasis, surgical bleeding, and transfusion. *In* Principles of Surgery, edited by S. I. Schwartz, Ed. 3, pp. 99–134. McGraw-Hill, New York, 1979.

60. Shapiro, S. S. Disorders of the vitamin K-dependent coagulation factors. *In* Hematology, edited by W. J. Williams, Ed. 2, pp. 1441–1447. McGraw-Hill, New York, 1977.
61. Sheldon, G. F., Lim, R. C., and Blaisdell, F. W. The use of fresh blood in the treatment of critically injured patients. J. Trauma, *15:* 670–677, 1975.
62. Sherry, S. Mechanism of fibrinolysis. *In* Hematology, edited by W. J. Williams, Ed. 2, pp. 1294–1305. McGraw-Hill, New York, 1977.
63. Shires, G. T. Principles and management of hemorrhagic shock. *In* Care of the Trauma Patient, Ed. 2, pp. 3–51. McGraw-Hill, New York, 1979.
64. Slichter, S. J., and Harker, L. A. Preparation and storage of platelet concentrates. II. Storage variables influencing platelet viability and function. Br. J. Haematol., *34:* 403–419, 1976.
65. Storb, R., Thomas, E. D., Buckner, C. D., *et al.* Marrow transplantation in thirty "untransfused" patients with severe aplastic anemia. Ann. Intern. Med., *92:* 30–36, 1980.
66. Thomas, E. D., Sanders, J. E., Fluornoy, N., *et al.* Marrow transplantation for patients with acute lymphoblastic leukemia in remission. Blood, *54:* 468–476, 1979.
67. Trunkey, D. D., Sheldon, G. F., and Collins, J. A. The treatment of shock. *In* The Management of Trauma, edited by G. D. Zuidema, R. B. Rutherford, and W. F. Ballinger, II, Ed. 3, pp. 80–101. W. B. Saunders, Philadelphia, 1979.
68. Tullis, J. L. Albumin. I. Background and use. J.A.M.A., *237:* 355–360, 1977.
69. Tullis, J. L. Albumin. 2. Guidelines for clinical use. J.A.M.A., *237:* 460–463, 1977.
70. Valeri, C. R. Blood components in the treatment of acute blood loss: use of freeze-preserved red cells, platelets, and plasma proteins. Anesth. Analg. (Cleve.), *54:* 1–14, 1975.
71. van der Sande, J. J., Veltcamp, J. J., Boekhout-Mussert, R. J., and Bouhuis-Hoogerwerf, M. L. Head injury and coagulation disorders. J. Neurosurg., *49:* 357–365, 1978.
72. Vecht, C. J., Smit Sibinga, C. T., and Minerhoud, J. M. Disseminated intravascular coagulation and head injury. J. Neurol. Neurosurg. Psychiatry, *38:* 567–571, 1975.
73. Weiss, H. J. Congenital qualitative platelet disorders. *In* Hematology, edited by W. J. Williams, Ed. 2, pp. 1368–1377. McGraw-Hill, New York, 1977.
74. Weiss, H. J. Acquired qualitative platelet disorders. *In* Hematology, edited by W. J. Williams, Ed. 2, pp. 1377–1384. McGraw-Hill, New York, 1977.
75. Weiss, H. J. von Willebrand's disease. *In* Hematology, edited by W. J. Williams, Ed. 2, pp. 1434–1440. McGraw-Hill, New York, 1977.
76. Williams, W. J. Sequence of coagulation reactions. *In* Hematology, edited by W. J. Williams, Ed. 2, pp. 1266–1275. McGraw-Hill, New York, 1977.
77. Williams, W. J. Control of coagulation reactions. *In* Hematology, edited by W. J. Williams, Ed. 2, pp. 1276–1285. McGraw-Hill, New York, 1977.
78. Williams, W. J. Structure and function related to hemostasis. *In* Hematology, edited by W. J. Williams, Ed. 2, pp. 1306–1310. McGraw-Hill, New York, 1977.
79. Williams, W. J. General effects of disorders of hemostasis. *In* Hematology, edited by W. J. Williams, Ed. 2, pp. 1313–1316. McGraw-Hill, New York, 1977.
80. Zucker, M. B. Platelet function. *In* Hematology, edited by W. J. Williams, Ed. 2, pp. 1200–1209. McGraw-Hill, New York, 1977.

CHAPTER

3

Anticoagulant in Cerebrovascular Disease

J. DONALD EASTON, M.D., JOHN A. BYER, M.D., and DAVID G. SHERMAN, M.D.

INTRODUCTION

Anticoagulant therapy in the form of heparin and dicumarol was introduced into clinical practice 40 years ago, and shortly thereafter it was held beneficial in the treatment of stroke. Carotid endarterectomy was introduced about 15 years later, and 10 years ago antiplatelet-aggregating agents were reported to be useful in transient ischemic attack (TIA). We will review the data regarding the effectiveness of anticoagulation in cerebrovascular disease. The focus will be on those conditions that produce most of the focal cerebral infarctions in adults (Fig. 3.1). It is desirable to classify ischemia-infarction in pathophysiologic terms. Since it is generally not possible to determine whether atherogenic cerebral ischemia is embolic or thrombotic, most investigators have categorized these disorders according to their clinical presentation (Fig. 3.2). We will use this classification and present the data which supports our views regarding the role of anticoagulant in cerebrovascular disease.

TRANSIENT ISCHEMIC ATTACK

A TIA is a focal disturbance of neurological function that lasts less than 24 hours, usually less than 1 hour, and is confined to an area of brain irrigated by a specific artery. Fisher (36) states that "70% of TIAs last less than 10 minutes." There is certainly more than one mechanism for TIA (*e.g.*, vasculitis, hyperviscosity states, fibromuscular dysplasia, presumably vasospasm in migraine, etc.), but we will focus on atherosclerotic disease (27). The primary problem may be hemodynamic obstruction of the artery with a transient regional decrease in cerebral blood flow below a critical level. Alternatively, the primary cause of the ischemia may be embolic. When an atherosclerotic plaque on the arterial wall ulcerates, the necrotic material (cholesterol crystals, calcified connective tissue debris, etc.) may dislodge and embolize distally. Additionally, platelets may adhere to the exposed arterial wall connective tissue, and further aggregation of platelets may occur. These platelet masses may dislodge and serve as emboli, or they may provide a surface on which

Atherogenic Cerebral Ischemia

embolic or thrombotic disease

Cardiogenic Cerebral Ischemia

embolic

FIG. 3.1. The commonest pathophysiologic types of cerebral ischemia-infarction.

Atherogenic Cerebrovascular Disease

Transient Ischemic Attack

Progressing Stroke

Completed Stroke

Cardiogenic Cerebral Embolism

FIG. 3.2. Ischemic cerebrovascular disease categorized by its usual clinical presentation.

coagulation of fibrin occurs. This clot may also dislodge into the arterial circulation, or it may grow into a major thrombosis with resultant complete occlusion of the artery. Whether vasospasm or other factors play a significant role in the cause of the cerebral ischemia or infarction is not known.

While the exact cause of reversible ischemia and fixed infarction in brain is not known, the primary abnormality is clearly atherosclerosis with its complicating lesion, the fibrous plaque.

Systemic hypotension is probably an infrequent cause of TIA. Some years ago, Kendell and Marshall (55) produced hypotension in 37 TIA patients with hexamethonium, and all but one had syncope, not a focal TIA.

With the above concepts in mind regarding the pathophysiology of cerebral ischemic disease, one can visualize the potentially beneficial role of anticoagulation, antiplatelet aggregation agents, and extracranial vascular surgery in treatment. Treatments aimed at lowering blood viscosity, increasing cerebral blood flow, and increasing blood oxygenation above normal levels have gained limited acceptance (15).

ANTICOAGULATION IN TIA

Four randomized prospective studies (7, 8, 70, 72) comparing anticoagulant-treated TIA patients to controls showed no significant difference in the incidence of stroke or death in the two groups (Table 3.1). The number of patients was small, and the follow-up period was short for most of the studies. Only the Pearce study (70) was double-blind. The data favors the view that anticoagulants reduce the number of TIA recurrences, but the evidence is weak. Several nonrandomized studies (33, 34, 42, 68, 76, 80) also showed no reduction in mortality (Table 3.1). However, all but one of them demonstrated a decreased incidence of stroke, and one showed a reduced number of TIA recurrences.

These data have been discussed in detail and interpreted quite differ-

TABLE 3.1
Anticoagulant Therapy in Transient Ischemic Attack

AUTHOR	YEAR	PATIENTS	FOLLOW-UP MONTHS	CEREBRAL INFARCTS	CEREBRAL HEMORRHAGE	TRANSIENT ISCHEMIC ATTACK
			RANDOMIZED			
Cooperative Study VA (72)	1961					
Control		15	13	0	?	8
Treated		22	9	1	?	1
Baker et al (7) (Cooperative Study)	1962					
Control		20	20	5	0	23
Treated		24	18	1	2	5
Pearce et al (70)	1965					
Control		20	11	2	?	9
Treated		17	11	1	?	10
Baker et al (8)	1966					
Control		30	41	7	?	14
Treated		30	38	2	0	10
			NON-RANDOMIZED			
Fisher (34)	1958					
Control		23	?	8	0	4
Treated		29	30	1	0	1*
Siekert et al (76)	1963					
Control		160	60	51	7	?
Treated		175	60	7	13	?
Fezekas et al (33)	1963					
Control		7	14	0	0	2
Treated		3	22	0	0	0
Friedman et al (42)	1969					
Control		23	27	8†	1	?
Treated		21	27	0	0	?
Toole et al (80)	1975					
Control		56	46‡	7	?	?
Treated		21	46	6	?	?
Olsson et al (68)	1976					
Treated		163	25	0	1?	24

* The other 28 treated patients had "cessation of transient ischemic attack (except for occasional attack)."

† One patient had been on anticoagulant, but it was discontinued before the cerebral infarction.

‡ The average duration of anticoagulation was 27 months during the 46-month average follow-up.

ently by different writers (14, 20, 64, 71, 74, 84). Much of the difference of opinion centers on whether one attributes meaning to trends or only to statistically significant data and whether one attributes meaning to nonrandomized studies or only randomized and controlled ones. It is very important to note that most of the studies have involved too few patients, the follow-up period has been too short, and the controls have been inadequate to determine the definitive role of anticoagulation in the treatment of TIA. On balance, however, when properly used, we believe it may reduce the risk of further TIA and subsequent cerebral infarction.

PROGRESSING STROKE

In this condition, the focal ischemia worsens from minute to minute or hour to hour. There are usually stepwise incremental increases in neurological deficit occurring over a period of several hours, though in the posterior circulation the stroke may evolve over 2, or even 3 or more days. It is not always possible to be certain if the deficit is progressing, and careful observation during the early hours of ischemia is important. Occasionally this category of patients is difficult to distinguish from that with an intracerebral hemorrhage, although in that with hemorrhage, the patients are usually obtunded or comatose. A CT scan and/or a lumbar puncture may be valuable in this situation, but sometimes the urgency of the clinical situation dictates that therapy be started immediately based on clinical judgement. Many clinicians would include crescendo TIA in this category.

In studying the temporal profile of both carotid system and vertebrobasilar system infarction, Jones *et al.* (50, 51) reported their observation (Fig. 3.3), that progressing stroke is common. While there may be several pathogenic mechanisms producing a progressing stroke, one appears to be a thrombus-in-evolution with a progressive thrombus extending from its site of origin in a primary artery and obliterating collateral branches,

Carotid		Vertebrobasilar
39%	stable (unchanged)	11%
35%	improved	35%
19%	progressed	43%
3%	remitting-relapsing	11%
4%	late worsening (>48h)	0%
10.6%	mortality	27%

FIG. 3.3. Temporal profile of cerebral infarction (clinical course over 7 days). Adapted from refs. 50 and 51, by permission of the American Heart Association.

thereby interfering with anastomotic vessels. Hence, the rationale for anticoagulation.

ANTICOAGULATION IN PROGRESSING STROKE

Three randomized (7, 16, 35) and three nonrandomized (34, 63, 83) studies strongly suggest, but don't conclusively prove, that anticoagulation benefits patients with progressing stroke (Table 3.2). The patients were generally heparinized at the time of diagnosis and then switched over to oral anticoagulant for a period of weeks or months thereafter. The evidence is considerably more favorable for anticoagulation preventing stroke progression than it is for preventing death. Little information is provided regarding the outcome after the first few days and weeks when the likelihood of benefit would seem to be maximal.

Whisnant (83), in discussing vertebrobasilar system infarction, emphasized the need for accurate diagnosis in selecting patients for comparing treatment and control groups because he noted that patients with well-localized infarctions in the distribution of a single small artery, as com-

TABLE 3.2

Anticoagulant Therapy for Progressing Stroke

AUTHOR	YEAR	PATIENTS	FOLLOW-UP MONTHS	CEREBRAL INFARCTS (LETHAL)	CEREBRAL HEMORRHAGE (LETHAL)	PROGRESSIVE INFARCTS	TOTAL PROGRESSIVE	ALL DEATHS
				RANDOMIZED				
Carter (16)	1961							
Control		38	6	7	0	12	19	7
Treated		38	6	3	0	9	12	3
Fisher (35) (National Study)	1961							
Control		49	7.4	7	0	14	20	10
Treated		51	5.7	4	1	7	8	9
Baker et al (7) (Cooperative Study)	1962							
Control		67	15	10	0	21	31	17
Treated		61	12	5	1	8	14	13
				NON-RANDOMIZED				
Fisher (34)	1958							
Control		14	?	0	0	9	9	7
Treated		14	?	0	0	3	3	0
Millikan (63)	1965							
Control		60	12	25	0	8	33	--
Treated		181	12	12	0	25	37	--
Whisnant (83)	1961							
Control		39	--	--	--	--	--	23
Treated		140	--	--	--	--	--	12

pared to those with major vertebral or basilar distribution ischemia, have a generally good prognosis with or without anticoagulant (83).

In spite of the limited evidence that anticoagulant is beneficial in treating progressive stroke, most clinicians favor immediate heparinization. Then, depending on the circumstances, a choice must be made regarding evaluation for immediate or delayed vascular surgery, more prolonged anticoagulation with warfarin, institution of antiplatelet aggregation therapy, or discontinuation of therapy at some point.

ANTICOAGULATION IN COMPLETED STROKE

There are substantial data to indicate that anticoagulant is not beneficial in the management of completed stroke. In fact, there is evidence to suggest that it is detrimental in this condition. Data from 7 randomized studies are shown in Table 3.3 (6, 7, 31, 47, 49, 59, 61). There is no significant evidence that early treatment is hazardous, in the sense that it will convert a white into a more serious hemorrhagic infarct. Rather, anticoagulant therapy simply does not prevent subsequent stroke, and in patients treated for several months, it adds to morbidity and mortality. While this risk is not excessively high, it does outweigh the benefit in the best studies available.

CARDIOGENIC CEREBRAL EMBOLISM

The commonest causes of cardiogenic cerebral embolism are listed in Fig. 3.4. This discussion will be confined to rheumatic heart disease (RHD), coronary heart disease, and nonvalvular atrial fibrillation (AF) (28).

Most rheumatic hearts have mitral stenosis, and the thrombi form in the left atrium, about half in the atrial appendage, the size of which has no clear relationship to the likelihood of systemic embolization (1, 25, 38, 53, 77, 78). Only two-thirds of these hearts are in AF or obviously changing rhythm at the time of embolization (44, 66, 82). Approximately 20% of RHD patients will experience a major embolism in their lifetime (19, 24–26, 30, 38, 57, 66, 67, 73, 79, 85, 88), about one-half of them to the brain (2, 25, 66). Between 30 and 75% of those with one systemic embolism will have at least one recurrence (11, 17, 25, 26, 38, 67, 73, 79, 82), with 75% reported by Carter's long-term follow-up series (17). Darling *et al.* (26) reported that one-third of the recurrences occur within 2 weeks, and Daley *et al.* (25) and Szekely (79) found that 35 to 40% of recurrences occur within 1 month (Fig. 3.5).

Data collected from several major series (9, 13, 43, 52, 56, 60, 81) indicate that mural thrombi are found in 44% of hearts in patients who die of myocardial infarction (MI) and in 75% of those with a ventricular aneurysm (54). It will be less in those patients with less serious infarcts.

TABLE 3.3

*Anticoagulant Therapy for Completed Stroke**

AUTHOR	YEAR	PATIENTS	FOLLOW-UP MONTHS	LETHAL STROKES	ISCHEMIC STROKES	ALL DEATHS	SEVERE BLEEDING
Marshall, Shaw (59)	1960						
Control		25	1.5	--	--	3	--
Treated		26	1.5	--	--	6	--
Baker (6) (VA Study)	1961						
Control		62	13	2	4	7	3
Treated		56	9	6	6	12	10
Baker et al (7) (Cooperative Study)	1962						
Control		60	11	5	6	15	0
Treated		72	11	6	12	18	7
Hill et al (47) (Phase I)	1962						
Control		71	10	0	4	1	0
Treated		71	9	4	9	8	5
(Phase II)							
Control		65	31	1	19	4	0
Treated		66	28	5	22	12	4
Howard et al (49)	1963						
Control		15	12	--	--	3	0
Treated		15	12	--	--	3	0
McDowell, McDevitt (61)	1965						
Control		99	34	7	22	57	2
Treated		92	42	4	20	53	11
Enger, Boyeson (31)	1965						
Control		49	23	3	10	6	0
Treated		51	23	1	5	6	3

* All 7 studies were randomized.

While peripheral emboli that come to clinical attention occur in only 2 to 12% of patients, with the higher incidence in those with the biggest infarcts, peripheral infarcts were found in 45 to 60% of autopsied patients in the series' of Hellerstein and Martin (45) and Garvin (43). About 85% of all systemic emboli will occur within 1 month of the MI. Bean (9) and Darling *et al.* (26) reported recurrence rates of one-fourth and one-third, and Darling found that 71% of the recurrences occurred within 2 weeks of the previous one (Fig. 3.6).

A matter of some importance and controversy is the issue of whether thrombi are prone to form in the left atrium of patients with AF not due to RHD or other identifiable valvular disease. We will use the terms "arteriosclerotic AF," "idiopathic AF," and "nonvalvular AF" inter-

Rheumatic Heart Disease

mitral stenosis $\pm$ AF*

Coronary Heart Disease

myocardial infarction

Non-valvular AF

Other

cardiomyopathy
atrial myxoma
fat emboli
septic material
non-bacterial thrombotic endocarditis
mitral valve prolapse
congenital heart disease
venous clots/intracardiac shunt
mitral annulus calcification

FIG. 3.4. The commonest causes of cardiogenic cerebral embolism. **AF*, atrial fibrillation.

virtually all have mitral stenosis	
thrombi: on atrial wall	1/2
: in atrial appendage	1/2
majority, but not all, in AF*	2/3
peripheral arterial emboli (half of them cerebral)	20%
recurrent embolization	30-75%
recurrences within 2 weeks	1/3
recurrences within 1 month	35-40%

FIG. 3.5. Major characteristics of cerebral embolism in rheumatic heart disease. **AF*, atrial fibrillation.

changeably. Until recently, many authors used the term arteriosclerotic AF because the patients were in the arteriosclerotic age group without evidence of RHD, rather than because of clear evidence of an arteriosclerotic basis for the arrhythmia.

Friedberg (40) states that emboli are rarely caused by a fibrillating heart without RHD, and he advises against anticoagulating such patients. Beer and Ghitman (10) concluded that peripheral embolization is uncommon in patients with atherosclerotic heart disease without myocardial infarction, regardless of the cardiac rhythm. These authors excluded another 8 emboli from an atrial source because they discovered atrial infarction or abnormal heart valves. These patients should not be discarded from the overall statistics when one is managing patients only with clinical data, that is, with a *clinical* diagnosis of nonrheumatic AF. There is other evidence to suggest that "arteriosclerotic" and idiopathic AF may cause systemic emboli. Aberg (1) reported an autopsy study on 506 patients with AF but no valvular disease or congenital heart lesions. Half of them had myocardial infarction, and the other half had other manifestations of atherosclerotic or hypertensive heart disease, or some other illness. Of these patients, 13.7% had left atrial, not ventricular, thrombi. Also, 41.7% had systemic emboli, half of them to the brain. Thus 20% of these patients with AF and no valvular disease had cerebral emboli. Darling *et al.* (26) reported a clinical series of 260 consecutive patients with arterial emboli, and 97 had arteriosclerotic AF. One-third of these 97 patients had associated myocardial infarction, and two-thirds had only atherosclerotic heart disease and fibrillation. Thus, nearly 20% of all systemic emboli occurred in patients with atherosclerotic heart disease with AF but without myocardial infarction. They noted that about 70% of their patients had AF, with atherosclerosis being the commonest cause. It is noteworthy, and surprising, that they had no patients with RHD and normal sinus rhythm. This may mean that some of their "arteriosclerotic fibrillators" in fact had RHD with left atrial thrombi. Nevertheless, these patients were in the atherosclerotic age group (average age 72 years), and *clinically* they had arteriosclerotic AF.

In an autopsy study of 333 patients with AF, Hinton and coworkers (48) found embolism to be nearly as common without RHD (59 of 171, or

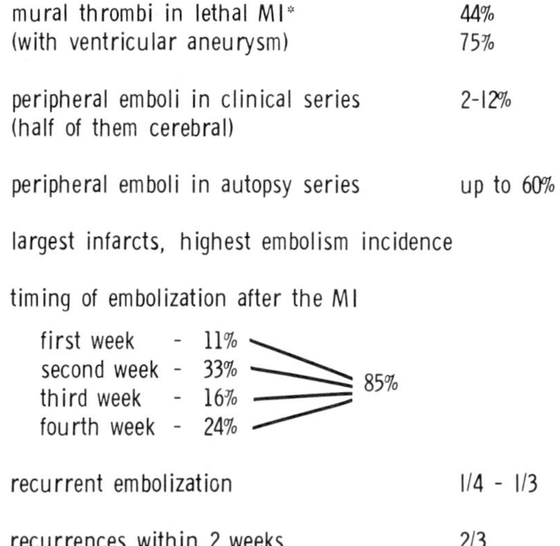

FIG. 3.6. Major characteristics of cerebral embolism in coronary heart disease with myocardial infarction. **MI*, myocardial infarction.

35%) as with mitral valve disease (29 of 70, or 41%). In 20% of the non-RHD patients they found thrombus in the left atrium.

Wolf and colleagues (86) recently provided valuable prospective epidemiological data from the Framingham Study assessing the risk of embolic stroke in patients with chronic AF. While patients having AF with RHD had a 17-fold increased risk of stroke, compared to the general population, patients having chronic idiopathic AF had a 5.6-fold increase.

Fogarty (39) found that of 300 consecutive patients with systemic emboli, 183 had arteriosclerotic AF as the source. That is, 61% of all emboli were due to arteriosclerotic AF. Fisher (37) reported 100 patients with AF and cerebral embolism. The underlying heart disease was nonvalvular in 83. He also described another group of 48 unselected patients with AF, though it is not clear how many had nonvalvular disease who were followed prospectively for 4 years. Thirty-five percent of them suffered a typical embolic stroke. Friedman and associates (41) also showed that " . . . atrial fibrillation in the absence of myocardial infarction, congestive heart failure, or rheumatic heart disease was strongly associated with stroke."

Fairfax and associates (32) described 100 patients with chronic sinoatrial disorder. Sixteen of them had evidence of systemic emboli, and multiple episodes occurred in 6. Fifteen of the 16 patients had the bradycardia-tachycardia syndrome. An additional 41 patients with chronic ventricular bradycardia and atrial flutter or fibrillation had an embolic prevalence rate of 7.3%. These authors believe that "impaired atrial function appears to be a key factor in predisposing to intracardiac thrombosis, and paroxysmal supraventricular tachycardia increases the risk of subsequent embolization."

Systemic embolism is a particular risk when the atrial rhythm is changing. One to two percent of patients undergoing cardioversion for AF will experience an embolus in the first few days (2). The risk exists whether the AF is rheumatic or idiopathic in origin. Bjerkelund and Orning (12) noted fewer emboli in those patients anticoagulated at the time of cardioversion. Other investigators cite the low incidence of cardioversion-associated emboli and recommend anticoagulating only high risk patients (2, 58).

We believe that nonvalvular AF is a significant source of systemic embolism in our population; however, these data are not conclusive.

ANTICOAGULATION IN CARDIOGENIC CEREBRAL EMBOLISM

The combined available data (3, 4, 17, 18, 22–24, 29, 38, 69, 79, 82, 88) suggests that anticoagulation benefits patients with cardiogenic cerebral embolism and those at high risk of such emboli. In RHD, the recurrence rate is reduced to approximately 30 to 40% of the natural recurrence rate

(18, 79). In MI, the occurrence rate is reduced to approximately 25% of the natural occurrence rate (29, 62, 89, 90). While the effect of anticoagulation in patients with nonrheumatic AF is not known, in part because these patients are usually not given anticoagulants, 40% of Darling's patients with arteriosclerotic AF and systemic emboli had atrial thrombi present at autopsy (26). This observation suggests that these patients also may benefit from anticoagulation. Consequently, we believe that anticoagulation is beneficial treatment in the prevention of cardiogenic cerebral embolism.

While there is little question about the efficacy of anticoagulation in the prevention of cerebral embolism in "at risk patients," there is considerable debate about when anticoagulation should be initiated and how long it should be continued. Because it was recognized that cerebral embolism often produced hemorrhagic infarcts, many clinicians feared that early treatment with anticoagulant after a cerebral embolism would result in grossly hemorrhagic infarcts with worsening of the morbidity and mortality.

There are a modest amount of experimental animal data showing that immediate anticoagulation probably makes the infarct more hemorrhagic but probably doesn't affect mortality (65, 75, 87). Meager human studies (18, 90) probably show a beneficial effect on both morbidity and mortality when anticoagulant is used immediately following embolization (in spite of a few anecdotal reports of patients on anticoagulant dying with grossly hemorrhagic infarcts). This issue is discussed in detail elsewhere (28).

ANTICOAGULATION IN PERSPECTIVE

While it is somewhat unfair to summarize our personal views about antiplatelet aggregation agents and carotid endarterectomy without reviewing the data, we think it is worth doing briefly in order to put these two treatment modalities in perspective with anticoagulation (15). Data providing for the selection of specific therapy in ischemic cerebrovascular disease are incomplete by modern methodological and epidemiological criteria. Consequently, the definitive role of anticoagulation, antiplatelet aggregation agents, surgery, and some other forms of therapy is controversial. Nevertheless, if a patient with a carotid system TIA or small infarct has a surgically correctable arterial lesion appropriate to the deficit, such as a large ulcerated plaque or a stenosis greater than 60%, is in otherwise good health, and is neurologically stable, carotid endarterectomy can be recommended. Cardiac disease, multiple or inaccessible arterial disease, moderate or severe neurological deficit, and other factors diminish the indication and increase the risk of endarterectomy.

In patients having TIA who are not candidates for endarterectomy, aspirin may be recommended indefinitely. Alternatively, warfarin sodium may be given for a period of 3 to 6 months, followed by aspirin. Some clinicians believe that aspirin is more effective than anticoagulant while others prefer anticoagulant over aspirin. Definitive data are not available regarding the relative efficacy of these two agents.

For progressing stroke or a flurry of TIAs, most clinicians favor immediate heparinization in spite of the limited evidence that anticoagulant is beneficial in this situation. A choice must then be made regarding evaluation for immediate or delayed vascular surgery, more prolonged anticoagulation, institution of antiplatelet aggregation therapy, or discontinuation of therapy at some point. While some physicians recommend surgery in the acute stroke period, *i.e.*, within 12 hours of onset of symptoms, most believe that the patient should be neurologically stable prior to endarterectomy.

With respect to cardiogenic cerebral embolism, virtually all patients with moderate to severe RHD or large myocardial infarcts, those patients who have had one systemic embolism, and many patients with nonvalvular AF should be prophylactically anticoagulated indefinitely.

A physician skilled in the use of anticoagulant medication, with access to a reliable coagulation laboratory, can properly manage selected patients with an acceptably low morbidity and mortality (5, 7, 21, 46, 76).

REFERENCES

1. Aberg, H. Atrial fibrillation. Acta Med. Scand., *185:* 373–379, 1969.
2. Abernathy, W. S., and Willis, P. W. Thromboembolic complications of rheumatic heart disease. Cardiovasc. Clin., *5:* 131–175, 1973.
3. Adams, G. F., Merrett, J. D., Hutchinson, W. M., and Pollock, A. M. Cerebral embolism and mitral stenosis: survival with and without anticoagulants. J. Neurol. Neurosurg. Psychiatr., *37:* 378–383, 1974.
4. Askey, J. M., and Cherry, C. B. Thromboembolism associated with auricular fibrillation. J.A.M.A., *144:* 97–100, 1950.
5. American Heart Association. Committee on Anticoagulants. Myocardial infarction, its clinical manifestations and treatment with anticoagulants: a study of 1,031 cases, by I. S. Wright (Chairman), C. D. Marple, and D. F. Beck. Grune & Stratton, New York, 1954.
6. Baker, R. N. An evaluation of anticoagulant therapy in the treatment of cerebrovascular disease: report of the Veterans Administration cooperative study of atherosclerosis (Neurology Section). Neurology (Minneap.), *11:* 132–138, 1961.
7. Baker, R. N., Broward, J. A., Fang, H. C., Fisher, C. M., Groch, S. N., Heyman, A., *et al.* Anticoagulant therapy in cerebral infarction. Neurology (Minneap.), *12:* 823–835, 1962.
8. Baker, R. N., Schwartz, W. S., and Rose, A. S. Transient ischemic attacks. A report of a study of anticoagulant therapy. Neurology (Minneap.), *16:* 841–847, 1966.
9. Bean, W. B. Infarction of the heart. III. Clinical course and morphological findings. Ann. Intern. Med., *12:* 71–94, 1938.
10. Beer, D. T., and Ghitman, B. Embolization from the atria in arteriosclerotic heart disease. J.A.M.A., *177:* 287–291, 1961.
11. Belcher, J. R., and Somerville, W. Systemic embolization and left auricular thrombosis

in relation to mitral valvulotomy. Br. Med. J., *2:* 1000–1003, 1955.

12. Bjerkelund, C. J., and Orning, O. M. The efficacy of anticoagulant therapy in preventing embolism related to D.C. electrical conversion of atrial fibrillation. Am. J. Cardiol., *23:* 208–216, 1969.
13. Blackwood, W., Hallpike, J. F., Kocen, R. S., and Mair, W. G. P. Atheromatous disease of the carotid arterial system and embolism from the heart in cerebral infarction: a morbid anatomical study. Brain, *92:* 897–910, 1969.
14. Brust, J. C. M. Transient ischemic attacks: natural history and anticoagulation. Neurology (Minneap.), *27:* 701–707, 1977.
15. Byer, J. A., and Easton, J. D. Therapy in ischemic cerebrovascular disease. Ann. Intern. Med., *93:* 742–756, 1980.
16. Carter, A. B. Anticoagulant treatment in progressing stroke. Br. Med. J., *2:* 70–73, 1961.
17. Carter, A. B. Prognosis of cerebral embolism. Lancet, *2:* 514–519, 1965.
18. Carter, A. B. The immediate treatment of cerebral embolism. Q. J. Med., *26:* 335–348, 1957.
19. Casella, L., Abelmann, W. H., and Ellis, L. B. Patients with mitral stenosis and systemic emboli. Arch. Intern. Med., *114:* 773–781, 1964.
20. Cervantes, F. D., and Schneiderman, L. J. Anticoagulants in cerebrovascular disease. A critical review of studies. Arch. Intern. Med., *135:* 875–877, 1975.
21. Coon, W. W., and Willis, P. W. Hemorrhagic complications of anticoagulant therapy. Arch. Intern. Med., *133:* 386–392, 1974.
22. Cosgriff, S. W. Chronic anticoagulant therapy in recurrent embolism of cardiac origin. Ann. Intern. Med., *38:* 278–287, 1953.
23. Cosgriff, S. W. Prophylaxis of recurrent embolism of intracardiac origin. J.A.M.A., *143:* 870–872, 1950.
24. Coulshed, N., Epstein, E. J., McKendrick, C. S., Galloway, R. W., and Walker, E. Systemic embolism in mitral valve disease. Br. Heart J., *32:* 26–34, 1970.
25. Daley, R., Mattingly, T. W., Holt, C. L., Bland, E. F., and White, P. D. Systemic arterial embolism in rheumatic heart disease. Am. Heart J., *42:* 566–581, 1951.
26. Darling, R. C., Austen, W. G., and Linton, R. R. Arterial embolism. Surg. Gynecol. Obstet., *124:* 106–114, 1967.
27. Discussion. *In* Cerebrovascular Diseases, Tenth Princeton Conference, edited by P. Scheinberg, pp. 47–54. Raven Press, New York, 1976.
28. Easton, J. D., and Sherman, D. G. Management of cerebral embolism of cardiac origin. Stroke, *11:* 433–442, 1980.
29. Ebert, R. V. Anticoagulants in acute myocardial infarction. Results of a cooperative clinical trial. J.A.M.A., *225:* 724–729, 1973.
30. Ellis, L. B., and Harken, D. E. Arterial embolization in relation to mitral valvuloplasty. Am. Heart J., *62:* 611–620, 1961.
31. Enger, E., and Royesen, S. Long-term anticoagulant therapy in patients with cerebral infarction. A controlled clinical study. Acta Med. Scand. [Suppl.], *438:* 1–6, 1965.
32. Fairfax, A. J., Lambert, C. D., and Leatham, A. Systemic embolism in chronic sinoatrial disorder. N. Engl. J. Med., *295:* 190–192, 1976.
33. Fazekas, J. F., Alman, R. W., and Sullivan, J. F. Vertebrobasilar insufficiency. Arch. Neurol., *8:* 215–220, 1963.
34. Fisher, C. The use of anticoagulants in cerebral thrombosis. Neurology, *8:* 311–332, 1958.
35. Fisher, C. M. Anticoagulant therapy in cerebral thrombosis and cerebral embolism. A national cooperative study, interim report. Neurology (Minneap.), *11:* 119–131, 1961.
36. Fisher, C. M. Discussion. *In* Cerebrovascular Diseases, Tenth Princeton Conference, edited by P. Scheinberg, p. 50. Raven Press, New York, 1976.
37. Fisher, C. M. Reducing risks of cerebral embolism. Geriatrics, *34:* 59–66, 1979.

38. Fleming, H. A., and Bailey, S. M. Mitral valve disease, systemic embolism and anticoagulants. Postgrad. Med. J., *47:* 599–604, 1971.
39. Fogarty, T. J. Sudden arterial occlusion: surgical aspects. Cardiovasc. Clin., *3:* 173–182, 1971.
40. Friedberg, C. K. Diseases of the heart. Ed. 3. W. B. Saunders, Philadelphia, 1966.
41. Friedman, G. D., Loveland, D. B., and Ehrlich, S. P. Relationship of stroke to other cardiovascular disease. Circulation, *38:* 533–541, 1968.
42. Friedman, G. D., Wilson, S., Mosier, J. M., Colandrea, M. A., and Nochaman, M. Z. Transient ischemic attacks in a community. J.A.M.A., *210:* 1428–1434, 1969.
43. Garvin, C. F. Infarction in heart disease. Am. J. Med. Sci., *203:* 473–476, 1942.
44. Harris, A. W., and Levine, S. A. Cerebral embolism in mitral stenosis. Ann. Intern. Med., *15:* 637–643, 1941.
45. Hellerstein, H. K., and Martin, J. W. Incidence of thromboembolic lesions accompanying myocardial infarction. Am. Heart J., *33:* 443–452, 1947.
46. Hilden, T., Iversen, K., Raaschou, F., and Schwartz, M. Anticoagulants in acute myocardial infarction. Lancet, *2:* 327–331, 1961.
47. Hill, A. B., Marshall, J., and Shaw, D. A. Cerebrovascular disease: trial of long-term anticoagulant therapy. Br. Med. J., *2:* 1003–1006, 1962.
48. Hinton, R. C., Kistler, J. P., Fallon, J. T., Friedlich, A. L., and Fisher, C. M. Influence of etiology of atrial fibrillation on incidence of systemic embolism. Am. J. Cardiol., *40:* 509–513, 1977.
49. Howard, F. A., Cohen, P., Hickler, R. B., Locke, S., Newcomb, T., and Tyler, H. R. Survival following stroke. J.A.M.A., *183:* 921–925, 1963.
50. Jones, H. R., and Millikan, C. H. Temporal profile (clinical course) of acute carotid system cerebral infarction. Stroke, *7:* 64–71, 1976.
51. Jones, H. R., Millikan, C. H., and Sandok, B. A. Temporal profile (clinical course) of acute vertebrobasilar system cerebral infarction. Stroke, *11:* 173–177, 1980.
52. Jordan, R. A., Miller, R. D., Edwards, J. E., and Parker, R. L. Thromboembolism in acute and in healed myocardial infarction. Circulation, *6:* 1–6, 1952.
53. Jordan, R. A., Scheifley, C. H., and Edwards, J. E. Mural thrombosis and arterial embolism in mitral stenosis. Circulation, *3:* 363–367, 1951.
54. Juergens, J. L., *et al.* Prognosis of patients surviving first clinically diagnosed myocardial infarction. Arch. Intern. Med., *105:* 444–450, 1960.
55. Kendell, R. E., and Marshall, J. Role of hypotension in the genesis of transient focal cerebral ischemic attacks. Br. Med. J., *2:* 344–348, 1963.
56. Levine, J., and Swanson, P. D. Nonatherosclerotic causes of stroke. Ann. Intern. Med., *70:* 807–816, 1969.
57. Loew, D. E., Harken, D. E., and Ellis, L. B. Valvular heart disease: undiagnosed valvular involvement, concomitant coronary artery disease and systemic embolization. Am. J. Cardiol., *30:* 222–228, 1972.
58. Lown, B. Electrical reversion of cardiac arrhythmias. Br. Heart J., *29:* 469–489, 1967.
59. Marshall, J., and Shaw, D. A. Anticoagulant therapy in acute cerebrovascular accidents. A controlled trial. Lancet, *1:* 995–998, 1960.
60. McDonald, G. S. A., and McCaughey, W. T. E. Mural thrombosis and myocardial infarction. J. Irish Med. Assoc., *67:* 173–176, 1974.
61. McDowell, F., and McDevitt, E. Treatment of the completed stroke with long-term anticoagulant. Six and one-half years experience. *In* Cerebrovascular Diseases, Fourth Princeton Conference, edited by R. G. Siekert and J. P. Whisnant, pp. 185–199. Grune & Stratton, New York, 1965.
62. Medical Research Council Report. Assessment of short-term anticoagulant administration after cardiac infarction. Br. Med. J., *1:* 335–342, 1969.

63. Millikan, C. H. Anticoagulant therapy in cerebrovascular disease. *In* Cerebral Vascular Diseases, Fourth Princeton Conference, edited by C. H. Millikan, R. H. Siekert, and J. P. Whisnant, p. 183. Grune & Stratton, New York, 1965.
64. Millikan, C. H., and McDowell, F. H. Treatment of transient ischemic attacks. Stroke, *9:* 299–308, 1978.
65. Moyes, P. D., Millikan, C. H., Wakim, K. G., Sayre, G. P., and Whisnant, J. P. Influence of anticoagulants on experimental canine cerebral infarcts. Proc. Mayo Clin., *32:* 124–130, 1957.
66. Neilson, G. H., Galea, E. G., and Hossack, K. F. Thromboembolic complications of mitral valve disease. Aust. N.Z. J. Med., *8:* 372–376, 1978.
67. Olesen, K. H., Hansen, J. F., and Lauridsen, P. Systemic arterial embolism after mitral valvulotomy. Scand. J. Thorac. Cardiovasc. Surg., *6:* 52–56, 1972.
68. Olsson, J. E., Muller, R., and Berneli, S. Long-term anticoagulant therapy for TIAs and minor strokes with minimum residuum. Stroke, *7:* 444–451, 1976.
69. Owren, P. A. The results of anticoagulant therapy in Norway. Arch. Intern. Med., *111:* 240–258, 1963.
70. Pearce, J. M. S., Gubbay, S. S., and Walton, J. Long-term anticoagulant therapy in transient cerebral ischemic attacks. Lancet, *1:* 6–9, 1965.
71. Report of the Joint Committee for Stroke Resources. XIV. Cerebral ischemia: the role of thrombosis and of antithrombotic therapy. Stroke, *8:* 148–175, 1977.
72. An evaluation of anticoagulant therapy in the treatment of cerebrovascular disease. Report of the Veterans Administration Cooperative Study of Atherosclerosis, Neurology Section. Neurology (Minneap.), *11:* 132–138, 1961.
73. Rowe, J. C., Bland, E. G., Sprague, H. B., and White, P. D. The course of mitral stenosis without surgery: ten- and twenty-year perspectives. Ann. Intern. Med., *52:* 741–749, 1960.
74. Sandok, B. A., Furlan, A. J., Whisnant, J. P., and Sundt, T. M. Guidelines for the management of transient ischemic attacks. Mayo Clin. Proc., *53:* 665–674, 1978.
75. Sibley, W. A., Morledge, J. H., and Lapham, L. W. Experimental cerebral infarction: the effect of dicumarol. Am. J. Med. Sci., *234:* 663–677, 1957.
76. Siekert, R. G., Whisnant, J. P., and Millikan, C. H. Surgical and anticoagulant therapy of occlusive cerebrovascular disease. Ann. Intern. Med., *58:* 637–641, 1963.
77. Soderstrom, N. Myocardial infarction and mural thrombosis in the atria of the heart. Acta Med. Scand. [Suppl.], *217:* 1–114, 1948.
78. Somerville, W., and Chambers, R. J. Systemic embolism in mitral stenosis: relation to the size of the left atrial appendix. Br. Med. J., *2:* 1167–1169, 1964.
79. Szekely, P. Systemic embolism and anticoagulant prophylaxis in rheumatic heart disease. Br. Med. J., *1:* 1209–1212, 1964.
80. Toole, J. F., Janeway, R., Choi, K., *et al.* Transient ischemic attacks due to atherosclerosis. Arch. Neurol., *32:* 5–12, 1975.
81. Towbin, A. Recurrent cerebral embolism. Arch. Neurol. Psychiatry, *73:* 173–192, 1955.
82. Wells, C. E. Cerebral embolism. Arch. Neurol. Psychiatry, *81:* 667–677, 1959.
83. Whisnant, J. P. Discussion of progressing stroke: anticoagulant therapy. *In* Cerebral Vascular Diseases, Third Princeton Conference, edited by C. H. Millikan, R. G. Siekert, and J. P. Whisnant, pp. 156–157. Grune & Stratton, New York, 1961.
84. Whisnant, J. P., Matsumoto, N., and Elveback, L. R. The effect of anticoagulant therapy on the prognosis of patients with transient cerebral ischemic attacks in a community. Mayo Clin. Proc., *48:* 844–848, 1973.
85. Wilson, J. K., and Greenwood, W. F. The natural history of mitral stenosis. Can. Med. Assoc. J., *71:* 323–331, 1954.
86. Wolf, P. A., Dawber, T. R., Thomas, H. E., and Kannel, W. B. Epidemiologic assessment

of chronic atrial fibrillation and risk of stroke: the Framingham Study. Neurology (Minneap.), *28:* 973–977, 1978.

87. Wood, M. W., Wakim, K. G., Sayre, G. P., Millikan, C. H., and Whisnant, J. P. Relationship between anticoagulants and hemorrhagic cerebral infarction in experimental animals. Arch. Neurol. Psychiatry, *79:* 390–396, 1958.
88. Wood, P. An appreciation of mitral stenosis. Br. Med. J., *1:* 1051–1063, 1113–1124, 1954.
89. Wright, I. S., Marple, C. D., and Beck, D. F. Report of the committee for the evaluation of anticoagulants in the treatment of coronary thrombosis with myocardial infarction. Am. Heart J., *36:* 801–815, 1948.
90. Wright, I. S., and McDevitt, E. Cerebral vascular diseases: their significance, diagnosis and present treatment, including the selective use of anticoagulant substances. Lancet, *2:* 825–830, 1954.

CHAPTER

4

Antibiotic Therapy in Neurosurgical Infections

JAMES P. LUBY, M.D.

Infections in neurosurgical patients represent some of the most difficult and challenging problems in antibiotic therapy. This article reviews the present therapy of such infections and points to the near future when new drugs will become available that are capable of entering the cerebrospinal fluid (CSF) and having a broader antibacterial spectrum. Drugs presently available that are effective in central nervous system (CNS) infections are listed in Table 4.1. The drugs included are the penicillin derivatives, chloramphenicol, and the aminoglycosides. The penicillin derivatives are effective because the therapeutic ratio is high, and hence doses of drug can be large enough so that sufficient quantities of antibiotic may move across the blood-brain barrier. Toxicity in the form of convulsions occurs when major excretory routes are blocked, as in renal failure, and modifications of the dose have not been made. Representative of penicillinase-resistant semisynthetic penicillins (PRSP) are methicillin and nafcillin. Chloramphenicol CSF/serum ratios approximate 30 to 50%. The aminoglycosides are necessary drugs because of the problem of hospital-acquired meningitis in neurosurgical patients. These drugs are effective against hospital acquired Gram-negative bacteria, but in order to be effective they must be administered both parenterally and directly into the CSF. A major problem related to the administration of these drugs is the route wherein they are best placed into the CSF. The controversy revolves around whether the drug should be placed into the CSF at the lumbar space or whether intraventricular administration is necessary, and data concerning this controversy will be presented later.

Methicillin-resistant *Staphylococcus aureus* and *Staphylococcus epidermidis* infections are not treated by the listed drugs and may require therapy with vancomycin alone or in combination with an aminoglycoside or a drug such as rifampin. Although newer penicillins and cephalosporins may answer part of the problems posed by Gram-negative bacteria, resistance may develop to these agents with use. The aminoglycosides remain under such circumstances as necessary antibiotics with which the therapist must remain familiar.

TABLE 4.1
Antibiotics Presently Effective in CNS Infections

Penicillin derivatives
Penicillin G
Ampicillin
Methicillin
Nafcillin
Carbenicillin
Ticarcillin
Chloramphenicol
Aminoglycosides
Gentamicin
Tobramycin
Amikacin

What types of infections appear most prevalent at the present time? To look at the problem, 50 consecutive consultations involving infectious disease complications were reviewed. These consultations involve an active Neurosurgical Service at Parkland Memorial Hospital (Table 4.2). The major diagnoses arrived at during the consultation are listed, the total being greater than 50 because of multiple conditions in the same patient. Of non-CNS infections, urinary tract infections were most common, followed by pneumonia. Urinary tract infections were explainable on the basis of foley catheterization in patients unable to void. All the urinary tract infections were symptomatic and occurred despite use of a closed bag drainage system where the closest attention was given to maintaining the integrity of each junction. Pneumonia was common, as these patients were often comatose and could not clear their pulmonary secretions and were prone to aspirate organisms from the nasopharynx into the lung. In sick hospitalized patients, it must be assumed that the nasopharynx has lost its native "mucosal immunity" and that hospital acquired Gram-negative bacteria have established residence at that site. Empiric antibiotic therapy of hospital-acquired urinary tract infections involves use of an aminoglycoside with or without the concomitant administration of a cephalosporin. Hospital acquired pneumonia can best be treated empirically again with an aminoglycoside coupled with a PRSP or a cephalosporin to cover the infrequent but definite occurrence of *S. aureus* in these infections.

The most common neurosurgical infection encountered in these 50 consultations was posttraumatic or postneurosurgical meningitis. Gram-positive organisms, *S. aureus*, *S. epidermidis*, and *Streptococcus fecalis* (*Enterococcus*) were encountered in 5 patients, Gram-negative organisms in 7 patients *Klebsiella pneumoniae*, *Escherichia coli*, *Pseudomonas aeruginosa*, *Haemophilus influenzae*, *Enterobacter cloacae*, and *Serratia marcescens*. Empiric treatment of such infections is difficult, requires expert use of the Gram-stain of the CSF and, most importantly, adequate culturing to guide subsequent therapy (4–7, 10). If an organism cannot be ascertained with certainty on Gram-stain, therapy with a PRSP and parenteral aminoglycoside, along with the administration of the latter drug into the lumbar space, will be necessary. If a Gram-positive coccus is found on Gram-stain, a PRSP is indicated. Care must be taken that a dual infection is not missed, and to avoid that problem, the most cautious approach would also be to administer an aminoglycoside until cultures return. If a Gram-negative organism is seen, chloramphenicol plus an aminoglycoside should be started. If the patient has previously been on chloramphenicol or if *P. aeruginosa* is a likely pathogen, carbenicillin or ticarcillin should be substituted for chloramphenicol. Empiric therapy for an epidural abscess involves a PRSP. In drug addicts and hospitalized patients with a previous lumbar puncture, a Gram-negative bacillus should be suspected, and an aminoglycoside should be instituted. Brain abscesses and subdural empyemas commonly contain anaerobic organisms and require chloramphenicol plus a PRSP to cover the possibility of *S. aureus* (2, 8). Empiric therapy of osteomyelitis necessitates a PRSP. In cervical osteomyelitis, anaerobic organisms may play a role, particularly if a fragment such as a bullet has penetrated the nasopharynx and lodged in or near the vertebral body. In such instances, chloramphenicol should also be instituted. Adequate cultures from bone in osteomyelitis are essential since the etiologies of nontraumatic vertebral body infection may involve *S. aureus*, urinary tract

TABLE 4.2

A Summary of Infectious Diagnoses Made in 50 Consecutive Consultations on the Neurosurgical Service of Parkland Memorial Hospital

	No. of cases*	% cases
Meningitis	12	24
Gram-positive	5	10
Gram-negative	7	14
Epidural abscess	5	10
Brain abscess	4	8
Osteomyelitis	4	8
Cervical spine	2	4
Cranium	2	4
Subdural empyema	2	4
Orbital cellulitis	1	2
Cryptococcoma	1	2
Cysticercosis	1	2
Urinary tract infection	13	26
Pneumonia	8	16
IV catheter-associated bacteremia	1	2
Transfusion-associate hepatitis	1	2

* Total is greater than 50 because of multiple conditions in the same patient.

organisms such as Gram-negative bacteria and *S. faecalis* or *Mycobacterium tuberculosis.* In orbital cellulitis, a predisposing cause such as sinusitis must be searched for, and empiric antibiotic therapy usually requires both a PRSP and chloramphenicol. Treatment of fungal organisms necessitates amphotericin B. In entities like a cryptococcoma, 5-fluorocytosine can be added. With the last disease, diagnosis and consequent therapy can best be made, often through combined medical and surgical approaches.

The organisms isolated in these 50 patients are listed in Table 4.3. They comprise a variety of Gram-positive, Gram-negative, anaerobic, and nonbacterial etiologies. Subtracting the organisms causing urinary tract infections and pneumonia does not diminish the variety of etiologies. Neurosurgical infections at the present time are caused not only by the classical pathogens, but also by organisms resident in the hospital that contribute to and complicate these infections.

Fig. 4.1 lists representative organisms found in the series matched

TABLE 4.3

A Summary of the Organisms Isolated from 50 Neurosurgical Patients Seen in Consultation

	No. of cases*	% cases
Gram-positive organisms		
S. aureus	9	18
S. epidermidis	2	4
S. faecalis	2	4
Viridans streptococci	2	4
S. pneumoniae	1	2
Group B streptococci	1	2
Gram-negative organisms		
K. pneumoniae	4	8
E. coli	3	6
P. aeruginosa	2	4
H. influenzae	2	4
E. cloacae	2	4
E. aerogenes	1	2
S. marcescens	1	2
Eikenella corrodens	1	2
Nonfermentative Gram-negative rod	1	2
Anaerobic organisms (including Bacteriodes sp.)	5	10
Miscellaneous organisms		
Blastomyces dermatididis	1	2
Cryptococcus neoformans	1	2
Taenia solium	1	2
NA-NB hepatitis	1	2

* Total is less than 50 because the organism was not identified in some cases.

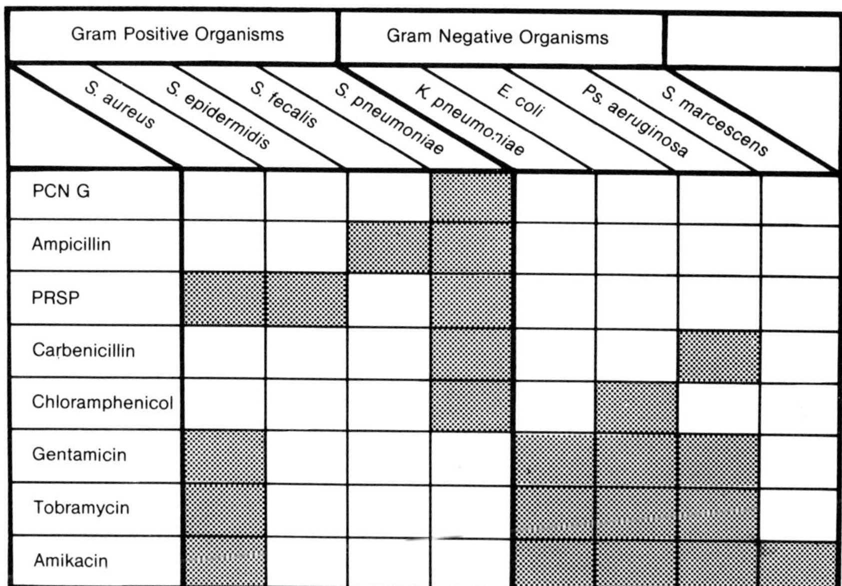

	Gram Positive Organisms				Gram Negative Organisms			
	S. aureus	S. epidermidis	S. fecalis	S. pneumoniae	K. pneumoniae	E. coli	Ps. aeruginosa	S. marcescens
PCN G				X				
Ampicillin			X	X				
PRSP	X	X		X				
Carbenicillin				X			X	
Chloramphenicol				X		X		
Gentamicin	X				X	X	X	
Tobramycin	X				X	X	X	
Amikacin	X				X	X	X	X

Marked box indicates 90% of strains susceptible to the antibiotic tested.

FIG. 4.1. Susceptibility data relating antibiotics presently effective in CNS infection to organisms commonly isolated from these infections.

against the antibiotics effective presently in CNS infections. The susceptibility data was accumulated from the Bacteriology Laboratory of Parkland Memorial Hospital under the direction of Dr. Paul Southern. *S. aureus* can be treated by a PRSP; aminoglycosides are effective *in vitro* but should not be considered primary drugs for infections due to this organism. Of concern is a probable increasing incidence of methicillin-resistant *S. aureus* isolates. Such infections are now endemic in certain hospitals. A recent burn ward epidemic of methicillin-resistant *S. aureus* infections occurred at Parkland and spilled over to involve one neurosurgical patient who expired with bacteremia and meningitis. It is essential to attempt to control such infections by epidemiological methods, and in the epidemic mentioned it was possible to accomplish this. Otherwise, sufficient therapy must necessitate the use of vancomycin with or without the use of an aminoglycoside. Another alarming trend is the emergence of gentamicin-resistant *S. aureus*. Just under 10% of *S. aureus* isolates tested at Parkland are resistant to gentamicin. *S. epidermidis* infections are an increasing problem, with approximately 10% of such isolates being resistant to methicillin. Although these resistant organisms may be sensitive to cephalosporins, these antibiotics cannot be relied upon to enter the CSF. Therapy of resistant *S. epidermidis* in CNS infections must depend upon vancomycin with or without the addition of an aminoglycoside. Rifampin has been used with vancomycin to treat these infections, but tests must be performed in the laboratory to determine whether this combination is synergistic and to exclude antagonism. *S. faecalis* is an occasional cause of posttraumatic or postneurosurgical meningitis. Initial therapy involves the use of penicillin G or ampicillin plus an aminoglycoside. If the organism is sensitive to ampicillin at a low concentration, ampicillin alone may be continued as therapy. *Streptococcus pneumoniae* is effectively treated with penicillin G. In penicillin allergic patients, chloramphenicol should be used. *P. aeruginosa* infections require combined therapy with carbenicillin or ticarcillin plus an aminoglycoside. Unless the isolate is sensitive to carbenicillin or ticarcillin at low concentrations, combined therapy is essential since the penicillin derivative may not reach CSF levels of sufficient magnitude to handle the infection alone. *P. aeruginosa* isolates are sometimes more sensitive to tobramycin than to gentamicin. Some isolates are resistant to both gentamicin and tobramycin and require the use of amikacin. *S. marcescens* is an example of an organism that may be resistant to all antibiotics except amikacin. The laboratory should also test such isolates to determine if carbenicillin-ticarcillin and aminoglycoside synergy may exist. If such can be documented, combined therapy may be the most beneficial approach. The increasing resistance of Gram-negative bacteria to the aminoglycosides is a matter of concern. Many Infection Control committees limit the use of amikacin in the hospital so that sensitivity to that antibiotic can be maintained. Since tobramycin, at least in some hospitals, has maintained its utility against *P. aeruginosa*, an argument can be advanced for the selective use of that antibiotic in closed ward settings in those hospitals so that the effectiveness of that antibiotic can continue.

Selective aspects of the pharmacology of the antibiotics under discussion are summarized in Table 4.4. For illustrative purposes, adult doses are given. A major problem related to penicillin administration is allergy to the drug. If the organism is susceptible to another antibiotic, that drug can be given, *e.g.*, chloramphenicol in *S. pneumoniae* infections. If an alternative antibiotic is less likely to reach the therapeutic goal in the penicillin allergic patient, skin testing should be undertaken. It has been determined that an immediate reaction to penicillin, such as anaphylaxis, is very unlikely if the patient is skin test negative to 3 testing materials: benzylpenicilloyl-poly-L-lysine (Pre-Pen), benzylpenicillin G, and penicilloic acid. The penicillin derivative can be administered if the skin tests are negative. Approximate skin testing and the interpretation of the tests can sometimes best be accomplished by consultation with the Allergy

TABLE 4.4

Pharmacological Data on Drugs Presently Effective in CNS Infections

	Usual dose	Dose Interval	Total daily dose	Maximum daily dose in renal failure		Dose adjustment in hepatic and renal failure	Usual solute load per day
				Moderate	Severe		
Penicillin	3 to 4 × 10^6 u	4	20 × 10^6	10 × 10^6	5 × 10^6		34 mEq K^+
Ampicillin	2 g	4	12	Unchanged	6		36 mEq Na^+
Methicillin	2 g	4	12	Unchanged	6		
Nafcillin	2 g	4	12	Unchanged	Unchanged	+	
Carbenicillin	5 g	4	30	15	5	+	141 mEq Na^+
Ticarcillin	3 g	4	18	9	3	+	94 mEq Na^+
Chloramphenicol	1 g	6	4	Unchanged	Unchanged	+	
Gentamicin	$\frac{1.5\ mg}{kg}$	8	$\frac{4.5\ mg}{kg}$	"Rule of 8's"			
Tobramycin	$\frac{1.5\ mg}{kg}$	8	$\frac{4.5\ mg}{kg}$	"Rule of 8's"			
Amikacin	$\frac{7.5\ mg}{kg}$	8	$\frac{15\ mg}{kg}$	"Rule of 9's"			

* For illustrative purposes, adult doses of the drugs are given.

Service of the hospital. If such testing cannot be performed or if one of the skin tests is positive, desensitization can be performed. This involves the administration of penicillin G or the required derivative in an intensive care setting. If desensitization cannot be accomplished or if some hypersensitivity response occurs that is progressive and unresponsive to symptomatic medication, an alternate antibacterial regimen is necessitated. This may involve vancomycin with or without an aminoglycoside for *S. aureus*, *S. epidermidis*, or *S. faecalis* infections.

Since the penicillin derivatives have such a high therapeutic ratio, the dosages must have only a moderate modification in the face of renal failure. Modified doses are listed in Table 4.4. Moderate renal failure is denoted by creatinine clearances of 10 to 40 ml/minute or by serum creatinines of 4 to 10 mg/dl. Patients with severe renal failure have creatinine clearances less than 10 ml/minute or serum creatinines greater than 10 mg/dl. Nafcillin has a predominantly hepatic route of excretion, and its dosage is unaffected in renal failure but needs to be altered with significant hepatic disease. The doses of carbenicillin and ticarcillin need further downward adjustment with combined hepatic and renal insufficiency. Significant solute loads are encountered predominantly with the use of carbenicillin and ticarcillin. Since these antibiotics are the sodium salts of weak bases and since the sodium load per day may approximate that of a liter of normal saline, hypokalemic alkalosis may occur with the use of these antibiotics. The administration of methicillin may be accompanied by an interstitial nephropathy in an estimated 5 to 10% of patients. Clinically, this is manifest by microscopic hematuria, eosinophiluria, eosinophilia, and azotemia. Prompt withdrawal of the drug results in an amelioration of the abnormalities. If such a reaction occurs, it is necessary to change to an antibiotic from another family of drugs since cases of progressive azotemia have been reported with the institution of another penicillin derivative. Nafcillin usage may be complicated by leukopenia with white blood cell counts falling below 3000 in approximately 20% of patients on high dose therapy for prolonged periods. The drug has been continued in patients without further fall, but the decrease may be progressive reaching WBC values of 1500. Restoration of the white blood cell count is rapid upon withdrawal of the drug. In patients with renal failure, the use of carbenicillin and ticarcillin may be associated with platelet aggregation defects.

Chloramphenicol is associated with a dose-dependent effect on the bone marrow. Long-term therapy may result in anemia and may be particularly prominent in patients who may have an associated hemolytic process. The idiosyncratic response of bone marrow aplasia is unpredictable and, although rare, has been reported with the intravenous administration of the drug. Since the drug is conjugated by the liver before renal excretion, combined hepatic and renal insufficiency may result in excessively high serum levels, and its use is probably best avoided in such patients.

Aminoglycoside dosage should be adjusted to dry weight in edematous patients. Adjustments must also be made downward in obese persons. Nomograms have been constructed to guide dosage. These nomograms give dose approximations, and serum levels of the antibiotic must be ascertained at a peak and trough point in a therapeutic steady state so that actual long-term doses may be adjusted accurately. Peak values of gentamicin and tobramycin should approximate 5 to 8 μg/ml. Trough values should always be below 2 μ/ml. Perhaps the simplest guide for adjustment of dosage of the aminoglycosides is the "rule of 8's" for gentamicin and tobramycin and the "rule of 9's" for amikacin. These rules require an adjustment of the interval between successive doses of the aminoglycoside. For gentamicin and tobramycin, the maintenance dose is given at a time interval in hours of 8 times the serum creatinine and for the amikacin the interval is 9 times the serum creatinine. Worsening renal function or its improvement requires further adjustment. Serum levels must be ascertained to determine whether the dosage alterations given by the rules are, in fact, correct. The dosage of gentamicin in the normal adult given at the lumbar space should approximate 8 mg/day. A gentamicin preparation is available without preservative for delivery of the drug into the CSF and contains 2 mg/ml. Its use is indicated because of the possible development of arachnoiditis or radiculopathy with the usual form of parenteral gentamicin (1). The dose of amikacin delivered at the lumbar space in the adult approximates 15 to 20 mg/day.

Evidence has been presented indicating that in humans, gentamicin is more nephrotoxic than tobramycin (11). Contrary evidence has also been presented. Nevertheless, it appears prudent to use tobramycin where nephrotoxicity may become a problem. Most importantly, this would pertain to patients with some degree of renal dysfunction at the start of therapy. If gentamicin is more nephrotoxic than tobramycin, the actual clinical effect of such a difference is probably slight. There would appear to be no difference in ototoxic potential between the two drugs. The most important problem related to aminoglycoside is the route employed to deliver the antibiotic into the CSF. Cures of Gram-negative bacterial meningitis have been reported both with the administration of the drug into the lumbar space and intraventricularly via an Ommaya or Rickham reservoir (3, 4, 6, 7). There are no controlled random trials testing the efficacy of either route of administration in consecutive patients with Gram-negative bacterial meningitis unresponsive to other forms of therapy. The data of Kaiser and McGee (3) suggest that ventriculitis as assessed by positive bacterial cultures is almost invariable in Gram-negative bacterial meningitis. Their pharmacological data show that delivery of the aminoglycoside at the lumbar space results in adequate CSF levels at the point of delivery at the cisternal space, but that intraventricular levels may not be detectable. Occasionally, administration of the aminoglycoside at the lumbar space may not be actually delivered into the CSF. Intraventricular administration of the drug via a reservoir results in more predictable levels throughout the CSF. These investigators have experienced few complications with the use of such a reservoir in these infections. Prudence would dictate against any unnecessary procedure being performed in such desperately ill patients where the case-fatality ratio may reach 40%. In the absence of controlled trials assessing the delivery of aminoglycoside by either method, the wisest course would appear to be, in a stable patient, to begin therapy parenterally and by injection at the lumbar space. Chloramphenicol or carbenicillin-ticarcillin can be begun simultaneously. If the clinical course worsens or if the patient is moribund at the initiation of therapy, intraventricular administration of the aminoglycoside appears warranted.

With the advent of methicillin-resistant *S. aureus* and *S. epidermidis*, further experience with parenteral vancomycin with or without an aminoglycoside or an antibiotic such as rifampin must be obtained. Pediatric experience with shunt infections indicates that in a therapeutic steady state, vancomycin CSF levels may approximate 15 to 20% of serum levels (9). The penetration of vancomycin into the CSF is most pronounced with inflammation, but accumulation of the drug into the CSF does occur with prolonged administration, even with the improvement of the inflammatory changes. Intravenous sulfatrimethoprim preparations soon will become available and may be useful in susceptible Gram-negative bacterial infections because of the ease of the penetration of the drug combination into the CSF. Finally, newer penicillins and cephalosporins are on the horizon promising effective therapy of many Gram-negative bacterial infections formerly only susceptible to the aminoglycosides. Prominent among the cephalosporins include moxalactam, cefotaxime, cefoperazone, and cefsulodin. Although promising agents, their eventual role in the treatment of CNS infections will have to be established by clinical trials. If these newer antibiotics do prove to be effective, we need to use them wisely in the ensuing years to get off a treadmill where the problem of the emergence of resistance of Gram-positive and Gram-negative bacteria seems always several steps ahead.

REFERENCES

1. Buckley, R. M., Watters, W., and MacGregor, R. R. Persistent meningeal inflammation associated with intrathecal gentamicin. Am. J. Med. Sci., *274:* 207–209, 1977.

2. Heineman, H. S., and Braude, A. I. Anaerobic infections of brain. Am. J. Med., *35:* 682–697, 1963.
3. Kaiser, A. B., and McGee, Z. A. Aminoglycoside therapy of Gram-negative bacillary meningitis. N. Engl. J. Med., *293:* 1215–1220, 1975.
4. Mangi, R. J., Holstein, L. L., and Andriole, V. T. Treatment of Gram-negative bacillary meningitis with intrathecal gentamicin. Yale J. Biol. Med., *50:* 31–41, 1977.
5. Murphy, F. K., Mackowiak, P., and Luby, J. P. Management of infections affecting the nervous system. *In* Treatment of Neurological Diseases, edited by R. N. Rosenberg, pp. 249–376. Spectrum Publications, Inc., New York, 1979.
6. Rahal, J. J., Jr. Treatment of Gram-negative bacillary meningitis in adults. Ann. Intern. Med., *77:* 295–302, 1972.
7. Rahal, J. J., Jr., Hyams, P. J., Simberkoff, M. S., and Rubinstein, E. Combined intrathecal and intramuscular gentamicin for Gram-negative meningitis. Pharmacologic study of 21 patients. N. Engl. J. Med., *290:* 1394–1398, 1974.
8. Samson, D., and Clark, K. Current review of brain abscess. Am. J. Med., *54:* 201–210, 1973.
9. Schaad, U. B., McCracken, G. H., Jr., and Nelson, J. D. Clinical pharmacology and efficacy of vancomycin in pediatric patients. J. Pediatr., *96:* 119–126, 1980.
10. Schoenbaum, S. C., Gardner, P., and Shillito, J. Infections of cerebrospinal fluid shunts: epidemiology, clinical manifestations, and therapy. J. Infect. Dis., *131:* 543–552, 1975.
11. Smith, C. R., Lipsky, J. J., Laskin, O. L., Hellmann, D. B., Mellits, E. D., Longstreth, J., and Lietman, P. S. Double-blind comparison of the nephrotoxicity and auditory toxicity of gentamicin and tobramycin. N. Engl. J. Med., *302:* 1106–1109, 1980.

CHAPTER

5

Agents for Cerebral Edema

R. A. DE LOS REYES, M.D., J. I. AUSMAN, M.D., PH.D., and F. G. DIAZ, M.D., PH.D.

Cerebral edema may be defined as an abnormal accumulation of fluid in the brain (27). There are two basic forms of brain edema: vasogenic and cytotoxic (27, 44). Vasogenic edema is associated with injury to the walls of cerebral blood vessels leading to an escape of water and plasma constituents into the surrounding parenchyma. It is chiefly extracellular and is the type of edema associated with brain tumors, head injury, and brain inflammation. An important aspect of this is that, although there is blood-brain barrier (BBB) disruption at the site of injury, the blood-brain barrier remains intact in the areas into which the edema spreads (10, 19). Cytotoxic edema is associated with injury produced by noxious factors directly affecting the structural elements of the parenchyma, producing intracellular swelling. Vascular permeability remains essentially intact, at least as evidenced by conventional blood-brain barrier indicators. This type of edema is associated with water intoxication and triethyl tin poisoning. While realizing that the two types of edema may coexist, the vasogenic type is much more common and is the type most frequently encountered in neurosurgery. Thus, the following review will address itself to agents for the control of vasogenic cerebral edema, either not amenable to or following surgical therapy.

Pharmacologic agents for the control of cerebral edema include the various types of diuretics, corticosteroids, barbiturates, and miscellaneous other drugs.

DIURETICS

The diuretics include the osmotic diuretics (hypertonic glucose, urea, mannitol, and glycerol), the loop diuretics (furosemide and ethacrynic acid), and the carbonic anhydrase inhibitors (acetazolamide).

Osmotic Diuretics

Osmotic diuretics effect a decrease in intracranial pressure through dehydration of *normal* cerebral tissue. Since there is no membrane across which water may be osmotically withdrawn (edema) in areas of BBB disruption, no reduction in the water content of these areas is seen (41). In fact, the reverse may occur, with accumulation of the osmotic diuretic in these areas of BBB disruption, leading to a "rebound" increase in the water content of the lesion, and thus a subsequent rise in intracranial pressure (ICP) (24).

Hypertonic glucose, in 50% concentration, was one of the first agents used for reduction of intracranial pressure. Due to reversal of the osmotic gradient as the serum glucose concentration fell to less than that of the brain and CSF, this agent was found to have a short duration of action and prominent "rebound" increases in ICP (29). This resulted in its abandonment as a therapeutic agent for cerebral edema.

Urea was first introduced clinically for the reduction of increased ICP by Javid (25). Though a potent diuretic, its effect in decreasing ICP is not dependent on diuresis, as evidenced by equal or better pressure reduction in nephrectomized monkeys (26). Like the other osmotic diuretics, it decreases ICP by dehydration of normal brain (41). Urea is a nonpolar, un-ionized, water-soluble agent. While much slower to equilibrate with brain and CSF than hypertonic glucose, it nevertheless does cross the blood-brain barrier and can lead to "rebound" increases in ICP by the same mechanism (28, 37). Furthermore, particularly at high concentrations, urea can lead to headache, nausea, vomiting, hemoglobinuria, alteration of the prothrombin time, and tissue necrosis at sites of subcutaneous extravasation (2, 50). As a result, urea has been replaced by mannitol in most institutions as the cerebral dehydrating agent of choice, due to the latter's reduced propensity for "rebound" increases in ICP and relative lack of toxicity (2, 29, 50).

Mannitol, a 6-carbon hexahydric alcohol with a molecular weight of 182, is commonly used intravenously in a 20% concentration in solutions of water or 0.3 to 0.45% sodium chloride (2, 23). Since its introduction by Wise and Chater (50), doses of 1.0 to 1.5 g/kg have been considered standard and are quite effective in reducing acute ICP elevations. Because of disturbances in serum osmolarity and electrolytes as well as "rebound" ICP elevations due to accumulation of the drug at the site of the lesion after repeated usage, it has been proposed that lower dosage schedules be used for more prolonged (1 to 20 days) treatment of intracranial hypertension (24, 31, 36). This consists of dosages on the order of 0.25 g/kg every 4 hours as a fixed dosage schedule or by giving 20-g boluses PRN, titrated to the patient's intracranial pressure as measured by an ICP monitor.

While concurring in general with the above management in adults, Bruce *et al.* (8) advocate a more restricted use for mannitol in severely head-injured children. They postulate that a large percentage of head-injured children have intracranial hypertension as a result of severe diffuse brain swelling that seems to be due to hyperemia, rather than edema. Having previously demonstrated that mannitol increases cerebral blood flow in adults irrespective of the ICP, they suggest that it be used cautiously and in reduced doses, if at all, in intracranial hypertension not due to mass lesions in children (9).

In recent years, there has been interest in the intravenous use of glycerol as an osmotic agent. While the oral route has long been used for such conditions as pseudotumor cerebri, the intravenous route has not been commonly used due to reports of associated hemoglobinuria and renal failure. Certain authors, however, contend that these complications are a function of the concentration of the administered glycerol solution, and cite such theoretical advantages as less "rebound" and the provision of usable calories in favor of intravenous glycerol as an osmotic diuretic (49). Further investigations along these lines would seem to be indicated.

Loop Diuretics

The loop diuretics furosemide (Lasix) and ethacrynic acid (Edecrin) act primarily by inhibition of sodium and chloride reabsorption in the ascending limb of the loop of Henle, thus producing a potent diuresis (23). It has been suggested that these diuretics also have a separate, direct action on the reduction of cerebral edema by suppressing sodium transport and decreasing CSF production (1, 42). Clasen *et al.* (12), working with a cold-injury model of cerebral edema in the monkey, demonstrated significant reductions in the water content of the damaged hemispheres using extremely high (50 mg/kg) doses of furosemide (12). In a study comparing furosemide and mannitol for intraoperative ICP reduction, Cottrell *et al.* (13) found the two drugs to be roughly equal in this regard. However, the patients in this study were undergoing craniotomies for clipping of aneurysms, repair of arteriovenous malformations (AVMs), or resection of tumors, and had no preoperative evidence of intracranial hypertension. We are not aware of any controlled, randomized studies comparing furosemide with mannitol in traumatic cerebral edema in humans, and in our experience the main benefit of the loop diuretics is in the treatment of patients with concomitant cerebral and pulmonary edema, or in those patients prone to the development of congestive heart failure, given approximately 15 minutes prior to mannitol infusion.

Other Diuretics

Acetazolamide (Diamox), a carbonic anhydrase inhibitor, has likewise been used in the treatment of cerebral edema associated with pseudotumor cerebri. It has been postulated that this drug decreases CSF formation through inhibition of choroid plexus carbonic anhydrase activity

(35). While experience in the literature with the use of this drug for acute cerebral edema has not been extensive, studies both supporting and refuting its effectiveness have been reported (6, 30). We believe further studies are necessary to delineate the role of acetazolamide in acute cerebral edema.

CORTICOSTEROIDS

The action of corticosteroids, mainly dexamethasone and methylprednisolone, in reducing cerebral edema associated with brain tumors is well-known (7, 20). Their use in the management of traumatic cerebral edema, however, remains quite controversial. Advocates of corticosteroid therapy cite various hypotheses to explain their beneficial effects. These include reduction of CSF production, stabilization of cell membranes leading to preservation of intracellular-extracellular water and electrolyte gradients, preservation of the blood-brain barrier, increasing brain glucose availability, and others (17, 24, 40, 45). Working with a cranial-impact model in the cat, Tornheim and McLaurin (48) failed to demonstrate a significant reduction of brain edema in cats treated with dexamethasone 1 hour postimpact, as compared to controls (48). Likewise, Ransohoff (43) failed to demonstrate a statistically significant difference in outcome in head-injured patients treated with corticosteroids as opposed to those who were not.

Recent studies suggest that "high dose" (in the range of 150 to 400 mg dexamethasone/day) steroid therapy may significantly improve outcome when compared to the more traditional "low dose" (16 mg dexamethasone/day) therapy or no steroid groups.

Faupel *et al.* (18), in a well-controlled double-blind study on patients with severe closed head injury, demonstrated a reduction in mortality from 57% in his placebo group to 30% in his low-dose (16 mg/day) and 18% in his high-dose (100 mg initially and at 6 hr, then 16 mg/day) dexamethasone groups. Gobiet (21, 22), having previously obtained similar results with high-dose corticosteroid therapy, further demonstrated significant reductions in post-traumatic brain edema as evidenced by fewer pathologic increases in ICP as measured by a pressure transducer. The timing of steroid administration also appears to be important, with better response in patients treated sooner (within 6 hours) after their injury (18). Bremer (6), working with an ischemic cerebral edema model in primates, was able to demonstrate reduction of edematous changes in the cortex, putamen, and white matter with high-dose dexamethasone and methylprednisolone therapy. There does not appear to be any higher incidence of steroid-related complications (gastrointestinal ulceration or hemorrhage, wound infection, hyperglycemia, etc.) with high-dose than with low-dose therapy (33).

We presently use high-dose corticosteroid therapy on our closed head injury patients. They are given dexamethasone (100 mg IV) on arrival to the Emergency Department and maintained on 100 mg IV every 6 hours for 3 days (coinciding with the peak rise in cerebral edema formation). The steroid is then decreased to 4 mg IV every 6 hours and tapered over the next 4 days, or as the patient's clinical status permits. We have not had sufficient experience to determine whether this high-dose regimen is indeed superior to the standard dosages. Further investigations to compare high *vs.* low-dose therapy, the different corticosteroids (*e.g.*, dexamethasone vs methylprednisolone), and different brands of the same corticosteroid (*e.g.*, Hexadrol *vs.* Decadron) appear warranted.

BARBITURATES

The barbiturates, chiefly pentobarbital and thiopental, are the newest therapeutic agents for the control of intracranial hypertension. Introduced clinically about 5 years ago by Shapiro and Marshall, the results obtained by these investigators in reducing the mortality and improving the outcome from severe closed-head injury have been quite impressive (31, 32, 45, 46).

The mechanisms of action of the brain-protective effects of barbiturates remain speculative. Barbiturates do decrease the brain's metabolic requirements, but this seems to be of insufficient magnitude to fully explain their effects (32). A better explanation might be their direct constrictive effects on the cerebrovasculature, thus lowering ICP by decreasing cerebral blood volume. This is supported by the fact that in a recent study, most of the barbiturate nonresponders also had no change in ICP to variations in $PaCO_2$ (45). Decreased edema formation and various mechanisms of action at the cellular level have likewise been suggested (11, 31).

Iatrogenic barbiturate coma involves the administration of anesthetic doses of barbiturates, over a period of days or weeks, to patients with intracranial hypertension refractory to the more "standard" therapeutic modalities of controlled hyperventilation, ventricular drainage, osmotic diuretics, and corticosteroids. The technique presupposes capability for and familiarity with intracranial and intraarterial pressure monitoring as well as cardiovascular monitoring in a well-equipped intensive care setting.

Using loading doses of pentobarbital (3 to 5 mg/kg IV) followed by 100 to 200 mg every 30 to 60 minutes, titrated to the patient's measured ICP, Marshall *et al.* (32) obtained an initial response rate (lowering of ICP to less than 15 torr) of 76% and an overall mortality rate of 36% in patients with an initial ICP of 400 torr refractory to standard therapy. Previous studies had demonstrated a mortality rate of 100% in a similar group of patients (38).

Our own experience with barbiturate therapy, using both pentobarbital and thiopental (thiopental loading dose 20 mg/kg IV followed by continuous infusion of 10 mg/kg/hr × 6 hr followed by 3 mg/kg/hr) suggests an age-related response to barbiturates: of 21 patients with intracranial hypertension, 5 of the 6 (83%) with fair or good outcome were under the age of 35 years (16). While the bulk of experience in humans has been with cerebral edema and intracranial hypertension secondary to trauma, animal studies have demonstrated increased tolerance to global as well as focal cerebral ischemia with the administration of barbiturates before or soon (within 1 hour) after the onset of ischemia (4, 47). There has been some limited human experience with the use of barbiturates in encephalitis, focal cerebral ischemia (stroke), and global cerebral ischemia (drowning, cardiac arrest). Marshall *et al.* (34) report 100% survival in their series of 7 children with Reye's syndrome. Conversely, their limited experience with global and focal ischemia has been uniformly dismal, with no survivors in 3 cases of drowning or 4 cases of acute cerebrovascular occlusion (45). While we agree with their results with regard to global ischemia, our admittedly small experience with barbiturate therapy *followed by acute revascularization* for focal cerebral ischemia has been more encouraging. The first patient underwent emergency carotid thromboendarterectomy following acute internal carotid occlusion, and was beginning to respond to verbal commands when he suddenly expired due to a pulmonary embolus. The second patient underwent emergency superficial temporal to middle cerebral artery anastomosis following acute middle cerebral artery occlusion, and she made a good recovery. Both patients were placed on barbiturates within 6 hours of their event. While these results are far from conclusive, we would encourage further investigation into barbiturate therapy in combination with cerebral revascularization procedures for acute focal cerebral ischemia.

Despite these encouraging initial results, we must agree with J. Douglas Miller's (39) assertion that the jury is still out on barbiturate therapy. While there is little doubt that they can lower intracranial pressure, to date there are no controlled randomized trials to prove that they make a difference in the final outcome in closed head injury or focal or global cerebral ischemia. On the other hand, the cost, both in terms of equipment and manpower, the emotional drain on the patient's family, and the potential for systemic as well as neurologic complications in this therapy lead us to believe that, at the present time, barbiturate therapy outside of a major center should be undertaken under only the most unusual circumstances (15).

TABLE 5.1
Dosage Recommendations

Mannitol	
	Acute: 1 g/kg IV
	Chronic: 0.25 g/kg IV q 4h > 15 torr
Dexamethasone	
	100 mg IV q 6h × 72 h, then 4 mg IV q 6h and taper by 4 mg every 24 hrs
Pentobarbital	
	5 to 7 mg/kg IV initially, then 3 to 5 mg IV q 4h
Thiopental	
	20 mg/kg IV over 1 hour, then 10 mg/kg/hr IV × 6 hr, then 3 mg/kg/hr IV continuous infusion

OTHER DRUGS

Miscellaneous other drugs, such as phenytoin and dimethylsulfoxide (DMSO), have been proposed as having an anticerebral edema action (3, 6, 14). Though quite interesting, the use of these drugs for cerebral edema is, at present, strictly experimental.

SUMMARY

Hyperventilation, ventricular drainage, and mannitol remain the mainstays of the treatment of cerebral edema not amenable to or following surgical therapy. There appears to be good therapeutic rationale for the use of "low-dose" mannitol in more prolonged treatment of intracranial hypertension (Table 5.1). The beneficial effects of steroids, either in "standard" or "high" doses, is less clear but, pending evidence to the contrary, we favor the use of "high-dose" corticosteroid therapy.

Barbiturates appear to hold promise, but pending controlled, randomized trials to confirm or refute their efficacy, the logistics of their use, as well as their potential complications, precludes their widespread use outside of major centers. Certainly, the "ideal" agent for the treatment of cerebral edema, one that would selectively mobilize and/or prevent the formation of edema fluid with a rapid onset and prolonged duration of action, and with minimal side effects, remains to be discovered. In the meantime, research to refine the use of the older agents and determine the usefulness of the newer ones should be encouraged.

REFERENCES

1. Albin, M. Neuroanesthesia—intracranial neurosurgical procedures in the adult. Contemp. Neurosurg., *8:* 1–5, 1979.
2. AMA Drug Evaluations, 2 Ed. pp. 66, 685–686. Publishing Sciences Group, Inc., Acton, Mass.
3. Artru, A. A., and Michenfelder, J. D. Cerebral protective, metabolic, and vascular effects of phenytoin. Stroke, *11:* 377–382, 1980.

4. Bleyaert, A. C., Nemoto, E. M., Safar, P. *et al.* Thiopental amelioration of brain damage after global ischemia in monkeys. Anesthesiology, *49:* 390–398, 1978.
5. Bouzarth, W. F., and Shenkin, H. A. Possible mechanisms of action of dexamethasone in brain injury. J. Trauma, *14:* 134–136, 1974.
6. Bremer, A., Yamada, K., and West, C. Ischemia cerebral edema in primates: effects of acetazolamide, phenytoin, sorbitol, dexamethasone, and methylprednisolone on brain water and electrolytes. Neurosurgery, *6:* 149–154, 1980.
7. Brock, M., Wiegand, H., Zillig, C., *et al.* The effect of dexamethasone on intracranial pressure in patients with supratentorial tumors. *In* Dynamics of Brain Edema, edited by H. Pappius and W. Feindel, pp. 330–336. Springer Verlag, New York, 1976.
8. Bruce, D., Gennarelli, J., and Langfitt, J. Resuscitation from coma due to head injury. Crit. Care Med., *6:* 254-269, 1978.
9. Bruce, D. A., Langfitt, T. W., and Miller, J. D. Regional cerebral blood flow, intracranial pressure, and brain metabolism in comatose patients. J. Neurosurg., *38:* 131–144, 1973.
10. Bruce, D. A. The pathophysiology of increased intracranial pressure. *In* Current Concepts. The Upjohn Co., Kalamazoo, Mich., 1978.
11. Clason, R. A., Pandolfi, S., and Casey, D. Furosemide and pentobarbital in cryogenic cerebral injury and edema. Neurology, *24:* 642–648, 1974.
12. Clasen, N. A., Pandolfi, S., and Casey, D. Furosemide and pentobarbital in cryogenic cerebral injury and edema. Neurology, *24:* 642–648, 1974.
13. Cottrell, J., Robustelli, A., Post, K., *et al.* Furosemide and pentobarbital in cryogenic cerebral injury and edema. Neurology, *24:* 642–648, 1974.
14. de la Torre, J. C., Rowed, D. W., Kawanaga, H. M., *et al.* Dimethyl sulfoxide in the treatment of experimental brain compression. J. Neurosurg., *38:* 345–354, 1973.
15. de los Reyes, R. A., Babcock, R. A., Malik, G. M., *et al.* Silent duodenal perforation: a difficult diagnosis in iatrogenic barbiturate coma. Crit. Care Med., in press, 1981.
16. Diaz, F. G., Quandt, C., de los Reyes, R. A., *et al.* The use of an ultrashort acting barbiturate in the treatment of intracranial hypertension. Presented at the 1980 Annual Meeting of the American Association of Neurological Surgeons, New York, New York, April 1980.
17. Eisenberg, H. M., Barlow, C. F., and Lorenzo, A. V. The effect of dexamethasone on altered brain vascular permeability. Arch. Neurol., *23:* 18–22, 1970.
18. Faupel, G., Reulen, H. J., Miller, D. *et al.* Double blind study on the effects of steroids on severe closed head injury. *In* Dynamics of Brain Edema, edited by H. M. Pappius and W. Feindel, pp. 337–343, Springer Verlag, New York, 1976.
19. Fishman, R. A. Brain edema. N. Engl. J. Med., *293:* 706–711, 1975.
20. French, L. A., and Galicich, J. H. The use of steroids for control of cerebral edema. Clin. Neurosurg., *10:* 212–223, 1964.
21. Gobiet, W. The influence of various doses of dexamethasone on intracranial pressure in patients with severe head injury. *In* Dynamics of Brain Edema, edited by H. M. Pappius and W. Feindel, pp. 351–355. Springer Verlag, New York, 1976.
22. Gobiet, W., Bock, W. J., Liesegang, J. *et al.* Treatment of acute cerebral edema with high dose dexamethasone. *In* Intracranial Pressure III, edited by J. W. F. Becks, D. A. Bosch, and M. Brock, pp. 231–235. Springer Verlag, New York, 1976.
23. Goodman J., and Gilman, A. The Pharmacologic Basis of Therapeutics, Ed. 5. Macmillan, New York, 1975.
24. Hooshmand, H., Dove, J., Houff, S., *et al.* Effects of diuretics and steroids on CSF pressure. Arch. Neurol., *21:* 499–509, 1969.
25. Javid, M. Urea—new use of an old agent. Reduction of intracranial and intraocular pressure. Surg. Clin. North. Am., *38:* 907–928.

26. Javid, M., and Anderson, J. The effect of urea on cerebrospinal fluid pressure in monkeys before and after bilateral nephrectomy. J. Lab. Clin. Med., *53:* 484–489, 1959.
27. Klatzo, I. Neuropathological aspects of brain edema. J. Neuropathol. Exp. Neurol., *26:* 1–14, 1967.
28. Langfitt, T. W. Possible mechanisms of action of hypertonic urea in reducing intracranial pressure. Neurology, *11:* 196–209, 1961.
29. Langfitt, T. W. Increased intracranial pressure. *In* Neurological Surgery, edited by J. Youmans, pp. 477–481. W. B. Saunders Co., Philadelphia, 1973.
30. Long, D. M., Maxwell, R. E., Choi, K. S. *et al.* Multiple therapeutic approaches in the treatment of brain edema induced by a standard cold lesion. *In* Steroids and Brain Edema, edited by H. J. Reulen, and K. Schurmann, pp. 87–94. Springer-Verlag, New York, 1972.
31. Marsh, M. L., Marshall, L. F., and Shapiro, H. M. Neurosurgical intensive care. Anesthesiology, *17:* 149–163, 1977.
32. Marshall, L. F., Smith, R. W., and Shapiro, H. M. The outcome with aggressive treatment in severe head injuries. Part II. Acute and chronic barbiturate administration in the management of head injury. J. Neurosurg., *50:* 26–30, 1979.
33. Marshall, L. F., King, J., and Langfitt, J. W. The complications of high-dose corticosteroid therapy in neurosurgical patients: a prospective study. Ann Neurol., *1:* 201–203, 1977.
34. Marshall, L. F., Shapiro, H. M., Rauscher, A., *et al.* Pentobarbital therapy for intracranial hypertension in metabolic coma: Reye's syndrome. Crit. Care Med., *6:* 1–5, 1978.
35. McCarthy, K. D., and Reed, D. J. The effect of acetazolamide and furosemide on cerebrospinal fluid production and choroid plexus carbonic anhydrase activity. J. Pharmacol. Exp. Ther., *189:* 194–201, 1974.
36. McGraw, C. P., Alexander, E., and Howard, G. Effect of dose and dose schedule on the response of intracranial pressure to mannitol. Surg. Neurol., *10:* 127–130, 1978.
37. McQueen, J. D., and Jeanes, L. D. Dehydration and rehydration of the brain with hypertonic urea and mannitol. J. Neurosurg., *21:* 118–128, 1964.
38. Miller, J. D., Becker, D. P., Ward, J. D., *et al.* Significance of intracranial hypertension in severe head injury. J. Neurosurg., *47:* 503–516, 1977.
39. Miller, J. D. Barbiturates and raised intracranial pressure. Ann. Neurol., *6:* 189–193, 1979.
40. Miller, J. D., Sakalas, R., Ward, J. D., *et al.* Methylprednisolone treatment in patients with brain tumors. Neurosurgery, *1:* 114–117, 1977.
41. Pappius, H. M., and Dayer, L. A. Hypertonic urea: its effect on the distribution of water and electrolytes in normal and edematous brain tissues. Arch. Neurol., *13:* 395–402, 1965.
42. Pappius, H. M. Effects of steroids on cold injury edema. *In* Steroids and Brain Edema, edited by H. Reulen and K. Schurmann, pp. 57–62. Springer-Verlag, New York, 1972.
43. Ransohoff, J. The effects of steroids on brain edema in man. *In* Steroids and Brain Edema, edited by H. J. Reulen, and K. Schurmann, pp. 211–218. Springer-Verlag, New York, 1972.
44. Reulen, H. J. Vasogenic brain oedema. Br. J. Anaesth., *48:* 741–751, 1976.
45. Rockoff, M. A., Marshall, L. F., and Shapiro, H. M. High-dose barbiturate therapy in humans: A clinical review of 60 patients. Ann. Neurol., *6:* 194–199, 1978.
46. Shapiro, H. M., Wyte, S. R., and Loeser, J. Barbiturate-augmented hypothermia for reduction of persistent intracranial hypertension. J. Neurosurg., *40:* 90–100, 1974.
47. Smith, A. L., Hoff, J. T., Nielsen, S. L., *et al.* Barbiturate protection in acute focal cerebral ischemia. Stroke, *5:* 1–7, 1974.

48. Tornheim, P. A., and McLaurin, R. L. Effect of dexamethasone on cerebral edema from cranial impact in the cat. J. Neurosurg., *48:* 220–227, 1978.
49. Tourtellotte, W., Reinglass, J., and Newkirk, T. Cerebral dehydration action of glycerol. Clin. Pharmacol. Ther., *13:* 159–171, 1972.
50. Wise, B., and Chater, N. The value of hypertonic mannitol solution in decreasing brain mass and lowering cerebrospinal fluid pressure. J. Neurosurg., *19:* 1038–1042, 1962.

CHAPTER

6

The Practical Management of Pituitary Replacement Therapy Related to Sellar and Parasellar Surgery

EDWARD R. LAWS, JR., M.D., CHARLES F. ABBOUD, M.D., and ALVIN B. HAYLES, M.D.

It was in 1951 that the efforts of Kendall and Hench, working at the Mayo Clinic, resulted in the isolation, synthesis, and general availability of compound F or cortisone. This discovery resulted in the Nobel Prize for Kendall and Hench, and a major advance in the care and welfare of neurosurgical patients. As the science of pituitary endocrinology has become ever more precise, the management of pituitary deficiency states of all kinds has become increasingly effective. This discussion will include those disruptions of pituitary function associated with surgery involving the gland itself and its neighboring structures, both vascular and neural. We must therefore consider the correction of deficiency states and/or hyperfunction states produced by pituitary neoplasms and other forms of sellar and parasellar pathology, the need to anticipate relative pituitary insufficiency in patients with borderline pituitary function who are subjected to the stress of surgery, the management of acute pituitary failure produced by surgery in and around the gland, and the need for long-term replacement of pituitary function lost either as a result of the primary disease or the surgical procedure. Although this appears complex, a systematic approach based on pituitary physiology allows very effective management of each of these problems.

Our goals at all times are to assure the safety of the patient, to avoid unnecessary discomfort and expense, and to achieve a normal endocrine state as rapidly and as efficiently as possible. The principles of management to be discussed have evolved as a result of experience with nearly 900 surgically treated patients with pituitary and parapituitary disorders, and are the product of a great deal of careful thought and constant reassessment of the results. In each instance, many alternative schemes of replacement therapy might be equally suitable or nearly so, and our recommendations are not to be considered as exclusive or mandatory.

Replacement therapy will be considered for each of the important known pituitary trophic hormones and their respective target organs.

Replacement for chronic preoperative deficiency, acute surgical insufficiency, and subacute or chronic postoperative loss of function will be addressed, along with the means of assessing the adequacy of replacement therapy.

HYPOTHALAMIC-PITUITARY-ADRENAL AXIS

Adrenal function and endogenous cortisol production are among the most essential homeostatic mechanisms under pituitary control. The overall mechanisms involved in this axis are illustrated in Fig. 6.1. ACTH mediates pituitary control to the target organ, the adrenal cortex. For practical purposes, assessment of function is best performed by measuring blood corticosteroid levels in the morning and in the afternoon, with the patient withdrawn from any steroid medication. Assays for ACTH may be done, but are costly, time consuming, and not reliable for determination of hypofunction.

Preoperative pituitary-adrenal insufficiency must be treated before subjecting the patient to any significant stress. Because most patients with severe preoperative adrenal insufficiency will not regain function postoperatively, it is reasonable in these cases to use the traditional "long steroid prep" of cortisone acetate 100 to 200 mg IM daily for 3 days prior to surgery. These patients, and all other patients with normal pituitary-adrenal function, are also given short-term steroid coverage for the day of surgery and the immediate postoperative period. This "short steroid prep" consists of prednisolone sodium phosphate (Hydeltrasol), 40 mg IM q 8 hours on the day of surgery, and the same dose the following day.

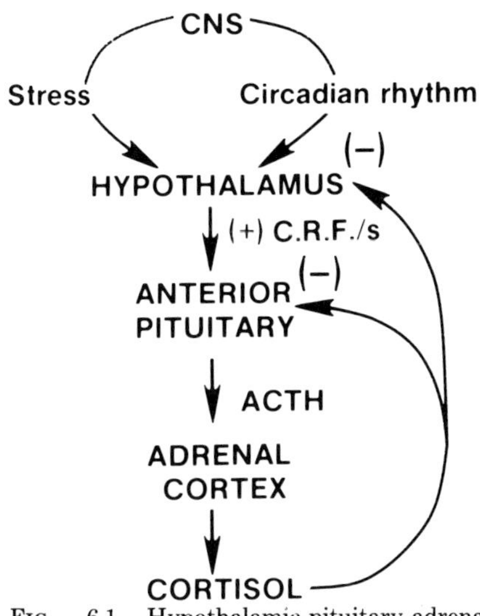

FIG. 6.1. Hypothalamic-pituitary-adrenal axis.

This is rapidly decreased to 20 mg b.i.d. on the second postoperative day and 10 mg b.i.d. on the third. In patients who are alert, well, and taking food and drink normally, parenteral steroid medication may then be discontinued. We prefer prednisolone to the more neurosurgically traditional dexamethasone because the former is shorter in duration of action.

In patients with normal preoperative pituitary-adrenal function, when ample amounts of normal anterior pituitary gland are left in place at surgery, no replacement is given after the 4th postoperative day, and blood corticosteroid levels are measured morning and afternoon on the 5th and 6th postoperative days. With this routine, the need for cortisol replacement can be assessed prior to dismissal of the patient from hospital.

Those patients with Nelson's syndrome who have had prior adrenalectomies, are maintained on fluorocortisone acetate (Florinef), 0.1 mg daily throughout.

When pituitary-adrenal insufficiency on a long-term basis is anticipated, either because of the preoperative findings or the operative procedure, oral steroid replacement therapy is instituted. Our usual recommendation is 5 mg of prednisone in the morning and 2.5 mg in the afternoon. Steroid dosage is increased during periods of stress. Each patient is given a syringe of dexamethasone, 4 mg injectable for emergency use and is asked to obtain an identification bracelet (Medic Alert) indicating potential need for cortisone. Florinef is not given to these patients with intact adrenal glands as the renin-angiotensin system is intact.

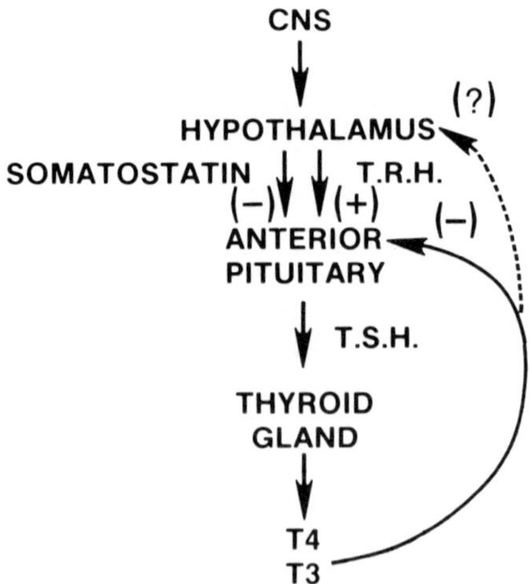

FIG. 6.2. Hypothalamic-pituitary-thyroid axis.

HYPOTHALAMIC-PITUITARY-THYROID AXIS

Factors influencing thyroid control are indicated in Fig. 6.2; the pituitary trophic hormone is TSH. The measurement of serum thyroxine (T_4), total and free, provides the most reliable and practical guide to normal function of this axis. Those patients who are significantly hypothyroid preoperatively should be brought to a euthyroid state. This can be accomplished rapidly, if needed through the use of intravenous infusions of L-thyroxine.

Patients who have normal preoperative thyroid function will usually not show signs of deficiency for at least 3 months postoperatively. If endocrine testing reveals thyroid insufficiency at this time, replacement is provided by L-thyroxine (Synthroid), with average dosage of 0.15 mg daily.

HYPOTHALAMIC-PITUITARY-GROWTH HORMONE AXIS

Growth hormone has a number of actions, many of which, particularly in the adult, are incompletely understood. The control mechanisms are shown in Fig. 6.3. Insufficiency of growth hormone is best detected by provocative testing, with assay of serum hGH levels in response to insulin-induced hypoglycemia. Adequacy of growth hormone action may also be assessed by measurement of Somatomedin-C.

Because growth hormone deficiency in the adult is without known

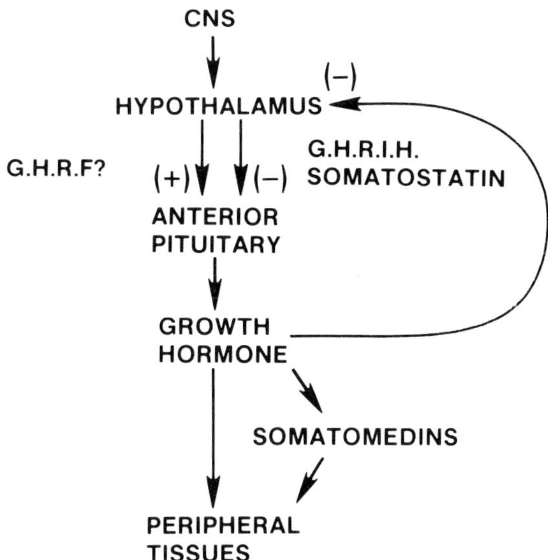

FIG. 6.3. Hypothalamic-pituitary-growth hormone axis.

serious side effects, replacement is not considered. In the child, growth hormone replacement should be attempted in an effort for the patient to achieve near-normal stature. Growth hormone is available from the National Pituitary Agency, and commercial sources are developing as well. The Agency has strict requirements which include: documentation of pituitary failure; limited growth potential (5′4″ in the male and 5′2″ in the female); a protocol on file; Somatomedin-C response; and progress reports every 3 months. The recommended dose of growth hormone is 0.1 international unit/kg IM, three times a week. The medication has been free of adverse effects, but a "waning effect" occurs, so that it becomes less clinically effective over time. Patients with Cushing's disease do not respond to growth hormone, but physiologic doses of cortisol replacement agents do not interfere with the effect.

HYPOTHALAMIC-PITUITARY-GONADAL AXIS IN THE FEMALE

The factors influencing this axis are shown in Fig. 6.4. The history is of particular importance here, as primary failure must be distinguished from secondary, so it is important to determine whether spontaneous menses have ever occurred. The pelvic examination provides helpful information as normal vaginal epithelium and cervical mucus are dependent on normal endocrine function. Measurements of prolactin and gonadotropins

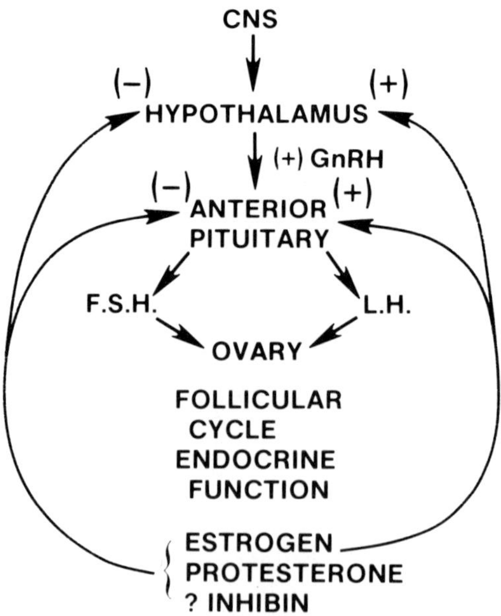

FIG. 6.4. Hypothalamic-pituitary-gonadal axis in the female.

(FSH and LH) in the serum are the most practical laboratory means of assessing function of this axis (Fig. 6.5).

In most patients, surgery offers a chance of restoration of function, so replacement therapy is usually delayed for about 3 months. If insufficiency is documented then and recovery is not anticipated, women between age 12 and 45 are treated with a cyclical program of replacement. This consists of conjugated estrogens (Premarin) 0.125 mg daily, 3 of each 4 weeks, and medroxyprogesterone acetate (Provera) 10 mg daily during the 3rd week. Menstrual flow occurs during the 4th week when the patient receives no medication. Ordinarily, replacement is not recommended for menopausal women. If fertility is desired in a pituitary deficient woman, gonadotropes can be given as replacement therapy, but this is expensive and difficult to manage. If prolactin is abnormally elevated postoperatively, it may be suppressed when suppression is indicated with bromocriptine (Parlodel), 2.5 mg twice or three times a day.

HYPOTHALAMIC-PITUITARY-GONADAL AXIS IN THE MALE

The control mechanisms involved are given in Fig. 6.6. Semen analysis and serum testosterone analysis are practical guides to insufficiency. If preoperative deficiency is present and is not expected to return, replacement therapy may be instituted at any time. The most convenient method is to give a depot preparation of testosterone enanthate (Delatestryl) 200 to 400 mg IM every 3 to 4 weeks. As with the female, if

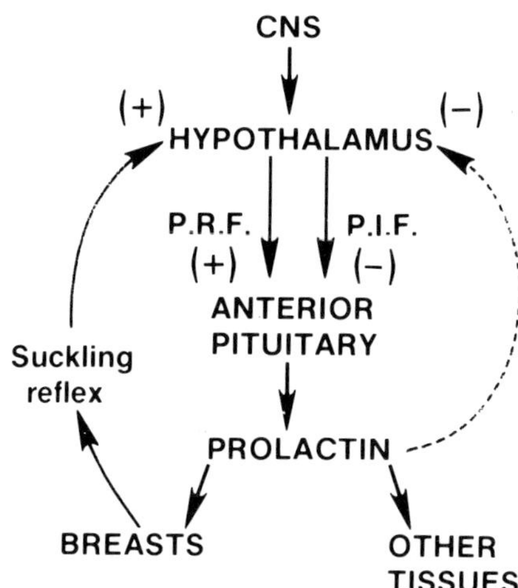

FIG. 6.5. Hypothalamic-pituitary prolactin axis.

fertility is desired, gonadotropins may be given as replacement, but success is difficult and expensive to achieve.

HYPOTHALAMIC-NEUROHYPOPHYSEAL-RENAL AXIS

Homeostatic control of extracellular fluid and blood volume are both mediated to a significant degree by ADH, as indicated in Figs. 6.7 and 6.8. Documentation of diabetes insipidus is provided by measurements of

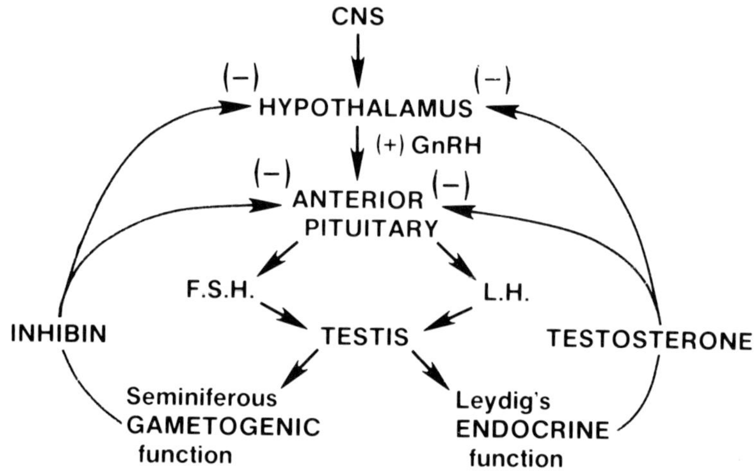

Fig. 6.6. Hypothalamic-pituitary-gonadal axis in the male.

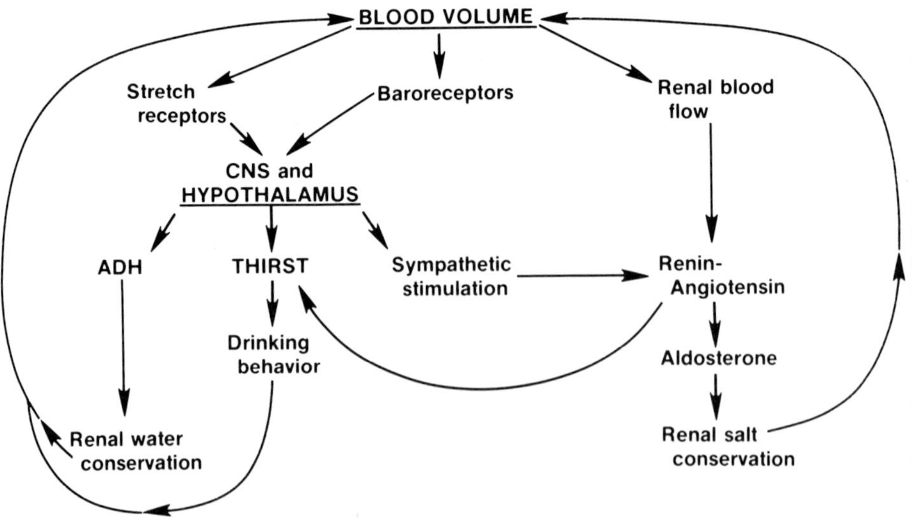

Fig. 6.7. Homeostatic control of blood volume.

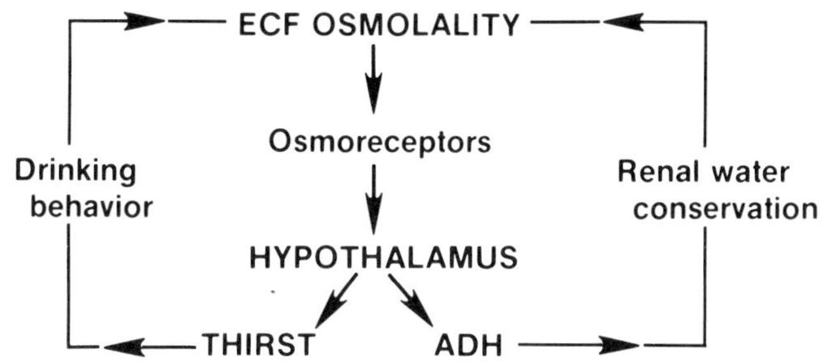

FIG. 6.8. Homeostatic control of extracellular fluid osmolality.

intake and output and of serum and urine osmolality. Patients with preoperative diabetes insipidus may be expected to continue to have this problem following surgery and we usually manage them through surgery with pitressin tannate in oil, 1.0 ml IM every 24 to 48 hours as needed.

In those cases where postoperative diabetes insipidus may be a transient phenomenon, aqueous pitressin 5 units given subcutaneously every 4 to 6 hours, as necessary, is utilized.

Once a patient with clinically significant diabetes insipidus is alert, awake, and taking food and drink normally, therapy with dDAVP (Desmopressin) may be started, usually 0.05 ml nasally b.i.d. Patients who have undergone transsphenoidal surgery must wait until nasal packing is removed.

Mild diabetes insipidus may be managed with other agents as well, and in certain cases these are equally effective and less expensive. We believe the most suitable agents are chlorpropamide (Diabinase), 100 mg daily or thiazide diuretics (*e.g.*, Dyazide), 500 mg daily. Patients taking chlorpropamide must be monitored for the possibility of hypoglycemia.

These therapeutic recommendations serve us well in our current management of pituitary replacement therapy. Further progress in the field undoubtedly will occur, and will allow such therapy to become even more effective in the future.

REFERENCES

1. Abboud, C. F., and Laws, E. R., Jr. Clinical endocrinological approach to hypothalamic-pituitary disease. J. Neurosurg., *51:* 271–291, 1979.
2. Laws, E. R., Jr., Abboud, C. F., and Kern, E. B. Perioperative management of patients with pituitary microadenoma. Neurosurgery, *7:* 566–570, 1980.

CHAPTER

7

Neuropharmacology of Depression, Anxiety, and Pain

ROBERT B. KING, M.D.

INTRODUCTION

Behavioral neuropharmacology has moved through 3 phases in its recent development (11). Initially, drugs were correlated with behavior and the level of neurotransmitters or their metabolites in the central nervous system (50). Some drugs, however, which induced marked behavioral changes caused minimal changes of transmitter levels, such as lysergic acid, the amphetamines, tricyclic antidepressants, and some antipsychotics. The second phase was thus introduced in which changes in behavior were linked to changes in the turnover rates of neurotransmitters. It was then possible to relate the decreased turnover of serotonin to the actions of LSD (1) and the increased turnover of dopamine to the acute actions of neuroleptics (12). Behavioral changes, however, occurred over weeks, while neurochemical processes were altered in minutes or hours, and neurone firing rates changed in seconds or milliseconds, suggesting that behavioral changes reflected secondary CNS events rather than those at a primary site of action. Thus, changes in neurotransmitter kinetics and the behavioral changes associated with drug treatment may be correctly correlated but may not be related as cause and effect. A third phase began to focus attention on adaptive changes within the central nervous system which had been initiated by chronic pharmacologic manipulations. Tricyclic antidepressants, for instance, require treatment periods of weeks—well in excess of any measured neuropharmacologic or neurophysiologic event.

Hence, new concepts have been introduced which indicate new mechanisms of action. None of these is clearly defined nor applied in a universally accepted fashion.

Neurotransmitters classically were released by presynaptic terminals, produced excitation or inhibition, and operated by inducing a change in membrane potential of the postsynaptic neurone.

Neurohormones were initially identified with the peptide-secreting cells of hypothalamo-hypophysial circuits. They received synaptic information from the central nervous system and released their transmitters to the blood stream. Yet neurosecretory hypothalamic neurons have been found with efferent connections on neurons of the brainstem and spinal cord (9, 68). There is no evidence in this circumstance that the neurohormones oxytocin and vasopressin are secreted either into the vascular system or diffuse extracellular spaces.

Neuromodulators (25) have been defined as having nonsynaptic sites of origin. They influence the excitability of neurons by changing their responsiveness to transsynaptic actions of presynaptic neurons. They may also alter spontaneous neural activity. Neuromodulators alter neuronal excitability without producing changes in membrane potential or ionic conductance. They change the ability of neurotransmitters to elicit receptor-coupled conductance changes (6). Adrenal corticosteroids, adenosine, and prostaglandins, even CO_2 and ammonia, may be included in this category.

Neuromediators include substances such as cyclic AMP and cyclic GMP. They participate in the target cell response to a transmitter or modulator, as in the second messenger role at specific synaptic transmission sites (10, 64).

Behavioral neuropharmacology is further complicated by dose-dependent and time-related response studies. Injecting normal animals with amphetamine or apomorphine, for instance, induces a variety of behaviors: increased locomotion, rearing, gnawing, biting, and rhythmic head motions. Some believe these responses are dose related on a continuum (72). It is clear, however, that the multiple behavioral patterns consume different portions of a time sample. With apomorphine, rats first increased locomotion and an hour later increased gnawing. Different neuroleptic drugs have reverse effects on the two behaviors. Clozapine, a strong antipsychotic with mild extrapyramidal effects, suppressed locomotion without affecting the gnawing pattern. Conversely, haloperidol, a weak antipsychotic with pronounced extrapyramidal effects, suppressed gnawing without affecting locomotion. These responses may also be dependent on the delivery rate of a drug. A rapid intravenous injection may induce locomotion without gnawing. A very slow rate of injection may reverse this effect on the two behavior patterns. Sequential injections of the drug, *i.e.*, a very small priming injection, followed by a subcutaneous injection, reversed the effect of the second injection on the two behaviors. The priming treatment evidently sensitized the system controlling gnawing but desensitized the system evoking locomotion. Such observations suggest separate dopaminergic receptor systems for the two sets of behavior; one, perhaps the nigrostriatal tract, the other, the mesolimbic system. Different sets of receptors, specific to a particular behavior, would then be dose- and time-dependent with respect to a common agonist but blocked by selective antagonists.

It must also be recognized that a drug which may alter synthesis, degradation, uptake, release, or turnover of a neurotransmitter will not necessarily lead to increased or decreased activity in the neural system utilizing that transmitter. There are a number of ways in which a drug may alter firing rates of neurons. It can act directly on a nerve cell body, on other neurons which then influence impulse flow in the neuron under study, or at the postsynaptic receptor, causing excitation or inhibition which may result in a feedback influence on the presynaptic neuron. The feedback may be either transsynaptically or biochemically mediated. It also may enhance or suppress further release of a neurotransmitter from the presynaptic terminal.

Many neurotransmitters may also function as a neurohormone, modulator, or mediator, depending on their source. Pharmacologic manipulations of a presumed neurotransmitter may be effective by changing its characteristics to those of a neuromodulator. This feature may in part explain the dichotomy between the very rapid action of many drugs in neurophysiologic parameters as opposed to the long time period they require to induce behavioral changes.

The clinical implications of these observations are complex, but suggest that drug effects such as tolerance and rebound, as seen with amphetamine, may reflect behavioral manifestations of receptor adaptation to altered aminergic input. Biochemical adaptation may be as important to neural plasticity as synaptic events or anatomic remodeling.

Despite the fragmentary evidence, metafacts, and possible epiphenomena we have at out disposal, some would suggest that the neuropharmacology of depression, of anxiety, and of pain are to some degree separable.

I shall consider first some changes in catecholamines which may relate to depression; second, neurotransmitters which may be related to anxiety; and third, some pharmacologic changes associated with pain-signaling neural pathways.

CATECHOLAMINE THEORY OF DEPRESSION

The catecholamine theory of depression states in general that depression may be associated with a deficiency of catecholamines, particularly norepinephrine, while mania is associated with an increase in this neurotransmitter.

The impetus for the theory came from the observation that monoamine oxidase inhibitors, specifically iproniazid, acted clinically as a mood elevator. Brain amine levels increased with the use of this compound. Reserpine, a potent tranquilizer, depleted brain amines, and amphetamine caused a temporary increase in norepinephrine at receptor sites. DOPA, 3,4-dihydroxyphenylalanine, a precursor of catecholamine biosynthesis, could reduce most of the reserpine-induced symptoms.

The two general classes of drugs most commonly used to treat depressive disorders are the monoamine oxidase inhibitors and tricyclic antidepressants.

The tricyclic antidepressants inhibit catecholamine reuptake, particularly norepinephrine, and potentiate the peripheral autonomic effects of exogenous norepinephrine and the central effects of DOPA and amphetamine. In depression, they function presumably by blocking the reuptake of norepinephrine into presynaptic terminals.

The noradrenergic system arises from the locus ceruleus, a compact cell group in the pons. While containing relatively few neurons (1500 in the rat), they project widely in the central nervous system through five major well-defined tracts: the central tegmental tract, dorsal longitudinal fasciculus, and the ventrotegmental medial forebrain bundle tract. These three are primarily, but not exclusively, ipsilateral. They innervate all of the medullary layers of the cerebral cortex, specific thalamic and hypothalamic nuclei, and the olfactory bulb. Another component projects to the cerebellar cortex, and the fifth descends into the mesencephalon and spinal cord in the ventrolateral column.

Some noradrenergic neurons lie outside the locus ceruleus scattered through the lateroventrotegmental fields of the brainstem. These intermingle with neurons of locus ceruleus and contribute mainly descending fibers within the mesencephalon and spinal cord.

Cells in the dopamine-containing system are more complex in their organization. There are several dopamine-containing nuclei and specialized dopamine neurons. They project primarily to basal forebrain and brain stem but not to cortex.

An ultrashort system links plexiform layers in the retina and periglomerular cells of olfactory bulb.

An intermediate-length system, such as the tuberohypophysial dopamine cells, projects from arcuate and periventricular nuclei to the intermediate lobe of the pituitary and median eminence; incertohypothalamic neurons link dorsal and posterior hypothalamus with the dorsal anterior hypothalamus and lateral central nuclei; the medullary periventricular group includes cells of the dorsal motor nucleus of the vagus, tractus solitarius, and periaqueductal grey matter.

Long projections link the ventral tegmental and substantia nigra with the neostriatum, limbic cortex, and other limbic structures.

Iontophoretic administration of dopamine indicates a predominant inhibitory function in this system, but there are exceptions such that when electrical stimulation is applied to the ventral tegmentum and substantia nigra, the response in the caudate may be either excitatory or inhibitory. Unambiguous pharmacologic and electrophysiologic analyses

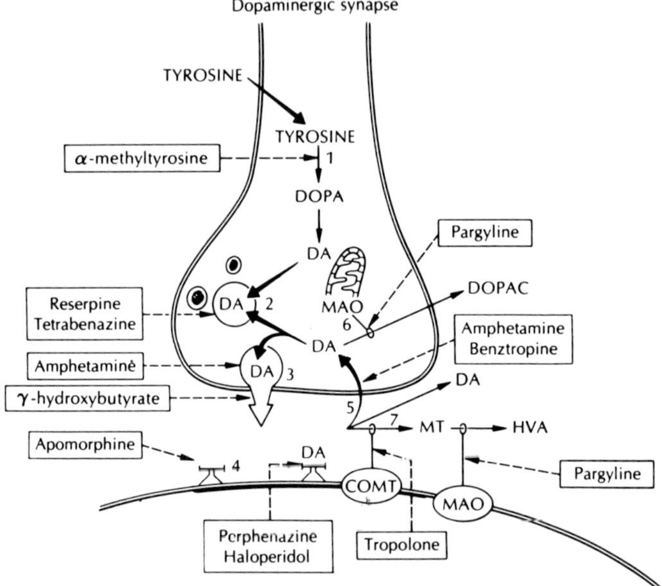

FIG. 7.1. Schematic model of a central dopaminergic neuron indicating possible sites of drug action. *Step 1:* Enzymatic synthesis. Tyrosine hydroxylase reaction blocked by the competitive inhibitor α-methyltyrosine (*MT*) and other tyrosine hydroxylase inhibitors. *Step 2:* Storage. Reserpine and tetrabenazine interfere with the uptake-storage mechanism of the amine granules. The depletion of dopamine (*DA*) produced by reserpine is long-lasting, and the storage granules appear to be irreversibly damaged. Tetrabenazine also interferes with the uptake-storage mechanism of the granules, except that the effects of this drug do not appear to be irreversible. *Step 3:* Release. Gamma-hydroxybutyrate effectively blocks the release of *DA* by blocking impulse flow in dopaminergic neurons. Amphetamines administered in high doses release dopamine, but most of the releasing ability of amphetamine appears to be related to its ability to effectively block *DA* reuptake. *Step 4:* receptor interaction. Apomorphine is an effective *DA* receptor-stimulating drug, with both pre- and postsynaptic sites of action. Perphenazine and haloperidol are effective *DA* receptor blocking drugs. *Step 5:* Reuptake. *DA* has its action terminated by being taken up into the presynaptic terminal. Amphetamine, as well as the anticholinergic drug benztropine, are potent inhibitors of this reuptake mechanism. *Step 6:* Monoamine oxidase (*MAO*). *DA* present in a free state within the presynaptic terminal can be degraded by the enzyme *MAO*, which appears to be located in the outer membrane of the mitochondria. Dihydroxyphenylacetic acid (*DOPAC*) is a product of the action of *MAO* and aldehyde oxidase on *DA*. Pargyline is an effective inhibitor of *MAO*. Some *MAO* is also present outside the dopaminergic neuron. *Step 7:* Catechol-*O*-methyltransferase (*COMT*). *DA* can be inactivated by the enzyme COMT, which is believed to be localized outside the presynaptic neuron. Tropolone is an inhibitor of COMT. *HVA*, homovanillic acid (From J. R. Cooper *et al.* (16). Published with permission.)

of this system have not been reported, although the bulk of the evidence favors an inhibitory role for dopamine (Fig. 7.1).

Electrical stimulation of noradrenergic neurons in locus ceruleus activates tyrosine hydroxylase and an increased turnover of norepinephrine which is frequency-dependent. Interruption of impulse flow in these neurons decreases the turnover of norepinephrine with little or no effect on the steady state level of the transmitter.

Acute stress causes an increase in the turnover of norepinephrine in the central nervous system thought to be the result of an increase in impulse flow in noradrenergic neurons. If the noradrenergic neurons projecting to the cerebral cortex are acutely interrupted by destruction of locus ceruleus, the increase in norepinephrine turnover and accumulation of its biproducts which are characteristically induced by stress are completely blocked. Monoamine oxidase inhibitors block the degradation of norepinephrine. Tricyclics block the reuptake of norepinephrine, allowing increasing accumulation of the neurotransmitter in the synaptic cleft (Fig. 7.2).

Dopaminergic neurons, however, have other characteristics. An increase of nerve impulse flow in the nigroneostriatal system does lead to both an increase in dopamine synthesis and turnover in a frequency-dependent fashion. However, if the impulse flow is interrupted in the nigrostriatal or mesolimbic system, the concentration of dopamine rapidly increases in the nerve terminals with an increased rate of dopamine synthesis. This peculiar response suggests that a decrease of impulse flow has resulted in a change in the physical properties of tyrosine hydroxylase, making it insensitive to feedback inhibition by endogenous dopamine, thus removing a normal regulatory feedback influence, which continues until endogenous concentrations of dopamine are sufficiently elevated that a second significant inhibitory influence on tyrosine hydroxylase supersedes. This phenomenon may be dependent on the availability of intracellular calcium and calmodulin (51).

In a fashion similar to that which occurs with norepinephrine, the monoamine oxidase inhibitors block the degradation of dopamine and to a lesser extent, the tricyclics block reuptake, augmenting its accumulation in presynaptic terminals and in the synaptic cleft. In each instance, reserpine reduces the release of the neurotransmitter into the synaptic cleft.

The monoamine oxidase inhibitors, while they inhibit an enzyme responsible for the breakdown of norepinephrine and dopamine, also inhibit the metabolism of 5-hydroxytryptamine, tyramine, and tryptamine (16). They also block other enzymes unrelated to monoamine oxidase, including succinic dehydrogenase, dopamine β-hydroxylase, 5-hydroxytryptophan decarboxylase, choline dehydrogenase, and diamine oxidase.

The catecholamine theory of depression then does not rule out the participation of dopamine, 5-hydroxytryptamine, or other putative neurotransmitters in the full expression of depression.

Berger and Barchas (5) have noted that this hypothesis does not

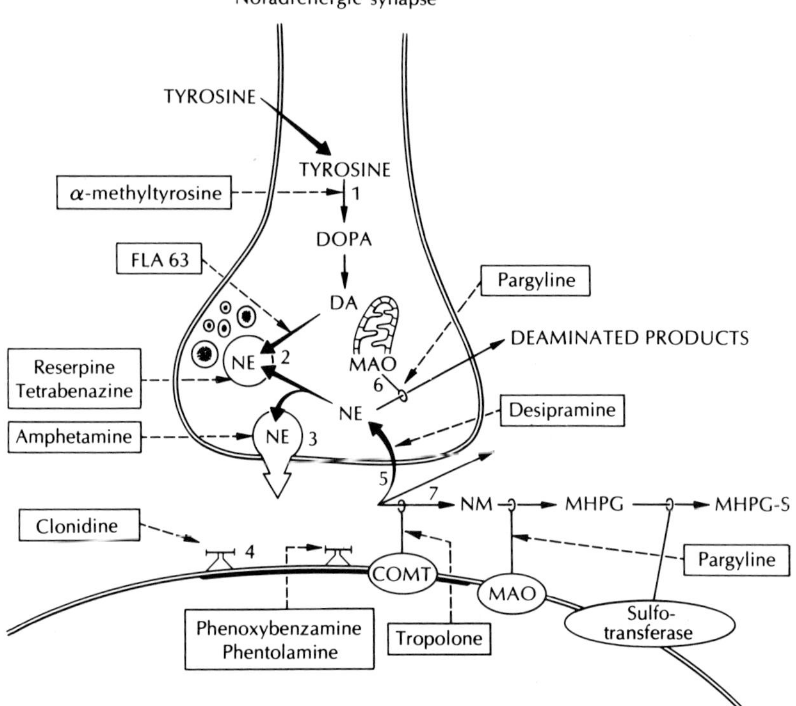

FIG. 7.2. Schematic model of central noradrenergic neuron indicating possible sites of drug action. *Step 1:* Enzymatic synthesis. Tyrosine hydroxylase reaction blocked by the competitive inhibitor, α-methyltyrosine; dopamine (*DA*) β-hydroxylase reaction blocked by a dithiocarbamate derivative, FLA-63, bis-(1-methyl-4-homopiperazinyl-thiocarbonyl)-disulfide. *Step 2:* Storage. Reserpine and tetrabenazine interfere with the uptake-storage mechanism of the amine granules. The depletion of norepinephrine (*NE*) produced by reserpine is long-lasting, and the storage granules are irreversibly damaged. Tetrabenazine also interferences with the uptake-storage mechanism of the granules, except the effects of this drug do not appear to be irreversible. *Step 3:* Release. Amphetamine appears to cause an increase in the net release of *NE*. Probably the primary mechanism by which amphetamine causes release is by its ability to block effectively the reuptake mechanism. *Step 4:* Receptor interaction. Clonidine appears to be a very potent receptor stimulating drug. Phenoxybenzamine and phentolamine are effective α-receptor blocking agents. Recent experiments indicated that these drugs may also have presynaptic site of action. *Step 5:* Reuptake. *NE* has its action terminated by being taken up into the presynaptic terminal. The tricyclic drug desipramine is a potent inhibitor of this uptake mechanism. *Step 6:* Monoamine oxidase (*MAO*). *NE* or *DA* present in a free state within the presynaptic terminal can be degraded by the enzyme MAO, which appears to be located in the outer membrane of mitochondria. Pargyline is an effective inhibitor of MAO. *Step 7:* Catechol-O-methyltransferase (*COMT*). *NE* can be inactivated by the enzyme *COMT*, which is believed to be localized outside the presynaptic neuron. Tropolone is an inhibitor of *COMT*. The normetanephrine (*NM*) formed by the action of *COMT* on *NE* can be further metabolized by *MAO* and aldehyde reductase to 3-methoxy-4-hydroxyphenylglycol (*MHPG*). The *MHPG* formed can be further metabolized to *MHPG*-sulfate by the action of a sulfotransferase found in brain. (From J. R. Cooper *et al.* (16). Published with permission.)

resolve important clinical discrepancies. For example, cocaine is a very potent inhibitor of catecholamine reuptake, similar to tricyclic antidepressants, but does not possess any significant antidepressant activity. Iprandole, a tricyclic compound, has no significant effect on catecholamine uptake, but is an effective antidepressant. Both the tricyclic antidepressants and monoamine oxidase inhibitors elevate brain catecholamines soon after their administration, but clinically they require several weeks of continuous administration to produce therapeutic effects.

The use of lithium to treat mania by an effect almost opposite to that of the tricyclics would seem to fit the catecholamine theory of affective disorders, except that lithium is also reported by some to be effective in treating patients with bipolar depression.

Several clinical studies suggest that depressed patients excrete less 3-methoxyl-4-hydroxyphenol (MHGP) and that urinary levels of MHGP may be predictive of the therapeutic response to be expected with amitriptyline or imipramine. Large amounts, however, of this byproduct come from peripheral sources. These clinical findings hinge on the degree to which urinary MHGP reflects central as opposed to systemic norepinephrine metabolism. Clinical trials are not consistent in reporting the effectiveness of any therapeutic regimen intended to relieve depression.

There may be some relation of the monoamine oxidase inhibitors and tricyclic antidepressants to depression, but the neuropharmacologic events in support of the catecholamine theory of depression are both fragmentary and incomplete.

Depression today, like anemia 60 years ago, may be the clinical expression of a vast array of neuropharmacologic perturbations.

ANXIETY AND THE BENZODIAZEPINES

Antianxiety drugs, minor tranquilizers, and the benzodiazepines, have been studied extensively and have received particularly popular use. In 1960, chlordiazepoxide (Librium) received rapid clinical acceptance, as did its more potent analog diazepam (Valium), and in 1970 flurazepam (Dalmane). They have been used as muscle relaxants, anticonvulsants, anxiolytics, and hypnotics. It has been estimated that 8,000 tons of the benzodiazepines were consumed in the United States in 1977 alone (69).

These drugs accumulate preferentially in adipose tissue and brain and are primarily metabolized by the liver and excreted by the kidneys. Active metabolites are frequently present for weeks. Cumulative dose effects, psychological dependence, and physical withdrawal symptoms have been reported. Interactions with alcohol have been a major problem in clinical practice. Nevertheless, there is a wide safety margin between therapeutic and toxic doses.

Benzodiazepines have the impressive effect of positively reinforcing behaviors which have been suppressed by punishment (15, 27). In "conflict" situations, untreated experimental animals will normally respond to punishment and suppress responses for a rewarding stimulus. The administration of a benzodiazepine characteristically increases behavioral responses which promote rewarding stimuli even during conditions of punishment. From such studies, these drugs have been considered as disinhibitors of suppressed behavior.

At a clinical level, they reduce manifestations of unfavorable behavior induced by frustration, fear, and punishment. Hence, they are viewed as anxiolytic drugs.

Their neuropharmacology is certainly not related to a single neurotransmitter. They affect the concentrations of many putative neurotransmitters, including norepinephrine, dopamine, 5-hydroxytryptamine, acetylcholine, glycine, and γ-aminobutyric acid (GABA). There is no known effect of these drugs on glycine-mediated transmission, on strychnine sensitivity, or on microiontophoretically applied 5-hydroxytryptamine or norepinephrine. Picrotoxin, a reasonable blocker of GABA, however (18, 57, 67), also blocks the clinical manifestations of the benzodiazepines.

Combined iontophoretic and electrophysiologic studies have suggested that the clinical effects of benzodiazepines are related to their specific interactions with GABA (18, 32). Diazepam can potentiate postsynaptic inhibition (62) in the spinal cord (14, 49), where GABA is presumed to be the neurotransmitter (23). Similar observations have been reported with studies of the cuneate nucleus, sympathetic ganglia, dorsal raphe nucleus (26), cerebral cortex (44), substantia nigra, hippocampus, and cerebellar cortex (24, 28, 32, 52, 55, 58, 70, 78).

By way of contrast, these drugs have been reported to antagonize GABA inhibition in Deiters' nucleus, cerebellum, and cultured Purkinje cells, but these studies may require further evaluation with respect to dose dependence. Low doses of these drugs may enhance GABA-mediated inhibition, whereas higher doses may antagonize the same responses (49) (Fig. 7.3).

Some properties of the benzodiazepines are not potentiated by GABA, *i.e.*, their anticonvulsant effects, their sedative effects, and even their relation to chlorpromazine. Since GABA may mediate transmission in as many as 30% or more of the brain synapses, it is likely that variations either in its release or reuptake mechanisms or even its effect on active as opposed to reserve receptor sites may contribute to these variations. There is growing evidence that these drugs and GABA share a common pathway and that relevant doses of these drugs at least potentiate GABA-mediated inhibition in the central nervous system. At a molecular level, this potentiation is not well understood. It might occur by direct activa-

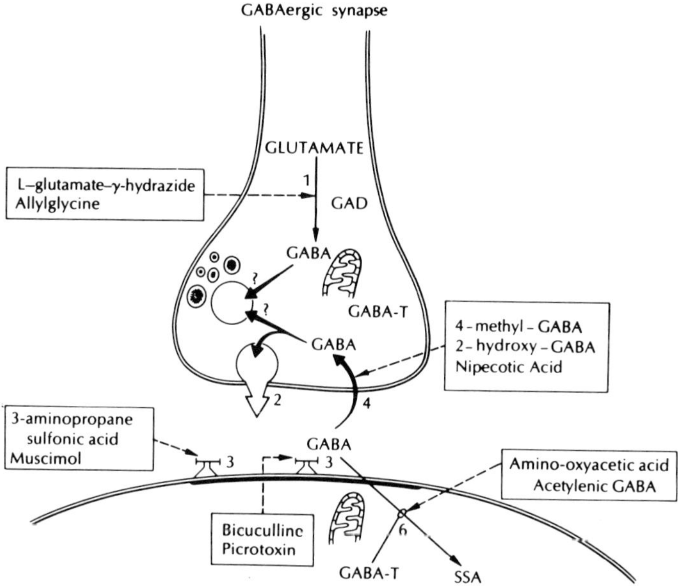

FIG. 7.3. Schematic illustration of a *GABA*ergic neuron indicating possible sites of drug action. *Site 1.* Enzymatic synthesis. Glutamic acid decarboxylase (*GAD*) is inhibited by a number of various hydrazines. These agents appear to act primarily as pyridoxal antagonists and are therefore very nonspecific inhibitors. L-glutamate-γ-hydrazide and allylglycine are more selective inhibitors of *GAD*, but these agents are also not entirely specific in their effects. *Site 2.* Release. *GABA* release appears to be calcium dependent. At present no selective inhibitors of GABA release have been found. *Site 3.* Interaction with postsynaptic receptor. Bicuculline and picrotoxin block the action of *GABA* at postsynaptic receptors; 3-aminopropane sulfonic acid and the hallucinogenic isoxazole derivative muscimol appear to be effective *GABA* agonists at postsynaptic receptors. *Site 4.* Reuptake. In brain, GABA appears to be actively taken up into presynaptic endings by a sodium-dependent mechanism. A number of compounds will inhibit this uptake mechanism, such as 4-methyl-*GABA* and 2-hydroxy-GABA, but these agents are not completely specific in their inhibitory effects. *Site 5.* Metabolism. *GABA* is metabolized primarily by transamination by *GABA*-transaminase (*GABA-T*), which appears to be localized primarily in mitochondria. Amino-oxyacetic acid and acetylenic *GABA* are effective inhibitors of *GABA-T*. (From J. R. Cooper *et al.* (16). Published with permission.)

tion of GABA receptors, an increase in presynaptic GABA release, an inhibition of GABA removal from its receptor site, or an alteration in the postsynaptic response to GABA. The latter seems most likely. There is a close relation between these drugs and GABA receptor sites.

GABA, one of four inhibitory amino acids, is unique in that it is found in highest concentration only in the brain. It has been implicated either directly or indirectly in the pathogenesis of many disorders, including Huntington's disease, Parkinsonism, epilepsy, schizophrenia, and senile dementia, but in the context of today's discussion we will consider it as it relates to the pharmacology of the benzodiazepines (17).

The mechanisms whereby GABA functions as an inhibitory neurotransmitter are uncertain. Its precursor, glutamic acid, and glutamic acid decarboxylase are widely distributed throughout the central nervous system, and the three correlate well in their regional distribution. The degradation enzyme, GABA transamynase, however, does not precisely correlate in its distribution with that of GABA.

There is sufficient evidence to support GABA as a neurotransmitter so far as its production, storage, and pharmacologic activity are concerned, but it has not been demonstrated in association with *specific* inhibitory pathways of the cortex. Most analytic studies concerned with the mechanism of GABA's depressive action have been directed at spinal cord motor neurons. More recently, stronger evidence suggesting that GABA raises the membrane potential of cortical neurons and increases their conductance tends to support its role as a major inhibitory neurotransmitter in the cerebral cortex.

Benzodiazepine receptors in the brain, as demonstrated by radioactively labeled compounds, interact with GABA receptor sites (41, 42, 74). The magnitude of GABA potentiation of benzodiazepine binding varies regionally in the brain (41, 42). This variation may represent heterogeneity of the receptors for either agent or variations in the interactions between the two and the many functions they may subserve.

Neural membranes treated so as to remove GABA-modulin inhibit GABA binding and also inhibit competitive benzodiazepine binding. When GABA-modulin is reintroduced to these treated membranes, it enhances the high affinity GABA binding which is stereospecifically antagonized by the benzodiazepines. This model constructs the notion that a GABA modulin interacts with both GABA and benzodiazepine at receptor sites as part of a postsynaptic GABA-benzodiazepine-ionophore complex which produces hyperpolarization (31).

Further attempts to purify the receptor sites and their proteins for GABA (30), GABA-modulin (31), and benzodiazepine (77) have indicated that for the latter, the receptor is a 200,000-dalton protein; for GABA-modulin it is a thermostable acidic protein of 15,000 daltons (31), and the GABA receptor itself has a molecular weight of 900,000 (30). The temperature-dependent characteristics of these suggest that binding appears in part to be entrophy-driven (77). Further clarification of these protein molecules may resolve some discrepancies in benzodiazepine-DOPA interactions.

Such features as the effects of endogenous GABA modulators, the relative density of occupation of receptor sites, modulation of inputs to the receptor neuron, and the effective long-term sensitization or desensitization of the receptor sites by medication remain controversial or unknown issues.

Even genetic factors may modify the binding sites for benzodiazepine. For instance, the "nervous mouse" (46, 65) which undergoes spontaneous degeneration of Purkinje cells has a normal complement of receptors at birth but loses them by the time the disorder is manifest at 60 to 70 days. A mutant mouse known as "staggerer" lacks synaptic spines on Purkinje cell dendrites and has a reduced number of benzodiazepine cerebellar binding sites (66). The "weaver" mutants undergo granule cell degeneration (59) and have a relative enrichment in cerebellar benzodiazepine binding sites (13). In each of these groups there is no change in the affinity of the remaining receptors for tritiated benzodiazepines.

If an endogenous agent other than GABA which interacted with the benzodiazepine receptors could be identified, it would have important implications, both therapeutically and in neurobiology. None of the data as yet confirms a particular candidate, but the purines and nicotinamide do have similar properties and bind competitively with benzodiazepine receptors. It is clear that these or similar endogenous substances may be physiologic modulators of the GABA-benzodiazepine receptors. An additional possibility suggests that receptor occupation by GABA or benzodiazepine, or both, directly changes adjacent ionophores of the membrane, which could alter the permeability changes of the membranes and regulate neuronal activity (33). GABA-modulin may participate in this construct.

Observations such as these have had almost immediate and practical application. By using the techniques required for these studies, potential antianxiety drugs can be screened in large numbers by radioreceptor assays, before behavioral studies are undertaken. New drugs have already emerged from such studies (7, 75). One such study suggests less hazard in its crossover potential with alcohol and other side effects (triazolopyridazine). These techniques can also be used for rapid assays of biological samples, including blood, in circumstances suggesting toxicity or abuse.

NEUROPHARMACOLOGY AND PAIN

The neuropharmacology of pain is burgeoning with observations and conjecture, but little concrete understanding has yet emerged. Spurred by the observation that brainstem stimulation induced analgesia which was reversed by naloxane, Hughes (39) began to look for endogenous materials which bound to opiate receptors and identified two pentapeptides, Met^5- and Leu^5- enkephalin, in 1975. Their distribution was similar to opioid receptors, though not identical. The difference indicates that these, like other neurotransmitters and neuroregulators, may serve many functions. Soon α-endorphin, γ-endorphin, and β-endorphin were also identified as components of β-lipotropin, a pituitary hormone. Although enkephalins have not usually been demonstrated in the cerebral and cerebellar cortices, they are clearly evident in many areas which are related to pain signaling systems (substantia gelatinosa and nucleus caudalis of the trigeminal nuclei, nuclei raphe of the medulla, ventrolateral aspects of the periaqueductal gray, lateral septal nucleus, amygdala, dorsomedial and intralaminar nuclei of the thalamus, hypothalamus, caudate nucleus, locus ceruleus, and nucleus reticularis gigantocellularis). They are probably present in interneurons, but leucine enkephalin has also been reported in parasympathetic preganglionic motoneurons (29). They usually exhibit axoaxonic presynaptic terminals on other neural systems.

They induce excitation in the hippocampus but generally reduce neural firing when injected iontophoretically. In substantia gelatinosa, the enkephalins primarily reduce cell responses to noxious, though not to nonnoxious stimuli, an effect which is reversed by naloxone. They also reduce the spontaneous firing rate and the glutamate-enhanced firing rate of cells in the periaqueductal gray and caudate.

β-endorphin has not been shown to be particularly effective when introduced intraventricularly in man in an attempt to relieve pain. On the other hand, during stimulation of the posteroinferomedial thalamus and relief of pain, β-endorphin-like materials have increased as much as 30-fold in human third ventricle spinal fluid (4, 38).

Substance P is found in high concentration in the central nervous system, except for neocortex and cerebellar cortex (20, 22, 36, 47, 48), and is clearly evident in pain signaling systems (posterior root ganglia, raphe pallidus, and raphe magnus of the medulla, ventroperiaqueductal gray, laminae I to VI of the posterior horn of the spinal cord, dorsal and medial raphe nuclei, and medial amygdaloid nucleus and septal area).

That substance P is related to pain signaling mechanisms is suggested (34) by an increase in spontaneous firing rate of cells responding to noxious stimuli following the iontophoretic application of this material. It has only been identified in A delta and C fiber sizes of primary neurons which are related to pain signaling mechanisms.

It may operate as a neurotransmitter (56) in that it is concentrated in synaptosomal fractions of brain (60) and within synaptic vesicles of nerve terminals (21), but it has not yet been demonstrated to fulfill other criteria for a neurotransmitter. Some have suggested that it may operate as a neuromodulator because its time course of action is far too long for it to be considered a neurotransmitter (8, 53).

GABA, norepinephrine, serotonin (Fig, 7.4), and an enkephalin analog have all been shown to inhibit a potassium-evoked release of substance P, suggesting that each of these may have a presynaptic inhibitory action

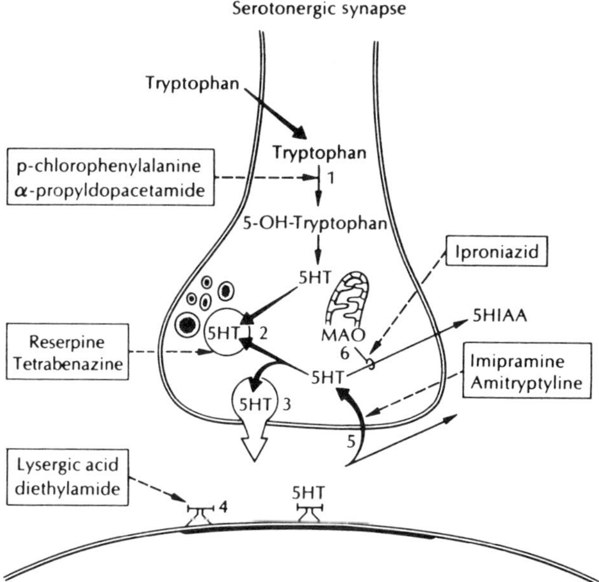

FIG. 7.4. Schematic model of a central serotonergic neuron indication possible sites of drug action. *Site 1:* Enzymatic synthesis. Tryptophan is taken up into the serotonin-containing neuron and converted to 5-OH-tryptophan (*5HT*) by the enzyme tryptophan hydroxylase. This enzyme can be effectively inhibited by ρ-chlorophenylalanine and α-propyldopacetamide. The next synthetic step involves the decarboxylation of *5HT* to form serotonin. *Site 2: Storage.* Reserpine and tetrabenazine interfere with the uptake-storage mechanism of the amine granules causing a marked depletion of serotonin. *Site 3: Release.* At present there is no drug available which selectively blocks the release of serotonin. However, lysergic acid diethylamide, because of its ability to block or inhibit the firing of serotonin neurons, causes a reduction in the release of serotonin from the nerve terminals. *Site 4:* Receptor interaction. Lysergic acid diethylamide acts as a partial agonist at serotonergic synapsess in the CNS. A number of compounds have also been suggested to act as receptor blocking agents at serotonergic synapses, but direct proof of these claims at the present time is lacking. *Site 5:* Reuptake. Considerable evidence now exists to suggest that serotonin may have its action terminated by being taken up into the presynaptic terminal. The tricyclic drugs with a tertiary nitrogen such as imipramine and amitryptyline appear to be potent inhibitors of this uptake mechanism. *Site 6:* Monoamine oxidase (*MAO*). Serotonin present in a free state within the presynaptic terminal can be degraded by the enzyme MAO, which appears to be located in the outer membrane of mitochondria. Iproniazid and clorgyline are effective inhibitors of MAO. *5-HIAA*, 5-hydroxyindoleacitic acid. (From J. R. Cooper *et al.* (16). Published with permission.)

on axonal terminals of substance P fibers but that their interrelated and selective characteristics are unknown (35, 43).

In general, the enkephalins suppress and substance P promotes pain signaling mechanisms. However, the issue is not entirely clear. Depletion of substance P from primary sensory neurons elevates an animal's threshold to thermal and chemical pain, but not to intense mechanical stimuli (76).

Whether substance P produces analgesia or hyperalgesia may be dose dependent or reflect the tested individual's threshold for pain. Intravenously administered substance P in mice (using a hot plate jump latency test) caused analgesia at high doses, but hyperalgesia at lower doses. The effect of substance P in this circumstance also depended on the individual mouse's control response latency. Analgesia was produced in mice with a high sensitivity to thermal stimuli whereas hyperalgesia occurred in animals with prolonged control latencies. These observations have suggested that substance P may "normalize responsiveness to pain" and operate as a regulatory peptide stabilizing behavior toward a steady state (54).

Angiotensin II, cholecystokinin, and somatostin have all been found in anatomic regions which imply a potential relationship to pain signaling mechanisms, but no clear evidence relating them specifically to pain signaling mechanisms has been reported. Not all forms of analgesia need be opioid dependent (37, 71).

It has been shown that some forms of stress may induce analgesia, and the role of endogenous opioids has not been established in that setting (45). Some studies have indicated that a cross tolerance develops between opioid and stress analgesia while others indicate that stress analgesia neither manifests cross tolerance with morphine nor is antagonized by naloxone. A recent investigation has indicated that depending on the temporal characteristics of inescapable foot shock stimuli, the stimulus may cause either an opioid- or nonopioid-related analgesia. In matching experimental groups using dexamethasone and naloxone to block stress-induced analgesia, studies reinforced the view that there exists an opioid-mediated system with inputs which may be activated by stress and modified by dexamethasone. It has been pointed out, however, that plasma concentrations of β-endorphin after stress are well below those needed to produce analgesia with systemic β-endorphin administration. Hence, stress may be effective in triggering either opioid or nonopioid dependent analgesia.

Sodium glutamate injected into the periaqueductal gray of rat has produced a short-lived analgesia if it was injected 30 minutes but not 5 minutes before testing (73). Paradoxically, higher doses of naloxone potentiated the glutamate analgesia, depending on the time of injection. These observations have suggested that the glutamate-induced analgesia may not depend on processes underlying morphine analgesia and that dose-related naloxone antagonism may not be an essential criterion for assessing endogenous opioid activity.

Several neurotransmitters or regulators participate in pain signaling systems. Analgesia induced by stimulation of the periaqueductal gray is augmented by increased levels of dopamine and serotonin and is suppressed by norepinephrine (3). Serotonin is released at the dorsal horn from terminals of cells in nucleus raphe magnus in the medulla. A norepinephrine-dependent descending pain-suppressing system has also been described (61, 76). Substance P probably operates within this system at terminals of primary afferents within the spinal cord but may function as a neuromodulator rather than a neurotransmitter. The enkephalins and endorphins participate in opioid-dependent analgesia by binding with opioid receptors, but not all analgesia need be opioid dependent. Angiotensin, cholecystokinin, and releasing factors for somatostatin and neurotensin may enter the field as neuroregulators related to pain. The criteria for their being classified as specific neuroregulators have not been established, and their regional distribution suggests they may serve many functions.

Despite the apparent conceptual advantages which have been added to our notions regarding neurotransmitters, modulators, mediators, and hormones and to the experience of pain and the relative clarification which was introduced with the concepts of descending endogens opioid-dependent pain-suppressing mechanisms from the brainstem, the issue has again become increasingly complex. There are, for instance, at least 9 neurotransmitters (GABA, epinephrine, substance P, enkephalin, angiotensin II, thyrotropin-releasing hormone, vasoactive intestinal peptide, serotonin, and neurotensin) represented in afferent systems to locus ceruleus, the central locus of noradrenergic neurons. Each of these may be brought into play under different though unidentified circumstances. Each may subserve separate behavioral counterparts, and each may modify the others. This complex interplay of multiple factors modulating the perception and behavioral consequences of pain clearly indicates that profound homeostatic mechanisms, neuroplasticity, and neuroadaptation may follow any operative procedure or pharmacologic manipulation which, while initially effective in alleviating pain, may yet fail with the passage of time. Hence, while a great deal of new information and much new conjecture regarding the neuropharmacology of pain and analgesics have emerged in the last 10 years, we have learned mostly that new vistas are opening rapidly and that much of what we think we know today will be revised tomorrow.

CONCLUSION

The recognition that neuroreceptor regulatory mechanisms are influenced by stress, genetic, biochemical, and pharmacologic homeostatic controls is a conceptual turning point in the understanding of drug effects in the nervous system. Neuroreceptor sensitivies compensate according to the amount, the time sequence, and the combinations of agonists and antagonists to which they are exposed. Their sensitivity is reduced by prolonged treatment with drugs which enhance transmitter concentration on postsynaptic receptors (by increasing its available precursor, exposing it to long-acting agonists, displacing endogenous transmitters, and inhibiting reuptake (40, 63). Conversely, manipulations which decrease transmitter concentration (as with long-term depletion of storage, inhibition of synthesis, or denervation with anatomic lesions or neurotoxins) may lead to an increase in postsynaptic sensitivity.*

Incorporating these concepts of neuropharmacology into therapeutic reality will be a monumental task. We must shift gears from thinking in terms of milliseconds to weeks; from neurotransmitters to neuroregulators; from simple excitation or inhibition to homeostatic tides or currents; from electrical communication systems to biochemical determinants of neural activity; from static states to molecular kinetics; from organ anatomy to subcellular, even molecular, anatomy. With such conceptual changes, however, will come new insights and the assurance of more effective therapeutic regimes for patients with depression, anxiety, and pain.

ACKNOWLEDGMENT

The author expresses appreciation to J. R. Cooper, F. E. Bloom, and R. H. Roth, authors of *The Biochemical Basis of Pharmacology*, and the Oxford University Press for their permission to reprint the illustrations used in this manuscript.

REFERENCES

1. Aghajanian, G. K. LSD and CNS transmission. Annu. Rev. Pharmacol. *12:* 157–168, 1972.
2. Aghajanian, G. K. Tricyclic antidepressants long term treatment increases responsivity of rat forebrain neurons to serotonin. Science, *202:* 1303–1305, 1978.
3. Akil, H., and Liebeskind, J. D. Monoaminergic mechanisms of stimulation-produced analgesia. Brain Res., *94:* 279–296, 1975.
4. Akil, H., Richardson, D. E., Barchas, J. D., and Li, C. H. Appearance of β-endorphin-like immunoreactivity in human ventricular cerebrospinal fluid upon analgesic electrical stimulation. Proc. Natl. Acad. Sci., *75:* 5170–5172, 1978.
5. Barchas, J. D. Psychopharmacology, edited by J. D. Barchas, P. A. Berger, R. D. Ciaranello, and G. R. Elliot. Oxford University Press, New York, 1977.
6. Barker, J. L., Neale, J. H., Smith, T. G., Jr., and MacDonald, R. L. Opiate peptide modulation of amino acid responses suggests novel form of neuronal communication. Science, *199:* 1451–1453, 1978.

---

* As always, exceptions to such generalizations occur. For instance, in the central nervous system, opiate receptor density is not altered during long-term exposure to opiate alkaloids (19) and supersensitivity to serotonin but not to norepinephrine may occur with antidepressant compounds thought to inhibit reuptake of these two transmitters (2).

7. Beer, B., Klepner, C. A., Lippa, A. S., and Squires, R. F. Enhancement of 3H-diazepam binding by S Q 65, 396 a novel anti-anxiety agent. Pharmacol. Biochem. Behav., *9:* 849–851, 1978.
8. Belcher, G., and Ryall, R. W. Substance P and Renshaw cells: a new concept of inhibitory synaptic interactions. J. Physiol., *272:* 105–120, 1977.
9. Bliss, R. M. Intra- and extra-hypothalamic vasopressin and oxytocin pathways in the rat. Pathways to the limbic system, medulla oblongata, and spinal cord. Cell Tissue Res., *192:* 423–435, 1978.
10. Bloom, F. E. Neuropharmacology and the adaptive regulation of receptor sensitivity: an overview. Mechanisms of regulation of neuronal sensitivity. Neurosci. Res. Prog. Bull., *18:* 429–435, 1980.
11. Bloom, F. E. The role of cyclic nucleotides in central synaptic function. Rev. Physiol. Biochem. Pharmacol., *74:* 1–103, 1975.
12. Carlsson, A. Autoreceptors. *In* Pre- and Postsynaptic Receptors, edited by E. Usdin and W. E. Bunney, pp. 49–65. Marcel Dekker, New York, 1975.
13. Chang, R. S. L., Tran, V. T., and Snyder, S. H. Neurotransmitter receptor localizations and brain lesion induced alterations in benzodiazine, GABA, β-adrenergic and histamine H, receptor binding. Brain Res., *190:* 95–110, 1980.
14. Choi, D. W., Faub, D. H., and Fischbach, G. Chlordiazepoxide selectively augments GABA action in the spinal cord cell cultures. Nature, *269:* 342–344, 1977.
15. Cook, L., and Davidson, A. B. Effects of behaviorally active drugs in a conflict-punishment procedure in rats. *In* The Benzodiazepines, edited by S. Garattini, E. Mussini, and L. O. Randall, pp. 327–345. Raven Press, New York, 1973.
16. Cooper, J. R., Bloom, F. E., and Roth, R. H. The Biochemical Basis of Neuropharmacology. Oxford University Press, New York, 1978.
17. Cooper, J. R. *et al.* (16), p. 223.
18. Costa, E., Guidotti, A., Mao, C. C., and Suria, A. New concepts on the mechanism of action of benzodiazepines. Life Sci., *17:* 167–186, 1975.
19. Cox, B. M. Multiple mechanisms in opiate tolerance. *In* Characteristics and Function of Opioids, edited by J. M. VanRee and L. Terenius, pp. 13–24. Elsevier/North Holland Biomedical Press, Amsterdam, 1978.
20. Cuello, A. C., Del Fiacco, M. and Paximos, G. The central and peripheral ends of the substance P-containing sensory neurones in the rat trigeminal system. Brain Res., *152:* 499–509, 1978.
21. Cuello, A. C., Jessel, T. M., Kanazawa, I., and Iversen, L. L. Substance P: localization in synaptic vesicles in rat central nervous system. J. Neurochem., *29:* 747–751, 1977.
22. Cuello, A. C., and Kanazawa, I. The distribution of substance P immunoreactive fibers in the rat central nervous system. J. Comp. Neurol., *178:* 129–156, 1978.
23. Curtis, D. R., and Johnston, G. Amino acid transmitters in the mammalian central nervous system. Ergeb. Physiol. Biol. Chem. Exp. Pharmakol., *69:* 97–120, 1974.
24. Curtis, D. R., Lodge, D., Johnston, G., and Brand, S. J. Central actions of benzodiazepines. Brain Res., *118:* 344–347, 1976.
25. Florey, E. Neurotransmitters and modulators in the animal kingdom. Fed. Proc., *26:* 1164–1176, 1967.
26. Gallager, D. Benzodiazepines potentiation of GABA inhibitory response in the dorsal raphe nucleus. Eur. J. Pharmacol., *49:* 133–143, 1978.
27. Geller, I., Kulak, J. T., and Seifter, J. Effect of chlordiazepoxide and chlorpromazine on a punishment discrimination. Psychopharmacologia, *3:* 374–385, 1962.
28. Geller, H., Taylor, D. A., and Hoffer, B. J. Benzodiazepines and central inhibitory mechanisms. Naunyn Schmiedeberg's Arch. Pharmacol., *304:* 81–88, 1978.
29. Glazer, E. J., and Basbaum, A. I. Leucine enkephalin: localization in and axoplasmic

transport by sacral parasympathetic preganglionic neurons. Science, *208:* 1479–1480, 1980.

30. Greenlee, D. V., and Olsen, R. W. Solubilization of gamma-aminobutyric acid receptor protein from mammalian brain. Biochem. Biophys. Res. Commun., *88:* 380–387, 1979.
31. Guidotti, A., Toffano, G., and Costa, E. An endogenous protein modulates the affinity of GABA and benzodiazepine receptors in the brain. Nature, *275:* 553–555, 1978.
32. Haefely, W., Kulesan, A., Mohler, H., Pieri, L., Polc, P. and Schaffner, R. Mechanism of action of benzodiazepines. Adv. Biochem. Psychopharmacol., *14:* 131–151, 1975.
33. Heidmann, T., and Changeux, J. P. Structural and functional properties of the acetylcholine receptor protein in its purified and membrane-bound states. Annu. Rev. Biochem., *47:* 317–357, 1978.
34. Henry, J. L. Effects of substance P on functionally identified units in cat spinal cord. Brain Res., *114:* 439–451, 1976.
35. Hodge, C. J., Jr., and King, R. B. Medical modification of sensation. J. Neurosurg., *44:* 21–28, 1976.
36. Hokfelt, T. M., Elde, R., and Johansson, O. Distribution of peptide containing neurons. *In* Psychopharmacology: A Generation of Progress, edited by M. Lipton, A. Dimascio, and K. Killam, pp. 39–66. Raven Press, New York, 1978.
37. Hosobuchi, Y., Rossier, J., and Bloom, F. E. Oral loading with L-tryptophan may augment the simultaneous release of ACTH and beta-endorphin that accompanies periaqueductal stimulation in humans. *In* Neural Peptides and Neuronal Communication, pp. 563–570. Raven Press, New York, 1980.
38. Hosobuchi, Y., Rossier, J., Bloom, F. E., and Guillemin, R. Periaqueductal gray stimulation (PAGS) for pain suppression in humans. Adv. Pain Res. Ther. *3:* 515–523, 1979.
39. Hughes, J. Isolation of an endogenous compound from the brain with pharmacologic properties similar to morphine. Brain Res., *88:* 295–308, 1975.
40. Kahn, C. R. Membrane Receptors for hormones and neurotransmitters. J. Cell Biol., *70:* 261–286, 1976.
41. Karobath, M., Placheta, P., Lippitsch, M., and Krogsgaard-Larsen, P. Is stimulation of benzodiazepine receptor binding mediated by a novel GABA receptor? Nature, *278:* 748–749, 1979.
42. Karobath, M., and Sperk, G. Stimulation of benzodiazepine receptor binding by gamma-aminobutyric acid. Proc. Natl. Acad. Sci., USA, *76:* 1004–1006, 1979.
43. King, R. B. Pain and tryptophan. J. Neurosurg., *53:* 44–52, 1980.
44. Kozhechkin, S., and Ostrovskaya, R. Are benzodiazepines GABA antagonists? Nature, *269:* 72–73, 1977.
45. Lewis, J. W., Cannon, J. T., and Liebeskind, J. C. Opioid and nonopioid mechanisms of stress analgesia. Science, *208:* 623–625, 1980.
46. Lippa, A. S., Sano, M. C., Coupet, J., Klepner, C. A., and Beer, B. Evidence that benzodiazepine receptors reside on cerebellar Purkinje cells: studies with "nervous" mutant mice. Life Sci., *23:* 2213–2217, 1978.
47. Ljungdahl, A., Hokfelt, T., and Nilsson, G. Distribution of substance P-like immunoreactivity in the CNS of the rat. I. Cell bodies and nerve terminals. Neuroscience, *3:* 861–943, 1978.
48. Ljungdahl, A., Hokfelt, T., Nilsson, G., and Goldstein, M. Distribution of substance P-like immunoreactivity in the CNS of the rat. II. Light microscopic localization in relation to catecholamine-containing neurons. Neuroscience, *3:* 945–976, 1978.
49. MacDonald, R., and Barker, J. L. Benzodiazepines specifically modulate GABA-mediated postsynaptic inhibition in cultured mammalian neurones. Nature, *271:* 563–564, 1978.

50. Mandell, A. J. Redundant macromolecular mechanisms in central synaptic regulation. *In* New Approaches to Neurotransmitter Regulation, edited by A. J. Mandell, pp. 255–278. Raven Press, New York, 1974.
51. Marx, J. L. Calmodulin: a protein for all seasons. Science *208:* 274–276, 1980.
52. Montarolo, P., Raschi, F., Strata, P. Interactions between benzodiazepines and GABA in the cerebellar cortex. Brain Res., *162:* 358–362, 1979.
53. Mroz, E. A., and Leeman, S. E. Substance P. Vitam. Horm., *35:* 209–281, 1977.
54. Oehme, P., Hilse, H., Morgenstern, E., and Gores, E. Substance P: Does it produce analgesia or hyperalgesia? Science, *208:* 305–307, 1980.
55. Okamoto, K., and Sakai, Y. Augmentation by chlordiazepoxide of the inhibitory effects of taurine, beta alanine and gamma-aminobutyric acid on spike discharges in guinea pig cerebellar slices. Br. J. Pharmacol., *65:* 277–285, 1979.
56. Otsuka, M., and Knoishi, S. Substance P: an excitatory transmitter of primary sensory neurons. Cold Spring Harbor Symp. Quant. Biol., *40:* 135–143, 1976.
57. Polc, P., and Haefely, W. Effects of two benzodiazepines, phenobarbitone and baclofen on synaptic transmission of the cat cuneate nucleus. Naunyn-Schmiedeberg's Arch. Pharmacol., *294:* 121–131, 1976.
58. Raabe, W., and Gumwit, R. Anticonvulsant action of diazepine: increase of cortical inhibition. Epilepsia, *18:* 117–120, 1977.
59. Rakic, P., and Sidman, R. L. Sequences of development abnormalities leading to granule cell deficit in cerebellar cortex of weaver mutant mice. J. Comp. Neurol., *152:* 103–132, 1973.
60. Ryall, R. W. The subcellular distributions of acetyl choline, substance P, 5-hydroxytryptamine, δ-aminobutyric acid and blutamic acid in brain homogenates. J. Neurochem., *11:* 131–145, 1964.
61. Sasa, M., Munekiyo, K., Ikeda, H., and Takaori, S. Noradrenaline-mediated inhibition by locus coeruleus of spinal trigeminal neurons. Brain Res., *80:* 443–460, 1974.
62. Schmidt, R. F., Vogel, M. E., and Zimmermann, M. Die Wirkung von Diazepam auf die prasynaptische Hemmung und andere Ruckenmarksreflexe. Naunyn Schmiedebergs Arch. Pharmacol., *258:* 69–82, 1967.
63. Schwartz, J. C., Cosentin, J., Martres, M. D., Protais, P., and Baudry, M. Modulation of receptor mechanisms in the central nervous system: hyper- and hyposensitivity to catecholamines. Neuropharmacology, *17:* 503–513, 1978.
64. Siggins, G. R. Electrophysiological role of dopamine in striatum: excitatory or inhibitory. *In* Psychopharmacology: A Generation of Progress, edited by M. D. Lipton, A. DiMascio, and F. K. Killam, pp. 143–158. New York, Raven Press, 1978.
65. Skolnick, P., Syapin, P. J., Paugh, B. A., and Paul, S. M. Reduction in benzodiazepine receptors associated with Purkinje cell degeneration in "nervous" mutant mice. Nature, *277:* 397–399, 1979.
66. Speth, R. C., and Yamamura, H. I. Benzodiazepine receptors: alterations in mutant mouse cerebellum. Eur. J. Pharmacol., *54:* 397–409, 1979.
67. Stratten, W. P., and Barnes, C. D. Diazepam and presynaptic inhibition. Neuropharmacology, *10:* 685–696, 1971.
68. Swanson, L. Immunohistochemical evidence for a neurophysin-containing autonomic pathway arising in the paraventricular nucleus of the hypothalamus. Brain Res., *128:* 346–351, 1977.
69. Tallman, J. F., Paul, S. M., Skolnick, P., and Gallager, D. W. Receptors for the age of anxiety: pharmacology of the benzodiazepines. Science, *207:* 275–281, 1980.
70. Tsuchiya, T., and Fukushima, H. Effects of benzodiazepines and pentobarbitone on the GABA-ergic recurrent inhibition of hippocampal neurones. Eur. J. Pharmacol., *48:* 421–424, 1978.

71. Turnbull, I. M., Shulman, R., and Woodhurst, W. B. Thalamic stimulation for neuropathic pain. J. Neurosurg., *52:* 486–493, 1980.
72. Ungerstedt, U. Changes in central dopamine receptor sensitivity studied with behavioral models. Mechanisms of regulation of neuronal sensitivity. Neurosci. Res. Prog. Bull., *18:* 419–428, 1980.
73. Urca, G., Nahin, L. L., and Liebeskind, J. C. Glutamate-induced analysis: blockade and potentiation by naloxone. Brain Res., *192:* 523–530, 1980.
74. Wastek, G. J., Speth, R. C., Reisine, T. D., and Yamamura, H. I. The effect of gamma-aminobutyric acid on 3H-flunitrazepam binding in rat brain. Eur. J. Pharmacol., *50:* 445–447, 1978.
75. Williams, M., and Risley, E. A. Enhancement of the binding of 3H diazepam to rat brain membranes *in vitro* by SQ20009: a novel anxietolytic Gamma amino buteric acid (GABA) and muscinol. Life Sci., *24:* 833–841, 1979.
76. Yaksh, T. L., Farb, D. H., Leeman, S. E., and Jessel, T. M. Intrathecal capsaicin depletes substance P in the rat spinal cord and produces prolonged thermal analgesia. Science, *206:* 481–483, 1979.
77. Yousufi, M., Thomas, J. W., and Tallman, J. F. Solubilization of benzodiazepine binding site from rat cortex. Life Sci., *25:* 463–470, 1979.
78. Zakusov, V. V., Ostrovskaya, R. U., Markovitch, V. V., Molodavkin, G., and Bylayev, V. Electrophysiological evidence for an inhibitory action of diazepam upon cat brain cortex. Arch. Int. Pharmacodyn. Ther., *214:* 188–205, 1975.

CHAPTER

8

Current Concepts in the Management of Movement Disorders

C. WARREN OLANOW, M.D., F.R.C.P.(C)

An increased knowledge in our understanding of movement disorders has been one of the most exciting scientific advances of the past 20 years. A rational approach to the therapy of movement disorders is based upon a knowledge of the anatomy, biochemistry, and pharmacology of the basal ganglia. In the past, therapy was largely empirical. Recent advances now provide a scientific basis for designing therapeutic strategies to treat patients with movement disorders. These therapies are primarily symptomatic in nature and involve an attempt to manipulate a disordered neuropharmacological environment.

Clinically, movement disorders are comprised of a combination of involuntary movements, poverty of movement, and alterations of tone. They are frequently associated with pathology in the basal ganglia. The majority are the consequence of a neurotransmitter imbalance. In most cases, it is the imbalance which is treated and not the specific disease process. The disease may continue to progress with therapy becoming less effective. A more definitive approach to therapy awaits a clearer understanding of the basic pathogenetic and etiologic mechanisms responsible for these conditions.

ANATOMY AND PHARMACOLOGY

The basal ganglia are composed of massive subcortical nuclei derived from the telencephalon and consist of the caudate, putamen, globus pallidus, and amygdaloid nuclei. The globus pallidus is designated as the paleostriatum, as it is the oldest; the caudate and putamen are jointly referred to as the neostriatum. Collectively, the neostriatum and paleostriatum are referred to as the corpus striatum. The "extrapyramidal-system" groups are found together with the corpus-striatum with related brain stem nuclei which are felt to subserve somatic motor functions. While theoretically the term "extrapyramidal" includes the entire central nervous system with the exception of the pyramidal system, it is generally used to refer to the corpus-striatum plus the subthalamic nucleus, the substantia nigra, the red nucleus, the cerebellar outflow tracts, and the brain stem reticular formation. The extrapyramidal-system is considered to play an important role in the regulation of motor activity, but it does not project fibers to the spinal level, and its contribution to motor function is thought to be mediated via cortical motor neurons. The precise relationship between the pyramidal and the extrapyramidal system is not completely understood (42). Detailed descriptions of the anatomical connections of the basal ganglia system are available (21), and these are schematically represented in Fig. 8.1. It should be noted that the neostriatum (caudate and putamen) functions as the input system for the basal ganglia. The globus pallidus functions as the output system. Fibers from the globus pallidus are relayed to the thalamus and thence to the motor cortex, presumably to influence its output. The neostriatum is modulated by reciprocal connections with the substantia nigra. Similarly, the globus pallidus is modulated by reciprocal connections with the subthalamic nucleus. The thalamus and motor cortex, having received the output of the striatum, in turn provide afferent pathways to the basal ganglia. Thus, the extrapyramidal system is highly integrated with multiple feedback loops.

The major conceptual and anatomical advance of the past 20 years has been the appreciation that within these pathways lie neuropharmacological tracts which can be identified by their specfic neurotransmitter. Opposing pharmacologic transmitters within these tracts may modulate different effects. It is the balance of these various neurotransmitters within the extrapyramidal system which is essential for normal coordinated motor movement. The pharmacologic basis of a movement disorder is the result of a chemical imbalance between two or more opposing neurotransmitter systems.

The major basal ganglia neurotransmitters identified to date include norepinephrine (NE), dopamine (DA), γ-aminobutyric acid (GABA), acetylcholine (ACH), serotonin (5-HT), and probably glutamic acid (GLU) (20, 46, 56, 147). Most attention has focused on DA because of the demonstrated reduction of this neurotransmitter in the substantia nigra and the neostriatum of patients with Parkinson's syndrome. The synthesis and metabolism of DA are illustrated in Fig. 8.2. DA is formed in the substantia nigra and transferred by axonal transport to the neostriatum (4). Lesions in this pathway result in a reduction in striatal DA (122). DA-containing neurons are also found in the hypothalamus, limbic system, and diffusely throughout the cortex, but their relationship to motor activity is unknown.

DA receptors have been identified on the postsynaptic membranes and presynaptic membranes (autoreceptors) of DA neurons, as well as on other nerve terminals (1). Kebabian (79) has defined two classes of DA receptors based on their association or independence from a dopamine-

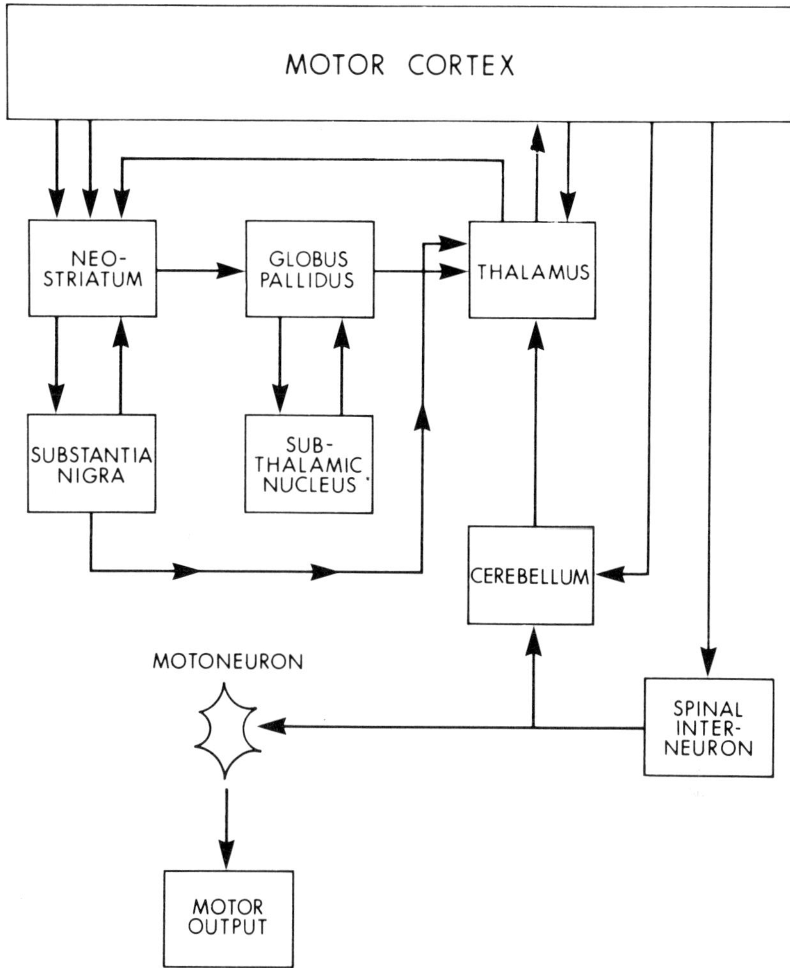

FIG. 8.1. A schematic representation of the anatomical connections of the basal ganglia. The interactions are complex but highly organized. The neostriatum functions as the input, and the globus pallidus functions as the output for the basal ganglia system. These are modulated by reciprocal connections with the substantia nigra and subthalamic nucleus, respectively. The interconnections among the basal ganglia, cerebellum, thalamus, motor cortex, and peripheral nervous system should be noted.

sensitive adenylcyclase. These are known as the D-1 (linked to adenylcyclase) and D-2 (unrelated to adenylcyclase) DA receptors (80). The ergot DA agonists specifically stimulate the D-2 receptors (143). Other DA agonists (apomorphine and DA) and their antagonists (phenothiazines and butyrophenones) affect both D-1 and D-2 receptors. There is evidence in humans to suggest that the beneficial effect of L-DOPA is

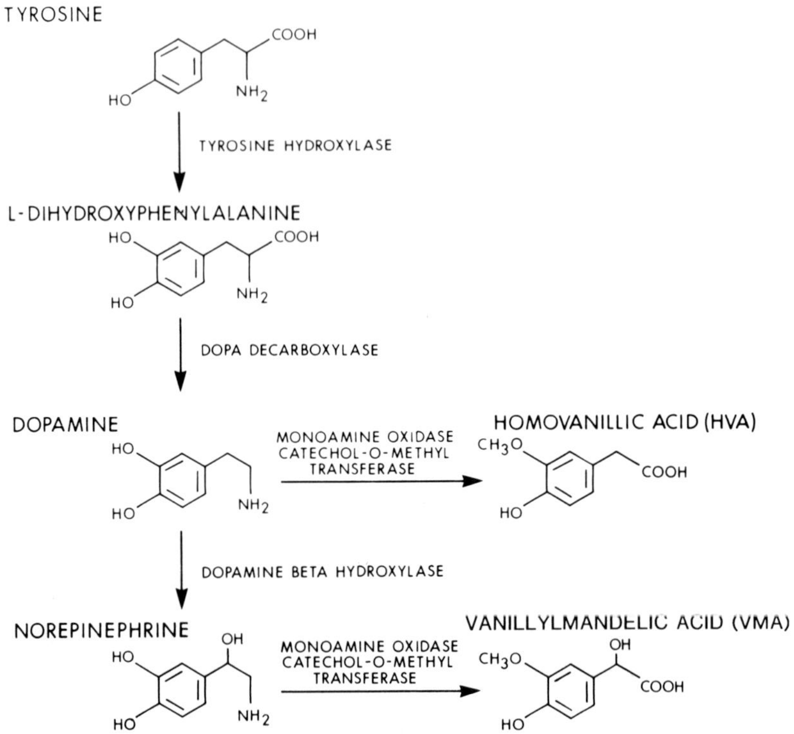

FIG. 8.2. Metabolic pathway of catecholamine synthesis and metabolism. A deficiency of tyrosine hydroxylase and *DOPA* decarboxylase has been reported in Parkinson's syndrome.

mediated through stimulation of the D-2 receptors (123). This hypothesis suggests the potential of stimulating selective DA mechanisms.

Within the nigrostriatal system, it is clear that normal function is the result of a complex interaction between several neurotransmitters, particularly DA, ACH, GABA, and GLU. A proposed mechanism for the interaction of these transmitters in the neostriatum and substantia nigra is illustrated in Fig. 8.3. DA fibers originating in the substantia nigra inhibit the firing of cholinergic neurons in the neostriatum (111). Cholinergic neurons stimulate GABA-aminergic neurons which are in turn inhibitory to nigral DA neurons. A reduction in DA activity results in uninhibited cholinergic firing. This leads to stimulation of GABA neurons and a further reduction in DA activity in the substantia nigra. By contrast, excessive DA activity inhibits striatal cholinergic neurons, resulting in reduced GABA stimulation and reduced inhibition of the dopaminergic neurons in the substantia nigra. Thus, transmitter alterations tend to be self perpetuating.

Within the neostriatum there is an intraneuronal pool which is excited by cortical afferents (GLU-ergic) inhibited by nigral afferents (DA-ergic) and possibly moderated by thalamic afferents (ACH-ergic) (68). Long-acting transmitters, such as substance P, may further influence the pharmacologic environment and facilitate DA release (70, 74).

DA deficiency in the nigrostriatal system results in a Parkinson-like syndrome. Drugs which block DA transmission (phenothiazines and butyrophenones) or which deplete basal ganglia DA (reserpine) may give rise to a Parkinson-like syndrome. Stimulation of the ACH system by injection of physostigmine aggravates DA deficiency and increases the features of Parkinsonism (49). Striatal injection of anticholinergic agents reduces Parkinson features. These observations have formed a rationale for the current treatment of Parkinsonism which is aimed at correcting the DA deficiency or blocking the unopposed ACH system.

Excessive DA activity, by contract, is felt to be the pharmacologic basis

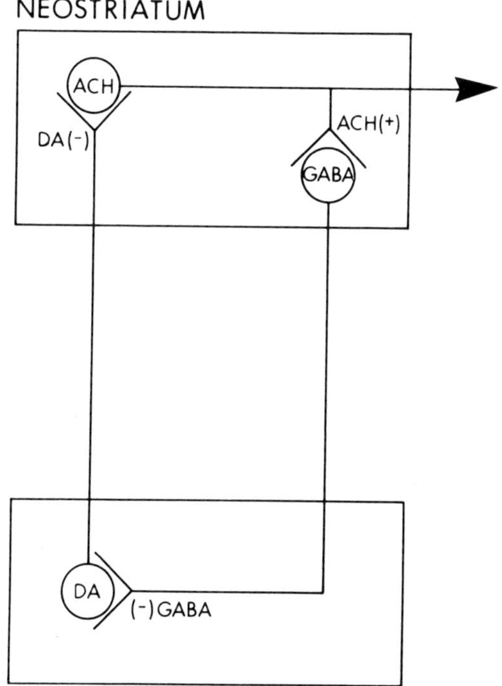

FIG. 8.3. Proposed neuronal interaction within the substantia nigra and neostriatum. DA neurons which originate in the substantia nigra are inhibitory to striatal cholinergic neurons. These in turn stimulate striatal GABA-aminergic neurons which are inhibitory to nigral DA neurons.

of chorea. A reduction in GABA or ACH transmission aggravates chorea, as do agents which increase DA activity. Therapy is aimed at blocking DA transmission or increasing ACH or GABA activity.

Fig. 8.4 illustrates that DA replacement therapy in Parkinson's syndrome may inadvertently result in excessive DA receptor stimulation which is clinically manifest as chorea. DA blocking agents which improve chorea may be complicated by DA deficiency which results in Parkinsonism. These drug-induced side effects are reversible with reduction in dosage. In disease states, however, a permanent neurotransmitter imbalance may exist and continue to progress despite therapy.

Animal models for the majority of movement disorders are not available. There are many conflicting reports as to the results of stimulation and destructive lesions within the basal ganglia system. The only consistent clinically recognized movement disorder which occurs spontaneously and following an experimental lesion in a basal ganglia nucleus is the hemiballismus which follows partial destruction of the subthalamic nucleus (22, 23). Small lesions of the caudate nucleus, globus pallidus, and substantia nigra cause no significant impairment in motor function. Bilateral destruction of the globus pallidus produces an akinetic state. Bilateral destructive lesions of the nigrostriatal pathways by 6-hydroxydopamine result in an immobile animal (144); however, bilateral radiofrequency destruction of these pathways results in hyperkinesia (18). Lesions in the ventromedial tegmentum of the midbrain of monkeys has been reported to produce a sustained tremor similar to that seen in Parkinson's syndrome (149). Neurons in the contralateral sensory-motor cortex and the ventrolateral (VL) nucleus of the thalamus fire in phase with the tremor, implying that a thalamocortical mechanism is involved (88). This is not effected by extensive dorsal rhizotomy (116), suggesting that the discharge originates within the cortex or within a thalamic "oscillator." The lesion in the brain stem may release the thalamus from inhibition, allowing a state of rhythmic bursting to develop, but the

	DOPAMINE ACTIVITY	CHOLINERGIC ACTIVITY	SYMPTOMATIC TREATMENT	SIDE EFFECT OF TREATMENT
Parkinsonism	DA deficiency	CH excess	a) DA replacement b) Ch blockade	Chorea
Chorea	DA excess	Ch deficiency	a) DA blockade b) Ch replacement	Parkinson

FIG. 8.4. A comparison of dopaminergic activity, cholinergic activity, therapeutic strategy, and side effect of treatment in parkinsonism and chorea. These clinical syndromes represent a pharmacologic state of dopaminergic-cholinergic imbalance. The therapy of the one condition has the other as its side effect.

anatomic basis for this is unknown. Marsden *et al.* (102) have reviewed the relationship between animal models and Parkinsonism.

Destruction of the nigrostriatal pathways by electrolytic lesions induces an animal to turn towards the side of the lesion (2). Similar results can be obtained with nigrostriatal lesions induced by 6-hydroxydopamine (145). This circling is correlated with a loss of DA in the substantia nigra and the neostriatum (3). Intrastriatal infusion of DA elicits contralateral circling which can be blocked by DA antagonists (146). It is hypothesized that rodents circle toward the side of the body with the less stimulated striatal "dopamine" system. This system has been used as a model to test the DA-stimulating or blocking properties of investigative drugs.

PARKINSON'S SYNDROME

Parkinson's syndrome is a degenerative brain disorder that affects 200,000 pepople in the United States. It generally affects adults over the age of 40 years, but a juvenile form occurs (112). Pathologically, there may be cellular loss throughout the basal ganglia and cerebral cortex. The characteristic alteration is depigmentation and neuronal loss within the substantia nigra (64). A reduction in the DA content of substantia nigra and neostriatum has been demonstrated (50). Homovanillic acid and DOPA decarboxylase (see Fig. 8.2) have also been found to be reduced in Parkinson's syndrome (99). These have provided the basis for the hypothesis that the clinical features of parkinsonism reflect a state of DA deficiency in the basal ganglia. The clinical picture was first described by James Parkinson in 1817 (119). The clinical features are:

(a) *Bradykinesia*—A slowness in performing voluntary and automatic movements. This may significantly interfere with activities of daily living and is the most disabling of the parkinsonian features. Bradykinesia may be seen as an isolated feature and is not simply a function of increased tone. The slowness is often most pronounced on initiating movements, and patients have a tendency to "freeze." There is, however, the potential for normal movement under circumstances of extreme stress. This is referred to as "kinesia paradoxica." Patients often have reduced facial expression with mask-like facies and decreased frequency of blinking. The voice tends to be monotonal and slurred with reduced amplitude. There is reduced arm swing when walking and synergic movements are lost. Bradykinesia is thought to be due to a diffuse DA deficiency.

(b) *Rigidity*—An increased resistance to passive movement. It is usually of the cogwheel or lead pipe type and may be so extensive as to limit the range of movement of a joint. Flexor and extensor muscles of the limbs or neck may be involved. Pathological alterations in tone may be exaggerated by the "Jendrassik maneuver," in which alternating contractions of the opposite limb result in increased tone. This may allow subclinical changes to be recognized. One must not confuse cogwheel rigidity with the underlying tremor. The mechanism responsible for rigidity is not known, but improvement following anticholinergic drugs or lesions of the VL nucleus globus pallidus suggests that it is related to a cholinergic-dopaminergic imbalance.

(c) *Tremor*—A regular, rhythmic tremor which is most pronounced at rest. It has a frequency of 3 to 5/second and usually involves the distal muscles (pill rolling). The face, tongue, and lips may also be involved. It is aggravated by emotional states and is occasionally present on intention and disappears during sleep. While it is the most clinically obvious feature of parkinsonism, it is generally the least disabling. The anatomic basis of tremor is unknown. Improvement following anticholinergic drugs and thalamotomy suggests, as with rigidity, that it is related to a cholinergic-dopaminergic imbalance.

(d) *Gait Disturbance*—A shuffling gait with postural instability and accompanying festination and retropulsion. Patients assume a flexed, stooped posture with arms held in internal rotation. A gait disorder may occasionally be the sole clinical feature of parkinsonism.

(e) *Dementia*—It is now appreciated that more than one-third of parkinsonian patients develop a dementia (93). The high incidence may reflect the longer life-span afforded parkinsonian patients by current therapy.

(f) *Miscellaneous*—These include: sialorrhea, seborrhea, micrographia, GI disturbances, and limitation of eye movements.

As discussed, parkinsonism is considered to represent a neuropharmacologic state of DA deficiency. There are many different mechanisms which may lead to an interference with DA regulation, and many syndromes of presumed degenerative origin which have parkinsonian features as a component. These are summarized in Table 8.1.

Therapy

The therapy of Parkinson's syndrome must include establishing the correct diagnosis and correcting any underlying disorder. Even "idiopathic parkinsonism" may be related to multiple etiologies which cannot

TABLE 8.1
Differential Diagnosis of Parkinson's Syndrome

Degenerative
Idiopathic parkinsonism, adult and juvenile forms
Striatonigral degeneration
Shy-Drager syndrome
Olivopontocerebellar degeneration
Supranuclear palsy
Parkinson-ALS-dementia complex
Infectious
Postencephalitic Parkinsonism
Creutzfeldt-Jakob disease
Toxic
Heavy metals (manganese)
Drugs
Phenothiazines
Butyrophenones
Rauwolfia alkaloids
α-methyldopa
Vascular
Stroke
Carbon monoxide
Neoplasm
Metabolic
Hypoparathyroidism
Wilson's Disease

currently be distinguished. Physical therapy, psychotherapy, and family counseling should be employed if appropriate. Current medical and surgical treatments are symptomatic and are classified in Table 8.2.

Anticholinergics, Antihistamines, and Antiviral Drugs

Historically, the therapy of Parkinson's syndrome has been based upon the empirical observation that anticholinergic and antihistaminic medications improve tremor and, to a lesser degree, rigidity. It has been postulated that the benefit is a consequence of blocking an unopposed striatal cholinergic system. Trihexyphenidyl (Artane) and benztropine (Cogentin) are the most widely used anticholinergic agents. Dosages range from 2 to 15 mg/day administered in divided doses. Small doses are used initially and are then gradually increased. The anticholinergic drugs have an atropine-like effect and may cause urinary retention, dry mouth, blurred vision, and constipation. The major limitations are confusion and psychotic behavior, which are dose related. While these medications have limited value in the treatment of parkinsonism, their sudden withdrawal may lead to a dramatic clinical deterioration (63). They must be tapered gradually when no longer desired. They are most often used for mildly affected patients, particularly when tremor is the

TABLE 8.2
Approach to Symptomatic Therapy of Parkinsonism

I. Minor Drugs
  A. Anticholinergics
  B. Antihistamines
  C. Amantadine hydrochloride (Symmetrel)
II. DA Replacement
  A. L-DOPA
  B. L-DOPA + peripheral decarboxylase inhibitor
III. Dopamine Agonists
IV. Surgery
V. Newer Approaches
  A. MAO-β inhibitors
  B. COMT inhibitors
  C. Long-acting DA agonists
  D. Membrane-stabilizing agents

major feature. They are also used as an adjunct to DA therapy in more advanced patients. Amantadine hydrochloride (Symmetrel), an antiviral agent, has also been noted to improve some symptoms of parkinsonism. A dosage of 200 to 300 mg/day is prescribed in divided doses in combination with L-DOPA. While definite benefit can be seen in some patients, it is usually transient, disappearing within 6 months (141). Side effects of confusion, a withdrawal syndrome, and minimal efficacy limit the usefulness of this medication as well.

Dopamine Replacement Therapy

The finding of a reduced dopamine content in the substantia nigra and neostriatum of patients with Parkinson's syndrome has prompted a therapeutic strategy based upon attempts to replace this neurotransmitter. Dopamine itself does not cross the blood-brain barrier, but its precursor, dihydroxyphenyalanine (DOPA), does. The levoform, L-DOPA, is the effective stereoisomer. In 1961, Berkmayer[12] and Barbeau,[6] in separate studies, reported that small doses of L-DOPA transiently improved the clinical symptoms of Parkinson's syndrome. It was 1967, however, before Cotzias et al.[34] demonstrated that large doses were required to obtain a sustained benefit. Double-blind studies confirmed this observation and ushered in a new therapeutic era (152). It is now widely recognized that L-DOPA is of great benefit in the treatment of parkinsonism, particularly for bradykinesia and rigidity (19, 33, 124). It has been postulated that bradykinesia and rigidity respond more dramatically because they are related to a diffuse striatal deficiency of DA. Tremor responds less strikingly because it is the result of an unopposed cholinergic output from the striatal system. This might account for the relatively select effect of thalamotomy and anticholinergic medications on tremor.

Since the introduction of L-DOPA, studies have demonstrated not only a marked clinical improvement, but also a longer life span (43, 75). Postmortem studies on the brains of L-DOPA-treated parkinsonian patients show evidence of increased DA formation in the striatum, suggesting that the therapeutic efficacy of L-DOPA is mediated through a correction of a DA deficiency (97).

Treatment is initiated with 250 mg of L-DOPA administered 1 to 3 times/day. It is slowly increased over weeks to months until the desired clinical response is obtained or intolerable side effects develop. Most patients can be maintained on a total daily dosage of 2 to 6 g divided into frequent intervals. Nausea and vomiting may be reduced by administering L-DOPA with meals or by dividing the dosage into more frequent intervals. Experimentation with frequency and timing of dosage is often useful in individual patients. Approximately 80% of patients will improve with L-DOPA, and it is not possible to predict which patients will fail to respond.

The incidence of nausea and vomiting and other peripheral side effects can be reduced by combining L-DOPA with a peripheral decarboxylase inhibitor (Fig. 8.5). This blocks the peripheral conversion of L-DOPA to DA, as the decarboxylase enzyme is present in both peripheral blood vessel walls and central nervous system. These inhibitors prevent the peripheral accumulation of DA, which is functionally ineffective, as it

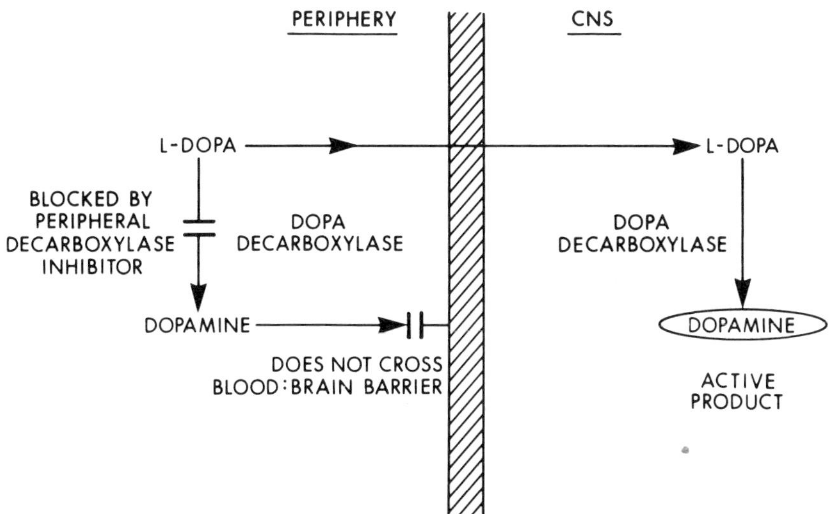

FIG. 8.5. Mechanism of action of a peripheral DOPA decarboxylase inhibitor. By blocking the peripheral conversion of L-DOPA to DA, a greater percentage of DOPA is available for entry into the CNS, and smaller doses can be employed. The accumulation of peripheral DA is prevented, and as a consequence peripheral side effects are reduced.

does not cross the blood-brain barrier. As a result a greater percentage of L-DOPA is available for central absorption, and dosage can be reduced by 75%. Furthermore, side effects which are related to circulating peripheral DA are reduced.

Carbidopa is the peripheral decarboxylase inhibitor which is most widely used in the United States. It is combined with L-DOPA and marketed as Sinemet. Carbidopa and L-DOPA are prescribed in a ratio of 10:1, in combination tablets of 10/100 mg and 25/250 mg. Recently a 25/100 mg tablet has been made available in order to provide adequate decarboxylase inhibition for patients who only require small quantities of L-DOPA. Patients are begun on 10/100 mg tid and increased to approximately 25/250 mg 3 to 6 times/day. Because of improved tolerance, the Sinemet dosage can be built up more rapidly than with L-DOPA alone. The same basic principles are employed when using Sinemet as L-DOPA—the drug is increased until the desired clinical response is obtained or until toxicity develops. The therapeutic efficacy of combined treatment is equal to or superior to that of L-DOPA alone (117). Because of reduced side effects and ease of administration, Sinemet is the preferred therapy (103). Side effects which relate to CNS DA, however, are similar to those of L-DOPA and may even be more severe. Benserazide, another decarboxylase inhibitor, has been widely employed outside the United States, and in combination with L-DOPA is marketed as Madopar. It is comparable to Sinemet.

Two to five years after initiating therapy with L-DOPA or Sinemet, there may be a loss of efficacy and clinical deterioration (71,100). This may be due to progression of the underlying disease but the possibility that it is related to the accumulation of toxic byproducts of DA metabolism must be considered. Free radicals and quinolines derived from DA metabolism are potentially toxic to nervous tissue.

There is a debate as to when to initiate DA replacement therapy. Many prefer to delay treatment until Parkinson's syndrome is relatively advanced, so that DOPA therapy will not be self limited and possibly toxic. Others argue that there has been reduced overall mortality since the introduction of L-DOPA, and they initiate treatment at the time of diagnosis. Some judgment must be used in prescribing therapy for the individual patient.

The side effects of DA replacement therapy are listed in Table 8.3 (8). Nausea and vomiting limit L-DOPA therapy in many patients. It is thought to be due to a high concentration of circulating DA stimulating the area postrema, which is not protected by the blood-brain barrier. Pyridoxine must be avoided, as it stimulates decarboxylation and reduces the amount of L-DOPA available for CNS penetration and is tantamount to reducing L-DOPA dosage. Postural hypotension is reported to occur in

TABLE 8.3

*Side Effects of DA Replacement Therapy**

Group A	Group B
Nausea, vomiting	Psychosis
Appetite suppression	Dyskinesia
Orthostatic hypotension	On-off effect
Cardiac arrhythmia	Loss of benefit
Pyridoxine reversal of L-DOPA effect	

* The combination of L-DOPA with a peripheral decarboxylase inhibitor eliminates the majority of side effects in Group A through a reduction in the accumulation of *peripheral* DA. Those side effects in Group B persist, however, as they are more directly related to *central* DA effects.

25% of L-DOPA-treated patients but it is rarely symptomatic (103). If it is severe, the possibility of the Shy-Drager syndrome with autonomic insufficiency needs to be considered (134). Cardiac arrhythmias (usually PVCs) are occasionally encountered but are rarely significant. Monoamine oxidase (MAO) inhibitors must be avoided with L-DOPA therapy, as they may precipitate a hypertensive crisis. The majority of these side effects can be reduced or abolished with combined DOPA and a peripheral decarboxylase inhibitor. The more important side effects are related to central DA activity and are identical for L-DOPA and Sinemet. They are the following.

PSYCHOSIS

Confusion and frank psychosis can develop in association with increasing doses of dopaminergic agents (138). They are most common in elderly and demented patients. They can be aggravated by concurrent drugs and underlying metabolic disorders. The basis of this mental change is believed to be an undesired stimulation of DA receptors in the limbic system (108). Ongoing studies are looking at agents which stimulate only DA receptors in the neostriatum, sparing those in the limbic system. L-DOPA is also known to inhibit 5-HT in the CNS (114). The 5-HT precursor L-tryptophan plus a peripheral decarboxylase inhibitor has occasionally prevented depression and psychosis in L-DOPA-treated patients.

DYSKINESIA

Abnormal involuntary movements are one of the most serious complications of DA replacement therapy and affect as many as 80% of patients. Chorea (particularly in the orofacial region) is the most frequent of these movements, but athetosis, dystonia, ballism, and myoclonus have all been described (9). These movements have also been classified according to when they occur following the dosage of L-DOPA (109). Occasionally, dyskinesia develops before adequate parkinson control is obtained, and a judgment must be made as to whether the patient can better tolerate the dyskinesia or the parkinsonian symptoms. Most patients prefer some degree of dyskinesia to the restricted movement associated with parkinsonism. With chronic DA therapy, a dosage which was previously well tolerated may cause dyskinesia. Reduction of dosage or a drug holiday with reintroduction of medication may provide an antiparkinsonian effect at a lower dosage which does not produce dyskinesia (44). Occasionally the therapeutic range of L-DOPA is so narrow that intolerable dyskinesia develops prior to any useful antiparkinsonian effect.

Dyskinesia is thought to be due to excessive DA receptor stimulation. In parkinsonism, the DA receptor is believed to be chemically denervated, resulting in a state of denervation hypersensitivity similar to that seen in the peripheral nervous system when a muscle is separated from its peripheral nerve (89). In this circumstance, exogenous DA overly stimulates the hypersensitive receptor, leading to dyskinesia (85). L-DOPA does not result in choreiform movements in nonparkinsonian patients, presumably because the receptors are not hypersensitive (26).

Experimentally, DA hypersensitivity can be induced by phenothiazines, butyrophenones, tyrosine hydroxylase inhibitors, reserpine, and 6-hydroxy-DA lesions of the nigrostriatal DA pathway (67, 145). Each of these results in an increased number of striatal DA receptors, as measured by increased DA agonist and antagonist binding sites. There is experimental evidence that lithium can stabilize the DA receptor and pevent the development of haloperidol-induced DA supersensitivity (59, 121).

Dyskinesia is one of the major limiting side effects of DOPA therapy. It is generally reversible by lowering the dosage of L-DOPA but usually with a loss in antiparkinsonian efficacy. Numerous agents, including choline, deanol, phenothiazines, etc., have been used in an attempt to reduce dyskinesia but appear to do so only by diminishing the therapeutic effect of L-DOPA (60, 86). There is currently no effective way of dealing with this side effect. It is reccomended that DOPA therapy be employed in as low a dosage as will provide an adequate therapeutic response in an effort to prevent this sometimes disabling side effect. Administering the total daily dosage at more frequent intervals may prevent the development of toxic peaks and consequent dyskinesia. Some DA agonists possess antidyskinesia function without loss of an antiparkinsonian effect and theoretically might be of value in combination with L-DOPA (48). Currently such agents (apomorphine) are too toxic for practical consideration. Pharmacologic attempts to augment GABA activity may also have theoretical benefit.

"ON-OFF" PHENOMENON

The on-off phenomenon has emerged as the major limitation of chronic DA therapy (54, 101). It consists of sudden and dramatic fluctuations in parkinsonian symptoms with periods of relative mobility ("on episodes") alternating with periods of severe akinesia and functional incapacity ("off episodes"). The on episodes are generally accompanied by dyskinesia of varying intensity. These stages may last minutes to hours, and the swing from one phase to the other may be very rapid, like turning a light switch on or off—hence, the name. Changes from one phase to the other may occur at any time and in an unpredictable manner. The on-off effect begins to occur 1 to 3 years after initiating L-DOPA therapy and earlier if a decarboxylase inhibitor is used. It is estimated that more than 50% of patients are affected who have been on treatment for longer than 5 years. Several variations of on-off episodes have been recognized, the most severe of which were not seen prior to L-DOPA therapy (104):

(1) *Early A.M. akinesia*—akinesia and rigidity on awakening that may represent parkinsonian features unrelieved by therapy and theoretically could be solved by long-acting L-DOPA preparations if they were available.
(2) *End of dose deterioration*—loss of clinical effectiveness associated with a reduction in the serum concentration of DOPA. Initially, this occurs 3 to 4 hours after administration, but with progression of the disease the latency may shorten. Doses of L-DOPA may initially reverse the off episode, but as time progresses, the drug is less effective, the swings more dramatic, and the dyskinesia during the "on" episodes more violent.
(3) *Peak dose akinesia*—the development of periods of akinesia in association with high serum concentrations of DOPA. This is a rare but important clinical syndrome, possibly equivalent to a cholinergic crisis in myasthenia gravis (28).
(4) *The yo-yo phenomenon*—the most severe type of on-off phenomena. There are wild swings between mobility and disability which may take place in a matter of seconds or minutes. These swings from one stage to the other occur in an unpredictable pattern without warning, and the oscillations are unrelated to the timing and plasma concentration of L-DOPA. This variation of the on-off phenomenon has only been described since the introduction of DA therapy. It is usually preceded by a state of progressive end-of-dose deterioration (7).

The mechanisms responsible for the on-off phenomena are unclear. Several theories have been proposed:

(a) Impaired GI or CNS absorption of L-DOPA due to competition with other amino acids. This may have relevance in the early stages of parkinsonism, but it is not a factor later on.

(b) Decreased availability of CNS DA due to a reduction in serum concentration of DOPA following administered dosage. The off episode is associated with a reduced serum concentration of DOPA while the on episode is associated with a high serum concentration. High blood levels of DOPA allow greater entry into the brain and presumably greater DA receptor activation. This does not, however, account for the more severe stages of the on-off effect where there is no relationship between the clinical stage and the serum concentration.

(c) Some DA metabolites may have an affinity for the DA receptor and function as pseudoagonists. It is postulated that the therapeutic effect of DOPA may be modulated by its own metabolites and that fluctuations in motor performance may be related to the accumulation of these metabolites. Tetrahydropapaveroline, for example, is a metabolite of L-DOPA, which is a DA antagonist (47). This theory fails to account for the persistence of an on-off effect with DA agonists which bypass DA metabolic pathways.

(d) Changes in striatal DA receptor sensitivity—this theory presumes that the development of on-off episodes relates to an alternating stage of hypersensitivity and hyposensitivity of the DA receptor. It has been postulated that denervation of striatal DA receptors results in receptor supersensitivity possibly mediated by increased numbers of DA receptors on the postsynaptic terminal (89). This is analagous to ACH hypersensitivity following denervation in the periphereal nervous system. Stimulation of supersensitive DA receptors might account for the combination of mobility and dyskinesia during the on phase. The off attack, by contrast, might reflect a relative state of receptor desensitization (89). Recent studies in humans and rats have demonstrated that hypersensitive receptors can be desensitized with chronic L-DOPA treatment (53, 67). A reduced number of DA receptors is found in treated as compared to nontreated patients as measured by haloperidol binding (89). If the postsnypatic DA receptor is desensitized below a critical level (becomes hyposensitive), it might result in an off spell. This theory would account for the relatively long latency before the development of the on-off phenomenon following the initiation of DOPA therapy. It is presumed that there is a critical threshold for DA receptor activation accounting for the sudden and often dramatic oscillations between akinesia and dyskinesia. The clinical appearance of being on or off may thus be related to the state of desensitization or supersensitization of the DA receptor coupled with DA availability.

A number of different approaches have been proposed to treat the on-off effect. These include increased L-DOPA dosage, more frequent administration of L-DOPA, decreased dietary protein, peripheral decarboxylase inhibitors, and DA agonists (76, 107, 118). These have generally failed to provide significant improvement. Their failure to influence the on-off effect suggests that pseudoagonists, fluctuations in absorption, and changing blood levels of L-DOPA are unlikely to be critical factors in its production. Long-acting L-DOPA preparations, which are currently not available, might theoretically help some cases with end-of-dose deterioration, but are unlikely to affect the more severe form of the on-off phenomenon.

More recently, reducing the dosage of DOPA or drug holidays (temporary cessation of medication) has been reported to improve the on-off effect in some patients (44, 45). It is postulated that lowering or discontinuing therapy may "resensitize" the DA receptor, allowing subsequent improvement. Agents such as lithium which may stabilize the DA receptor are currently under investigation (59). Chronic pretreatment with lithium prevents haloperidol-induced DA receptor supersensitivity as measured by behavioral stereotype to apomorphine and by reduced haloperidol binding (121). Stabilization of the membrane may prevent the supersensitization or densitization of the DA receptor, thus the oscillations of the on-off effect.

At the present time, there is no effective therapy for the on-off effect. It is currently recommended that L-DOPA or Sinemet therapy be employed in as low a dosage as possible in order to prevent receptor desensitization. Once the on-off phenomenon develops, there is no reliable treatment. Lowering the dosage of DOPA, increasing the dosage frequency, drug holidays, and DA agonists should all be tried. Membrane-stabilizing agents such as lithium warrant further investigation.

Dopamine Agonists

Dopamine agonists are drugs which directly stimulate the DA receptor but bypass the metabolic pathways which synthesize DA. They have diverse chemical structures but contain a DA-like moiety within their molecular configuration (Fig. 8.6). They provide several theoretical advantages to chronic L-DOPA therapy. Firstly, they avoid the accumulation of DOPA metabolites which may interfere with DA receptor stimulation. Secondly, a deficiency in the DOPA decarboxylase enzyme (found in some cases of parkinsonism) may be bypassed (99). Finally, these agents avoid fluctuations in DOPA absorption and serum concentration.

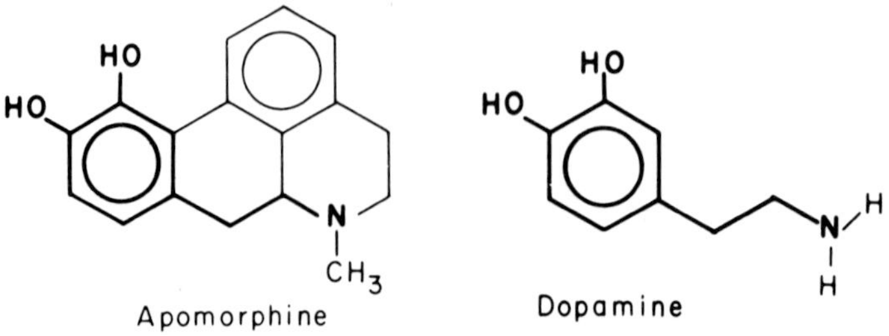

Fig. 8.6. A comparison of the molecular structures of DA and apomorphine. This illustrates the DA-like moiety within the molecular configuration of apomorphine. Many DA agonists, while chemically diverse, similarly contain a DA-like moiety within their molecular structure.

Many DA agonists have antiparkinsonian activity and also induce dyskinesia, presumably by stimulating hypersensitive DA receptors. Paradoxically, some DA agonists with antiparkinsonian activity may also reduce DA synthesis (148), and reduce dyskinesia (24, 142). This may be related to selective stimulation of different classes of DA receptors. Some DA agonists (apomorphine) stimulate DA-sensitive adenylcyclase (81) while others (bromocriptine) do not (143).

Several DA agonists have been studied in man including apomorphine (32), N-propylnoraporphine (35), lergotrile (95), piribedil (110), and bromocriptine (94, 140). Bromocriptine is the most widely studied and has a clinical efficacy comparable to that of L-DOPA. It has been employed for intolerable dyskinesia, dystonic cramps, late Sinemet failure, and the on-off phenomenon. While it has some antiparkinsonian efficacy when used alone, it is often short-lived (90), and it is questioned whether it offers any additional benefit to well-monitored Sinemet therapy. There may, however, be some additional antiparkinsonian benefit from combining bromocriptine with Sinemet. On-off fluctuations may be smoothed, but they are not eliminated. Dyskinesia and cramps are relieved in an occasional patient and only rarely does a patient respond to bromocriptine who did not respond to Sinemet. The side effects are similar to those of L-DOPA, but the psychosis and hypotension may be more pronounced (129). Furthermore, bromocriptine is extremely expensive and beyond the budget of many patients. In general, DA agonists have largely been relegated to the role of adjunct agents.

When bromocriptine is employed, it is generally used in combination with L-DOPA or Sinemet. Because the side effects are cumulative, we gradually taper the dosage of Sinemet while adding bromocriptine. In most patients, a daily dose of 20 to 60 mg in divided dosages is prescribed while the dosage of Sinemet is halved.

The failure of DA agonists to significantly influence the on-off phenomenon makes it unlikely that an accumulation of DOPA metabolites or a fluctuation in the serum level of L-DOPA is responsible for the on-off phenomenon. Ergoline derivatives which are long-acting DA agonists are currently being investigated in the hope that they will provide more constant and sustained DA receptor stimulation (92). Theoretically, they offer little more than further flogging of the DA receptor and do not address the problem of receptor desensitization. They are not likely to substantially improve upon our current level of therapy.

Surgery

Pedunculotomy was at one time performed for the tremor and rigidity of advanced parkinsonism. By serendipity, it was discovered that ligation of the anterior choroidal artery improved parkinsonian symptoms without inducing a hemiparesis (31). It has subsequently been recognized that lesions in the medial part of the globus pallidus or in the VL nucleus of the thalamus could improve tremor and to a lesser degree rigidity (82). The use of surgery has largely been supplanted by advances in medical therapy. It may still have a role in those patients in whom tremor, particularly if one sided, remains a persistent problem. Surgery has also been used in those patients where unilateral dyskinesia represents a dose-limiting side effect of dopaminergic therapy.

Newer Therapeutic Directions

Current therapeutic investigations involve three approaches (106):

(1) Drugs which potentiate DA activity—Dopamine is metabolized by catechol-*o*-methyltransferase (COMT) and MAO into homovanillic acid (HVA), and by dopamine β-hydroxylase (DBH) into norepinephrine (Fig. 8.2). Blockade of each of these enzymes has been attempted in an effort to enhance the L-DOPA effect so that dosage can be reduced. Inhibition of the MAO-β enzyme by deprenil (an MAO-β inhibitor) has been studied in humans and is reported to decrease the on-off phenomena (13).

(2) Selective DA receptor stimulation—an attempt to stimulate DA receptors in the neostriatum but not in the limbic system or elsewhere; an attempt to stimulate specific classes of striatal DA receptors in order to obtain a specific DA response.

(3) DA receptor-stabilizing agents—example, lithium.

All of these are currently under investigation in both laboratory and therapeutic trials. It seems unlikely that further stimulation of the DA receptor will significantly improve therapeutic efficacy. The development of dyskinesia, the risk of DA receptor damage due to the accumulation of toxic metabolic byproducts, and desensitization of the DA receptor all appear to be limiting factors to this approach. Selective DA receptor stimulation may be of value in preventing psychosis but is unlikely to relieve dyskinesia or the on-off effect. DA receptor-stabilizing agents are theoretically promising, but clinical trials are lacking.

It must be emphasized that all of these approaches deal with Parkinson's syndrome in a symptomatic manner. None prevent progression of the disorder or deal with the underlying etiology. An understanding of the different etiologies and pathogenetic mechanisms responsible for the state of DA deficiency and the dopaminergic-cholinergic imbalance is esential if the disease is to be arrested or eradicated.

CHOREIFORM DISORDERS

Chorea ("dance") is a disorder characterized by involuntary, nonpatterned, rapid, graceful, semipurposeful movements which interfere with coordinated movement. There is a predilection for involvement of the lips, mouth, and tongue (oro buccal lingual) in tardive dyskinesia and for the limbs in Huntington's chorea. Distal muscles tend to be more affected than proximal muscles but a generalized diffuse involvement can occur. Movements increase with agitation and disappear with sleep. Pathologically the basal ganglia may be diffusely affected with a particular dropout of small cells in the neostriatum. Chorea is analogous to Parkinson's syndrome in that clinical manifestations are a function of an altered neuropharmacologic state in which there is an imbalance between the dopaminergic and cholinergic systems. Where parkinsonism relfects a state of DA deficiency, chorea is related to excessive striatal DA activity. Chorea is characteristically diminished by DA blocking agents and increased by L-DOPA or DA agonists (25, 136). As with parkinsonism, it should be appreciated that chorea is a syndrome and not a disease process and that it may be a feature of numerous etiologies, as illustrated in Table 8.4.

Huntington's chorea is an autosomal dominant hereditary disorder of unknown etiology first described by George Huntington in 1872 (72). Chorea develops in association with a progressive dementia and emotional disturbances. Dysarthria, facial grimacing, and grinding of the jaw are commonly observed. Dementia or psychiatric problems may be the initial clinical manifestation, and there is a high incidence of suicide and criminal behavior in these patients. A juvenile "akinetic rigid" form of the disease has been described (14).

Degeneration of the basal ganglia, particularly the caudate nucleus, can be recognized radiologically and patholoIgically. A reduction in GABA and ACH, as well as their synthetic enzymes, glutamic acid

TABLE 8.4
Differential Diagnosis of Chorea

Genetic
Huntington's chorea
Infectious
Sydenham's
Postexanthematous chorea
Syphilis
Drug-induced
L-DOPA + DA agonists
Dilantin
Lithium
Anticholinergic
Oral contraceptives
Tardive dyskinesia
Phenothiazines and butyrophenones
Toxic
Mercury
Metabolic
Hypoparathyroidism + hypocalcemia
Hyperthyroidism
Hypomagnesemia
Porphyria
Hyponatremia
Addison's disease
Cirrhosis of liver
Wilson's disease
Vascular
Henoch-Schonlein purpura
Stroke
Systemic lupus erythematosis
Miscellaneous
Chorea gravidarum
Senile chorea
B_{12} deficiency
Thiamine deficiency

decarboxylase (GAD) and choline acetyltransferase (CAT), has been demonstrated in the neostriatum, substantia nigra, and globus pallidus (11, 98, 137). Reduced ACH and GABA activity results in uninhibited DA activity leading to a state of increased DA receptor stimulation and the clinical syndrome of chorea (5). This hypothesis is supported by the observation that kainic acid in an animal model of Huntington's chorea induces striatal degeneration with a loss of GABA binding sites (153). A loss of GABA receptors may explain the lack of efficacy of GABA mimetic agents.

Tardive dyskinesia is also worthy of special comment. This is a choreiform movement disorder which tends to specifically involve the mouth, lips, and tongue. It may become generalized, however, and be indistinguishable from Huntington's chorea. It is seen following prolonged use of antipsychotic drugs such as phenothiazines and butyrophenones (39, 58). It is more common in females and the elderly. Unlike the reversible chorea seen with L-DOPA, however, tardive dyskinesia may be permanent. Tardive dyskinesia is thought to be related to drug-induced damage of the DA receptor, leading to an increased synthesis of DA receptors and denervation hypersensitivity (83). Studies in rats and humans confirm that neuroleptic drugs can induce an increase in striatal DA receptors (17). The onset of dyskinesia may not be appreciated while patients are on phenothiazine or butyrophenone medications, since they simultaneously induce a DA blockade. Chorea may break through after long-term use of these medications (DA supersensitivity has progressed to critical point) or on discontinuing the drug (DA blockade removed). Reintroduction of these medications may transiently reduce dyskinesia but at the expense of further receptor damage possibly leading to a more severe chorea. The best therapy for tardive dyskinesia is prevention. When antipsychotic drugs are employed, the following guidelines should be observed:

(a) Always use as low a dose as will provide an adequate clinical response.
(b) Periodically assess the necessity of continuing therapy.
(c) Consider "drug holidays"—drugs are discontinued for days to weeks which allows the clinician to determine if chorea is developing. The "drug holiday" may reduce the likelihood of receptor damage and consequent denervation hypersensitivity.
(d) Don't employ concurrent antiparkinsonian drugs such as Artane, which may facilitate the development of tardive dyskinesia (16).

Treatment of Chorea

As with Parkinson's syndrome, treatment revolves around establishing the correct diagnosis, correcting any underlying disorder, psychotherapy, physiotherapy, educating the family, genetic counseling, and neuropharmacologic manipulation. Drugs used to treat chorea decrease DA availability (Fig. 8.7), or increase ACH activity. The major side effect of this form of therapy is a reversible Parkinsonian-like syndrome due to DA deficiency. It is analogous to the reversible choreiform syndrome due to excess DA stimulation seen as a complication of L-DOPA therapy in Parkinson's syndrome (Fig. 8.6). As with Parkinson's syndrome, drugs may modify the symptoms of chorea but do not affect the underlying

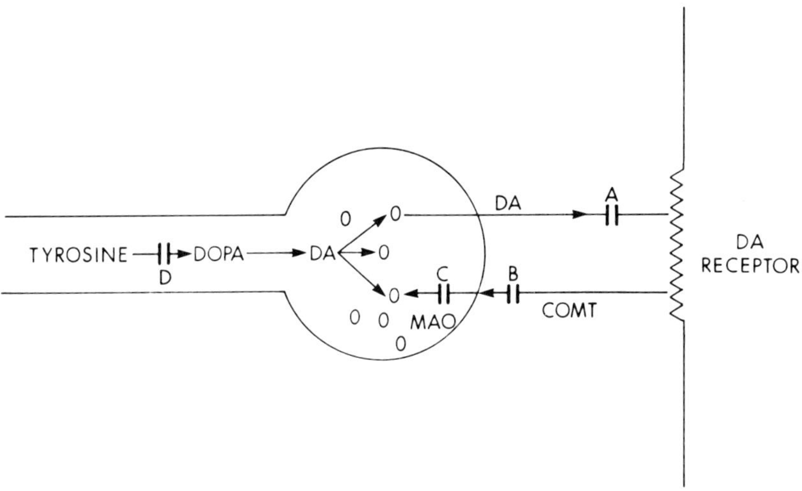

FIG. 8.7. Site of action of DA-blocking drugs. DA is stored in presynaptic granules and released to stimulate DA receptor. The majority of DA is taken back up into the presynaptic terminal by a membrane pump and ultimately restored in the presynaptic granules. *A*, block of receptor—phenothiazines, butyrophenones; *B*, block of membrane pump—phenothiazines, butyrophenones; *C*, block of uptake into presynaptic granules—reserpine, tetrabenazine; *D*, block of DA synthesis—α-methylparatyrosine.

disease process which, as in the case of Huntington's disease, continues to progress. The classes of drugs employed include:

(a) Phenothiazines and butyrophenones—block dopamine neurotransmission as well as the membrane pump which is necessary for the reuptake of DA. The disadvantage of these drugs is that they may damage DA receptors and lead to a tardive dyskinesia (59).

(b) Reserpine and tetrabenazine—block the uptake of DA into the presynaptic granules and deplete brain DA (77).

(c) α-methylparatyrosine—acts as a false transmitter to block catechol synthesis (55).

(d) Choline and lecithin—cholinergic stimulators (41, 65). They are presumed to increase ACH in the brain and restore the DA-ACH balance.

(d) GABA-minergic drugs (*e.g.*, valproic acid, muscimol, isoniazid, imidazoleacetic acid and GABA)—theoretically increase available GABA and thus inhibit the release of DA. They depend on intact GABA-minergic neurons to be effective, which limits their usefulness. They have failed to ameliorate Huntington's chorea (120, 131–133) but may benefit tardive dyskinesia (27, 96).

Each of the above therapeutic strategies, either singly or in combination, has been employed to treat chorea. The clinical response is a function of the underlying disease state, but generally is only of limited value. A common approach is to start the patient on haldol while reserpine is being introduced in gradual doses in order to avoid depression. Haldol is then discontinued, and reserpine is matained ether alone or in combination with α-methylparatyrosine (55). The observation that tardive dyskinesia is more prominent in postmenopausal women has led to trials of estrogen which are reported to be of some value (38). Of perhaps greater promise is the evidence previously described that lithium pretreatment may prevent neuroleptic-induced DA supersensitivity (121). While L-DOPA might be expected to aggravate chorea, it has been reported to desensitize the supersensitive DA receptor, and might be of value in tardive dyskinesia.

As with Parkinson's syndrome, therapy for chorea is symptomatic. Until such time as the etiology of the underlying disease state has been identified and the pathogenetic mechanisms have been defined, specific therapy cannot be designed.

DYSTONIA

Dystonic movements consist of slow, strong, sustained, torsional movements of somatic musculature. These involuntary movements may occur anywhere but there is a predilection for the trunk, neck, and proximal limb muscles. The movement resembles that of athetosis but is more sustained. The anatomic and pharmacologic basis of dystonia is unknown. As with other movement disorders, dystonia can be seen in association with multiple etiologies. It has been described as a feature of Wilson's disease, postencephalitic parkinsonism, encephalitis, Hallervorden-Spatz disease, hyperparathyroidism, tumors and other diseases of the basal ganglia, and as a complication of anoxia. A reversible dystonia may occur as a side effect of neuroleptic or L-DOPA therapy. Dystonia may be an isolated feature or may be associated with other neurological symptoms.

Dystonia musculorum deformans appears to be a specific entity. It is a rare hereditary disease reported with increased frequency in families of Russian-Jewish descent (52). The onset of symptoms is generally between 5 and 15 years and consists of abnormal movements and torsion spasms. These initially involve the lower extremities and pelvis, resulting in a gait disturbance. The muscles of the upper extremities, neck, and face may be involved later in the course of the disease. Dysarthria, facial grimacing, and torticollis may be features of this syndrome. The involuntary movements and spasms are increased by volitional movements or anxiety and disappear with sleep. The diagnosis is relatively easy in well-advanced cases but is often confused with hysteria and other psychological disorders in the early stages. The disease usually progresses to death within 5 to 10 years in the more severe forms. Minor changes in the basal ganglia and thalamus have been observed pathologically, but no specific lesion has been found to account for dystonia (154). Recently, serum levels of DA β-hydroxylase were found to be elevated, suggesting a possible disorder of DA metabolism (151).

There is no effective therapy for dystonia unless the primary disturbance can be corrected. Symptomatic therapy usually consists of trials of sedatives, phenothiazines, muscle relaxants, and antiparkinsonian drugs but those are rarely of significant benefit. L-DOPA has been reported to improve or aggravate dystonia. Surgical destruction of the globus pallidus and thalamus unilaterally and bilaterally is reported to benefit some patients, but may lead to pseudobulbar palsy (29). Physiotherapy and psychotherapy should not be ignored.

SPASMODIC TORTICOLLIS

Spasmodic torticollis is a localized form of dystonia involving muscles of the head and neck. It is characterized by paroxysmal stereotyped contractions of these muscles, resulting in a sustained deviation of the head to one side. Occasionally the head may be hyperextended (retrocollis) or flexed. Torticollis may be a fragment of a more generalized dystonic syndrome or a consequence of local disease in the neck. In the majority of cases, however, it is an isolated dystonic symptom of undetermined etiology. In some patients, there is an associated essential tremor (36). Psychological factors may adversely affect torticollis and personality disorders occur in 50% of studied cases. Unlike Parkinson's syndrome and Huntington's chorea, there is no rational basis for therapy. Focal lesions in the mesencephalic tegmentum of monkeys are reported to produce spasmodic torticollis (57), but no histological changes have been found in human patients (139).

Improvement has been reported after butyrophenones (32), phenothiazines (15), L-DOPA (128), bromocriptine (19), lithium (37), amantadine (60), diazepam (10), etc., but these have generally been of limited effectiveness. The various medical approaches are summarized in a review by Lal (87). Psychotherapy and biofeedback may be of value for an individual patient, but the response is often temporary and inconsistent. Despite the inadequacy of medical therapy, a conservative approach is recommended since patients frequently spontaneously improve or remit after 5 to 10 years of symptoms.

Various operative procedures have been tried. The most widely employed has been section of the first four anterior cervical roots bilaterally in combination with division of branches of the spinal accessory nerve to affected muscles in the neck (124). This approach is generally reserved for patients who are severely affected and functionally disabled. Stereotactic therapy has been reported to improve some patients but is not recommended since widespread bilateral destructive lesions are generally required (30).

ATHETOSIS

Athetosis is a movement disorder characterized by involuntary, irregular, slow, writhing, repeated movements first described by Hammond in 1871 (69). It consists of cramp-like and spasmodic movements which are slower than choreiform movements and less sustained than dystonia. There is a spectrum between the extremes of chorea and dystonia and athetotic movements may be combined with either of these. Athetosis is the result of relatively sustained, unequal contractions of agonist and antagonist muscle groups. Any part of the body may be involved, but the face and distal upper extremities are preferentially affected, often with an accompanying hemiplegia. Double athetosis refers to bilateral involvement and usually develops in infants as the result of developmental defects and birth trauma. Acquired athetosis may also be seen following infarction, hemorrhage, tumor, CNS storage diseases, Wilson's disease, and Hallervorden-Spatz disease. Like chorea and parkinsonism, athetosis is a symptom and not a specific disease process. When it is the result of a monophasic illness (*e.g.*, stroke), it does not progress.

Pathologically, athetosis is associated with lesions throughout the basal ganglia. In infantile cases, large myelinated fiber bundles crisscross throughout the striatum, resembling heavily grained marble. This is referred to as "status marmoratus." The pharmacologic and anatomic basis of this movement is unknown.

Therapy is symptomatic and not particularly effective. Physiotherapy, drugs, and surgery have been used. There are reports of improvement with L-DOPA (126) but this is of limited benefit. Thalamotomy has also been reported to help some patients (31). The prognosis is a function of the underlying disease.

ESSENTIAL TREMOR

Essential tremor is a benign familial disorder which is occasionally confused with parkinsonism. Unlike the resting tremor characteristic of parkinsonism, essential tremor is a postural tremor which is more pronounced on intention. It is aggravated by anxiety, reduced by rest, and disappears during sleep. Titubation of the head and tremor of the voice are frequent features. Symptoms usually progress with age. A few families have an associated torticollis (40), but in the majority of patients no other abnormalities are present. No consistent pathology has been observed.

Improvement often occurs with small doses of valium, possibly related to its sedative effect or its GABA-minergic activity. Alcohol can also improve tremor but may cause intoxication (66). Recently, β-adrenergic blockers such as propanolol have been found to induce a dramatic improvement in one-third of patients (150). They cannot be employed in patients with asthma or congestive heart failure, but a new β blocker, metopropolol, can be used for asthmatic patients.

HEMIBALLISMUS

Hemiballismus is a rare disorder consisting of extreme violent flinging movements of the arm and leg on one side of the body. It is due to partial destruction of the contralateral subthalamic nucleus which results in the loss of its inhibiting influence on the output of the globus pallidus (21). The lesion is usually due to hemorrhage or infarction, but may also occur as the result of tumor, abscess, or thalamic surgery. Unchecked, these movements may result in exhaustion and ultimately death. Fortunately, most cases remit spontaneously (73). Neuroleptic agents have been tried in large doses with some success (61). If there is no response, a surgical lesion in the VL nucleus of the thalamus or in the lateral portion of the globus pallidus is recommended (105).

GILLES de la TOURETTE SYNDROME

Gilles de la Tourette syndrome (tic convulsive) is a disease of unknown cause with onset in early childhood. It consists of multiple motor and vocal tics with occasional coprolalia. Personality disorder, sexual aberrations, and self-mutilation may be associated features. Seventy to 90% of cases occur in males. There is an increased likelihood of tics and vocalizations in family members, suggesting that there is a hereditary predisposition to this disorder (51, 62, 113).

As with other movement disorders, therapy is largely symptomatic. Haldol has been widely used and is generally effective (127). This suggests that DA receptor hyperactivity plays a role in the pathogensis. Paradoxically Tourette syndrome has been reported following long-term phenothiazine therapy (84). Lecithin, clonazepam, reserpine, tetrabenazine and α-methylparatyrosine have all been tried with some effectiveness, as have psychotherapy and behavioral modification.

LESCH-NYHAN SYNDROME

This is a sex-linked recessive disorder which has many similarities to the Gilles de la Tourette syndrome (135). Patients may have chorea, athetosis, dystonia, and tics as well as corticospinal tract signs. They are noted to have strikingly aggressive, compulsive, and self-destructive behavior. The latter is a much more prominent feature than in the Gilles de la Tourette syndrome and frequently involves chewing of fingers and lips and picking at wounds (115). This disorder is associated with a reduction in hypoxanthine-guanine-phosphoribosyl-transferase. There is an associated reduction in dopamine β-hydroxylase and an increased serum uric acid. Therapy has consisted of combinations of allopurinol, 5-hydroxytryptophane, phenothiazines, and diazepam.

REFERENCES

1. Aghajanian, G. K., and Bunney, B. S. Central dopaminergic neurons: neurophysiological identification and responses to drugs. In Frontiers in Catecholamine Research, edited by E. Usdin and S. Snyder, pp. 643–648. Pergamon Press, London, 1973.
2. Anden, N. E., Dahlstrom, A., Fuxe, K., and Larsson, K. Functional role of the nigro-neostriatal dopamine neurons. Acta Pharmacol., *24:* 263–274, 1966.
3. Anden, N. E., Dahlstrom, A., Fuxe, K., Larsson, K., Olson, L., and Ungerstedt, U. Ascending monoamine neurons to the telencephalon and diencephalon. Acta Physiol. Scand., *67:* 313–326, 1966.
4. Anden, N. E., Carlsson, A., Dahlstron, A., Fuxe, K., Hillard, N. A., and Larsson, K. Demonstration and mapping out of nigro-neostriatal dopamine neurons. Life Sci., *3:* 523–530, 1964.
5. Aquilonius, S. M., and Sjostrom, R. Cholinergic and dopaminergic mechanisms in Huntington's chorea. Life Sci., *10:* 405–414, 1971.
6. Barbeau, A. Biochemistry of Parkinson's disease. Excerpta Med. Int. Congr. Ser., *38:* 152–153, 1961.
7. Barbeau, A. The clinical physiology of side effects in long-term L-DOPA therapy. Adv. Neurol., *5:* 347–365, 1974.
8. Barbeau, A., Mars, H., and Gillo-Joffroy, L. Adverse clinical side effects of levo-dopa therapy. *In* Recent Advances in Parkinson's Disease, edited by F. H. McDowell, and C. H. Markham, pp. 203–237. Davis, Philadelphia, 1971.
9. Barbeau, A., Mars, H., Gillo-Joffroy, L., and Arsenault, A. A proposed classification of dopa-induced dyskinesias. In L-Dopa and Parkinsonism, edited by A. Barbeau, and F. H. MacDowell, pp. 118–120. Davis, Philadelphia, 1970.
10. Bianchine, J. R., and Bianchine, J. W. Treatment of spasmodic torticollis with diazepam. South. Med. J., *64:* 893–894, 1971.
11. Bird, E. D., and Iversen, L. L. Huntington's chorea. Brain, *97:* 457–472, 1974.
12. Birkmayer, W., and Hornykiewicz, O. Der L-Dioxyphenylalanin (L-Dopa—Effekt bei der Parkinson Akinese. Wien Klin. Wochenschr., *73:* 787–788, 1961.
13. Birkmayer, W., Riederer P., Youdim, B. H., and Linauer, W. The potentiation of the anti-akinetic effect after L-dopa treatment by an inhibitor of MAO-B, deprenil. J. Neural. Transm., *36:* 303–326, 1975.
14. Bittenbender, J. B., and Quadfasel, F. A. Rigid and akinetic forms of Huntington's chorea. Arch. Neurol., *7:* 275–288, 1962.
15. Blom, S., and Ekbom, K. A. Comparison between akathisia developing in treatment with phenothiazine derivatives and the restless leg syndrome. Acta Med. Scand., *170:* 689–694, 1961.
16. Burnett, G. B., Prange, A. J., Wilson, I. C., Jolliff, L. A., Creese, I. C., and Snyder, S. H. Adverse effects of anticholinergic anti-Parkinsonian drugs in tardive dyskinesia. Neuropsychobiology, *6:* 109–120, 1980.
17. Burt, D. R., Creese, I., and Snyder, S. Anti-schizophrenic drugs: chronic treatment elevates dopamine receptor binding in the brain. Science, *196:* 326–328, 1977.
18. Butcher, L. L., and Hodge, G. K. Selective bilateral lesions of pars compacta of the

substantia nigra: effects on motor processes and ingestive behaviors. Adv. Neurol., *24:* 71–82, 1979.

19. Calne, D. B., Stern, G. M., Spiers, A. S. D., and Laurence, D. R. L-Dopa in idiopathic Parkinsonism. Lancet, *2:* 973–976, 1969.
20. Carlson, A. Some aspects of dopamine in the basal ganglia. Res. Publ. Assoc. Rev. Nerv. Ment. Dis., *55:* 181–189, 1976.
21. Carpenter, M. B. Ballism associated with partial destruction of the subthalamic nucleus of Luys. Neurology, *5:* 479–489, 1955.
22. Carpenter, M. B. Anatomy of the basal ganglia and related nuclei: a review. Adv. Neurol., *14:* 7–48, 1976.
23. Carpenter, M. B., Whittier, J. R., and Mettler, F. A. Tremor in the Rhesus monkey produced by diencephalic lesions and studied by a graphic method. J. Comp. Neurol., *93:* 1–15, 1950.
24. Carroll, B. J., Curtis, G. C., and Kokmen, E. Paradoxical responses to dopamine agonists in tardive dyskinesia. Am. J. Psychol., *134:* 785–789, 1977.
25. Chase, T. N. Drug-induced extrapyramidal disorder. Res. Pub. Assoc. Res. Nerv. Ment. Dis., *50:* 448–471, 1972.
26. Chase, T. N., Holden, E. M., and Brody, J. A. Levodopa-induced dyskinesias: comparison in Parkinsonism—dementia and amyotrophic lateral sclerosis. Arch. Neurol., *29:* 328–330, 1973.
27. Chase, T. N., and Tamminga, C. A. Dopamine and GABA agonists in the treatment of hyperkinetic extrapyramidal disorders. Adv. Neurol., *24:* 379–386, 1979.
28. Claveria, L. E., Calne, D. B., and Allen, J. G. "On-off" phenomena related to high plasma levodopa. Br. Med. J., *11:* 641–643, 1973.
29. Cooper, I. S. Dystonia reversal by operation on basal ganglia. Arch. Neurol., *7:* 132–145, 1962.
30. Cooper, I. S. Effect of thalamic lesions upon torticollis. N. Engl. J. Med., *270:* 967–972, 1964.
31. Cooper, I. S. Involuntary Movement Disorders. Hoeber, New York, 1969.
32. Cotzias, G. C., Papavasiliou, P. S., Fehling, C., Kaufman, B., and Mean, I. Similarities between neurologic effects of L-Dopa and of apomorphine. N. Engl. J. Med., *282:* 31–33, 1970.
33. Cotzias, G. C., Papavasiliou, P. S., and Gellene, R. Modification of Parkinsonism: chronic treatment with L-dopa. N. Engl. J. Med., *280:* 337–345, 1969.
34. Cotzias, G. C., VanWoert, M. H., and Schiffer, L. M. Aromatic amino acids and modification of Parkinsonism. N. Engl. J. Med., *276:* 374–380, 1967.
35. Cotzias, G. C., Papavasiliou, P. S., Tolosa, E. S., Mensez, J. S., and Bell-Midura, M. Treatment of Parkinson's disease with aporphines—possible role of growth hormone. N. Engl. J. Med., *294:* 567–572, 1976.
36. Couch, J. R. Dystonia and tremor in spasmodic torticollis. Adv. Neurol., *14:* 245–258, 1976.
37. Couper-Smartt, J. Lithium in spasmodic torticollis. Lancet, *2:* 741–742, 1973.
38. Crane, G. E. Tardive dyskinesia in patients treated with major neuroleptics. A review of the literature. Am. J. Psychol. (Suppl.), *124:* 40–48, 1968.
39. Crane, G. E. Is tardive dyskinesia a drug effect? Am. J. Psychol., *130*(2)*:* 1043, 1973.
40. Critchley, M. Observations on essential (heredo-familial) tremor. Brain, *72:* 113–139, 1949.
41. Davis, K. L., Berger, P. A., and Hollister, L. E. Choline for tardive dyskinesia. N. Engl. J. Med., *293:* 152, 1975.
42. Delong, M. R. Putamen: activity of single units during slow and rapid arm movements. Science, *179:* 1240–1242, 1973.

43. Diamond, S. G., and Markham, C. H. Present mortality in Parkinson's disease: the ratio of observed to expected deaths with a method to calculate expected deaths. J. Neural. Transm., *38:* 259–269, 1976.
44. Direnfeld, L. K., Feldman, R. G., Alexander, M. P., and Kelly-Hayes, M. Is L-Dopa drug holiday useful? Neurology, *30:* 785–788, 1980.
45. Direnfeld, L., Spero, L., Marotta, J., and Seeman, P. The L-dopa on-off effect in Parkinson's disease: treatment by transient withdrawal and dopamine receptor resensitization. Ann. Neurol., *4:* 573–575, 1978.
46. Divac, I., Fonnum, F., and Storm-Mathisen J. High affinity uptake of glutamate in terminals of cortico-striatal axons. Nature, *266:* 377–378, 1977.
47. Dougan, D., Wade, D., and Mearrick, P. Effects of L-dopa metabolites at a dopamine receptor suggest a basis for "on-off" effect in Parkinson's disease. Nature, *254:* 70–72, 1975.
48. Duby, S. E., Cotzias, G. C., Papavasiliou, P. S., and Lawrence, W. H. Injected apomorphine and orally administered levodopa in parkinsonism. Arch. Neurol., *27:* 474–480, 1972.
49. Duvoisin, R. C. Cholinergic-anticholinergic antagonism in Parkinsonism. Arch. Neurol., *17:* 124–136, 1967.
50. Ehringer, H., and Hornykiewicz, O. Verteilung von Noradrenalin und Dopamin (3-Hydroxytyramin) im Gehirn des Menschen und ihr Verhalten bei Erkrankungen des extrapyramidalen Systems. Klin. Wochenschr., *38:* 1236–1239, 1960.
51. Eldridge, R., Sweet, R., Lake, C. R., Ziegler, M., and Shapiro, A. K. Gilles de la Tourette's syndrome: clinical, genetic, psychologic and biochemical aspects in 21 selected families. Neurology, *27*(1): 115–124, 1977.
52. Eldridge, R., Ryan, E., Brody, J. A., and Cooper, I. S. Dystonia musculorum deformans: evidence for two hereditary forms. Neurology, *18*(1): 287, 1968.
53. Ezrin-Waters, C., and Seeman, P. L-dopa reversal of hyperdopaminergic behaviour. Life Sci., *22:* 1027–1032, 1978.
54. Fahn, S. "On-off" phenomenon with levodopa therapy in Parkinsonism. Neurology, *24:* 431–444, 1974.
55. Fahn, S. Treatment of tardive dyskinesia with combined reserpine and alphamethyltyrosine. Ann. Neurol., *4:* 169, 1978.
56. Fahn, S., and Cote, L. J. Regional distribution of gamma ammino butyric acid (GABA) in brain of the Rhesus monkey. J. Neurochem., *15:* 209–213, 1968.
57. Foltz, E. L., Knopp, L. M., and Ward, A. A. Experimental spasmodic torticollis. J. Neurosurg., *16:* 55–72, 1959.
58. Food and Drug Administration Task Force, American College of Neuropsychopharmacology. Neurological syndromes associated with anti-psychotic drug use: a special report. Arch. Gen. Psychiatry *28:* 463–467, 1973.
59. Gallager, D. W., Pert, A., and Bunney, W. E., Jr. Haloperidol induced pre-synaptic dopamine supersensitivity is blocked by chronic lithium. Nature, *273:* 309–312, 1978.
60. Gilbert, G. J. The medical treatment of spasmodic torticollis. Arch. Neurol., *27:* 503–506, 1972.
61. Gilbert, G. J. Response of hemiballismus to haloperidol. J.A.M.A., *233:* 535–536, 1975.
62. Golden, G. C. Tourette syndrome: the pediatric perspective. Am. J. Dis. Child., *131:* 531–534, 1977.
63. Granger, M. Exacerbations in Parkinsonism. Neurology, *11:* 538–545, 1961.
64. Greenfield, J. G., and Bosanquet, F. D. The brain-stem lesions in Parkinsonism. J. Neurol. Neurosurg. Psychiatry, *16:* 213–226, 1953.
65. Growdon, J. H., Hirsch, M. J., Wurtman, R. J., and Wiener, W. Oral choline administration to patients with tardive dyskinesia. N. Engl. J. Med., *297:* 524–527, 1977.

66. Growdon, J. H., Shahani, B. T., and Young, R. R. The effect of alcohol on essential tremor. Neurology, *25:* 259–262, 1975.
67. Gudelsky, G. A., Thornburg, J. E., and Moore, K. E. Blockade of alpha-methyltyrosine induced supersensitivity to apomorphine by chronic administration of L-dopa. Life Sci., *16:* 1331–1338, 1975.
68. Hassler, R. Electromicroscopic differentiation of the extrinsic and intrinsic types of nerve cells and synapsis in the striatum and their putative transmitters. Adv. Neurol., *24:* 93–108, 1979.
69. Hammond, W. A. A Treatise on Diseases of the Nervous System. Appleton, New York, 1871.
70. Hong, J., Yang, H. Y. T., Racagni, G., and Costa, E. Projections of substance P containing neurons from neostriatum to substantia nigra. Brain Res., *122:* 541–544, 1977.
71. Hunter, K. R., Shaw, K. M., and Lawrence, D. R. Sustained levodopa therapy in Parkinsonism. Lancet, *2:* 929–931, 1973.
72. Huntington, G. On chorea. Med. Surg. Reporter, *26:* 317, 1872.
73. Hyland, H. H., and Forman, D. Prognosis in hemiballismus. Neurology, *7:* 381–391, 1957.
74. Jessell, T. M. Substance P release from the rat substantia nigra. Brain. Res., *151:* 469–478, 1978.
75. Joseph, C., Chassan, J. B., and Koch, M. L. Levodopa in Parkinson's disease: a long-term appraisal of mortality. Ann. Neurol., *3:* 116–118, 1978.
76. Kartzinel, R., and Calne, D. B. Studies with bromocriptine. I. "On-off" phenomena. Neurology, *26:* 508–510, 1976.
77. Kazamatsuri, H., Chien, C., and Cole, J. O. Treatment of tardive dyskinesia. I. Clinical efficacy of a dopamine depleting agent, tetrabenazine. Arch. Gen. Psychiatry, *27:* 95–99, 1972.
78. Kazamatsuri, H., Chien, C., and Cole, J. O. Treatment of tardive dyskinesia. II. Short term efficacy of dopamine blocking agents, haloperidol and thiopropazate. Arch. Gen. Psychiatry, *27:* 100–103, 1972.
79. Kebabian, J. W. Multiple classes of dopamine receptors in mammalian central nervous system: the involvement of dopamine-sensitive adrenyl cyclase. Life Sci., *23:* 479–484, 1978.
80. Kebabian, J. W., and Calne, D. B. Multiple receptors for dopamine. Nature, *277:* 93–96, 1979.
81. Kebabian, J. W., Petzold, G. L., and Greengard, P. Dopamine-sensitive adenylate cyclase in caudate nucleus of rat brain, and its similarity to the "dopamine receptor." Proc. Natl. Acad. Sci. USA, *69:* 2145–2149, 1972.
82. Kelly, P. J., Derome, P., and Guiot, G. Thalamic spatial variability and the surgical results of lesions placed with neurophysiologic control. Surg. Neurol., *9:* 307–315, 1978.
83. Klawans, H. L. The pharmacology of tardive dyskinesia. Am. J. Psychol., *130:* 82–86, 1973.
84. Klawans, H. L., Falk, D. A., Nausieda, P. A., and Weiner, W. J. Gilles de la Tourette syndrome after long-term chlorpromazine therapy. Neurology, *28:* 1064–1065, 1978.
85. Klawans, H. L., Goetz C., Nausieda, P. A., and Weiner, W. J. Levodopa-induced dopamine receptor hypersensitivity. Ann. Neurol., *2:* 125–129, 1977.
86. Klawans, H. L., Topel, J. L., and Bergen, D. Deanol in treatment of levodopa-induced dyskinesias. Neurology, *25:* 290–293, 1975.
87. Lal, S. Pathophysiology and pharmacotherapy of spasmodic torticollis: a review. Can. J. Neurol. Sci., *6:* 427–435, 1979.

88. Lamarre, Y. Tremorgenic mechanisms in primates. Adv. Neurol., *10:* 23–34, 1975.
89. Lee, T., Seeman, P., Rajput, A., Farley, I. J., and Hornykiewicz, O. Receptor basis for dopaminergic supersensitivity in Parkinson's disease. Nature, *273:* 59–61, 1978.
90. Lees, A. J., Haddad, S., Shaw, K. M., Kohout, L. J., and Stern, G. M. Bromocriptine in Parkinsonism—A long term study. Arch. Neurol., *35:* 503–505, 1978.
91. Lees, A. J., Shaw, K. M., and Stern, G. M. Bromocriptine and spasmodic torticollis. Br. Med. J., *1*(2)*:* 1343, 1976.
92. Lemberger, L., Crabtree, R., and Callaghan, J. T. Pergolide, a potent long-acting dopamine-receptor agonist. Clin. Pharmacol. Ther., *27:* 642–651, 1980.
93. Lieberman, A., Dziatolowski, M., Kupersmith, M., Serby, M., Goodgold, A., Korein, J., and Goldstein, M. Dementia in Parkinson disease. Ann. Neurol., *6:* 355–359, 1979.
94. Lieberman, A., Kupersmith, M., Estey, E., and Goldstein, M. Treatment of Parkinson's disease with bromocriptine. N. Engl. J. Med., *295:* 1400–1404, 1976.
95. Lieberman, A., Miyamoto, T., Battista, A., and Goldstein, M. Studies on the anti-Parkinsonian efficacy of lergotrile. Neurology, *25:* 459–462, 1975.
96. Linnoila, M., Viukari, M., and Hietala, O. Effect of sodium valproate on tardive dyskinesia. Br. J. Psychol., *129:* 114–119, 1974.
97. Lloyd, K. G., Davidson, L., and Hornykiewicz, O. The neurochemistry of Parkinson's disease: effect of L-Dopa therapy. J. Pharmacol. Exp. Ther., *195:* 453–464, 1975.
98. Lloyd, K. G., Dreksler, S., and Bird, E. D. Alterations in 3-H-GABA binding in Huntington's chorea. Life Sci., *21:* 747–754, 1977.
99. Lloyd, K. G., and Hornykiewicz, O. Parkinson's disease: activity of L-dopa decarboxylase in discrete brain regions. Science, *170:* 1212–1213, 1970.
100. Ludin, H. P., and Bass-Verrey, F. Study of deterioration in long-term treatment of Parkinsonism with L-dopa plus decarboxylase inhibitor. J. Neural. Transm., *38:* 249–258, 1976.
101. Markham, C. H. The "on-off" side effect of L-dopa. Adv. Neurol., *5:* 387–396, 1974.
102. Marsden, C. D., Duvoisin, R. C., Jenner, P., Parkes, J. D., Pycock, C., and Tarsy, D. Relationship between animal models and clinical parkinsonism. Adv. Neurology, Dopaminergic mechanisms, edited by D. B. Calne, T. N. Chase, and A. Barbeau, pp. 165–175, Vol. 9, Raven Press, New York, 1975.
103. Marsden, C. D., Parkes, J. D., Rees, J. E. A year's comparison of treatment of patients with Parkinson's disease with levodopa combined with carbidopa versus treatment with levodopa alone. Lancet, *2*(2)*:* 1459–1462, 1973.
104. Marsden, C. D., and Parkes, J. D. "On-off" effects in patients with Parkinson's disease on chronic levodopa therapy. Lancet, *1:* 292–296, 1976.
105. Martin, J. P., and McCaul, I. R. Acute hemiballismus treated by ventro-lateral thalamolysis. Brain, *82:* 104–108, 1959.
106. Marx, J. L. Parkinson's disease: search for better therapies. Science, *203:* 737–738, 1979.
107. Mena, I., and Cotzias, G. C. Protein intake and treatment of Parkinson's disease with levodopa. N. Engl. J. Med., *292:* 181–184, 1975.
108. Moskovitz, C., Moses, H., and Klawans, H. L. Levodopa-induced psychosis. A kindling phenomenon. Ann. Psychol., *135:* 6, 1978.
109. Muenter, M. D., Sharpless, N. S., Tyce, G. M., and Darley, F. L. Patterns of dystonia in response to L-dopa therapy for Parkinson's disease. Mayo Clin. Proc., *52:* 163–174, 1977.
110. McDellan, D. L., Chalmers, R. J., and Johnson, R. H. Clinical and pharmacological evaluation of the effects of piribedil in patients with Parkinonism. Acta Neurol. Scand., *51:* 74–82, 1975.
111. McLennan, H., and York, D. H. The action of dopamine neurons of the caudate nucleus. J. Physiol., *189:* 393–402, 1967.

112. Naidu, S., Wolfson, L. J., and Sharpless, N. S. Juvenile parkinsonism: a patient with possible primary striatal dysfunction. Ann. Neurol., *3:* 453–455, 1978.
113. Nee, L. E., Caine, E. D., Polinsky, R. J., Eldridge, R., and Ebbert, M. W. Gille de la Tourette syndrome: clinical and family study of 50 cases. Ann. Neurol., *7:* 41–49, 1980.
114. Ng, L. K., Chase, T. N., Colburn, R. W., and Kopin, I. J. L-dopa-induced release of cerebral monoamines. Science, *170:* 76–77, 1970.
115. Nyhan, W. L. Clinical features of the Lesch-Nyhan syndrome. Arch. Int. Med., *130:* 186–192, 1972.
116. Ohye, C., Bouchard, R., Larochelle, L., Bedard, P., Boucher, R., Raphy, B., and Poirier, L. J. Effect of dorsal rhizotomy on postural tremor in the monkey. Exp. Brain Res., *10:* 140–150, 1970.
117. Olanow, C. W., and Schwartz, A. M. A controlled blind double observer study of MK-486 (carbidopa) in Parkinson's Disease. In Current Concepts in the Treatment of Parkinsonism, edited by M. D. Yahr, pp. 69–86. Raven Press, New York, 1974.
118. Papavasiliou, P. S., Cotzias, G. C., and Mena, I. Short and long-term approaches to the "on-off" phenomenon. Adv. Neurol. *5:* 379–386, 1974.
119. Parkinson, J. An essay on the shaking palsy. Sherwood Neely and Jones, London, 1817.
120. Perry, T. L., Macleod, P. M., and Hansen, S. Treatment of Huntington's chorea with isoniazid. N. Engl. J. Med., *297:* 840, 1977.
121. Pert, A., Rosenblatt, J. E., Sivit, C., Pert, C. B., and Bunney, W. E., Jr. Long-term treatment with lithium prevents the development of dopamine receptor supersensitivity. Science, *201:* 171–173, 1978.
122. Poirier, L. J., and Sourkes, T. L. Influence of the substantia nigra on the catecholamine content of the striatum. Brain, *88:* 181–192, 1965.
123. Price, P., Debono, A., Kenner, P., Parkes, J. D., and Marsden, C. D. Is there evidence for different classes of cerebral dopamine receptors in man? Adv. Neurol., *24:* 423–431, 1979.
124. Putnam, T. S., Herz, E., and Glaser, G. H. Spasmodic torticollis. III. Surgical treatment. Arch. Neurol. Psychiatry, *61:* 240–247, 1949.
125. Rinne, U. K., Sonninen, V., and Siirtola, T. L-Dopa treatment in Parkinson's disease. Eur. Neurol., *4:* 348–369, 1970.
126. Rosenthal, P. K., McDowell, F. H., and Cooper, W. Levodopa therapy in athetoid cerebral palsy. Neurology, *22:* 1–11, 1972.
127. Shapiro, A. K., Shapiro, E., and Wayne, H. Treatment of Tourette's syndrome. Arch. Gen. Psychiatry, *28:* 92–97, 1973.
128. Shaw, K. M., Hunter, K. R., and Stern, G. M. Medical treatment of spasmodic torticollis. Lancet, *1:* 1399, 1972.
129. Shaw, K. M., Lees, A. J., and Stern, G. M. Bromocriptine in Parkinson's Disease. Lancet, *1*(2)*:* 1255, 1978.
130. Shimazu, H., Hongo, T., Kubota, K., and Narabayashi, H. Rigidity and spasticity in man. Arch. Neurol., *6:* 10–17, 1962.
131. Shoulson, I., Chase, T. N., Roberts, E., *et al.* Huntington's disease: treatment with imidazole-4 acetic acid. N. Engl. J. Med., *293:* 504–505, 1975.
132. Shoulson, I., Goldblatt, D., Charlton, M., and Joynt, R. Huntington's disease: treatment with muscimol, a GABA-minergic drug. Ann. Neurol., *4:* 279–284, 1978.
133. Shoulson, I., Kartzinel, R., and Chase, T. N. Huntington's disease: treatment with dipropylacetic acid and gamma-aminobutyric acid. Neurology, *26:* 61–63, 1976.
134. Shy, G. M., and Drager, C. A. A neurological syndrome associated with orthostatic hypotension: a clinical-pathological study. Arch. Neurol., *2:* 511, 1960.
135. Singer, H. S., Pepple, J. M., Ramage, A. L. and Butler, I. J. Gilles de la Tourette syndrome: further studies and thoughts. Ann. Neurol., *4:* 21–25, 1978.

136. Smith, R. C., Tamminga, C. A., Haraszti, J., Pandey, G. N., and Davis, J. M. Effects of dopamine agonists in tardive dyskinesia. Am. J. Psychol., *134:* 763–768, 1977.
137. Stahl, W. L., and Swanson, P. D. Biochemical abnormalities in Huntington's chorea brains. Neurology, *24:* 813–819, 1974.
138. Sweet, R. D., and McDowell, F. H. Five year's treatment of Parkinson's disease with levodopa. Ann. Int. Med., *83:* 456–463, 1975.
139. Tarlov, E. On the problem of pathology of spasmodic torticollis in man. J. Neurol. Neurosurg. Psychiatry *33:* 457–463, 1970.
140. Teychenne, P. F., Calne, D. B., Leigh, P. N., Greenacre, J. K., Reid, J. L., Petrie, A., and Bamji, A. N. Idiopathic parkinsonism treated with bromocriptine. Lancet, *2:* 473–476, 1975.
141. Timberlake, W. H., and Vance, M. A. Four year treatment of patients with parkinsonism using amantadine alone or with levodopa. Ann. Neurol., *3:* 119–128, 1978.
142. Tolosa, E. S., and Sparker, S. B. Apomorphine in Huntington's chorea: clinical observations and theoretical considerations. Life Sci., *15:* 1371–1380, 1974.
143. Trabucchi, M., Spano, P. F., Tonon, G. C., and Frattola, L. Effects of bromocriptine on central dopamine receptors. Life Sci., *19:* 225–232, 1976.
144. Ungerstedt, U. Adipsia and aphagia after 6-hydroxydopamine-induced degeneration of the nigro-striatal dopamine system. Acta Physiol. Scand. (Suppl.), *367:* 95–122, 1971.
145. Ungerstedt, U. Post-synaptic hyper-sensitivity after 6-hydroxygopamine-induced degeneration of the nigro-striatal system. Acta Physiol. Scand. (Suppl.), *367:* 79–93, 1971.
146. Ungerstedt, U., Butcher, L. L., Butcher, S. G., Anden, N. E., and Fuxe, K. Direct chemical stimulation of dopaminergic mechanisms in the neostriatum of the rat. Brain Res., *14:* 461–471, 1969.
147. Von Euler, U. S. A specific sympathomimetic ergone in adrenergic nerve fibers (sympathin) and its relationship to adrenaline and nor-adrenaline. Acta Physiol. Scand., *12:* 73, 1946.
148. Walters, J. R., Bunney, B. S., and Roth, R. H. Piribedil and apomorphine: pre- and post-synaptic effects on dopamine synthesis and neuronal activity. Adv. Neurol., *9:* 273–284, 1975.
149. Ward, A. A., Jr., McCulloch, W. S., and Magoun, H. W. Production of an alternating tremor at rest in monkeys. J. Neurophysiol., *11:* 317–330, 1948.
150. Winkler, G. F., and Young, R. R. Efficacy of chronic propanolol therapy in action tremors of the familial senile or essential varieties. N. Engl. J. Med., *290:* 984–988, 1974.
151. Wooten, F., Eldridge, R., Axelrod, J., and Stern, R. S. Elevated plasma dopamine-β-hydroxylase activity in utosomal dominant dystonia. N. Engl. J. Med., *288:* 284, 1973.
152. Yahr, M. D., Duvoisin, R. C., Schear, M. J., Barrett, R. E., and Hoehn, N. M. Treatment of parkinsonism with levodopa. Arch. Neurol., *21:* 343–354, 1969.
153. Zaczek, R., Schwarcz, R., and Coyle, J. T. Long-term sequelae of striatal kainic lesion. Brain Res., *152:* 626–632, 1978.
154. Zeman, W. Pathology of the torsion dystonias (dystonia musculorum deformans). Neurology, *20:* 79, 1970.

II

Scientific Communication

CHAPTER

9

Preparation of a Neurosurgical Manuscript, with Emphasis on Library Research

ROBERT H. WILKINS, M.D.

DISCLAIMER

Procrastination is the curse of medical writing. Writer's cramp and myopia pale by comparison.

I was reminded of this again today, when I began to prepare the present chapter. I had postponed the starting time to late on the last possible day. Then, when I saw that no natural disaster or major illness was going to remove me from this obligation, I began to assemble paper, pens, and dictionary. I welcomed the diversion of an hour-long telephone conversation with an insurance salesman, and I even straightened up the den before returning to my desk. The two preliminary paragraphs consumed an hour in the first draft. I rewarded myself with two trips to the refrigerator. Finally, after waiting in vain for additional inspiration, I stopped for the evening.

I can only offer advice about how to prepare a medical manuscript. I haven't yet been able to master the fine points myself. So, as preachers often tell their congregations, "Do as I say. Don't do as I do."

BEGINNING

The medical writer actually begins the manuscript long before he sits down to write. He starts with an idea or an assignment. For example, the clinician encounters a problem on the ward or in the operating room, the researcher is confronted by an unexplained phenomenon, or the teacher is asked to prepare an instructive review of a medical topic. Each of these individuals must then find out what is already known about the problem at hand.

The second step, that of consulting more experienced individuals and of reviewing the medical literature, is the biggest chore. But it is absolutely necessary! The same care must be spent in this phase as in creating the foundation of a building. Everything added on later rests on this background knowledge and in large part stands or falls according to the strength of the foundation blocks and their arrangement in respect to each other. And like the architect's reputation, the medical writer's reputation is the direct result of whether his work is functional, beautiful, and enduring, or whether it collapses because of inadequate preparation, flawed materials, or poor workmanship.

In most medical manuscripts the references are listed at the end. This gives the appearance that the references are an afterthought or have been tacked on for completeness. In actual fact, the references are of major importance. The medical author needs to begin his project by finding out the existing knowledge to gain the most informed approach to the topic and to avoid reduplication of effort. Just as no good lawyer comes to the courtroom without knowing all the background information on his case, a medical writer must spend the necessary time and effort to become an authority on his subject. There is just no substitute for doing one's homework!

As the medical writer reads on a topic, he finds out who has been working in that area. It is then worth writing or speaking to those individuals to find out their current or unpublished thoughts, which may be more pertinent than their published articles from previous years. In addition, consultation with experienced and respected individuals in the same general discipline of medicine is usually worthwhile regarding the perceived importance of the problem under discussion, the reputations of the key people working in the area, the recollection of unpublished presentations or discussions on the subject, etc. This may help the neophyte put his project in perspective and interpret the existing medical literature. It may also supply him additional sources of information.

KEEPING CURRENT

Before discussing how to search the medical literature, I will consider briefly a related topic—namely, how a neurosurgeon maintains and updates his general knowledge in his field. In this era of rapid scientific advancement, an individual quickly falls behind without a conscious effort to continue his education.

Source

By being at the source of new developments, the neurosurgeon theoretically could remain "on the cutting edge" of medicine in general and neurosurgery in particular. In practice, this is not possible because no single medical center pioneers in all areas, and the neurosurgeon would spend all of his time travelling and visiting, with no time left over for his ordinary activities. Still, regular attendance at weekly neurosurgical conferences and occasional trips to other neurosurgical centers are worthwhile ways to stay current. The neurosurgeon who does this is rewarded with new information, but he must realize that it is raw material that has not yet been adequately analyzed or received the test of time. It may be difficult for him to decide what has promise and what does not.

Meetings

Presentations at medical meetings and continuing education courses are usually more carefully prepared than those given at weekly conferences and, although the lag time is longer, the material has been analyzed more carefully by the time it is presented. Periodic attendance at medical meetings, especially those that permit discussion and audience participation, allows the neurosurgeon to hear about current developments and at the same time provides him some protection against erroneous or misleading information. Lists of upcoming meetings and courses of interest to neurosurgeons can be found in several general medical and neurosurgical journals (7). Each monthly issue of *Neurosurgery* contains such a calendar, with each January and July issue listing meetings for the subsequent 12 months.

Journal Articles

Journal articles have an even greater lag time than meeting presentations. Commonly, 6 to 12 months elapse between the completion of the project and the publication of the written report. However, the reader receives a more thoughtful and detailed presentation that has been subjected to peer review and editorial tailoring. The reader can refer back to it at any time, and the listed references permit the reader to find related material if he desires.

Over the years, I have found it helpful to scan the contents of a number of journals on a regular basis. The overall list of medical journals now published is overwhelming. For example, the Duke Medical Center Library receives 19 journals listed alphabetically between the *Journal of Nervous and Mental Diseases* and the *Journal of Neuro-Visceral Relations*, and 34 journals between *Neurochemical Research* and *Neurosurgical Review*. The list of journals scanned can be much smaller, of course, and Table 9.1 contains a list of journals that would be of interest to an American neurosurgeon.

I keep a checklist of the journals I scan and visit the library periodically to look at those to which I don't subscribe. Other papers come to my attention in various ways. I make an index card for each of the articles that is published in the *Journal of Neurosurgery*, *Surgical Neurology*, and *Neurosurgery*, and for any other interesting papers. I also obtain photocopies or reprints of a few papers each month that are of special value to me. I then file the cards and reprints by topic (Table 9.2). This system permits me to monitor the current neurosurgical literature. Fur-

TABLE 9.1

Journals of Interest to the North American Neurosurgeon

General Neurosurgery
1. *Acta Neurochirurgica*
2. *Journal of Neurosurgery*
3. *Journal of Neurosurgical Sciences*
4. *Neurochirurgia*
5. *Neuro-Chirurgie*
6. *Neurosurgery*
7. *Neurosurgical Review*
8. *Surgical Neurology*

Neurology or Several Disciplines
1. *Annals of Neurology*
2. *Archives of Neurology*
3. *Brain*
4. *Canadian Journal of Neurological Sciences*
5. *Journal of Neurology, Neurosurgery and Psychiatry*
6. *Journal of the Neurological Sciences*
7. *Neurological Research*
8. *Neurology*

Special Interest Areas
1. *Applied Neurophysiology*
2. *Child's Brain*
3. *Developmental Medicine and Child Neurology*
4. *Journal of Microsurgery*
5. *Journal of Trauma*
6. *Pain*
7. *Spine*
8. *Stroke*

thermore, the file cards and reprints accumulate like money in a savings account, and now after 20 years I have at hand a collection of references that provides me the basic material to prepare a talk or initiate a literature search on any neurosurgical topic without a lot of preliminary work. I recommend this or a similar system as a way of staying current and of facilitating the preparation of medical talks and manuscripts.

Recently the National Library of Medicine, through the MEDLINE system, has made available a monthly computerized search service called SDILINE. MEDLINE is the acronym given the on-line version of MEDLARS (Medical Literature Analysis and Retrieval System), and it provides computerized access to the articles in about 3000 current medical journals. The SDI in SDILINE stands for Selective Dissemination of Information. It provides a monthly printout of references in areas of an individual subscriber's interests. For a small fee (at the Duke Medical Center Library, this is $3.00 per month plus 15¢ for each page of references printed off-line), the individual's subjects are searched against the update portion of MEDLINE each month, and he is provided journal article and

TABLE 9.2

Topics for Neurosurgical Filing System

1. Neurosurgery in General; Neurosurgical Philosophy
2. History; Biography
3. Diagnostic Techniques; Neuroradiology
4. Operative Techniques
5. Neuro-ophthalmology
6. Neuro-otology
7. Cranial Nerves
8. Pain: Trigeminal Neuralgia
9. Pain: Other
10. Cerebellum and Posterior Fossa: Acoustic Neurinoma
11. Cerebellum and Posterior Fossa: Other
12. Third Ventricle: Pineal
13. Hypothalamus: Pituitary
14. CNS Infections
15. Craniocerebral Trauma
16. Intracranial Pressure; Cerebral Edema
17. Blood-Brain Barrier
18. Brain Tumors
19. Pseudotumor Cerebri
20. Cerebral Hemodynamics
21. Cranial Vascular Disorders: Cerebral Infarction; Cerebral Hemorrhage
22. Cranial Vascular Disorders: Microvascular Neurosurgery
23. Cranial Vascular Disorders: Angiomatous Malformations; Arteriovenous Fistulas
24. Cranial Vascular Disorders: Aneurysms; Subarachnoid Hemorrhage; Intracranial Arterial Spasm
25. Intracranial Venous Sinuses
26. Skull Base; CSF Rhinorrhea and Otorrhea
27. CSF Physiology and Cytology
28. Hydrocephalus
29. Congenital Anomalies: Dysraphism
30. Congenital Anomalies: Craniovertebral Junction Anomalies
31. Congenital Anomalies: Other
32. Degenerative Disc Disease and Spondylosis
33. Spine: Injuries
34. Spine: Tumors
35. Spine: Other
36. Peripheral Nerves
37. Autonomic Nervous System
38. Epilepsy
39. Functional Neurosurgery: Behavior
40. Functional Neurosurgery: Dyskinesias
41. Functional Neurosurgery: Other
42. Neurology
43. Neurophysiology, Neuroanatomy
44. Neuropathology
45. Neuroanesthesiology
46. General Surgery and Medicine

book chapter references from the most current issue of *Index Medicus* before that issue even arrives in the library.

Reviews, Tapes, Indexes, and Abstracts

Reviews, tapes, indexes, and abstracts may also be of value to the neurosurgeon. Review articles on specific topics appear from time to time in medical journals and can be found by scanning journal contents. In addition, the *Bibliography of Medical Reviews* appears in the *Index Medicus* and in the *Cumulated Index Medicus.* Audio tapes of a variety of individual presentations from neurosurgical meetings are made available commercially within a few months after these meetings. In addition, yearly reviews of the neurosurgical literature are given at the annual meetings of the American Association of Neurological Surgeons and the American College of Surgeons and at the Cook County Review Course in Neurological Surgery.

Various indexes of the medical literature have appeared over the years, and these will be discussed below. Two of these have dealt specifically with neurology and neurosurgery. Unfortunately, the *Concise Clinical Neurology Review: CCNR* stopped publication in June 1980. It had been the more current of the two. The other index, *Neurosurgical Biblio-Index,* is published quarterly as a supplement to the *Journal of Neurosurgery* in cooperation with the National Library of Medicine. Through the use of MEDLARS, the *Neurosurgical Biblio-Index* lists neurosurgically oriented articles that have appeared in recent issues of some 2300 journals published throughout the world. The index listing appears several months to a year or more after the original article has been published.

Abstracts of neurosurgical articles are published in *Neurosurgery, International Abstracts of Surgery* (published with *Surgery, Gynecology, and Obstetrics*), and *Excerpta Medica* (Section 8): *Neurology and Neurosurgery.* These appear 6 months to more than 1 year after publication of the original article. Similarly, abstracts are published each year in the hard-cover *Year Book of Neurology and Neurosurgery*; the lag time is generally 1 to 2 years between the publication of the original article and the appearance of the abstract.

Books

Reviews of neurosurgical topics also appear in book form. *Advances and Technical Standards in Neurosurgery* and *Progress in Neurological Surgery* are two such series of books that have been published in recent years. The proceedings of numerous continuing education courses and medical meetings are also published each year, and some of these provide useful topic reviews for the neurosurgeon. Many are single volumes, but some have appeared in series (*e.g., Advances in Neurology, Advances in Neurosurgery, Seminars in Neurological Surgery, Research Publications of the Association for Research in Nervous and Mental Diseases,* and *Cerebrovascular Diseases* (Princeton Conferences). *Clinical Neurosurgery* contains the invited papers that have been presented at the annual meeting of the Congress of Neurological Surgeons; each volume appears 1 year after the corresponding meeting.

Textbooks and encyclopedias (such as the *Handbook of Clinical Neurology*) are worthwhile as sources of basic information. However, these should not be viewed as current because of the greater than 1 year delay between preparation and publication.

Audiovisual Aids, Self-Assessment Examinations

Other sources of information for the neurosurgeon wanting to stay current include a variety of audiovisual materials and at least two self-assessment programs. The existing neurosurgical audiovisual aids have been catalogued by Dr. Courtland H. Davis, Jr., and plans are underway to have this Audio-Visual Index for Neurosurgery published. The Joint Committee on Education of the American Association of Neurological Surgeons and the Congress of Neurological Surgeons has also sponsored a self-assessment examination for neurosurgeons in conjunction with the Surgical Education and Self-Assessment Program Number 3 of the American College of Surgeons. This *SESAP-SANS III* examination has been subscribed to by more than 750 neurosurgeons. In addition, a commercially available continuing education series, *Contemporary Neurosurgery*, is now in its second year. Every 2 weeks the subscriber receives a review of a neurosurgical topic, with a self-assessment examination.

It is obvious from the foregoing presentation that a neurosurgeon has many avenues for staying current. These vary somewhat in format and timeliness, but all provide ongoing information about neurosurgical topics.

When he is faced with the need to find out more about a specific area, the neurosurgeon can begin with the material he has collected while keeping current. Then he needs to search the medical literature. During this process, the neurosurgeon will find pertinent references, and he may find it convenient to note these on previously prepared file cards (Tables 9.3 and 9.4). In this way, he will have the complete reference listing for later use in manuscript preparation (after he checks the citation against the original article for accuracy) and a notation of the source of the reference which is necessary if he wants to obtain the article through interlibrary loan. The compilers of indexes and abstracting journals may modify the original reference by omitting the names of authors after the

TABLE 9.3

Library Reference Card for Journal Article

Subject:
Authors:
Title:
Journal: Vol. ____, Inclusive Pages____-____, Year____
Reference Obtained From:
Notes:
(continue notes on back)

TABLE 9.4

Library Reference Card for Book Citation

Subject:
Authors:
Title:
Inclusive Pages:____-____
Book Title:
Book Editors:
Publisher: City: Edition____ Year____
Reference Obtained From:
Notes:
(continue notes on back)

third author, shortening the title, and occasionally making mistakes. Therefore, it is imperative that the neurosurgeon obtain a copy of the original work and verify the accuracy of the citation and the content of each reference he uses.

SEARCHING THE LITERATURE

William Beatty, Librarian and Professor of Medical Bibliography at Northwestern University Medical School, stressed an important point with the title of one of his papers, "Searching the Literature Comes Before Writing the Literature." In that 1973 article (3) and an updated version in 1979 (4), Professor Beatty summarized the methods available to the physician who wishes to search the medical literature. The following remarks are based in large part on those two useful papers.

Quick Current Search

Abridged Index Medicus. For a quick search for a few recent references, the neurosurgeon can consult the *Abridged Index Medicus* or request a MEDLINE search at a medical library. The *Abridged Index Medicus* indexes 118 of the most frequently used English language journals by subject and author.

MEDLINE. MEDLINE (MEDLARS plus "on line") provides computerized access to the articles in about 3000 medical journals for the current year and the 2 previous years. This search can be carried out in 15 to 30 minutes. Up to 25 references will be printed out for immediate use; a larger number can be printed out off-line at the National Library of Medicine in Bethesda, Maryland, and mailed to the searcher.

Other Computerized Lists. There are at least 38 other computerized data bases in the biomedical field, available through the National Library of Medicine (Bethesda, Maryland), BioSciences Information Service (Philadelphia, Pennsylvania), Chemical Abstracts Service (Columbus, Ohio), Excerpta Medica (Lawrenceville, New Jersey), Institute for Scientific Information (Philadelphia, Pennsylvania), Psychological Abstracts Information Service (Washington, D.C.), Smithsonian Science Information Exchange, Inc. (Washington, D.C.), Toxicology Information Response Center (Oak Ridge, Tennessee), and other organizations. In addition to those dealing with medical subjects such as epilepsy, several supply information about research grants (Table 9.5). Audiovisual materials catalogued by the National Library of Medicine can be found through AVLINE.

References Since 1960

The sources mentioned in the section "Keeping Current" can be used to start a search of the neurosurgical literature since 1960, and some of these sources also extend back before 1960. In addition to the *Neurosurgical Biblio-Index*, there are several other recurring bibliographies that might be helpful. *Parkinson's Disease and Related Disorders: Citations from the Literature* appears biweekly; *Epilepsy Abstracts* is published monthly; and both the *Cerebrovascular Bibliography* and

TABLE 9.5
*Computerized Grant Information**

I. For information on specific grants that are available	
A. FEDREG	On-line equivalent of *Federal Register Abstracts*, which summarizes the contents of the government's daily *Federal Register*. Includes announcements of available federal fellowships and grants as well as presidential proclamations and orders, proposed rules, new rules, notices, meetings, hearings, etc. File material dates from March 1977 to the present.
B. Grants	Describes over 1500 grants available from local, state, or federal governments, private foundations, associations, and commercial organizations. Grants are categorized under 88 broad subject fields (*e.g., medical education, medical research*, etc.) File is updated monthly to include notices of grants having application deadlines within the next 6 months.
II. For information on who awards the grants	
A. Foundation Directory	Gives data on more than 3000 foundations having assets of $1 million or more or which award, annually, grants of $100,000 or more. The foundations described represent 80% of all foundation giving in the U.S. Revised semiannually.
B. National Foundations	Covers more than 21,000 U.S. foundations. Supplements the Foundation Directory file. Revised annually.
III. For information on grants that have been awarded	
A. Foundation Grants Index	Lists grants awarded by over 400 major American philanthropic foundations. Grants less than $5000 and those to individuals are not included. File is updated with about 20,000 new awards each year and covers the period 1973 to the present.
B. Smithsonian Science Information Exchange (SSIE)	Contains summaries of research projects in all scientific areas funded by more than 1300 government, commercial, and private organizations. Projects described are being carried out currently or have been completed during the most recent two years. In addition to a brief report on the research, each record lists the investigators, agency performing the work, and the funding source and amount.

* Modified from Duke Medical Center Library listing.

Electroencephalography and Clinical Neurophysiology: Index to Current Literature appear quarterly.

Medical Subject Headings (MeSH). MeSH is published each January as a companion to the *Index Medicus.* It contains an alphabetical list of the words, normal and inverted phrases, cross-references, and symbols that are used to organize the *Index Medicus* and *Cumulated Index Medicus.* This list serves as a guide for the neurosurgeon who needs to look up material in the two indexes.

Index Medicus. Using the *MeSH* headings, the library researcher begins with the current monthly issue of *Index Medicus* and works back to the January issue. The *Index Medicus* covers both English and foreign-language journals. Under each topic heading, the English articles are listed first, in alphabetical order by journal title. Then the foreign language articles (set off by brackets) are arranged alphabetically by language. Within each language group the references are listed alphabetically by journal title. The *Index Medicus* contains numerous entries (there were approximately 245,000 citations in 1979), and it is an excellent source for references. However, only about 2600 of the more than 19,000 biomedical journals published throughout the world are indexed.

Cumulated Index Medicus. At the end of each year the *Index Medicus* listings are integrated and published together as the *Cumulated Index Medicus.* After the neurosurgeon has looked through the *Index Medicus* issues for the current year, he consults the *Cumulated Index Medicus* volumes in sequence back to 1960.

Science Citation Index. The *Science Citation Index* shows who is citing whom, and for this reason it is especially useful in finding out who has modified an operation, a diagnostic test, or some other procedure. It is published in bimonthly paperback issues and a hardbound annual cumulation each year. The *Science Citation Index* was begun in 1961 and now lists by author all the references cited in approximately 3000 journals and more than 1000 new books each year.

Meeting Guides. There are several guides that enable the neurosurgeon to locate papers presented at medical meetings. These include *InterDok (Directory of Published Proceedings), Index to Scientific and Technical Proceedings, Proceedings in Print,* and *Conference Papers Index.*

Guides to Books. Among the compilations of medical books in print, two are especially helpful. The *National Library of Medicine Current Catalog* is issued quarterly, with an annual cumulation. It indexes recently published books by subject and author. Bowker's *Medical Books and Serials in Print* is an annual list of English language medical books arranged by subject, author, and title. Since 1978, serials have been listed as well.

Translations. The neurosurgeon who wants to find an English abstract or translation of a foreign article can consult several sources. Many foreign journals include short English abstracts of their articles; this is noted in the *Index Medicus* and *Cumulated Index Medicus.* Abstracts of foreign neurosurgical articles appear periodically in *Neurosurgery* and in *International Abstracts of Surgery* (published with *Surgery, Gynecology and Obstetrics*). *Abstracts of World Medicine* was published between 1947 and 1971; *International Abstracts of Biological Science* has been published since 1954; and *Abstracts of Soviet Medicine* has appeared since 1957. *World Transindex*, currently in its third volume, has replaced the *World Index of Scientific Translations* (1967–1977).

The National Translations Center of The John Crerar Library in Chicago has some 200,000 translations on file, as well as the locations of more than 200,000 translations available from other sources. This center is the largest institution in the United States for information concerning English translations of foreign literature in the natural, physical, medical, and social sciences. A semimonthly magazine, the *Translations Register-Index*, lists the newly available translations by subject and source.

Guides to Audiovisual Materials. Until 1978, the *National Library of Medicine Current Catalog* contained information about films, cassettes, and other audiovisual materials. Since then, these have been listed in the *National Library of Medicine Audiovisuals Catalog.* In addition, AV-LINE offers a computerized access to the accumulated National Library of Medicine listings. As mentioned previously, Dr. Courtland H. Davis, Jr. has collected information about some audiovisual aids of interest to neurosurgeons.

References Before 1960

Many of the sources already mentioned in "Keeping Current" and "Searching the Literature: References Since 1960" extend back before 1960 and are helpful guides to the literature of that time. For example, *International Abstracts of Surgery* began in 1912; *Excerpta Medica*, in 1947; and *Bibliography of Medical Reviews*, in 1955. In addition, the following indexes are important guides to the medical literature before 1960.

Index Medicus. The first three series of the *Index Medicus* were published from 1879 to 1899, 1903 to 1920, and 1921 to 1927. *Bibliographia Medica* filled the gap from 1900 to 1902.

Quarterly Cumulative Index to Current Medical Literature. This was published between 1916 and 1926.

Quarterly Cumulative Index Medicus. This index replaced the *Index Medicus* and the *Quarterly Cumulative Index*, and was published between 1927 and 1956.

Current List of Medical Literature. The *Current List of Medical Literature* appeared between 1952 and 1959, and bridged the gap between the *Quarterly Cumulative Index Medicus* and the modern *Index Medicus* and *Cumulated Index Medicus.*

Index-Catalogue of the Library of the Surgeon General's Office, U.S. Army. This 61-volume series of books was published in five sets, from 1880 to 1895, 1896 to 1916, 1918 to 1932, 1936 to 1955, and 1959 to 1961. It indexed books as well as journal articles.

Developing the Reference Tree

After the diligent neurosurgeon has collected his references from the sources just discussed, he needs to obtain copies of these original papers and read them. It is surprising how many errors creep into the medical literature, and the surest way of keeping from perpetuating these errors is to consult the original articles.

Then the neurosurgeon needs to consult the references cited by these authors, and *their* references in turn. He repeats this sequence as often as necessary to follow each lead to its termination, like the branches on a tree. Only after he has read all of this material will the neurosurgeon have a reasonably complete background of information about his subject.

PLANNING THE PROJECT AND COLLECTING AND ANALYZING THE DATA

After he has researched his topic in the library (and not before!), the neurosurgeon can prepare his grant application, plan and execute his clinical or experimental research project, gather the facts about the technique or cases he wants to report, or write his subject review. If his project is thought out carefully from the beginning, it is likely to provide worthwhile information when it is completed. In fact, the project should be planned so that it *will* provide answers (positive or negative) to one or more questions. This is the best way to guard against equivocal results and indecisive conclusions. Careful planning will also make it easier for the neurosurgeon to later prepare any manuscripts or talks that grow out of his project.

Brilliant writing can't salvage a poorly planned experiment. Clarity and precision should be built into the project from the start—in the laboratory or on the ward. Based on the background knowledge gained from his search of the pertinent medical literature, the neurosurgeon must decide in the beginning what it is that he wishes to answer, solve, prove, or demonstrate. He must then decide how to accomplish his goal decisively, choosing the best methods, materials, statistical techniques, etc. for the purpose. After collecting the data carefully, he must analyze his results in the light of existing knowledge. He may then come to some conclusions about his work and make recommendations based on those conclusions.

Again, the key to success in this phase, just as in planning the project, is clear thinking.

WRITING THE MANUSCRIPT

Ethical Responsibilities

An author has several ethical responsibilities, as detailed by DeBakey and DeBakey (13). These responsibilities involve the areas of originality, scientific integrity, patient identification, copyright, authorship, literary form, and submission for publication.

Originality. In a strict sense, there is very little completely new material published in the medical literature each year. An author should avoid repeating something that is already known or that has already been done. Yet, an author may make a worthwhile contribution by extending our knowledge in some area, by altering a concept or technique, or by critically reviewing and interpreting existing information in a new way. He owes it to his reader not to waste his time. His material should contain at least some element of originality, just as it should be well worked up and well presented.

Scientific Integrity. The investigator-author has a duty to his patients and experimental animals, and also to his colleagues and to society. His research must be carried out in accordance with established ethical guidelines regarding patient safety, informed consent, avoidance of pain, etc. He also has the responsibility of reporting his own work, truthfully and accurately. He must not publish the work of another investigator without that individual's consent and without proper acknowledgment. He must be sure of the significance he attaches to his results, and should guard against premature publication.

Patient Identification. An author must protect the identity of the patients presented in his writings. Cases should be numbered consecutively in the report; patient initials and hospital numbers should be omitted. The author must obtain written consent from any person who can be identified in a photograph that is to be published.

Copyright. On January 1, 1978, a major statutory revision of United States copyright law became effective (17). It has expanded and clarified copyright practices. The new law clearly states that copyright in a work is held by the author or authors until it is transferred in writing. Journals such as *Neurosurgery* now require the transfer of copyright from the authors of a paper to the publisher before the paper is published. Also, written permission must be obtained from the original author and the original publisher for the use of previously published material such as illustrations, and for direct quotations of more than a certain length (*e.g.*, 6 printed lines or 50 words). Appropriate credit must be given in the figure legend or text for borrowed materials. Even if a previously published illustration has been modified, this fact and the source of the original illustration should be noted.

Authorship. The list of the authors of a paper should include only those who had a significant role in planning and conducting the project and in preparing the report. "According to DeBakey's law, as the number of names in the by-line increases, the likelihood decreases that any but the senior author has participated in the actual writing" (13). Individuals or organizations that have provided major assistance, financial or otherwise, should be acknowledged briefly at the end of the article.

Literary Form. The author has an obligation to the reader to present material that is well researched, accurate, complete, and easy to read.

Submission for Publication. The author should submit a manuscript to only one journal at a time for consideration of publication.

Beginning the Manuscript

There are basically two ways to begin a manuscript. One may prepare an outline and then add flesh to the skeleton, or one may simply start writing. In either case, after the first draft is done it is wise to put it aside for awhile before rewriting it. Cycles of thinking and rewriting should follow until the manuscript seems to need no further work. Then it should be given to a knowledgeable friend for an outside opinion before the final draft. At least one of the early revisions should be devoted to eliminating useless words, phrases, and sentences. One of the later revisions should be to put the manuscript into the specific form required by the journal to which it will be submitted.

Different types of articles have different forms (15), and the tyro would do well to use a standard format for the type of paper he is preparing. The usual research presentation contains, in order, the title, authors and institutions, abstract, key words, introduction, materials and methods, results, discussion, conclusions and/or summary, acknowledgments, and references. However, when the author is planning and conducting his project, he actually gathers his material in a somewhat different order: introduction, references, authors and institutions, materials and methods, results, discussion, conclusions and/or summary, abstract, key words, title, acknowledgments.

Style

Accuracy and detail are more important in a scientific manuscript than is literary style. However, style helps get the message across. There are a number of excellent sources available to the medical writer concerning basic grammar, English usage, synonyms, scientific writing, and literary style (1, 2, 5, 6, 8, 9, 12, 14, 16, 18–29, 32–42). These supply the guidelines, but the best teacher of medical writing is experience. Just as the neurosurgeon learns his operative technique mainly by operating, so he must learn to write by writing.

The successful neurosurgical author learns to write for a specific audience, choosing precise words and writing with words of action (nouns and verbs rather than adjectives and adverbs). He gives his words more impact if he uses the active instead of the passive voice. The reader's mind may wander if the author is redundant or writes with jargon (overuse of technical or scientific terms), clichés, or slang. Excessive wordiness, the use of multiple nouns as adjectives, and the use of nouns as verbs will also confuse and irritate the reader. To capture and hold the interest of the reader, the author should use short words and short sentences whenever possible, avoid technical terms when they are not necessary, and explain complex matters in such a way as to be educational but not patronizing (10, 11).

The writer should be as specific as possible. For example, "infarction in the right frontal lobe" is better than "cerebral infarction," which is better than "stroke," which is better than "CVA."

By all means, the writer should beware of making statements of priority. Palmer (31) has summarized this nicely in a letter to the Editor of the *Journal of the American Medical Association.* Palmer (31) concluded, "The point is that an author can *never* tell how many cases of any entity have previously been reported; no amount of library research will permit more than a rough guess." Furthermore, ". . . the author also must understand that, as important as the entity seems to him, others who have dealt with similar cases only rarely have bothered to write them up."

The writer must review his material to be certain that his word usage, spelling, and grammar are correct. DeBakey (10) tells the following story to emphasize the importance of punctuation. A visitor to a classroom observes for awhile and then writes on the blackboard, "The visitor thinks the teacher is a fool." The teacher replies simply by inserting two commas: "The visitor, thinks the teacher, is a fool." Just think what a difference it would make if you angrily replied to someone who was giving you a hard time, "Don't give me any of your lips!" Two commas or one letter can change things completely. The neurosurgical author must take the pains to write and rewrite carefully. He should take the same care in writing his papers as he does in treating his patients.

Specifics

Title. The title is the "name" of the final content of the manuscript. It is the guide for researchers scanning the literature and is the most widely circulated part of the article. It is the portion cited in indexes and in the reference lists of other authors. Therefore, the author should choose the title carefully, making sure that it captures the essence of his paper (6).

Abstract. Next to the title, this is the most widely read part of the paper. It should be a capsule version of the article, usually less than 250 words in length. It must inform, not merely indicate. "It should contain, in brief, all of the salient information in the report and should be written so that, standing alone, it makes sense to one who will not read the article itself" (6). It must not contain material not covered in the paper (30).

Opening Sentence. This sentence, and the first paragraph, introduce the problem. It should be written in such a way that it will entice the reader into reading the rest of the paper.

"The experienced writer knows that he must lead his reader *to*, *into*, and *through* his article. He leads the reader to the article by his choice of title and by his abstract; he leads the reader into the article by his introduction" (6).

References. For various reasons, the reference list is the portion of a scientific paper most likely to contain errors. The author may not have ready access to a first-rate medical library, he may be too lazy to consult the original references, or he may copy the information incorrectly onto his index cards. He may leave this portion of his work to the end, and may at that point be tired of the project or in a hurry to meet a publication deadline. Frequently an author will take great pains to plan, execute, and write up his project, only to turn over the job of preparing the bibliography to his secretary, who probably has had no training as a medical librarian and little experience with manuscript preparation. A medical writer should check original sources and should avoid perpetuating errors of content and citation. Invalid references naturally raise questions about the credibility of the entire paper. If the paper has gone through several drafts, the author must check the final draft to see if the reference numbers are still valid.

Special Instructions. Every journal has its own format for abbreviations, weights and measures, drugs, radioisotopes, equipment, microorganisms, etc. The writer should consult the instructions for authors in the specific journal for which his paper is being prepared.

Final Draft. In preparing the final draft of his paper, the writer would do well to reconsider the medical expositor's ten commandments:

"1. Thou shalt not, unless circumstances be extraordinary, release for publication a paper that neither contains anything new nor sheds new light on something old.
2. Thou shalt not allow thy name to appear as a coauthor unless thou hast some authoritative knowledge of the subject concerned, hast participated in the underlying investigation,

and hast labored on the report to the extent of weighing every word and quantity therein.

3. Thou shalt not fail to place within quotation marks the words of another, nor shalt thou fail to verify the accuracy of thy quotations.
4. Thou shalt not consider that to alter the words of another frees thee from the obligation to credit that other with an idea that thou hast borrowed from him.
5. Thou shalt not publish a reference in such manner that the reader will think thou hast read a certain article if thou hast read only an abstract or paraphrase thereof.
6. Thou shalt not write to please thyself but to meet the needs of thy reader.
7. Thou shalt not publish, as if thou wert sure of it, that of which thou art not sure.
8. Thou shalt not allow one part of thy paper to disagree with another part thereof.
9. Thou shalt not mix categories.
10. Thou shalt not fail to verify, again and yet again, thy arithmetic" (23).

Before the final copy is typed, the author and his typist should reread the instructions to authors from the journal to which the manuscript will be sent. Special attention should be paid to:

a. Placement and length of abstract
b. Style of heads and subheads
c. Style and numbering (Arabic or Roman) of tables
d. Style and numbering of figures and figure legends
e. Form of references and their citation
f. Typing instructions
g. Number of copies to submit

Remember that neatness counts!

CONCLUSIONS

The neurosurgeon has many ways to stay current. If he keeps appropriate files as he does so, he will develop an excellent base of information on neurosurgical topics. If he then decides to prepare a manuscript on some aspect of neurosurgery, he will have some appropriate material to consult. Many more sources of information are also available to him, and he should consult as many of these as possible. This detective work is done primarily in a medical library. Using the available guides, the researcher can find an amount of pertinent information that is proportional to his effort. With sufficient work, he can piece together the necessary foundation for his manuscript, and if he takes equal pains to plan and complete his own part of the project, he has the potential of producing a worthwhile report. Yet, that is not the end of it. He must continue to apply the same care to the preparation of his manuscript if he wants to finish with a paper that will be published and read, and that will be a source of pride to him.

To prepare a medical paper, the neurosurgeon must be able to think clearly, use resources, be creative, work under pressure, and make necessary changes to refine the finished product. These are the same attributes he relies on every day in his practice. Any neurosurgeon should be able to prepare a good manuscript. The raw materials and guides are all there. It just takes effort, time, and patience. Fortunately, the process gets easier with experience.

REFERENCES

1. Allbutt, T. C. Notes on the Composition of Scientific Papers, Ed. 3. Macmillan, London, 1923.
2. Baker, S. The Practical Stylist, Ed. 4. Thomas Y. Crowell, New York, 1977.
3. Beatty, W. K. Searching the literature comes before writing the literature: how clinicians can use printed bibliographies, tapes, and computers. Ann. Intern. Med., *79:* 917–924, 1973.
4. Beatty, W. K. Searching the literature and computerized services in medicine: guides and methods for the clinician. Ann. Intern. Med., *91:* 326–332, 1979.
5. Bernstein, T. M. The Careful Writer: A Modern Guide to English Usage. Atheneum, New York, 1965.
6. Comroe, J. H. Course on Scientific Writing, 1974. Unpublished.
7. Continuing Education Courses for Physicians. J.A.M.A., *244:* 873–1066, 1980 (see pp. 969–974).
8. Copperud, R. H. A Dictionary of Usage and Style. Hawthorn Books, New York, 1964.
9. Council of Biology Editors, Style Manual Committee. Council of Biology Editors Style Manual, Ed. 4. *In* Council of Biology Editors, Arlington, Va., 1978.
10. DeBakey, L. Competent medical exposition: the need and the attainment. Surgery, *60:* 1001–1008, 1966.
11. DeBakey, L. Language and the physician. Arch. Surg., *92:* 964–972, 1966.
12. DeBakey, L. The Scientific Journal: Editorial Policies and Practices. Guidelines for Editors, Reviewers, and Authors. C. V. Mosby, St. Louis, 1976.
13. DeBakey, L., and DeBakey, S. Ethics and etiquette in biomedical communication. Perspect. Biol. Med., *18:* 522–540, 1975.
14. DeBakey, L., and DeBakey, S. The art of persuasion: logic and language in proposal writing. Grants Magazine, *1:* 43–60, 1978.
15. DeBakey, S. Some types of medical papers: With suggestions on their preparation. South. Med. J., *52:* 1530–1535, 1959.
16. Dirckx, J. H. Dx + Rx: A Physician's Guide to Medical Writing. G. K. Hall, Boston, 1977.
17. Dobkin, D. S. Copyright law undergoes major face-lift. J.A.M.A., *241:* 1019–1020, 1979.
18. Fishbein, M. Medical Writing: The Technic and the Art, Ed. 4. Charles C Thomas, Springfield, Ill., 1972.
19. Follett, W. Modern American Usage: A Guide, edited by J. Barzun. Hill & Wang, New York, 1979.
20. Fowler, H. W. A Dictionary of Modern English Usage, Ed. 2, revised by E. Gowers.

Oxford Univ. Press, New York, 1965.

21. Gibson, W. Tough, Sweet & Stuffy: An Essay on Modern American Prose Styles. Indiana Univ. Press, Bloomington, Ind., 1966.
22. Gowers, E. A. The Complete Plain Words, revised by B. Fraser. H. M. Stationery, London, 1973.
23. Hewitt, R. M. Exposition as applied to medicine: A glance at the ethics of it. *In* A Group of Papers on Medical Writing: A Problem of Medical Education, edited by J. P. Gray, pp. 45–51. Parke, Davis, Detroit, 1955.
24. Hewitt, R. M. The Physician-Writer's Book: Tricks of the Trade of Medical Writing. W. B. Saunders, Philadelphia, 1957.
25. Kierzek, J. M., and Gibson, W. The Macmillan Handbook of English, Ed. 6. Macmillan, New York, 1977.
26. King, L. S. Why Not Say It Clearly: A Guide to Scientific Writing. Little, Brown, Boston, 1978.
27. King, L. S., and Roland, C. G. Scientific Writing. American Medical Association, Chicago, 1968.
28. Lambuth, D. The Golden Book of Writing. Penguin Books, New York, 1976.
29. O'Connor, M., and Woodford, F. P. Writing Scientific Papers in English: An ELSE-Ciba Foundation Guide for Authors. Elsevier/Excerpta Medica/ North-Holland, Amsterdam, 1975.
30. Orr, R. H., and deKoven, D. M. The summary—the most used and most neglected part of scientific papers. J. Einstein Med. Ctr., *8:* 270–275, 1960.
31. Palmer, E. D. Who was first? J.A.M.A., *239:* 1609–1610, 1978.
32. Roberts, F. Good English for Medical Writers. Charles C Thomas, Springfield, Ill., 1960.
33. Roget's International Thesaurus, Ed. 4, rev. by R. L. Chapman. Thomas Y. Crowell, New York, 1977.
34. Scientific Publications Division, American Medical Association. Stylebook/Editorial Manual. Publishing Sciences Group, Acton, Mass., 1976.
35. Soule, R. A Dictionary of English Synonyms and Synonomous Expression, rev. ed. Bantam Books, New York, 1974.
36. Southgate, M. T. Advice to Authors. American Medical Association, Chicago, 1964 (also, J.A.M.A., *190:* 1–24, 1964.)
37. Strunk, W., Jr., and White, E. B. The Elements of Style, Ed. 3. Macmillan, New York, 1979.
38. Thomas, P. E. L. A Guide for Authors: Manuscript, Proof and Illustration, Ed. 2, rev. 5th printing. Charles C Thomas, Springfield, Ill., 1975.
39. Thorne, C. Better Medical Writing. Pitman Medical, London, 1970.
40. Trelease, S. F. How to Write Scientific and Technical Papers. Williams & Wilkins, Baltimore, 1958; paperback edition, The M.I.T. Press, Cambridge, Mass., 1969.
41. University of Chicago Press. A Manual of Style. Ed. 12, revised. University of Chicago Press, Chicago, 1969.
42. Woodford, F. P. (ed.) Scientific Writing for Graduate Students: A Manual on the Teaching of Scientific Writing. Rockefeller Univ. Press, New York, 1968.

CHAPTER

10

Style, Final Draft, Submission or What I Wish I Had Known About How to Write

WILLIAM H. SWEET, M.D., D.Sc., D.H.C., F.A.C.S.

About a century ago, in a saloon in Leadville, Colorado, this notice was posted over the piano: "Please do not shoot the pianist. He is doing his best" (2). Words as well as music can ignite the passions leading to violent behavior. An even commoner response to words is profound somnolence. Here I shall suggest how to achieve by writing, responses intermediate between these two ends of the spectrum of human activity—suggestions based on several decades of my errors while on either the author's or the editor's side of the table.

The possibility of having one's thoughts and observations achieve the permanence of the printed word has become a probability for many of us. The current relative ease of securing publication somewhere has perhaps led authors to a more casual attitude toward the manuscript. *Time* magazine recently devoted three full pages to this problem under the rubric "The Decline of Editing" (31). Surely the primary fault lies with the writer, not the editor. It is, though, a relief to have nonscientific writers receiving some of the barbs so long thrust mainly into scientists. For example, Sir James Barrie around the turn of the century said, "The Man of Science appears to be the only man who has something to say just now—and the only man who does not know how to say it" (1). Appraisals of performance of the scientific and medical student in this country in recent decades have concentrated on machine graded examinations, and on general questions requiring the student to scribble as many relevant facts as he can in a sharply limited time. Our many systems usually have no counterpart to the expensive English custom in Oxford and Cambridge Universities of the student's weekly essay for a tutor. The scholar's task is to present a logical, readable development of of a topic, a consideration of which forms the basis for the tutorial hour. In our country one of the student's first encounters with such a criticism, including form of presentation, may be when his first scientific manuscript comes up for discussion. It is no wonder that this may bring rude surprises, and that some clinical teaching services actually hire an editor to rewrite the output both of resident and attending staff.

An even more serious problem is that the methods of education are leaning more and more toward primary teaching by pictures or images. This is not only a planned feature of formal education but the unplanned result of the incessant bombardment of the television screen. We are reversing the advice of Plato in his seventh epistle. He stated that "there are three things that are necessary if knowledge of a [real being] is to be acquired: first, the name; second, the definition; third, the image; knowledge comes fourth." "The fourth is science itself" (23, 24). As an example he selects the concept of a circle. He begins with the name; then he defines it as "the figure whose extremities are everywhere equally distant from its center." Only then does he move to the third step of the "image" or "resemblance." This placement of the word, the name, in the cardinal position of the process of thought becomes more convincing when we reflect that not only are words the most convenient means of describing the thought to someone else, we best develop our own uncommunicated thoughts by categorizing them in words upon whose meaning we are crystal clear. This basic reliance on words to develop thoughts not only about ideas but about things, and to tell others how we are doing on this score, is fundamentally threatened by the mesmerizing qualities of the ' "boob tube." ' I concede that we now know something Plato didn't know, namely that one entire hemisphere is devoted to the storage and analysis of images and patterns both visual and musical. We are undoubtedly well advised to utilize the resources of the hemisphere for picture-learning along with that for word-learning. But even if we all become accomplished artists—in the representational rather than the abstract mode—words will still dominate for interpersonal communication. There is no substitute for learning to use them in a sequential logical fashion.

In my title, the first four words of which were selected for me by Dr. Wilkins, the first word, style, is the crucial one. As applied to writing or speaking, style is defined almost identically by the unabridged Oxford and Webster dictionaries, as referring to "those features of literary composition which belong to form and expression rather than to the substance of the thought or matter expressed." However the innate content and the manner of its expression overlap and interact; there is no sharp boundary between the two. When I am writing I have at hand not only these two dictionaries but also Roget's Thesaurus, Fowler's Modern English Usage, and more recently Harper's Dictionary of Thought (8, 11, 25, 26, 32).

Before I continue with my assignment I wish to emphasize the importance of conviction by the author that the substance of what he is trying to say is worth saying. I have a close personal friend who decided a few years ago that his busy internist's clinical practice precluded his devoting the concentrated thought required to produce the valuable monograph or two he had in the nebulous recesses of his mind. So he carefully selected the right colleagues to whom to refer each of his patients, wrote to all concerned, and closed out his clinical practice in order to cap his career with some first class medical authorship. After he had laboriously completed and reread the first several chapters of opus no. 1 he came to the gloomy conclusion that the stuff was really not worth pursuing further. He decided that no amount of polishing or editing would make up for inadequate substance. Back he went into practice and says he is going to die with his stethoscope on.

The other side of the coin, too modest an appraisal of the substance, is exemplified by what happened to Dr. Paul Settlage. Around 1950 he submitted to the National Research Council (N.R.C.) a manuscript describing his animal experiments which showed the remarkable reduction in cerebrospinal fluid pressure from either high or normal levels which occurs when large doses of urea are given intravenously (28). Dr. Henry Schwartz and I were both on the specific committee of the N.R.C. charged with evaluating the accompanying request for research grant support. On our way into the meeting we commented to each other that the data and conclusions of this young Paul Settlage of Madison, Wis. seemed most intriguing. In the meeting, as soon as this proposal was brought up for consideration, a distinguished biochemist adduced a myriad of reasons why only a pathetic oaf would suggest anything so ludicrous. Putting back into the body the final waste product of protein metabolism could only be deleterious in his view. There were several experimental studies in dogs and rabbits, indicating that intravenous injections of urea are toxic. Dr. Schwartz and I were too cowed to utter a syllable in defense of the request, which was promptly voted down. Dr. Settlage was also apparently too intimidated to continue the work. So we all had to wait several years before publication of data on the first successful clinical agent to reduce cerebrospinal fluid pressure. Then the neurosurgeon Manucher Javid came to the Medical School in Madison. He recognized the potential of Settlage's early observations, and the two resumed work.

The next events bring into even sharper focus the necessity for a convincing manner of presentation. In June 1955 Javid and Settlage submitted a manuscript to the American Neurological Association. It was published in the Transactions but not deemed important enough for a place on the program (14). Two years later, by which time the two authors had used urea in 126 patients, their updated paper offered to the American Neurological Association suffered the same fate (15). I have recently reread both of these articles and can find no specific fault either in the work or in the manner in which it was written. In particular, the authors made it clear that they thought the work was important. For example, in the second paper they said, "Urea has been life saving in several instances." They then gave a case summary particularly convincing to me in retrospect, but obviously not convincing to that year's program committee of the American Neurological Association. After Settlage's death in 1957 Javid wisely kept hammering away at us obtuse practitioners of the art, selecting as his next major vehicle an issue of the Surgical Clinics of North America to which all the contributors were by prearrangement coming from the University of Wisconsin Medical School. His comprehensive 22-page article described the use of urea in a wide range of medical and surgical cases (13). The tactic at this juncture is worth keeping in mind. If you are having trouble securing adequate publication of an article whose data and style please you, select a volume to which you are an invited contributor. In this situation the editor may be only too pleased to get your manuscript and not subject it to the emasculation and maceration to which you have become so painfully accustomed.

In general, I fear that the more innovative the clinical concept, the more difficult it is to get it published or accepted by the medical community. The one idea I have had which came the closest to being truly original is that related to the giving of the neutron-capturing isotope boron 10 followed by irradiation with slow neutrons in the treatment of brain tumors. After my paper describing this concept with the supporting data had been declined by several journals, I presented it at a personal interview to the Editor of "Science." His gracious cordiality at the time was soon followed by another declination of the manuscript. After my further sales effort it was finally published by the New England Journal of Medicine (29).

The point in these two examples is that presumably meritorious substance alone may not suffice to win approval of your brain child. The more creative or inventive the presentation the more imperative it is for an editor to scrutinize it with special care in order to minimize the spread of nonsense. Correspondingly the newer your idea is, the more you may have to concentrate on your style or manner of presenting it, in order to convince the arbiter of its merit. A spectacular example of success on this score is the approach used by the late Dr. Alexander Sachs, the economist who had earlier persuaded Franklin D. Roosevelt of his perspicacity because so much of his advice had proven valuable. Several scientists including Einstein and Szilard had assembled the facts, discovered in Germany, relevant to the possibility of making an atomic bomb. In October 1939 they asked Dr. Sachs to present and explain to President Roosevelt the scientific rationale for research and development in this field. At an initial session Sachs read and interpreted selected portions of the scientific documents but made little headway convincing the President. Sachs was given one more chance at a breakfast session with F.D.R., in preparation for which he ruminated many hours. His telling lines recounted this historical episode. In the early part of the last century a young man urged on Napoleon that the Emperor finance his prototype of a species of ships which would enable the French army to cross the English channel powered independently of the vagaries of the winds. The French army would then not suffer the fate of the Spanish Armada, but would be able to deliver a surprise attack on the English coast at a precise time and place. Napoleon and his advisers dismissed this wild dreamer and England was spared an invasion. The world had to wait until Robert Fulton in 1807 returned to the U.S.A. and fulfilled his dream of building the first commercially successful steam-powered boat. Mr. Roosevelt got the point that "we had better not risk having the Nazis blow us up"; he decided at that breakfast session to go forward with the work on the atomic bomb (18). While we here may not be participating in such fateful decisions, the modus operandi of Dr. Sachs illustrates how decisive dramatization of an idea may be to its acceptance.

I have already indicated that we as writers must begin with, or develop as we proceed, confidence in the value of our effort. We may not necessarily seek with Oscar Wilde to "tread the sunlit heights and from life's dissonance strike some clear chord to reach the ears of God" (33). Even if we are not trying to communicate directly with the infinite sources of power and mercy, we have no less an obligation to communicate with maximal clarity to the scientific and medical world. The objectives are plain enough. We are striving for lucidity, succinctness, and simplicity. Ordinary conversation and even lectures delivered from memory or notes are an inadequate form of training for writing a good scientific article. A wordy, repetitious, casual speaking style may by its very redundancy drive home the speaker's points. Such a tactic is not likely to win over many editors or the subscribers to their journals. Moreover, when the spoken word is incomplete or misunderstood, subsequent questions may close the gap. Such supplementation is of course not available to the writer.

When Drs. Lester King and Charles Roland were on the editorial board of the Journal of the American Medical Association they gave a variety of courses on medical writing to residents and fully trained physicians (17). These varied in length from 1 day to 6 weeks. Dr. King thought the most satisfactory workshops lasted a week. I frankly would never have been willing to spend a week in such a course, even though I am in the position of the 90-year-old Vermonter who said, "If I'd known I was going to live this long I'd have taken better care of myself." If I had known I was going to write so much, I'd have tried to learn how to do it.

I do recommend to all of you the purchase of at least one of the following three books specifically addressed to helping the scientific writer (6, 12, 16). They all cover the subject systematically—which I shan't try to do here. I hope instead to persuade you to study and apply the teachings of a good book on this topic.

One of the most comprehensive, which in 1978 went into its 4th edition since 1960, is the *Style Manual of the Council of Biology Editors* (12). This volume is suggested by many medicoscientific journals, including the one with the largest voluntary subscription list in the world, the New England Journal of Medicine. The current text is the product of eight authors, six subcommittees, several dozen consultants, and much criticism of the previous editions. Its Chapter 12 refers to 20 other style manuals and 13 books on writing, prose style, and word usage. Its Chapters 2 and 3 deal with writing the article, from the first draft through revisions to the final draft—the crux of what you wish to know. Although you may find as revoltingly didactic as I do, a few of the pre- and proscriptions, these rules and guidelines present current widespread editorial opinions. Only 10 pages (18 through 27) are devoted to advice on prose style for scientific writing, although I fear that this is the main area requiring improvement. However, every other facet of aids to such writing is superbly covered. I wish I had been aware of this book 20 years ago. The use of prominent headings and subheadings throughout its text makes for prompt location of any desired detail. Both the general organization of the volume and its execution provide a first class model for us. In the chapters on general style conventions and on style in special fields are collected not only useful guides to common and uncommon punctuations but explanations of standard abbreviations and symbols of great help to naive readers such as me. Proper use of ellipsis, dieresis, and diacritical marks is described; statistical symbols are given and the terms for them defined. The write-up on special fields of basic science is particularly valuable for the clinician. Subdivided into microbiology, genetics, immunology, hematology, physiology, chemistry and biochemistry this section permits one to find quickly the newly adopted words and phrases—often for concepts developed since we were medical students. A chapter tells you the established customs for indicating your typographic preferences, *i.e.*, those relating to capital and small capital letters and to italic, roman, and boldface type. An important chapter on word usage defines precisely pairs of words often confused with each other, as well as other words often misused or misspelled. In short, the book is a treasure both for scientific writers and readers. It belongs in the library of every intellectually active physician.

My other two recommendations are by single authors: Lester King's "*Why Not Say It Clearly*" (16) and Robert Day's "*How to Write and*

Publish a Scientific Paper" (6). King's Volume has enough amusing illustrations and individual flair to make its short text on principles readable in a few evenings. Chapters 3 through 6 are the key portions of the book on how to achieve clarity and brevity. The whole book, though, elaborates on various aspects of achieving a better style and is complementary to rather than a short substitute for the fuller Style Manual.

Robert Day frankly says his advice is in cook book form with a few pages to each subsection of the task. There are chapters on how to write the title, the abstract, the introduction, the section on materials and methods, the results, the discussion, the tables etc. He rigorously prescribes one standard organization of the papers. The *introduction* describes the problem; the *materials and methods* indicate how it was studied; the *results* and the *discussion* of their significance then follow. If you would like to know one good way to get your efforts on paper and published in jig time, this is the book for you. Day's view is that a scientific paper is not "literature" and that its preparer is not really an "author" in the literary sense. He thinks that "if the ingredients are properly organized, the paper will virtually write itself." I doubt that this cheerful conclusion applies to many of us. In fact, on Day's final page (p. 133) he says "To learn to write well, you should read good writing. Read your professional journals, yes, but also read Shakespeare" (6). I would add as well, "Read Einstein" who said "The most beautiful thing we can experience is the mysterious. It is the source of all true art and science. He to whom emotion is a stranger, who can no longer pause to wonder and stand in awe, is as good as dead. His eyes are closed."

From the time of the initial concepts of the scientific method the notion was expressed that scientific writing should differ from usual literature. As early as 1661 Robert Boyle had stated: "Where our design is only to inform readers, not to delight or persuade them ... [we should not] ... affect needless rhetorical ornaments in setting down an experiment" (4). I say that the more we can delight the reader in the process of informing him, the more likely he is to finish the article, and the more we can persuade him the more likely he is actually to modify his future actions. Scientists may be almost as susceptible as the rest of the human race to influences other than a concise, orderly presentation of facts. However, it is pragmatically important for the medical scientist to be fully informed on such views as those of Mr. Day and to conform to them insofar as he can bear to do so. I suspect that they represent the views of most of our science editors, and in my less querulous moments I find many of the details of the advice worthwhile.

Almost every scientific journal prepares its own "Information for Authors." This includes all of the arbitrary points regarding format of title, authors' names, abstracts, references, tables, illustrations, abbreviations, drug names, permissions, units of measurements, typing directions, etc. These vary sufficiently from journal to journal so that one is well advised to select his first choice journal in advance of his final write-up so that the time of author and secretary will not be wasted on revisions of these technicalities.

Good scientific writing comes easily to virtually no one. I once overheard a conversation in which another physiologist was congratulating the Nobel Laureate Feldberg on the laboratory work involved in his experimentally proven new concepts. Feldberg replied, "Doing the experiments is just a pleasant form of indolence; the real work comes when you have to write them up." My chief, James C. White, came close to sustained skill on this latter score. We wrote two long monographs and many papers together. Each of us would prepare a draft of the section for which he was responsible and submit it to the other. Jim could always bring more conciseness and precision to what I had written; try as I would I could rarely improve on his effort. However, the knowledge that the other member of the pair was going to scrutinize every facet of the manuscript made each of us re-do his copy several times before turning it over to the other for dissection. If you are writing without a collaborator it is worthwhile to have a sympathetic friend subject your composition to an intellectual shredding. It may then have a better chance of surviving the same ordeal in a formal reviewer's hands. A new species of "text-editing typewriter" helps your secretary put up with your multiple revisions. It retypes automatically all unchanged portions of the previous version, leaving only to be retyped by hand your alterations. These are then automatically incorporated into the stored text.

Harvey Cushing was described after his death as "the most accomplished medical writer in our country" (7). One of his biographers, John Fulton, estimates that he wrote 5,000 to 10,000 words per day during the final 12 years of his active surgical career from 1920 to 1932 (9). Despite the fact that his biography of Sir William Osler published in 1925 had won a Pulitzer Prize (5), his scientific papers continued to go through four or five drafts. From his first days at the Peter Bent Brigham Hospital he "was a stern taskmaster when a manuscript prepared by one of his assistants was being made ready for publication." John Fulton further comments about Cushing, "He was especially particular about details of illustrations and bibliography. He also insisted that a scientific paper should have histrionic qualities, that the reader's attention should be engaged from the outset by having the problem presented in an interesting manner (9). Fulton thought that Cushing "tended at times to overdramatize, particularly his clinical reports, in an effort to make them interesting." However, to me this is one of the features that make them interesting 50 years later. Perhaps if Cushing's style had gone into the early articles on urea we might all have been wiser sooner.

Frequently Cushing's individual style brought him into conflict with journal editors, especially those of the American Medical Association who, he felt, had little imagination about writing. He said that after a paper had gone through their editorial mill, it came back sounding as though it had been written by a high school boy from the backwoods—in fact, all their papers he insisted, might have come from the same uninspired source" (9). One medical journal published this letter criticizing its copy editors. "Why must these obnoxious obscurantists be allowed to convert an interesting, well written and lively paper into an emasculated neutralized characterless tract?" (20). To this, at least when I am sitting on the author's side of the table, I say "Yea, man!" I am reminded of one famous writer's oft-quoted response to an editor who demanded that no sentence be terminated with a preposition. Winston Churchill replied that this was an interference with his style "up with which he would not put." Churchill's verbal mastery included scrupulous avoidance of the cliché and the creation of an incandescent phraseology from which he forged a victorious fighting nation.

To return to our professional problem I cannot overemphasize the point that for us the editors have the final say. The publication of the last monograph Jim White and I wrote was delayed for 6 months while we stupidly debated with the copy editor the use of hyphens. The variable mores with respect to titling the paper illustrate the need for accommodating to the bias of your editor as a matter of common sense. Thus, Joseph Garland, long the editor of the New England Journal of Medicine, said, "Of various forms of wordiness a particular bête noir is the edematous title of 3, 4, or even 5 lines, which gives us a preview of the entire paper to follow. It reminds me of the corner druggist obsessed with the idea of putting his entire stock in trade in the show window" (10). However the title guides not only the final reader but also the abstracting and indexing services upon whom many final readers rely. This initial component of the article is hence critical in determining the breadth of its readership. An example of an unusual title of no assistance to an indexer is one I chose some years ago, "The Difference Between Zero and One" (30). The title conveyed the nub of my message, but I should have included a subtitle to indicate the scientific content. French editors are likely to be sympathetic to a title length abhorred by Garland and the authors of the three books I recommended. An example is the heading of a recent article in *Neurochirurgie*, "Timing of Preoperative Investigations and Therapy with Special Reference to Diazepam in Ruptured Intracranial Saccular Aneurysms. Series of 250 Cases—Consciousness Grade I–II" (21). I'm happy with this much detail (in fewer words) to guide my decision about reading the article.* A recent compromise is the publication by many journals of a list of key words or descriptors selected by the author for use in indexes and information-retrieval systems. If you use descriptors chosen by the National Library of Medicine for its Medical Subject Headings (MESH), all are likely to be included in its Medical Literature Analysis and Retrieval System (MEDLARS) and in the Index Medicus.

The author is entitled to write for as miniscule an audience as he wishes. Thus the law secretary to the Supreme Court Justice Oliver Wendell Holmes said of one of the Justice's manuscripts, "Only one man in ten thousand will know what you're hitting at." To this Mr. Justice Holmes replied "Young fellow, that's the man I'm writing for . . . that man in ten thousand" (19). When my good friend, the chemist William Simpson, wrote a book on "Theories of Electrons in Molecules" I bought a copy to bring myself up to date on this important subject (27). The first two sentences of Chapter 1 are: "The Hamiltonian for a system of light and heavy particles has kinetic and potential energy terms referring to both kinds of particles, and interaction terms. We shall assume that the systems being considered have low nuclear charges so that magnetic and relativistic terms may be reserved as being the ultimate perturbations (LS-coupling), with the consequence that the first Hamiltonian has only the coulombic interactions." At the end of the first sentence I had concluded that I was not the one man in ten thousand, or perhaps a hundred thousand, Bill Simpson had in mind. When the second sentence provided overwhelming confirmation of this conclusion, I was spared the utter futility of ever reading another line of it. The more specialized the type of presentation the greater the obligation of the author to make this clear from the outset.

Most of us wish to inform a wider circle than the few dozen workers in a limited field. To do so we must define our highly technical words and phrases as we use them and keep these to a minimum. It also helps to introduce our subject with enough background data to indicate why we have done the work, and what its general value may be. Special consideration for the reader whose native tongue is not English is today an imperative for medical writers. The rest of the world has now graciously selected English as the lingua franca of science and medicine. The least

* I am not advocating the verbal profusion of this title or of "Protocol for the investigation of supratentorial cerebral tumors. (A propos a study of the comparative value of diagnostic C.A.T. scan, scintigraphy and angiography in 100 operatively verified supratentorial tumors)" (22). This is my literal translation of the original French. The 29 French words were actually reduced to 13 in the English translation published by *Neurochirurgie.* The verbal economy possible with our language and the insistence on this feature by editors of journals in English may be one of the main reasons that our medicoscientific "lingua franca" is no longer French.

we can do in return is to exclude local dialect, slang, and unnecessary scientific jargon from our output. The man of letters may take a word with a precise meaning such as "pregnant" and use it in many colorful senses unrelated to the female reproductive tract. We scientific writers do well to concentrate on the reverse tactic, to circumscribe the meaning of our terms in order to increase the precision of communication. Our words may not like those of Carlyle "come molten from the forge" (34). While we all recognize that the constant rapid evolution of English is one of its strengths, I would paraphrase a statement of Bolton to read "The state of the language in any age provides the basis from which a writer can work: the [scientist] cannot direct the language, he can only employ it . . . " (3)

In conclusion: 1. I urge you to study at least one book on scientific writing and to keep it at hand for reference. 2. The criticisms of the discriminating editor are designed to help you present your message. Try to thank him if you can; if not, please don't shoot him.

ACKNOWLEDGMENT

The author is grateful to the Neuro-Research Foundation for its support during the preparation of this paper.

REFERENCES

1. Barrie, Sir J. *In* How to Write and Publish a Scientific Paper, edited by R. A. Day, p. iii. iSi Press, Philadelphia, 1979.
2. Bartlett's Familiar Quotations, Ed. 14, p. 839. Little, Brown, Boston, 1968.
3. Bolton, W. F. The English Language. Essays by English and American Men of Letters 1490–1839, p. xi. Cambridge University Press, Cambridge, 1966.
4. Boyle, R. B. Certain physiological essays and other tracts. *In* The Works of the Honorable Robert Boyle (London 1772), edited by T. Birch, Vol. 1, p. 304. Georg Ohms, Hildesheim, 1966.
5. Cushing, H. The Life of Sir William Osler, Vol. 1 and Vol. 2. Oxford University Press, New York, 1940.
6. Day, R. A. How to Write and Publish a Scientific Paper. iSi Press, Philadelphia, 1979.
7. Editorial. Harvey Cushing. N. Engl. J. Med., *221:* 623–625, 1939.
8. Fowlers Modern English Usage. Second Edition revised by E. Gowers. Oxford University Press, New York, 1965.
9. Fulton, J. F. Harvey Cushing. A Biography, p. 375. Charles C Thomas, Springfield, Ill., 1946.
10. Garland, J. This Is How I See It. Harvard Med. Alum. Bull., *28:* 3–8, 1954.
11. The Harper Dictionary of Modern Thought, edited by A. Bullock and O. Stallybrass. Harper & Row, New York, 1977.
12. Huth, E. J., Chairman, CBE Style Manual Committee. Council of Biology Editors Style Manual. A Guide for Authors, Editors and Publishers in the Biological Sciences, Ed. 4, Council of Biology Editors, Inc., 1978.
13. Javid, M. Urea—new use of an old agent. Reduction of intracranial and intraocular pressure. *In* Surgical Clinics of North America, pp. 1–22. W. B. Saunders, Philadelphia, 1958.
14. Javid, M., and Settlage, P. Use of hypertonic urea for the reduction of intracranial

pressure. *In* Transactions of the American Neurological Association, pp. 204–206. William Byrd Press, Richmond, 1956.

15. Javid, M., and Settlage, P. Clinical use of urea for the reduction of intracranial pressure. *In* Transactions of the American Neurological Association, pp. 151–153. William Byrd Press, Richmond, 1958.
16. King, L. S. Why Not Say it Clearly? A Guide to Scientific Writing. Little, Brown, Boston, 1978.
17. King, L., and Roland, C. *In* Why Not Say It Clearly?, edited by L. S. King, p. vii. Little, Brown, Boston, 1978.
18. Lapp, R. E. The Einstein letter that started it all, p. 13. New York Times Magazine, August 2, 1964.
19. Lavery, E. The Magnificent Yankee. A Play in Three Acts. p. 60. Samuel French, New York, 1945.
20. Morgan, W. K. C. Verbal blemishes seen as virtues (letter to the editor). N. Engl. J. Med. *287:* 941, 1972.
21. Pertuiset, B., Lienhart, A., Metzgerk, J., Robert, G., and Gardner, A. Programmation des actes diagnostiques et thérapeutiques pré-opératoires et en particulier l'utilisation systématique du diazepam dans les ruptures anevrysmales intracraniennes (série de 250 cas—Conscience I et II). Neurochirurgie, *26:* 123–128, 1980.
22. Pertuiset, B., Nachanakian, A., Gardeur, D., Yacoubi, A., Ancri, D., Metzger, J., and Kujas, M. Protocole d'exploration des tumeurs cérébrales sus-tentorielles (A propos d'une étude de la valeur comparative des explorations tomodensitométrique, scintigraphique et angiographique dans 100 tumeurs sus-tentorielles vérifiées opératoirement. Neurochirurgie, *25:* 11–18, 1979.
23. Plato's Epistles. A Translation, with Critical Essays and Notes, translated by Glen R. Morrow, p. 238. Bobbs-Merrill, Indianapolis, 1962.
24. Plato's Works, Vol. IV. A New and Literal Version, Chiefly from the Text of Stallbaum, edited by George Burges, p. 525. G. Bell and Sons Ltd., London, 1912.
25. Roget's Thesaurus, revised and modernized by R. A. Dutch. St. Martin's Press, New York, 1967.
26. The Shorter Oxford English Dictionary on Historical Principles, 2 Volumes, prepared by W. Little. Clarendon Press, Clarendon, Tex., 1939.
27. Simpson, W. T. Theories of Electrons in Molecules. Prentice-Hall, Englewood Cliffs, N.J., 1962.
28. Smythe, L., Smythe, G., and Settlage, P. The effect of intravenous urea on cerebrospinal fluid pressure in monkeys. J. Neuropathol. Exp. Neurol., *9:* 438–442, 1950.
29. Sweet, W. H. The use of nuclear disintegration in the diagnosis and treatment of brain tumor. N. Engl. J. Med., *245:* 875–878, 1951.
30. Sweet, W. H. The difference between zero and one. Clin. Neurosurg., *23:* 32–51, 1976.
31. Time Books. The Decline of Editing, pp. 70–72. September 1, 1980.
32. Webster's Third New International Dictionary, Unabridged, edited by P. B. Gove. G. & C. Merriam, Springfield, Mass., 1971.
33. Wilde, O. Hélas. *In* Modern British Poetry, edited by L. Untermeyer, p. 66. Harcourt, Brace, New York, 1925.
34. Willey, B. Nineteenth Century Studies, p. 104. Columbia University Press, New York, 1964.

CHAPTER

11

Slide Concepts and Mechanics

ROBERT C. REEDER, M.D., F.A.C.S.

Visual aids can be a valuable adjunct to a scientific presentation. They must be chosen and prepared with care. Well-done visuals, no matter how attractive, will not improve a badly conceived paper. Poor visuals, on the other hand, can detract from our spoil an otherwise brilliantly executed presentation.

If you are fortunate enough to have access to either a medical center department of illustration or to a commercial firm which is familiar with medical topics, you can rely on these professionals to prepare your visuals. If these services are not available, all is not lost. You can make perfectly acceptable slides yourself with a little practice and attention to a few basics of technique, design, and legibility. Even if your do not prepare your own visuals, a knowledge of these facts will help you to describe your needs to the person who will prepare them.

Legibility

Legibility is a function of the size image projected on the screen, of the size of detail in the original artwork, of image contrast and of image brightness. As a speaker you have little control over the projected image size or the image brightness; these are the responsibility of the program chairman or the audiovisual supplier. A good chairman will insist that as large a screen as possible be used, that the projected image fill the screen, and that the projection equipment be such that maximum brightness of the image is achieved. Since you have no control over these factors, you must prepare your artwork to be maximally legible under any circumstances. If you do your preparation with the person in the last row in mind, then the projected image should be visible to all in the room.

The important factor in legibility is not the total height of the projected image, but the height of significant detail. This should be no less than 1/50 the vertical dimension of the screen. A height of 1/25 is even better. When the original artwork is prepared, keep this rule in mind.

When you prepare your original artwork, keep the dimension consistent with the format in which it will be photographed. Since the most commonly used format is the 35-mm slide, which has a length to width ratio of 2:3, prepare your artwork in the same proportion. Copying of the artwork is simplified if it is all prepared in not only the proper ratio but also the same size.

Try to limit each slide to one important point. Several simple slides are more effective than a single complicated or "busy" one. In general, use no more than 15 to 20 words or 25 to 30 elements on each slide. Use no more than 9 lines of copy and leave a space at least the height of a capital letter between lines.

The lettering on a visual should be simple and bold without ornamentation or small openings, which tend to fill in when copied and projected. Both printer's type and transfer letters come in a variety of styles and sizes. Size alone does not determine the legibility of a given type; some typefaces are significantly more legibile than others, even though the same size.

Type is measured in points, a point being roughly 1/72 inch. This must be kept in mind when preparing artwork so that the smallest lettering is no less than 1/50 (or 1/25) the vertical height of the artboard. Remember that the 1/50 rule applies to the height of the smallest letter, not capitals.

Lettering for slides can be produced by hand (not very good unless you are particularly talented), with a lettering guide, with transfer letters, or by having the information typeset. Transfer letters are simple to use and, if type style is properly chosen, produce clean, legible copy. With a little practice, anyone can learn to use them. If you have a lot of lettering to do, it may be simpler to have a typesetter "gang" the topics on a single sheet, then cut them apart and paste them on artboard to be photographed.

You can also use a typewriter to make slides. When doing this you must still maintain the 2:3 ratio, but use a smaller format. For most style types this should be 3 inches × 4 ½ inch. Use pica type or larger, limit information to 45 characters/line, double space between lines, and use a maximum of 9 lines/slide.

Graphs and charts must be carefully prepared for legible projection. The information lines should be the most prominent, and the axis lines clearly visible, but not distracting. If multiple lines are used, be sure that there is enough difference in design to avoid confusion.

A good way to test legibility of artwork is to view it from 8 times its vertical dimension. If you can read it easily, the graphics are suitable for copying and projection. Another way to test legibility is to hold the slide up to a lighted source. If you can read it at arm's length without assistance, chances are so can the audience when it is projected.

As important as the choice of lettering is the choice of a background for the artwork. To be legible, artwork must have a distinct contrast with the background. Choose colors which harmonize and work well together, yet which offer a good definition between the artwork and the background. Good combinations are black on yellow or orange; white on blue; green, red, black, or blue on white; or orange or white on black. Avoid black letters on dark blue, green, or red.

Photographing Artwork

After your original artwork has been prepared, it must then be converted to slides for projection. You can have this done by a professional or can do it yourself. Regardless of who does it, "come in tight" on the photograph so that the information fills the slide. In this step you also have the latitude to make various types of slides from your original work.

A 35-mm single lens reflex camera is the best to use for copying artwork. With this you can accurately frame the slide and can judge whether or not the lighting is balanced before making the exposure. A copy stand, while not essential, makes the task of copying easier and helps ensure that the slides are properly framed. Polarizing filters on the copy lights and camera lens will eliminate glare and produce brighter colors and deeper color saturation.

Many cameras have a built-in exposure meter from which proper exposure can be determined. If your camera does not have this type of meter, then use a separate hand-held meter. Regardless of the type used, exposure should be taken from a neutral (18% reflectance) grey card rather than from the artwork. After determining the proper exposure, it is still wise to "bracket" this by shooting additional pictures one stop above and below the recommended by the meter.

Most artwork will be copied on color film. This is true even if the original is black and white, since color reversal film produces an accurate reproduction of the original. Don't however, adhere to this slavishly. Many interesting variations can be reproduced from the artwork by various photographic techniques.

Black on white lettering or line artwork can be photographed on Kodalith or Kodaline high contrast black and white film. This gives a copy which is a negative of the original in which the black portions of the original are clear and the white parts are an opaque black. The clear portions can then be dyed with colored pens or a water soluble color such as Dr. Philip Martin's water colors to highlight certain areas. If you want to add color to all the cleared areas, sandwich the Kodalith with a colored gel in a slide mount.

Another way to enliven black-and-white artwork is to cover it with a color gel or to photograph it through a color filter over the camera lens.

The diazo slide is popular and effective. It has crisp white letters against a blue background. The technique of making these is complex and is best done by a professional, although the technique can be mastered by anyone who is willing to learn and who is willing to spend a bit of extra time in the processing.

Progressive disclosure is an effective method of presenting a series of ideas. If you have such a series to present, do it one at a time, rather than all at once, which may be distracting to the audience. On way to do this is to prepare the black and white artwork in full, then cover the unwanted material with white paper when making the photographs. Another is to shoot a number of the originals in full on Kodalith, then color the information line a light color, or leave it white, and dye the other lines a darker contrasting color.

Optical titling is another way to make your artwork interesting. To make this type of slide, start with a color slide for background and a Kodalith title slide. Using a slide box or copying device, first make an exposure of the background slide. Then, without advancing the film, expose (or double expose) the title slide. The resultant slide has white or clear letters "burned through" the background image. The background slide should, obviously, be dark enough to provide contrast with the white or clear lettering.

A good way to simulate optical titles is to use white transfer letters on clear acetate, then overlay this onto a suitable background and to photograph this "sandwich." This technique can also be used to make effective slides by using colored lettering on the acetate and overlaying this on a suitable background. White transfer letters can also be used on blue paper or card stock to simulate a diazo slide.

X-rays are often necessary in a scientific presentation. These should be copied on color reversal film so that the projected image is the same as that on a viewbox. If the pathology is either complex or not obvious, it can be demonstrated more effectively by making a drawing of the film on which the defect is emphasized, photographing this and mounting it in the film frame with the x-ray copy.

Coordinating Visuals and Text

Visual aids should amplify and illustrate, not duplicate, your scientific presentation. Their relationship to the text should be such that they match the flow of the presentation. Changes should be made at the appropriate point, but at the same time the change should not be distracting. It is preferable to make this change, for example, between sentences. The visuals should be so arranged that it will be necessary to dim the house lights but once and to bring them back up but once.

Effective correlation of slides and text demands not only an orderly approach to this task, but also a specific place in which to work. If you set aside such an area at the office (or at home), you will be better organized and accomplish the job with a minimum of confusion and wasted time. Such an area is essential if you plan to do your own artwork, but is still necessary for efficient compilation of text and slides, even if the visuals are made by someone else.

In the work area your should have, at a minimum, a large enough table to preview, sort, and arrange your slides. Some type of viewbox is necessary. This can be as simple as an x-ray viewbox on the tabletop or can be one which is constructed to flush mount in the table. You will also need a slide sorter on which to arrange your slides in order. Since the standard Carousel slide tray holds 80 slides, choose a sorter that has a similar capacity.

If you are going to make your own visual aids, you will need a drawing board, a cabinet for storage of supplies and equipment, and some means of photographing the artwork.

A planning board is a significant help to organize visuals and coordinate them with the text. This can be obtained commercially or can be constructed of plywood and cleared x-ray film. This, like the slide sorter, should have a capacity for 80 cards. A planning card should be made for each visual. The cards are then inserted into the appropriate slot on the board. They can be rearranged on the board as necessary until the proper sequence is determined. The cards are then used as instructions for the preparation of the visuals as well as a guide for arranging the completed slides in the proper order.

After the slides have been prepared, they should be sorted on view box, arranged in proper order on the sorter, then loaded into a projector tray. They should then be projected, since occasionally a slide which looks acceptable on the view box will be found to be slightly out of focus or poorly exposed when projected.

The slides which will be used for your presentation should be identified, numbered, and oriented. One way to identify them is to simply write your name on the mount. Another is to mark them with a rubber stamp. Avoid the temptation to use small gummed labels; these can pop loose from the heat of the projector lamp and catch fire or jam the projector. It is a good idea to number the slides so that if they are dropped or mixed up in some other way, they can be loaded into a projector tray in proper sequence with a minimum of confusion.

To orient a slide, place a dot in the lower left corner when it is viewed as it will be projected on the screen. Small gummed dots are commonly used for this. These, like the gummed identification labels, can become dislodged in a high intensity projector. A good way to mark the slide is to make the dot with a pencil eraser and stamp pad. When the slides are loaded into the projector tray, place the dot in the upper right corner. It will then project in the proper orientation.

If a group of slides is to be used frequently, have duplicates made, since the projector light will eventually cause the dyes in the film to fade. Try not to mix duplicate and original slides. The emulsion is on different sides of the film, which makes it necessary to refocus when changing from one type to the other.

A guaranteed way to drive an audience and a projectionist to distraction is to mix slide formats. Not all slides mounted in 2 × 2 inch mounts have the same film size. The standard 35-mm film has an aperture measuring 34.2 × 22.9 mm; the 126 format measures 26.5 × 26.5; the super slide measures 38 × 38 mm. Each of these will project a different size image on the screen. If all are the same format and if the projectionist is aware of this ahead of time, he can select the appropriate projection lens to fill the screen. If, however, you mix formats, the projected images will be of different size, with the smaller not filling the screen, while the larger overflow onto the wall.

Avoid glass and metal mounts. The metal ones can twist and deform and jam the projector gate. Glass mounts trap moisture, which appears to "broil" in the heat of the projector lamp. They also reduce image brightness. If you have any cardboard mounts which are dog-eared or frayed, remount them in plastic; otherwise they may fail to drop in the film gate or jam it. A good temporary fix for this is to simply cut off the bad corner with a pair of scissors.

CHAPTER

12

Presentation of a Medical Lecture

BRYCE WEIR, M.Sc., M.D.C.M., F.R.C.S.(C), F.A.C.S.

As Moses Was Saying

"My LORD, I am not eloquent, neither heretofore, nor since thou hast spoken unto thy servant; but I am slow of speech, and of a slow tongue. And the LORD said unto him, Who hath made man's mouth? or who maketh the dumb, or deaf, or the seeing, or the blind? have not I the LORD? Now therefore, go, and I will be with thy mouth, and teach thee what thou shalt say."

Exodus, Chapter II (11)

It follows, therefore, that those who seek to improve their abilities to speak in public are in good company, while those who aim to help are in the very best.

If I asked each one of you to take a few seconds and think of the finest medical talk you ever heard in your lives, probably one or two would spring into your stream of consciousness. What makes them memorable? If you knew why they were great lectures given by great lecturers, you would be in a position to emulate your heroes. I believe that we would make our selections on the basis that some neuroscientist, whom we admire, gave a carefully prepared talk which was of great intrinsic scientific merit. The actual way in which it was presented would be of lesser significance. This is an important point; that as neurosurgeons we should not be preoccupied with the methodology of behavioral modifers or supersalesmen. Our tasks in speaking to one another are, in one sense, easier in that no high theatrical standard is applied but in another sense, are more difficult because we have to lay our facts before a highly discriminating and critical audience. The price to be paid for being Princes among Greeks, Kings amongst Men!

Our fundamental aim is to transmit information to our listeners. If, coincidentally, the audience can be entertained and inspired, or its collective imagination can be stimulated, so much the better. To achieve this we must be convinced ourselves that information is worthwhile transmitting. When we have discovered the equivalent of cerebral angiography or the CT scanning, we have nothing to fear in presenting before a neurosurgical audience. The data will blaze a pathway for us. On the other hand, if we speak with the tongues of men and of angels and yet have no information, we become as sounding brass and tinkling cymbals.

At the very beginning, do not use excessive and flowery introductions. If reference is made to every officer, past and present of the organization, interest tends to drop off precipitously except for that small coterie to whom actual reference is made. I think it is adequate and polite to begin by acknowledging the senior officer or chairman of the meeting and "fellow doctors" or "ladies and gentlemen."

Our thoughts and our knowledge will only become useful to others if they are absorbed and that means they must be delivered with clarity, force, and elegance. The listener must be psychologically grasped with the first few words. Drive to the heart of your talk—don't ramble about at the onset. If you are quick and enthusiastic, the audience will be alert and responsive. Some techniques for use include: a recounting of an exciting case history, the posing of a question regarding a common clinical dilemma, the presentation of some arresting fact or statistic, or the employment of a dramatic visual aid. You will gain entrance to the minds of the audience if you begin with a specific image which relates directly to the dominant purpose of your talk. We should be aware of our aims and how to accomplish them (Table 12.1).

Is This Trip Really Necessary?

"They never open their mouths without subtracting from the sum of human knowledge."

Thomas Reed (1839–1902)
Speaker of the U.S. House of Representatives
on Members of Congress (6)

Times have perhaps changed with the advent of instant data processing and communication, and with the superabundance of technical journals. Perhaps something of the art and drama of communication at medical meetings has been lost. Is it really necessary to put any time and effort into improving one's communication skills? A group of surgeons from several major American institutions formally attempted to assess how frequently scientific presentations failed to transmit information effectively in the mid-70s. This was done at a meeting of the Association of Academic Surgery of the United States. They audited papers to see if a question was posed or a hypothesis stated, to assess whether or not the designs and strategy were clearly defined and explained to the audience, to assess the quality of the data whether pictorial, graphic, or tabular, and to note whether any conclusions were stated. This critical review concluded that more than 50% of the surveyed presentations failed to

TABLE 12.1
*Concepts of a Master Teacher**

Criteria by which speakers are evaluated
By what they do
By how they look
By what they say
By how they say it
Aims of a lecture
To make something clear
To impress and convince
To get action
To entertain
To train as a speaker
"Start with a strong and persistent desire
Know thoroughly what you are going to talk about
Act confident
Practice! Practice! Practice!"

* Dale Carnegie.

transmit scientific data effectively (5). Why should a neurosurgeon spend years or months on a project, weeks in writing up his results, and then fail to take more than a few minutes to ensure an effective delivery?

The first great medical lecturer in the United States was probably Daniel Drake (4). It was said of him that he was brilliant, with a splendid voice and possessed of a fiery eloquence which caused him to sway to and fro like a tree in a storm. When his work on the diseases of the interior valleys of North America was presented to the American Medical Association of 1850, he was greeted with prolonged demonstrations of enthusiasm and applause which caused him to cover his face with his hands and weep like a child. Such behavior might today be more likely to lead to one's certification than adulation. That fount of contemporary wisdom, Time Magazine, recently stated, "In America at least, a tradition of high rhetoric has always competed with a sentimental worship of the inarticulate.... It is possible that Adlai Stevenson lost the presidency twice in part because he spoke a little too well" (8). These thoughts should not be a source of anxiety to any neurosurgeon. A giant chasm of intelligence and education hopefully separates the average neurosurgeon from the average voter. We must never be afraid of gaining that improbable attainment—speaking too well.

If Training Is Hard, War Is Easy

"A speech must *grow* . . . think over it during odd moments, brood over it, sleep over it, dream over it. Discuss it with friends. Make it a topic of conversation.... It has been the method of almost all successful speakers."

Dale Carnegie (2)

If possible, the talk should be prepared in written form from dictated notes. The completed talk should probably be typed and then you should abstract it onto cards and rehearse it using simple cue words. This procedure will preserve the spontaneity and cadence of verbal speech which is indispensable in maintaining audience contact and interest. Your memories can be cued by small cards or by projected slides which accompany your talk. A dress rehearsal is absolutely mandatory to ensure a good sense of timing and an unhurried pace in your delivery.

Lincoln had only two weeks in which to prepare the Gettysburg Address. He was not even the principal orator at the event. The president's little talk was written in odd moments on scraps of paper which he filed in his top hat. He wrote one version after another using his spare time to give it "another lick". He read it to a member of his cabinet on one occasion to gauge audience reaction. It is astonishing that today, his 10 sentences, read in under 2 minutes, are the reason that those 7,000 fellow martyrs are immortalized—so much for the power of the word.

You cannot be overprepared. It is characteristic of Cushing's lectures that they were meticulously made ready. In 1922, when he gave the Cavendish Lecture to the West London Medico-Chirurgical Society, his formal presentation was on a new tumor type which he named 'meningioma'. His attention to detail paid dividends as " . . . the large audience, unusually responsive to the force of his personality, cheered him heartily at its conclusion" (13).

We Become What We Read

"I have given up newspapers in exchange for Tacitus and Thucydides, for Newton and Euclid, and I find myself much the happier."

Thomas Jefferson (2)

Get a dictionary, a thesaurus (10), and a book of quotations (1, 12) for general help—then search out the key papers on your subject and browse through the standard historical texts. Saturate yourself with the subject. Our diction is largely a reflection of the literary company we keep. May I give you two examples of what I consider to be beautifully lucid and important talks at medical meetings. Mixter and Barr (14), in 1933, spoke to the annual meeting of the New England Surgical Society as follows: "During the last few years, there has been a good deal written and a large amount of clinical work done stimulated by Schmorl's investigation of the condition of the intervertebral disc found at autopsy. . . . This work, however, is purely pathological and it now remains for the clinician to correlate it with the clinical findings and apply it for the relief of those patients who are disabled by the lesion. . . . The symptoms and signs of these so-called chondromata, which we believe, in most instances represent rupture of the intervertebral disc . . . depend entirely on the location and size of the lesion." These words changed the course of modern neurosurgery!

What excitement there must have been 3 months previously when Norman Dott (15) spoke to the Medico-Chirurgical Society of Edinburgh as follows, "The patient was a healthy man . . . of 53 . . . on the sixteenth day of illness, after three progressively severe attacks of haemorrhage, the aneurysm was exposed by operation on 22.4.31. The internal carotid artery was . . . closely followed upwards, outwards and backwards to its bifurcation into the middle and anterior cerebral arteries. As this point was being cleared of tenacious clot, a formidable arterial haemorrhage filled the wound. With the aid of suction apparatus held close to the bleeding point, we were able to see the aneurysm. . . . Meanwhile, a colleague was obtaining fresh muscle from the patient's leg. A small fragment of muscle was accurately applied to the bleeding point and held firmly in place, so that it checked the bleeding and compressed the thin-walled aneurysmal sac. This was steadily maintained for twelve minutes . . . no further bleeding occurred. The patient has so fully recovered that he is able for the responsible legal and social duties on which he was formerly engaged." This brief and exciting report conveyed the news that the first planned intracranial operation for a congenital aneurysm had been carried out successfully!

Those who are unaware of this type of history will be unlikely to repeat it.

Intention Tremor Fatigues

"Do the thing you fear the most and it will be the death of fear itself."
Ralph Waldo Emerson (7)

There are few speakers who are not aware of that fleeting uncertainty, that pang of self-doubt which assails anyone that instant they rise to their feet to begin a talk. It is the same sensation the runner has before the crack of the starter's pistol. If we are honest, we will admit it is the same feeling we have as we start the incision for a difficult aneurysm. However, as the catecholamine surge begins, we should use it for "fight," not "flight." The extra energy and excitement we feel can be harnessed to animate our voices and movements.

Practice Makes

"The ability to speak effectively is an acquirement rather than a gift."
William Jennings Bryan (2)

Having made clear, concise and brief notes, go over them "live" as often as you can. The most simple technical aid is a mirror. If you bore yourself, you are unlikely to be able to excite anyone else. All of us have dictaphones and it is a useful technique to tape a recording of your own talk and then listen to it in playback. If you are at a university centre, there is almost always a videotaping facility which can be used to advantage. When we get to our feet with a paper at a national meeting, it should not be for the first time. At the very least, local rounds should have been the site of a trial run. Some habits to avoid are listed in Table 12.2.

Right On!

"For I have neither wit, nor words, nor worth, Action, nor utterance, nor power of speech, To stir mens' blood; I only speak right on; I tell you that which you yourselves do know."

William Shakespeare (12)

If your introduction has captured your audience, you must build on that initial interest. Orient them to your main theme. Tell them what you're going to tell them. Lay the ground work for the actual data presentation. Review the essential definition and concepts for your talk. Establish a common ground with the audience. After that, you can proceed to direct their attention to your main findings, stressing new findings and priorities.

The inspirational influence of a good lecture on the young mind is given in the reminiscences of Louis Pasteur. He wrote on the eloquence of one of his early teachers—Dumas (the chemist), who taught at the Sorbonne. "You cannot imagine what a crowd of people come to these lectures. The room is immense, and always quite full. We have to be there half an hour before the time to get a good place, as you would in a theatre; there is also a great deal of applause; there are always six or seven hundred people" (9). In motivating young Pasteur and channelling

TABLE 12.2

Ten commandments for a speaker

Do not apologize for anything
Do not learn "on the job" the use of the microphone, projector, and light pointer
Do not fidget with coins, keys, or other distractions
Do not perseverate in the use of any single word, phrase, or noise such as "Uhm". To err–rr is human
Do not blame the projectionist if your slides are backwards, upside down, or in the wrong order
Do not use slang or the latest local acronym
Do not read your entire talk
Do not say you have insufficient time to cover some topic in detail—you will waste time
Do not continue beyond your allotment
Do not finish with "I guess I will end here" or a similar phrase calculated to uninspire

his energies and genius into the world of science, Dumas himself made an enormous contribution: "At first thought it would seem that the spirit of science is completely alien to the spirit of oratory.... But when the patient inquirer passes beyond his technical demonstrations to the sublime reaches of science and the social obligations of the scientist ... he inspires awe even as he communicates understanding" (9).

Mumbling Turns on the REM Switch

"Nor do not saw the air too much with your hand, thus; but use all gently:. . . . Be not too tame neither, but let your own discretion be your tutor: suit the action to the word, the word to the action. . . . "

William Shakespeare (12)

Have an animated facial expression when you talk—somewhat between petit mal status and a tonic-clonic seizure. Vary the speed, volume, and spacing in your speech. Our tone should consciously try to convey enthusiasm, seriousness, and confidence. Avoid speech fads and slovenly argot.

The podium of a meeting is not the best place for name dropping. Using the nicknames or first names of world authorities as we discuss a subject will not draw the audience into a bond with us; it tends to exclude them from our own narcissistic reminiscences and intimations of grandeur by association.

Our deportment during a lecture should be calculated not to interfere with our ability to gain the attention and sympathy of your audience. Sartorial excesses or gross inadequacies are distracting. Nervous tics and mannerisms similarly reduce the level of attentiveness of our listeners.

When in doubt, do not mumble. Make sure you can be heard in the back of the room. On the other hand, avoid yelling into a microphone. This can decompensate borderline equipment and cause that grotesque hum which eats words.

Excessively stylized deliveries are probably counterproductive with the neurosurgical audience, which is primarily interested in learning the facts relevant to the practice of its craft. The graduate of a public speaking course is likely to earn antipathy if his gestures are too theatrical or perfect. An appropriate movement can, however, direct attention. All movements should be deliberate.

Project Your Fancies

"One seeing, is better than a hundred times telling about" and, from the other edge of the East China Sea, "One picture is worth ten thousand words."

Proverbs (2)

Keep your slides off the screen until you are ready to use them and don't talk to the slides, talk to the audience. When projecting slides, avoid total darkness. This permits the audience to slip away psychologically and sometimes physically. If the slides only show up under these circumstances, they should be abandoned anyway. Most people need some element of photic stimulation to stay awake. Depending on the content of the slides, some can be projected rapidly, others require longer.

It is unworthy to apologize for errors in our slides as we project them. We should either ignore the errors if we have not previously seen them or, better still, check them carefully enough so as to catch them before the talk. Failure to attend to a detail such as this makes people wonder if other aspects of our work are also riddled with mistakes. It is not the projectionist's fault if the slides are improperly mounted in the carousel. Blaming him makes the speaker look like a bully as well as an incompetent.

The pointer must never be used to demonstrate Brownian movement. Turn the light on and off and point to the part of the slide that the audience should look at. Hold the pointer with both hands or support it on the podium and flick it on and off as required. Otherwise, one is in danger of precipitating collective rotatory nystagmus.

It is only a common courtesy to our potential listeners to familiarize ourselves with the hall in which we will be delivering our talk. Learn to use the slide control before the actual moment of truth. The speaker who demonstrates that he cannot master the intricacies of a light pointer in front of his peers is not likely to impress them with his ability to solve a complex clinical or experimental problem. If you have the misfortune to be speaking in a room which is too large, it is best to accept the fact stoically. An attempt to relocate the audience is sure to arouse their hostility; still, the greatest boon a speaker can have is an optimal face-to-chair ratio (which is somewhere just over 1). A brilliant lecture can be blighted by the appearance of endless rows of deserted seats.

Poetic and Other Licenses

> "Wilde (after a bright remark by Whistler): I wish I had said that!
> Whistler: "You will, Oscar, you will!" (6)

Do not hesitate to pick up a verbal gem and make it your own. Every good speaker does this whether he is aware of it or not. Lifting all your talk from the same source is plagiarism, from many is scholarship. I was once terribly impressed by a chairman who congratulated his panel at an epilepsy meeting on condensing so many words into so few ideas. Years later, I came across a virtually identical quotation from the works of Abraham Lincoln. He probably heard it from a backwoods Illinois teacher. Nihil novum sub sole!

To a certain extent, we can be pardoned for mild excesses in order to stress a point or imprint an idea. Consider this example from Horsley's address to the Medical-Surgical Society in 1888, " . . . I think I have shown reason for regarding the operation of trephining the spine as a comparatively easy one, safe and justifiable . . . the avoidance of (septic meningitis) is well understood and provided for in 999 cases out of 1000 . . . " (16) or Cushing's lecture to the St. Louis Surgical Society 19 years later, "In something over 350 craniotomies, I have never seen an infection, even a superficial stitch absess, and have ceased to regard the chance of sepsis as a possible complication of these operations" (17). They had to be optimists to get our embryonic specialty safely delivered from the womb of fear and ignorance. Would that their dismissal of the risk of infection in neurosurgery have been fully justified!

If I Have Told You Once

" . . . New ideas . . . must be repeated. Not in exactly the same language . . . but if the repetition is couched in fresh phraseology, if it is varied, your hearers will never regard it as repetition at all."

Dale Carnegie (2)

A good lecture usually has carefully limited objectives. A vivid impression is made upon the audience if it is told what is going to be said, if this is actually said to them, and if it then hears what has been said. Repetition is almost indispensable in the hammering home of a critical point.

One point should flow from another, and there should be a logical transition between them. Use point-to-point buildup and many summaries throughout the body. Napoleon himself declared that repetition was the only serious principle of rhetoric (2).

The Best Laid Plans

The Gettysburg Address was " . . . an offensive exhibition of boorishness and vulgarity."

Chicago Times, 1863 (6)

Psychologically, the speaker should prepare himself for the worst. His slides may get lost, dumped on the floor, or incinerated in the projector, all the lamps may blow simultaneously, the pointer may not point. The previous speaker may conclude his remarks with a convulsion or a coronary. The roof may fall in, a war or assassination may be announced in whispers from the rear of the hall—there are some contingencies which no one can surmount or anticipate. On the other hand, relative disadvantages such as being the first speaker the morning after the banquet or the last speaker on the last day of the meeting are relative only and should be looked upon as additional and welcome challenges. The ultimate disaster—to be avoided at all costs—is for a speaker to lapse into petrified silence as his hippocampal mechanism seizes. This happens when we discover that page 15 of our talk is missing as we glance up from the bottom of page 14. Some form of failsafe mechanism should be present in the form of cue cards or a typed manuscript which has been carefully checked. We should not burden ourselves with the impossible task of memorizing our entire talks. This is self defeating if we know we don't have to remember every last word or figure, we will have greater confidence in our ability to carry through with our lecture in a spontaneous and uneventful fashion.

Things can sometimes go wrong with even the most distinguished speaker. Cushing attended a talk by Paget during which a senior surgeon in the balcony fell asleep and dropped his umbrella on the head of a hapless spectator to the intense amusement of everyone except Sir James. Even the founder of modern neurosurgery had his difficulties. Following his oration in surgery for the American Medical Association on the "Hypophysis Cerebri," he wrote to his wife that it had gone off "O.K." but he didn't think many people there knew what he was talking about. It had been a large crowd and there had been much coming in and going out so that several times he'd had to wait for quiet and, as a result, his talk was disjointed. He sounded somewhat disconsolate when he wrote to Mrs. Cushing, "Still it was a good paper, wasn't it? And someday they will find . . . I helped straighten out the hypophysis question in the winter of 1908–09" (13).

If you have done your best and given a good talk, be content. We should be our own harshest critics. The occasional unresponsive audience is inevitable. To paraphrase Schopenhauer, a good paper is like a mirror: if an ass looks in, you cannot expect an angel to look out.

A Little Nonsense Now and Then

"The sublime and the ridiculous are often so nearly related, that it is difficult to class them separately. One step above the sublime, makes the ridiculous; and one step above the ridiculous, makes the sublime again."

Thomas Paine (12)

Humor should be used sparingly and only if it is relevant and brief. Spontaneous humor in a clash between medical personalities is generally well appreciated and livens the audience considerably. It is not astonishing, but perhaps mildly depressing, that there is so little genuine humor recorded in the neurosurgical literature. A nice example was Professor Dott's follow-up paper on his aneurysm experience to your society in Toronto in 1969. He told a story overheard in the hospital waiting room, "Aye the professors dae marvellious operations noo!" "Our Jenny's awa until Professor Broon's ward fer a gastero-something." "Hoots! That's naethin'! Oor Jock's in under Professor Dott for a post-mortem!" (3). In the context of his talk, this was appropriate, gently self-deprecating, and it was genuinely funny.

Sir William Osler's abilities as a speaker were as much legend as his skill as an author. Yet even he came a terrible cropper when he overestimated the intelligence of his audience and the decency of the press. In his valedictory address, as he left the United States, he made joking reference to Anthony Trollop's suggestion (in one of his plays) that those over 60, having fulfilled their usefulness, should be chloroformed. This was taken out of context and given such publicity by certain unscrupulous newsmen that many of the pledges to his farewell tribute (which had been painfully raised by Harvey Cushing and others) were subsequently withdrawn. It cast a pall over the final moments of his medical life in the United States (13).

Our Paper Should Be Read—But Not By Us

"How can they tell?"

Dorothy Parker, on hearing of Calvin Coolidge's death (6).

Under the exquisitely rare circumstances, of such solemnity and gravity, that every word is of the essence, one can justify reading a speech. In the vast majority of cases, including neurosurgical national meetings, it is a form of intellectual hara-kiri to regurgitate verbatim what has been prepared for a journal. No matter how impressive the prose or content, I have yet to hear a speaker who can truly retain the undivided attention of his audience if he reads. Contrast this to the fact that almost no one falls asleep during an ordinary conversation, no matter how mundane or tedious the topic or company. There is something hypnotic about the measured cadence which creeps into our voices when we use our brains as simple transducers between optic afferents and phonetic efferents.

On Verbal Jousting

"In controversial speaking, aim to anticipate your adversaries argument. Reply to his jests seriously and to his earnestness by jest. Always reflect beforehand upon the kind of audience you are likely to have ... never, if you can help it, be dull."

Lord Bryce (2)

The structured or spontaneous debate is an excellent technique for bringing out different controversial aspects of a topic. In the history of neurosciences, there has probably never been a more exciting battle of minds and ideas than at the 1881 International Medical Congress in London. David Ferrier felt he had proved cortical localization in a primate, and Goltz of Germany felt he had disproved it in a dog. There was enormous suspense generated as the meeting repaired to Professor Yeo's laboratory to study the pathology of the animals presented. An ad hoc committee was formed to adjudicate. They came down on the side of Ferrier's conclusions. Few meetings could compete with the sense of drama engendered by those speakers and by the importance of the new concepts advanced at that time (18). The cut and thrust of a good debate is an effective means of advancing knowledge.

A Crescendo of Clarity

"If truth were self-evident, eloquence would not be necessary."

Cicero (9)

We should prepare for a talk the way we prepare for a craniotomy. The work-up should be accurate and complete. Mentally, we should have run through the entire procedure in our minds, anticipating difficulties and clarifying for ourselves our major aims. A logical sequence should be followed from the opening to the closure. All extraneous activity should be consciously suppressed. There should be a practiced economy of effort. In every danger there is opportunity. We should look forward to success because we have prepared well, and our final emotion will be a feeling of satisfaction. It is not surprising to me that the finest neurosurgeons generally give the finest talks. They carry from the operating room to the podium a methodical approach and an obsessive insistence upon perfection. Table 12.3 summarizes some hopefully useful hints.

End on a high note. Do not run downhill in either the tone of your voice or enthusiasm for your message. If fatigue is overcoming you, it will most assuredly annihilate the listener's attention.

Neque Te Excusa

"Never make a defense of apology before you be accused."

Charles I (12)

We must never beg indulgence for our presentation. The easiest way to turn off a group is to begin with a rambling account of what it is we had hoped to accomplish but did not. It bodes ill to use the old line that we are sure the people whom we are addressing know more about the subject than we do—this obsequious fawning is bound to irritate the discriminating listener. If we make any intimation of inadequacy, our audience will hasten to agree with us.

Time

"No speech can be entirely bad if it is short enough."

Irvin S. Cobb

"To make a speech immortal you don't have to make it everlasting."

Lord Leslie Hore-Belisha (1)

TABLE 12.3
Helpful Hints

Look your audience in the eye
Talk so they can hear you in the back row
Drive to the heart of your subject immediately
Tell the audience what your are going to say, say it, and tell them what you said—all in different words
Use plain terms and give the nonexpert an instant refresher course so he can stay with you, strive to be clear
Tie the topic to the vital interests of the listener
Tell extraordinary facts about ordinary things
Relate your talk to the work and lives of the listeners
Scatter phrases that create vivid images
If you are seeing further than others, admit which giant's shoulders you are standing upon
Enjoy yourself, be proud of your work, smile
Try to build associations in the minds of the audience between what is new and what they already know
Consciously cover introduction, method, results, discussion, and conclusions but do not read a paper which is ready for the journal—delete minutiae and the obvious
Do not try to cover every point, emphasize the important, synthesize a concept to cover the facts, summarize your conclusions
If the worst comes to the worst—remember—many great neurosurgeons have given abysmal talks

A detailed explanation of what you will not be covering because of time constraints is another self-defeating ploy. This uses up your valuable time and imparts nothing useful to the audience. Let the facts you present speak for themselves. Remember, also, that anything you say when your time is up will be taken down and used in evidence against you. I have never heard a lecturer yet who provided information of such burning importance that it was required to go beyond the flashing red light stage. At a blood flow meeting in Northern Scotland, a tape recording of the bagpipes came on at extreme volume if the speaker showed the slightest inclination to ignore the red light. This had a most salutory effect on the proceedings.

All Our Trials Will Soon Be Over

"Say what you have to say and when you come to a sentence with a grammatical ending, sit down."

Winston Churchill (1)

It is unwise to telegraph the end of a talk. The phrase "in conclusion" usually causes massive ascending cortical inhibition in the assembled telencephalons. By all means, we should give our conclusion but by summarizing, simplifying, and dramatizing our key points in the closing moments. If the average listener can recall a single point we sought to make one month after we have made it, success will have been achieved by almost any standard. If we finish with, "I think I will stop there . . . ", the implication is that the energy to carry on has simply left us or that our management of time has been so inept that we are unable to present the remaining important data. We can see the finish line and should press on! Reach a stunning denouement, a masterful synthesis, say thank you and retire.

"It is a good divine that follows his own instructions; I can easier teach twenty what were good to be done, than be one of the twenty to follow mine own teaching."

William Shakespeare (12)

REFERENCES

1. Braude, J. M. Braude's Handbook of Stories for Toastmasters and Speakers. Prentice-Hall, Englewood Cliffs, N. J., 1975.
2. Carnegie, D. Public Speaking and Influencing Men in Business. Association Press, New York, 1955.
3. Dott, N. M. Intracranial aneurysmal formations. Clin. Neurosurg., *16:* 1–16, 1969.
4. Garrison, F. H. An Introduction to the History of Medicine. W. B. Saunders, Philadelphia, 1929.
5. Kraft, A. R., Saletta, J. D., Moss, G. S., Herman, C. M., and Tomkins, R. K. A critical appraisal of the effectiveness of scientific presentations. J. Surg. Res., *20:* 377–379, 1976.
6. McPhee, N. The Book of Insults. Penguin Books, New York, 1978.
7. Montgomery, R. L. Effective Speaking for Managers. Four Audio Cassettes. Amacon. A Division of American Management Associations, New York, 1975.
8. Morrow, L. The decline and fall of oratory. Time, *116:* 55–56, 1980.
9. Peterson, H. A Treasury of the World's Great Speeches. Simon & Schuster, New York, 1965.
10. Roget, P. M. Roget's International Thesaurus. Crowell, New York, 1962.
11. The Holy Bible. Mark and Charles Kerr, His Majesty's Printers, Edinburgh, MDCCXCV.
12. The Oxford Dictionary of Quotations. Oxford University Press, London, 1959.
13. Thomson, E. H. Harvey Cushing: Surgeon, Author, Artist. Collier Books, New York, 1961.
14. Wilkins, R. H. Neurosurgical Classics. XV. J. Neurosurg., *21:* 73–81, 1964.
15. Wilkins, R. H. Neurosurgical Classics. XXIV. J. Neurosurg., *21:* 892–905, 1964.
16. Wilkins, R. H. Neurosurgical Classics. XI. J. Neurosurg., *20:* 814–824, 1963.
17. Wilkins, R. H. Neurosurgical Classics. V. J. Neurosurg., *20:* 267–270, 1963.
18. Wilkins, R. H. Neurosurgical Classics. XXII. J. Neurosurg., *21:* 724–733, 1964.

CHAPTER

13

Graphics in Medical Illustration*

FRANK H. NETTER, M.D.

I am sometimes asked, "What is the function of medical illustrations? What are they good for, anyway?" And, in reply I like to tell the story about the eminent British barrister who was invited to the African interior to study the judicial system there. On arrival in this hinterland he was told, "You know we have never been to London, but we have studied the British judicial records very carefully, and we believe that our judicial system, the operation of our courts, is very much like, in fact we think it is identical to, what it is in London." The next day he went to observe a trial and surely, everything was exactly as it was in London. The courtroom was arranged in the same way, the judge and the barrister wore the same wigs and robes, and the procedure was exactly as it was in London except for one detail. Along one wall of the courtroom there was a line of native girls all nude to the waist. As the trial proceeded, every once in a while, a man would run in, palpate the breast of one of these girls, and then run out again. This continued all through the trial. After the trial he was asked, "What did you think of our judicial system." "Well," he said, "I must say it was in most details, exactly as in London except for this one item. I don't understand why you had those girls along the wall there and why the man would run in and feel their breasts at intervals." They said, "Well we are surprised that you asked that question, because we said we have never been to London but we have studied those judicial records very carefully. And, we noted that every once in awhile, there is inserted a phrase "And a titter ran through the courtroom!"

Now, I am sure that if the British judicial records had been properly illustrated this grave mistake would not have taken place. I have given quite a little thought to the function of medical illustrations and what they should accomplish, because I feel that if I understand their function, I may be able to make them a little more useful and functional. And, it occurred to me, that comprehension, or the understanding of a subject, consists largely of being able to visualize it. We say we understand the

* Editor's note: This paper was edited from a presentation recorded during the 30th Annual Meeting of the Congress of Neurological Surgeons, Houston, Texas, October 5–10, 1980

anatomy and the function of the knee joint, for example. We mean that we can visualize the condyles of the femur and the tibia, the semilunar cartilages, the cruciate ligaments, the quadriceps tendon in flexion and extension, and so forth. We say we understand the pathology of acute cholecystitis. We mean that we have a mental image of an acutely inflamed gallbladder.

Based upon this, I think we can say that medical illustrations have three main functions. First, they help the individual who is studying a subject to gain comprehension of it. Second, they serve to transmit ideas from one mind to another, as in a lecture or published article. And third, they serve to transmit ideas from one generation to another, that is, to preserve ideas for posterity.

Now, consider the first of these—helping an individual gain comprehension of a subject. As he sketches the thing out on paper or he studies an illustration made by someone else, he is helped in gaining a mental image of the subject. But, more than this, illustrations are hard taskmasters. They force us to think clearly and logically. One can write around a subject of which one is not quite sure. But, it is hard to leave holes or blank spaces in a picture. I have, on occasion, been asked to make an illustration of a subject which some author has described in his writing. But, when I sketch the subject out, I find it just does not fit. Something is wrong. Then I go back to the author and we find out where he has gone astray, because it must fit together if it is true.

Sometime ago I was planning to make some illustrations on the autonomic innervation of the gastrointestinal tract and as is my usual practice, I first studied the literature very thoroughly and very carefully. But, the more I read and the more I studied, the more confusing the subject became because different authors use the same words to mean different things and different words to mean the same thing, etc. But I came across the writing of one man, Professor George Mitchell in Manchester, England, that really made sense to me. I felt I could not make these pictures without talking to Doctor Mitchell. So, I went to England and we spent three very nice days together discussing the subject quite thoroughly. Then I returned home and made the illustrations.

It just so happened, a few months later Professor Mitchell was in the United States and he called me up and I asked him if he would review the pictures. He came to my studio and after the usual amenities I sat him down and spread out the pictures before him. He sat there in absolute silence for 10 or 15 minutes and I thought to myself, "My goodness I must have made some terrible blunders and he's just too embarrased to tell me about them." But then he looked up and he said, "You know, it's very interesting. I know every fact you have in these pictures. In fact, I told most of them to you, but, when I see them organized graphically in this way, I have a different overall concept of the subject."

Now the second function of medical illustrations I mentioned was the transmission of ideas from one mind to another. In this sense they are a teaching shortcut. They obviate the necessity for the lecturer, or the teacher, or the author to translate the mental image which is in his mind into words and for the student or the reader to translate those words back into a mental image. But, more than this, pictures are much easier to remember.

I read a book once on memory training and it said that if you wanted to remember something you should try to relate it to a mental image of some familiar object. For example, if you wanted to remember a man's name, say Mr. Swanson, you might visualize him as a swan with his little son swimming along side of him. Or, if his name was Mr. House, you might visualize him as a house with windows on his chest, a doorway at his navel and possibly a chimney coming out of his head. The images are easy to remember, but words may not be so easy.

When I was in the Army during World War II, I received, one day, a call from a General in the Pentagon and he said, "I understand you have some special qualifications for a certain job we want done." And with that he took out a paperback book and dropped it on the desk and said, "There, that's the *Army First Aid Manual*, 420 pages; tells you what to do for sunburn and chigger bites, and gives you 27 different kinds of splints to use for a broken arm, none of which are available in the battlefield. We have just 8 hours in which to teach the boys combat first aid—what to do for themselves or their companions if they are wounded. We would like you to prepare something practical for us that we can teach these boys in that amount of time."

Well, I was delighted. I really felt now that I had something to do. Something important that I could tackle. And I thought, well, the best way to do this in that short of time, would be to do it pictorially, that is, to show the different types of wounds that a soldier might suffer and what he should do about it, in a step-by-step manner. Quickly, however, I found I had bitten off a pretty large order. I knew nothing about combat or the types of wounds an individual might receive, or even the situations a soldier might find himself in. So, as is the proper first step in making pictures, I had to find these things out. I went around and talked to different people and I found out a great deal about this problem. I found out, for example, that first aid is a different process, depending upon the situation a soldier finds himself in. It is quite a different thing in the midst of an assault from what it would be in an artillary placement miles behind the lines. I eventually made the illustrations, and the Army found that it could teach these boys this subject in the amount of time they had; furthermore, the soldiers could remember under the stress of combat what they had seen in the pictures.

I like to think that I was instrumental in the medical department of the Army discovering the value of pictures as a teaching aid because after that I was transferred to the Surgeon General's office and placed in charge in what was known as "Graphic Training Aids of the Training Division of the Medical Department." The orders for pictures became thick and fast. We did things like survival in the artic, survival in the tropics, sanitation in the field, and so forth. But, we also produced many strictly medical and scientific manuals. Among the former was one on roentgenology technique. In civilian life it takes 2 to 3 years to train an x-ray technician, but the Army wanted to do this in a matter of a few months. So, we prepared a manual of about 1,000 pictures showing for each different x-ray, each part of the body, and each exposure the position of the patient, the position of the x-ray, the direction of the beam, and so forth. The Army found that it could train these men in the shorter time with the aid of these illustrations.

Now the third function of illustrations which I mentioned was the transmission of ideas from one generation to another, or the preservation of ideas for posterity. It's interesting that many of the great men whose names have practically become part of our medical nomenclature today, people like Eustachi, Varolio, Santorini, Scarpa, Bartholinus, and many others found it desirable, even necessary, to make illustrations to express their ideas. And upon the early, basic original illustrations of these men, amplified, improved upon, and modified in many ways, much of our present day anatomical and medical knowledge has been based. Medical progress, after all, has been a step by step process—a process in which blocks of knowledge have been added upon foundations which may have been layed in another part of the world by people speaking different languages, by people of previous generations, even previous centuries. This has been made possible by communication from one mind to another. The media of communication are the written or spoken word and pictures of one sort or another. But whereas the written word can sometimes be misinterpreted, pictures are much more precise and specific.

Now, I said previously that the transmission of ideas from one mind to another is a basic function of medical illustration. In this sense, pictures are a means of communication and I believe it is instinctive in all of us to make illustrations, drawings, sketches, scribbles of some kind in attempting to communicate. They are a natural means of communication, just as are speech and writing. It is unfortunate that children are sometimes told by their teachers or by their parents, who may know nothing about art or illustration, "you have no talent, you cannot draw." The child believes this and goes through life convinced he or she cannot draw, so does not try. It is almost like telling a child "you cannot speak, so he therefore does not try to talk. This is wrong because I believe everyone can make drawings to some extent, some better than others, some very poorly, but one should try because drawings are a natural means of communication.

I wish that in the schools, in college, and even in medical school, the students would be encouraged to make drawings because it would help them both in learning their subjects and in expressing themselves. When I was an intern at Bellvue Hospital, our professor of gynecology insisted that all the interns and residents make drawings, on the chart, of their findings. It was interesting to see how greatly their artistic ability improved in a short time.

One of the first steps, the first step in fact, in making a medical illustration is for the physician or author to get across to the artist what he has in his mind. It would be most helpful if he could put down on paper some sort of a sketch, a scribble if you will, of what he has in mind. It is the up to the artist to make those scribbly lines recognizable for what they are intended to be—arteries, veins, muscles, nerves, bones, or whatever and to place them in proper relationship to each other. The artist, on the other hand, has his problems. He must decide from what angle shall the view be—from the front, from the back, from the top, from the side, and so forth. He must decide how much should be included in the picture, enough to make the area recognizable but not so much to obscure the essentials. How deep a dissection must be shown in order to clarify the subject and in what plane must that dissection be? For some situations a "see-through" or phantom type of illustration might serve the purpose best, or if it is a rather abstruse physiologic concept he is trying to put across he may resort to a purely schematic approach or even a flow chart of some kind. But, in any event the artist must have enough medical knowledge to understand basically what the doctor is trying to express and he must have the artistic ability to portray it recognizably and to put the various structures in their current relationships. This latter, the artistic ability, is quite important in a medical artist because if he has to struggle too much with drawing a hand or a head or some internal organ as seen from a certain angle, he cannot concentrate adequately upon the subject matter.

I studied art quite extensively and was a successful commercial artist before I became a doctor. I studied at the National Academy of Design and at other outstanding art schools and I learned to draw the figure realistically and academically, I learned perspective composition, proportions, harmony, color, drapery, and all the other elements that an artist should know. I had some teachers, however, who were more creative and more imaginative than others. I had one in particular who taught us that making a drawing involved not just the eye and the hand but the eye, the brain, and the hand. In other words he wanted us to understand what we were trying to draw, to have a mental concept of the form and structure of what we were portraying rather than copy it blindly as a camera would.

He would give us exercises like this: "Now I want the students on this side of the room to draw that model as she would appear if you were sitting on the opposite side of the room and vice versa, or as she would appear if you were looking down at her from the skylight. At other times he would have the model pose for 15 minutes without anyone drawing. Then he would ask the model to step down and he would tell us to draw what we had seen. He said, "before you can learn to draw you must learn to see."

This training has stood me in good stead to this day. When I go to the operating room or dissecting room or a laboratory of some kind, I seldom, if ever, make sketches on the spot. I prefer to digest what I am looking at, to understand it, to correlate it with what I have learned from my studies and my reading and then go back to my studio and sometimes days later, make the drawing. By that time my mind has automatically filtered out all the unessentials, and only the important factors remain. That's what I want to put into the picture.

Now about media. Many young artists, budding medical illustrators, come to see me and want to get my advice about their work and how they should proceed in this career. Invariably the first questions they ask are: "What sort of brushes shall I use?" "What kind of paint shall I get?" "What sort of paper shall I paint on?" and so forth. And, I say, "I will tell you all these things, in fact I will show you just what I use, but this will not make you a good medical illustrator. The questions you are asking are like asking an author what sort of typewriter should I use."

"The important thing" I tell them, "is that you must learn to grasp what you are trying to portray, to have an understanding of the subject matter and keep in mind what you are trying to put into the picture. And, also make yourself into a good enough artist so that you can draw respectably well. Good illustrations can be made in any medium, and a person should use the medium with which he is most familiar and with which he feels he can work most freely and most easily." Most of my drawings are made in water color, not because I think it is better than any other medium but just because I feel more at home with it and I seem to be able to work more directly and freely with it (Fig. 13.1).

Max Brödel was a pioneer medical illustrator in this country. He came from Germany just before the turn of the century and he founded the first school for teaching medical illustration at Johns Hopkins. He also originated what was known as the scratch board technique. This is a technique of making a drawing with chalk dust upon a special clay-coated

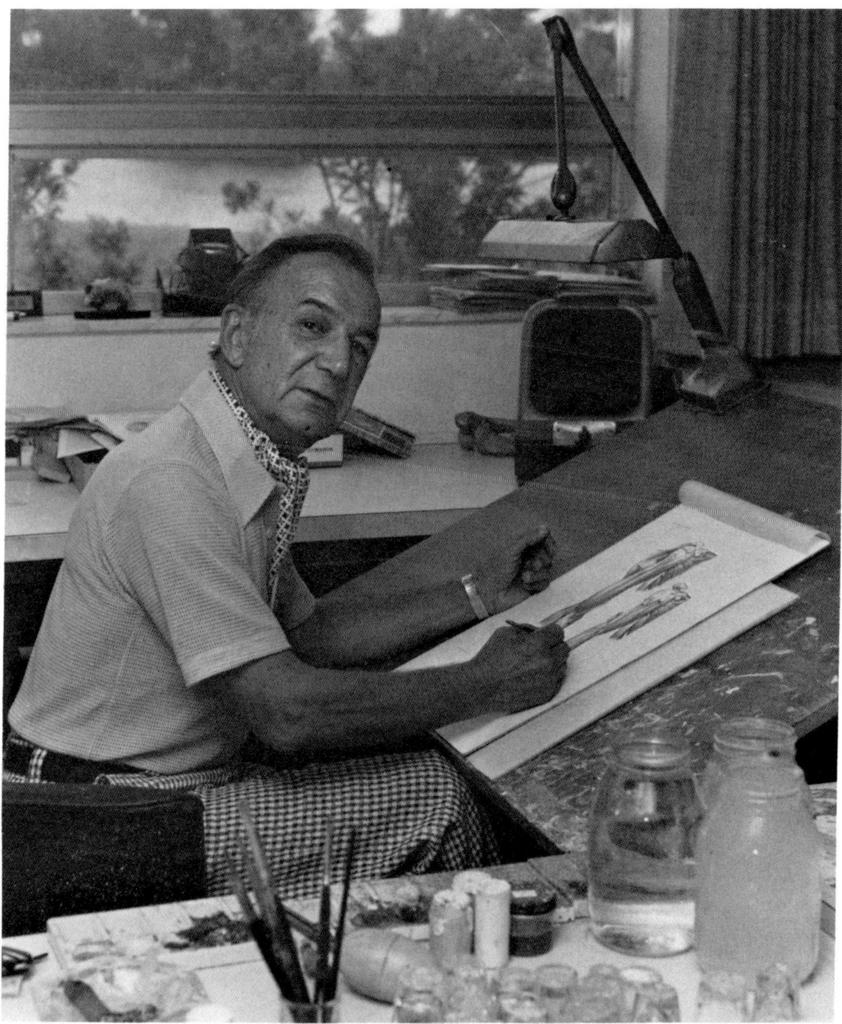

FIG. 13.1. The author at work in his studio.

board and then scratching out the highlights to give a very brilliant and illuminous effect. Brödel and some of his students made some very beautiful and highly instructive illustrations with this medium. Unfortunately to some of those who came later it became a fettish. They seemed to have gotten the idea that all that was necessary to make a good medical illustration was to use this technique, and it did not matter how well or how clearly one depicted the essential subject matter of the picture. Now I have no argument with this technique, in fact I have used it myself on occasion and still do once in a while. But I think it is a mistake to let any medium become more important than the subject matter of the illustration itself. Pen and ink is a very practical and important medium for illustrations for reproduction for the very simple reason that it is the cheapest medium to reproduce. Additionally when it is reproduced, the reproduction is practically identical with the essential drawing. It loses very little or nothing in its reproduction. So, I think that for practical purposes, in most medical publications, the medical artist should become facile with the pen.

CHAPTER

14

Neurosurgical Photography through the Microscope

LEONARD I. MALIS, M.D.

The basic requirements for photography of microneurosurgery include the following:

1. proper exposure
2. absence of movement blur
3. sharp focus with adequate depth of field
4. total simplicity for the surgeon—no photographic thinking
5. no interference with the microscope or accessories
6. constant format and relation to viewed field

All of the above may be achieved with some minor compromises.

The author's photographs are taken through the microscope optics using the existing microscope light without supplementation. The original Zeiss system is illustrated in Fig. 14.1. The beam splitter is interposed between the magnification changer and the binocular. At this point the light paths are parallel, and so no change is introduced in the visual system except for the division of the light in the beam splitter. Only the 50-50 beam splitter should be used. The 70-30 or 7-1 beam splitters further reduce the light for the surgeon to provide a slight increase for the camera and are absolutely unacceptable. To the right hand port of the beam splitter, a Zeiss 220 mm photographic adapter is attached. An adapter ring is then fastened to the photographic adapter to provide the proper focal spacing, and the 2× auxiliary objective is fastened to the adapter ring. The camera back is then attached to the 2× auxiliary objective.

The original camera had no built-in automatic film advance or powered shutter. While accessory devices were available, they seemed too bulky and cumbersome. Our draping technique simply allowed the corner of the camera with the film advance lever and the shutter release to be exposed (Fig. 14.2). For film advance, I originally used a sterile Kocher clamp. This had a number of disadvantages, such as slipping off and scarring the rewind handle. A special rewind clamp was made which has been quite satisfactory. The ridges on the inner surface of a large clamp were ground off and a pin attached near the tip of one blade, closing

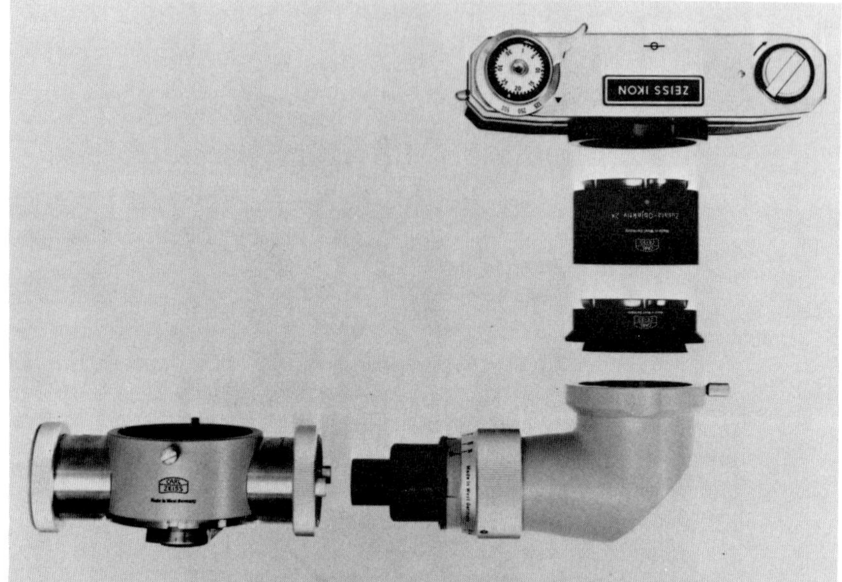

FIG. 14.1. Clockwise from the right upper corner: the camera back, the 2× expander, the spacing separator, the 220-mm photoadapter, and, finally, the beam splitter.

through a hole in the other blade of the reformed clamp. A hole was drilled through the camera rewind handle into which the pin can be set. In use, the clamp is part of the instrument tray. It is snapped in place after draping and then can be swiveled without falling off or damaging the camera. It provides an easily used rewind lever for either the surgeon or his assistant.

A cable release is used for the shutter both to provide a sterile connection and to prevent camera shake. Standard cable releases inexpensively available at most camera stores have stood up under repeated autoclaving unexpectedly well. Electrically driven shutter solenoids were available, but they introduced significant vibration on this camera unit.

Other cameras may be substituted for the old Zeiss back. Specifically supplied by Zeiss is the new Zeiss CONTAX RTS which provides a motor drive and power shutter rewind, as well as the choice of infrared or electrical push button triggering instead of a mechanical shutter release (Fig. 14.3). Both the powered system and the shutter release are real advantages. This is a single lens reflex camera, yet mirror bounce, theoretically a source of motion blur, really appears to produce no detectable degradation. The camera provides automatic exposure control which I do not use. Since our distance and light levels are fixed, the correct exposure for the same view of the tissues should be unchanged whether a bright object or instrument is in the center of the field or not; the automatic shutter, however, will react to the reflected brightness, reduce the exposure, and underexpose the tissue (Fig. 14.4). The new cameras are directly usable for photography and have a high public demand and resale value. They, therefore, tend to disappear from the operating room too easily. In most operating rooms, this will necessitate removing the camera from the microscope at the end of each case and locking it away. On the other hand, our old backs remain undisturbed, always in place on the microscopes, year after year.

The photographic adapter used for 35-mm photography has a focal length of 220 mm. Other photoadapters are available with shorter focal lengths which are suitable for motion pictures or television. As the photoadapter is attached to the port of the beam splitter, four possible positions 90° apart are available. Rotating the adapter rotates the direction of the photographed field, as does rotating the camera back on the photoadapter, so that the field can be placed vertically or transversely by rotating either section. I always have the adapter in the position shown in Fig. 14.5. This makes the photographic field always horizontal no

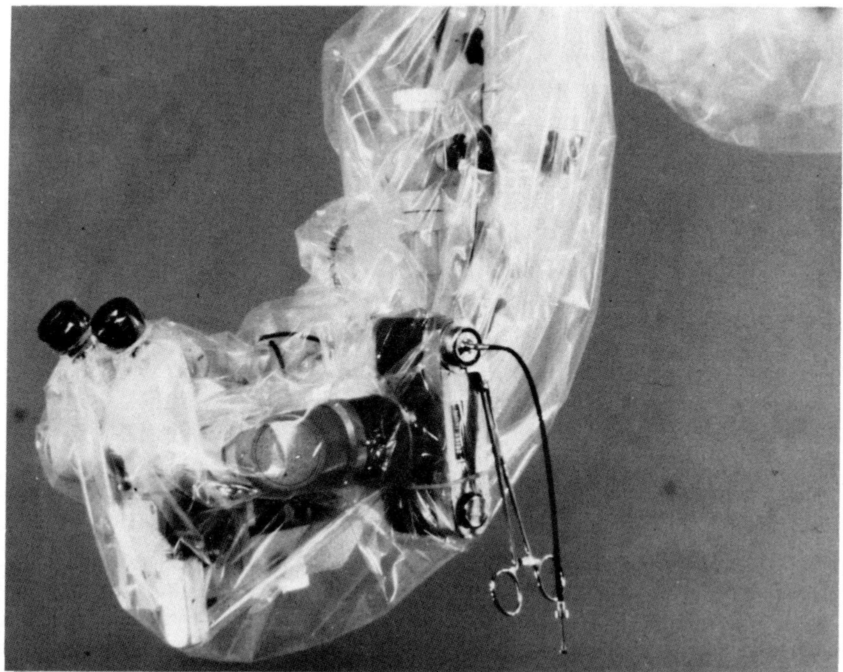

FIG. 14.2. The draped microscope showing the modified clamp used as a rewind lever and the sterile cable release used for shutter triggering.

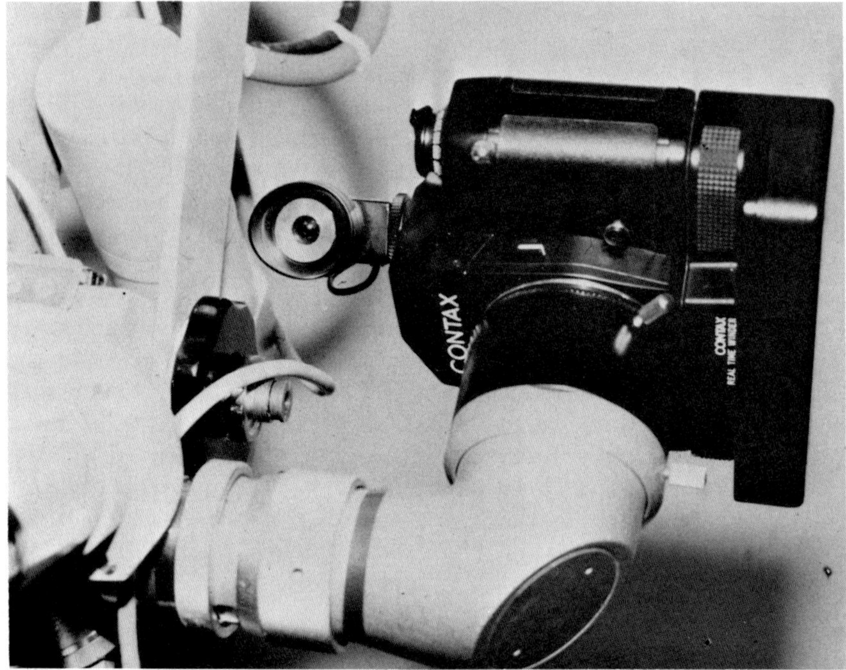

FIG. 14.3. The Zeiss CONTAX RTS with motorized autowinder and the infrared shutter trigger.

matter whether the microscope is used for a patient sitting up or lying down and corresponds to the movie frame direction or the TV screen position. It need never be removed or altered and is out of the surgeon's way.

In the photographic system described, the optical components used for 35-mm photographs are the primary microscope objective (always 300 mm in my operating room), the magnification changer, the beam splitter, the 220-mm photoadapter, and the 2× auxiliary photographic objective. The binocular tubes and the oculars are not part of the photographic optics. While these elements determine the surgeon's viewed field, they do not affect the photograph in any way, including magnification or area photographed.

The 220-mm photographic adapter, used without the 2× auxiliary photographic objective, provides a real image 22 mm in diameter at a distance of 38 mm from the end of the adapter. The film plane of the camera was to be placed at this point. While this covers a half frame 35-mm system, it is not satisfactory for regular full frame slides, where the 22-mm circular photograph has a large black surround. The 2× auxiliary objective enlarges this 22-mm circle to 44 mm, giving complete coverage of the 35-mm standard film frame. Accordingly, this 2× auxiliary lens is an invariable part of our system.

The 2× auxiliary lens is a well corrected concave lens which reduces the power of the 220-mm lens of the photoadapter making it effectively

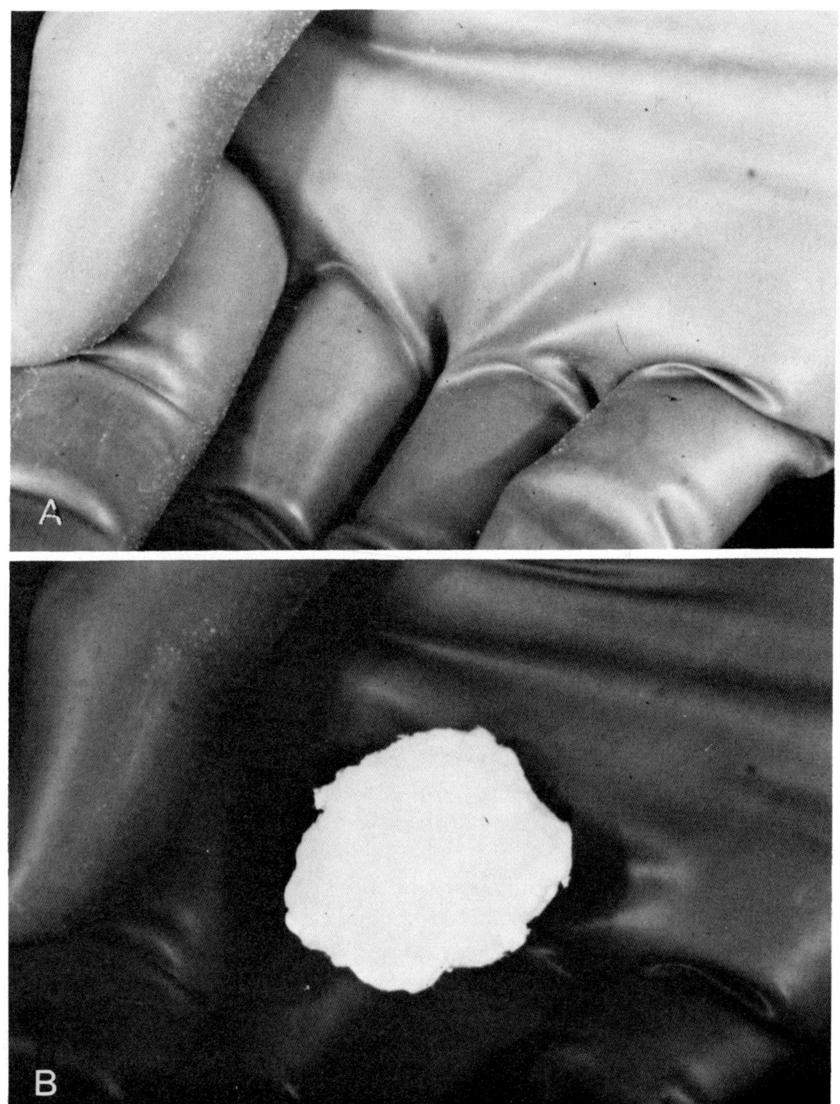

FIG. 14.4. (*A*) Automatic exposure gives correct exposure of the gloved hand. (*B*) Placement of a white cotton ball in the center of the field shifts the automatic exposure toward the correct exposure for the cotton ball and so produces underexposure of the glove.

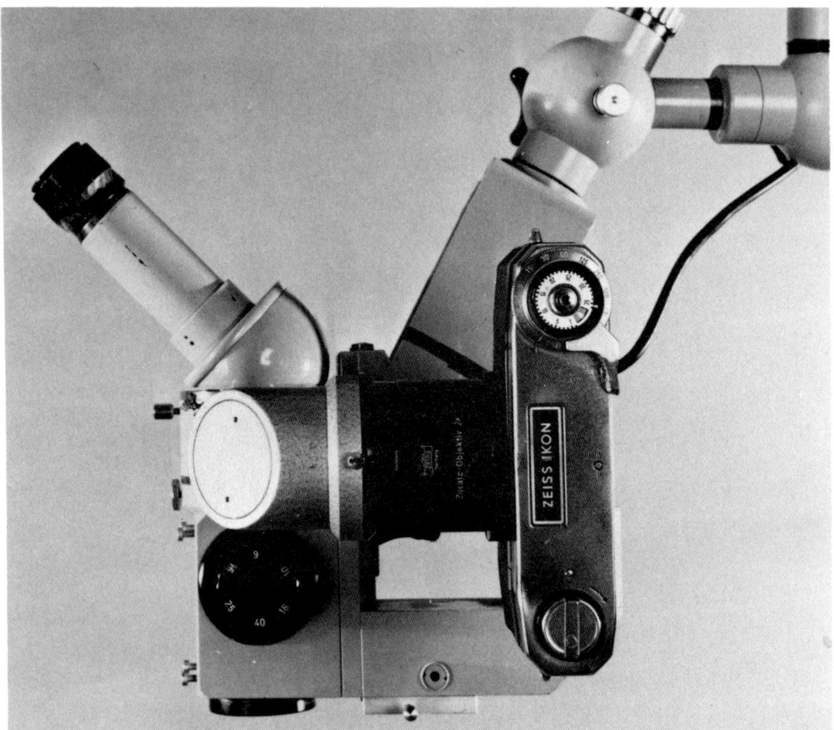

FIG. 14.5. The illustrated position and orientation of the photoadapter and the camera produces a horizontally framed field without interfering with the surgeon.

a 440-mm lens, so that a real image twice as large is produced at a new more distant focal plane. The camera body is moved to the new plane by the thickness of the lens mount and a coupling ring adapter. The only remaining variable determining photographic magnification is the setting of the magnification changer. Basically, if one remembers simply that with the standard arrangement I use for neurosurgery, when the microscope is set at 10×, the photograph is a true one-to-one reproduction, and the other photographic magnifications can be simply read off the magnification changer by dividing its marking by ten.

As noted above, I have standardized on one single relationship between the circular viewed field and the photographed area. This is shown in Fig. 14.6. The same relationship is maintained on television by use of a 137-mm photoadapter for the color vidicons. The 107-mm adapter provides the same coverage for 16-mm film, and the 74-mm adapter for the Super 8. The viewed circle size is determined by the microscope objective and magnification changer (both the same as for the photographic area) plus the binocular and oculars which affect only the viewed field. To achieve the aspect ratio shown in Fig. 14.6, we use the 125-mm length binoculars with 20× oculars, or the 160-mm binoculars with 16× oculars. Again, these combinations are permanently fixed to each other to prevent inadvertent change. With this standardized arrangement, the circular viewed field and the photographic field have the same diameter, altered only by the magnification changer setting. At 6×, this diameter is 60 mm; at 10×, 36 mm; at 16×, 22 mm; at 25×, 14 mm; and at 40×, 9 mm.

Focusing Accuracy

Before taking photographs through the microscope, one must be certain that the film will be in sharp focus when the observer's eye is seeing sharply through the ocular. When an ocular with a reticle is used, with the ocular correctly adjusted, the eye accommodation must be relaxed to infinity to bring the reticle into sharp focus. The microscope optics will then have the camera film in sharp focus, assuming that everything has been correctly assembled and there is no defect. When correctly chosen and matched to the objective and the camera setup, the reticle will also show the limits of the rectangular frame of the photographic field.

I do not use a reticle, but it is still necessary that the eyepiece focus matches the surgeon's eye. This assumes that the surgeon is either emmetropic or that he wears corrective glasses which make him the equivalent of emmetropic. If he is hyperopic or myopic and refuses to wear his glasses with the microscope, the correction which would make him emmetropic can be set on the focusing scale of the eyepiece. For example, a myope who required −3 diopters of sphere for his correction

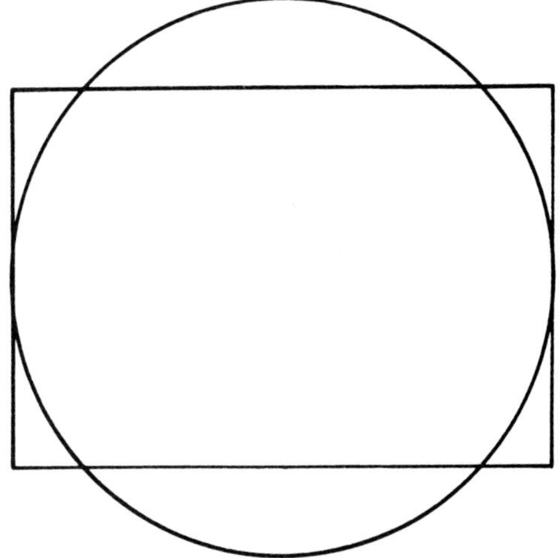

FIG. 14.6. The constant relationship of the viewed field and the photograph field. This format is retained for all procedures and for motion picture as well as television.

and does not wear his glasses to operate would set the eyepiece at −3. The final assumption required in working without a reticle is that the surgeon is able to totally relax his own accommodation.

Whether basically emmetropic or with a corrected defect or with the eyepiece correction, it is still essential that the surgeon relax his own accommodation to infinity if he expects his picture to be sharp. If he has difficulty in doing this, then he must use a reticle to focus on. This is one of the few areas where advancing presbyopia can be a considerable help.

I consider it preferable to keep the eyepieces at zero, use no reticle, and to have each surgeon wear whatever corrective eyeglasses make him emmetropic. In our operating rooms, all oculars are permanently set at zero and permanently fastened into the binoculars to prevent displacement or adjustment. All of us wear our corrective glasses so no changes need ever be made in the microscopes for different operators. This assures correct parfocality of photographs, television cameras, and the surgeon's viewed field.

In evaluating the relationship between ocular field of view and the photographic field, the fact that the two oculars see slightly different fields at different angles must be noted. If the photographic adapter is attached to the right side of the beam splitter, then the right ocular view only must be used in composing the photograph. Alternately closing one eye or the other while looking through the microscope will quickly demonstrate the considerable difference. Many disappointing photographs have resulted from consideration of a stereo view in which the area of primary interest was partially obscured on the photographed side, while being clearly seen from the other side of the binoculars. A slight repositioning of the microscope while looking through the ocular only on the camera side will correct this difficulty.

Stereoscopic photographs can also be taken, and when these paired films are properly viewed, can be very much of an improvement over single views. Particularly in reviewing cases done some time ago, the availability of stereo permits identification of questionable structures when their relationships otherwise may have been forgotten.

I simply take a photograph, advance the film, shift the microscope right or left 2 or 3 cm, recenter the field, and take another picture. The two pictures form a surprisingly adequate stereo pair, considering the crudity of the system. Care should be taken not to raise or lower or rotate the microscope and to move it directly laterally. The distance moved is also surprisingly noncritical (Fig. 14.7). I use this method routinely. It takes only a few seconds longer per photograph, and theorectically uses twice as much film, but these seem trivial objections. Prior to taking routine stereo photographs, I usually took duplicate photographs in order to be certain that vibration, movement, or some chance fault did not ruin

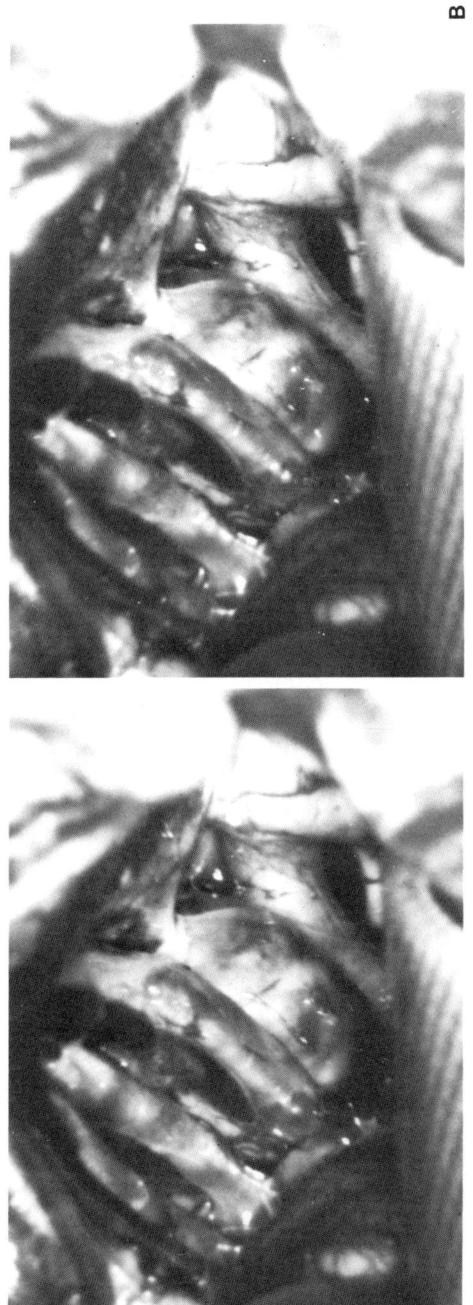

FIG. 14.7. A stereo pair visualizing an arteriovenous malformation and aneurysm dissected out in the Sylvian fissure. The challenge of vigorous pulsation as well as the requirement of great depth of field has been met. *A* is to be viewed at with the right eye and *B* with the left eye for stereoscopic visualization.

an important photograph wanted for reproduction. Now I have a choice between the two views of the stereo pair, so that nothing is lost; not even time or film.

Photographic Exposure

For all practical purposes, photography through the microscope is restricted to color film. While black and white panchromatic films may be used, the loss of color information is so great that it is for most purposes not desirable. While it is true that a black and white reproduction made from a color transparency is not as good as a black and white original, the results are generally acceptable. We use Eastman Kodak 35-mm ASA 160, Ektachrome ET 135 film, rated at 3200° K, which gives excellent color balance. Daylight film requires a blue filter and the loss of light involved and the marked increase in exposure required (4×) would make this unwarranted, even with a superior daylight film rated at ASA 400. Photographers confidently expect release of an ASA 400 3200° K film with higher acutance and better overall quality from Kodak in the near future. This is a much to be desired innovation.

Shutter speeds would obviously seem to have to be quite fast to avoid motion blur. Respiratory pulsation of the brain or spinal cord can produce a major displacement, and cardiac pulsation transmitted as vessel movement is, of course, a major problem as well. Since all of our operative procedures are carried out under endotracheal intubation with the use of a muscle-paralyzing drug and controlled respiration provided by a mechanical respirator, we have the anesthetist stop respirations for the instant of the photograph. On the other hand, this would be no solution for the cardiac vascular pulsation nor for microscope vibration. Nevertheless, it is here on the question of shutter speed that the greatest compromise is made. We actually take our pictures with a 1-second exposure with the respiration cut off. For vessel movement, 1-second exposures or longer will give sharper pictures than ¼ or ½ second. The apparent paradox occurs since most of the vessel motion will be a rather brief systolic pulsation. During a 1-second exposure, this will occupy a small fraction of the second and, therefore, the picture will appear essentially as sharp as though taken with a very short exposure carefully timed to occur during diastole. The long exposure averages out fast movements. This long exposure also permits the smallest possible aperture in order to improve depth of field.

The larger the aperture (the smaller the f number), the less depth of field is present. This means that the area in sharp focus can be a very, very narrow range. Particularly in the higher magnifications, the depth of field is already severely limited and even reasonably acceptable photographs must show only a relatively flat area. If a considerable depth of field is required, small apertures such as f44 can provide depth of field which will be satisfactory. In any case, the choice between depth of field and speed is always a compromise. If the light were bright enough or the film fast enough, shutter speeds of 1/250 of a second and an f stop of f64 would always be used. Unfortunately, this would require 1000 times the light brightness or film speed in combination, a situation not likely to be achieved in the reasonable future. The compromise is met with the 1-second shutter speed.

Depth of field varies inversely with magnification. It also varies directly with the number of the f stop which, of course, means inversely with the size of the lens opening. F stops are marked on the iris diaphragm setting ring of the 220-mm photographic adapter and are calibrated as f14, f16, f22, f32, f44, and f64. Except for their relationship to each other, they could be considered as arbitrary numbers because of the other components in the optical path.

All of my photographs are taken with the factors as noted in Table 14.1.

If a separate assistant's binocular viewing tube is placed on the beam splitter, the other port can carry either the television camera or the 35-mm still camera. Since the 35-mm camera is used for so few seconds at a time, a combination unit can be used (Fig. 14.8). My original unit used a 137-mm primary lens and a movable mirror to direct the beam 90° to the vidicon. With the mirror flipped out of the way (a separate hand movement to remember), the light path went through an additional 3.5× expander lens to provide full coverage of the 35-mm film. A new Zeiss-Urban dual camera adapter (Fig. 14.9) has fixed beam splitter to divide the light and so requires either twice the exposure time or one stop larger aperture. I prefer the 2-second exposure, keeping the f stop unchanged. This new unit uses a 137-mm lens, correct for the vidicon, and a 2.5× expander, which gives a photographic circle 27 mm in diameter. A 1.5×

TABLE 14.1

Factors Used for Photography of Microneurosurgery

300-mm objective
220-mm photoadapter
2× expander
Ektachrome ET 135 Tungsten, ASA 160
Standard development
1-second exposure
6×, 10× f32
16×, 25× f22
Hold the respiration

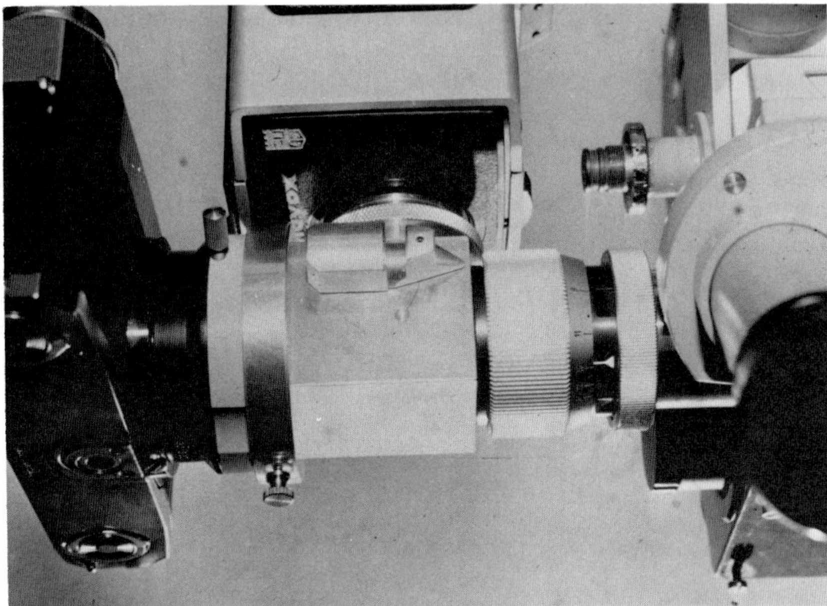

FIG. 14.8. A photoadapter with movable mirror and expander lens to alternate between television camera and 35-mm camera.

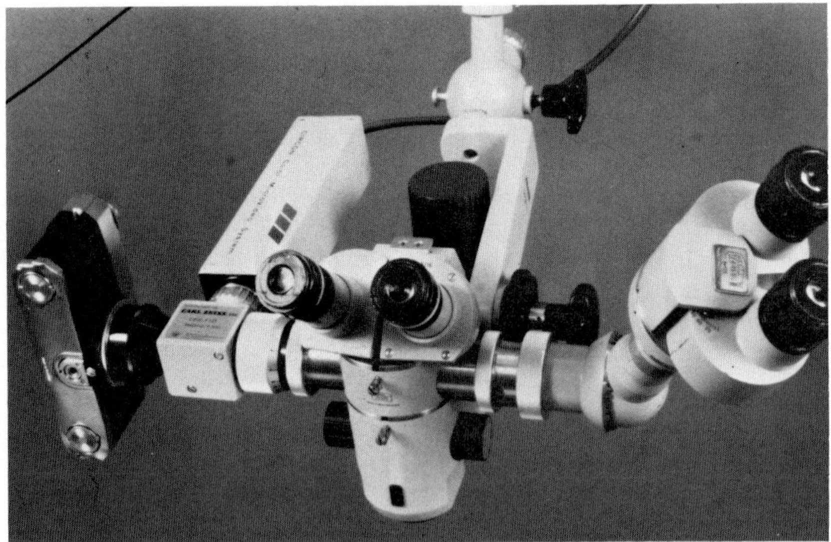

FIG. 14.9. Photoadapter with beam splitter and expander to permit simultaneous use of television and 35-mm camera.

additional expander has to be added to get full coverage. A 3.5× built-in expander has been promised by Zeiss, which would be a far better arrangement. When the new ASA 400 color film is made available, a 1-second exposure will still permit an f stop selection small enough to provide excellent depth of field.

CHAPTER

15

Neurosurgical Applications of Video Techniques

RONALD I. APFELBAUM, M.D.

INTRODUCTION

The rapid development of video technology in the last decade has allowed increasing utilization of this modality of "electronic photography" in many fields of medicine and specifically in our own specialty of neurosurgery. This technology is especially applicable to microneurosurgical procedures because the operative field, in such cases, is well defined and demarcated, and well lighted. Video equipment can be easily attached to the side port of the beam splitter on the operating microscope so that no camera operator is needed to aim and focus the video camera.

The use of video techniques offers many advantages. The foremost of these advantages is to allow the entire operating room staff to see the operative field and thereby participate in the operation. Because we often operate through narrow apertures and at significant depths, it is usually difficult or impossible for anyone other than the surgeon and perhaps his immediate assistant to visualize the operative field. As such, it is difficult for the scrub nurse and others to appreciate what is being accomplished and to focus a high level of attention on the operation to most effectively assist the surgeon. When video equipment is available, all in the operating theater can visualize the operative field. The staff's attention is thereby accentuated rather than diminished and they are able to better assist the surgeon by being better able to anticipate his needs.

Additional advantages of videotaping (which, of course, applies as well to other forms of documentation) is the ability to record portions of the operative procedure for individual review and critique. This applies equally well whether it is used for self criticism, for teaching purposes, or in a conference setting. We have found this function extremely valuable and routinely show videotapes of our cases at our departmental weekly conferences utilizing a number of monitors and a video projector for this purpose.

Videotaped material, of course, is instantly available, unlike photographic media, and the videotapes can be reused if desired.

Technical Details

While I believe most of us are familiar with the basic concepts of how photography works, namely, the alteration via a photochemical reaction of silver containing salts in a photographic emulsion, and can understand how color photography is merely an extension of this through more complicated chemical wizardry, most of us will probably never know how an artist like Dr. Netter can so vividly and accurately capture intimate anatomic details in a manner which makes them readily apparent to all. We should, however, be able to understand, at least in rudimentary form, the basic principles behind the generation of a video image and its recording so that we might better apply this technology.

The video camera is the first component in the system. Illumination is provided by the integral light source within the operating microscope and perhaps is supplemented by additional illumination aimed at the field from accessory sources. This light is reflected from the field and converted to essentially parallel rays of light by the objective lens on the microscope (Fig. 15.1). This parallel light path allows the insertion of various lenses

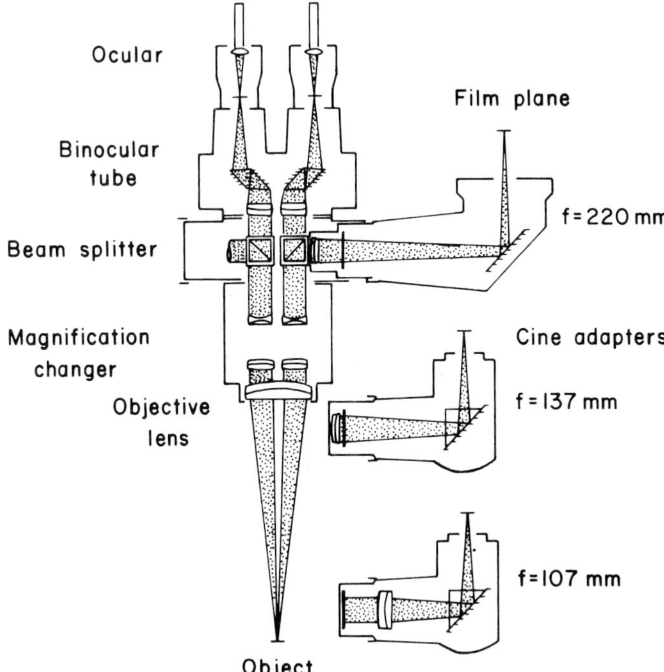

FIG. 15.1. Light path in Zeiss operating microscope demonstrating interposition of beam splitter in the light path and various focal length photoadapters to accommodate different types of photo documentation devices. (Modified and used with permission of Carl Zeiss).

to change the magnification and also allows the insertion of a beam splitter to divert part of the light beam to side ports to which are connected observer tubes and photodocumentation devices.

For several years now, we have been employing an optical switch* to allow the use of both a 35-mm camera and a video camera on the same port of the beam splitter (1). It always seems a bad compromise to have to monopolize one port of the beam splitter for a 35-mm camera which would only be used for moments during an entire operation. With the use of the switch, the video camera is only switched off momentarily when it is desirable to take a 35-mm picture. The 35-mm and video images are identical, so one can compose and focus the picture on the TV monitor and then take a picture after setting the f-stop.

The optical switch or photo adaptor has a lens system to focus the light on the face of a special sensing element within the video camera. This is known as the camera tube or vidicon (Fig. 15.2). It contains a photosensitive target plate which changes resistance in inverse proportion to the intensity of light falling on its surface. An electron beam is swept across the target, in a controlled manner, scanning its surface. The variations in resistance of individual areas on the target screen are thereby detected and converted to a video signal after appropriate electronic amplification and processing. This processing includes combining the video signals and appropriate synchronizing pulses.

In color systems, individual colors are formed by using an *additive* color process combining red, blue, and green to form any shade of color in the spectrum. More expensive color cameras, such as those used for broadcast work, include individual vidicon tubes to sense each of these individual colors. In the type of cameras that we will be using, however, compromises are effected and a single tube system is used with various means of obtaining the individual color components through the use of electronic filtration and special processing circuitry. Much of this circuitry is included in the camera control unit, separate from the camera itself, and connected by an interconnecting multiconductor cable. Most of the control circuitry functions automatically and, on the type of equipment that is usually used in neurosurgery, does not require individual adjustment.

The processed signal from the TV camera can then be connected directly to a video monitor. This is really nothing more than a color television receiver which has been modified to accept the video signal directly, bypassing the tuner in the set. (The tuner is used to take the radiofrequency signal transmitted over the airwaves and process this to extract the video information.) Within the monitor, the video signal is

* Manufactured by the Designs for Vision Corporation, New York, N.Y.

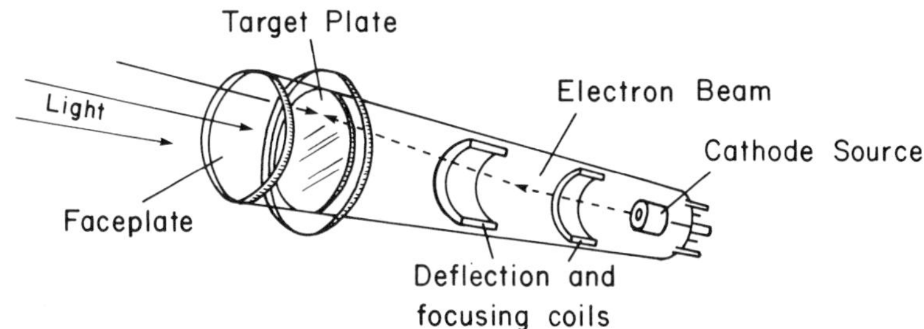

FIG. 15.2. Diagram of essential components of vidicon tube, the photo receptor device within the TV camera. (Modified from and used with permission of Charles Bensinger, The Video Guide, Video-Info Publications, 1977).

again processed and ultimately controls the deflection and intensity of the electron beam within the cathode ray tube (picture tube). The phosphores on the face of the tube glow in proportion to the intensity of the electron beam. This beam scans the face of the tube in a similar manner and synchronized to the beam in the vidicon tube in the video camera. Its intensity is modulated in proportion to the light intensity received on a target in the vidicon tube, resulting in the duplication of the image focused on the vidicon tube.

The video image is made up of 525 horizontal lines in the NTSC† system. The electron beams in both the camera and monitor scan one half of these lines (every other one) in 1/60th of a second, then scan the other half in the next 1/60th of a second. Each of these sets of 262½ lines is called one field and the two fields are combined (interlaced) to produce one 525 line frame each 1/30th of a second (Fig. 15.3). Thirty complete frames are scanned every second so that the human eye does not see individual frames or scan lines but perceives a complete and moving picture.

In practical use, most often the TV signal from the TV camera will be connected first to a videotape recorder. Videotape recorders work in a similar fashion to audiotape recorders in that the video signal is recorded on a thin plastic tape coated with a magnetically sensitive oxide. The requirements, however, for video recording are significantly more stringent then for audio recording. Very precise speed control of the tape is required in addition to the precise tracking of the tape. The tape path is such that the tape wraps around a recording head drum (Fig. 15.4).

† National TV Standards Committee of the Electronic Industries Association. This system (NTSC) is used exclusively in American systems and for the most part in the Western hemisphere. A different system is used in Western Europe where a 625 line scan system called PAL is used. France and the Soviet Union use still a different separate system called SECAM. None of these systems are intercompatible, and videotapes made on one of these will not play back on another, although equipment is available to copy a tape and convert it to another system.

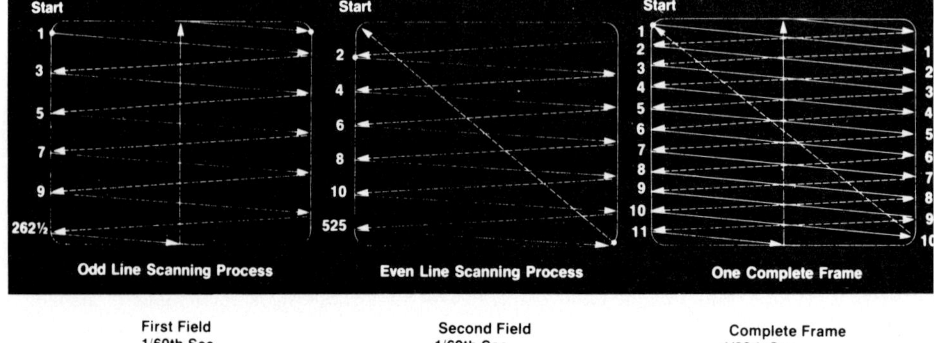

FIG. 15.3. TV scanning process. Diagram of scanning pattern to detect and reproduce the video picture (see text). (From Charles Bensinger, The Video Guide, Video-Info Publications, 1977).

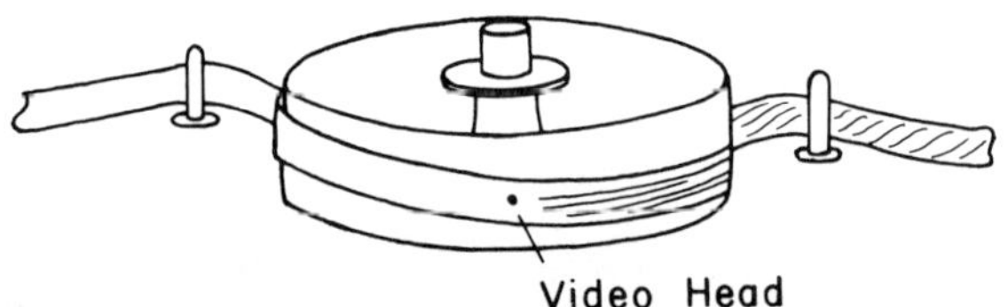

FIG. 15.4. Helical scanning. Diagram of tape path used in a helical scan videotape recorder. The videotape is wrapped in a helical fashion around the drum containing the video heads to record a diagonal band of information. (Modified from and used with permission of Charles Bensinger, The Video Guide, Video-Info Publications, 1977).

Within this drum, two recording heads rotate at 1800 revolutions/minute so that each head passes over the tape every 1/60th of a second. In addition, the supply reel is on a higher plane then the take-up reel, resulting in an angulated tape path. The tape thus contacts the rotating head in a helical fashion, resulting in the video signal being laid down in a diagonal band (Fig. 15.5). Each individual band contains the video information for one field of the picture (262½ lines). You recall that an individual picture or video image is composed of two fields or 525 separate lines. Combined within the video signal are the horizontal and vertical sync pulses which control the electronic beam in the CRT. Also recorded on the videotape is a control track which serves as an electronic sprocket to regulate and precisely control the speed of the tape transport via a servo mechanism. In addition, audio tracks are laid down in a similar manner to our standard audio tape. On playback, the material is extracted by a similar process and then supplied to the video monitor.

The Use of Video Techniques

To employ video techniques one must have available the video camera with a suitable photo adaptor or optical switch to connect it to the microscope. (To record macrosurgical procedures a tripod to support the camera and an appropriate zoom lens will also be required.) In addition, as a bare minimum, a video monitor as described above is required, though most users will also want to have available a videotape recorder. Some specific details are provided to help guide those who do not already possess this equipment in an addendum to this chapter. Many hospitals, of course, already have video equipment which can be employed in neurosurgery. It is our procedure to place the video camera, mounted on the optical switch, on the side of the beam splitter closest to the scrub nurse (Fig. 15.6). This allows the surgeon free access to the scrub nurse

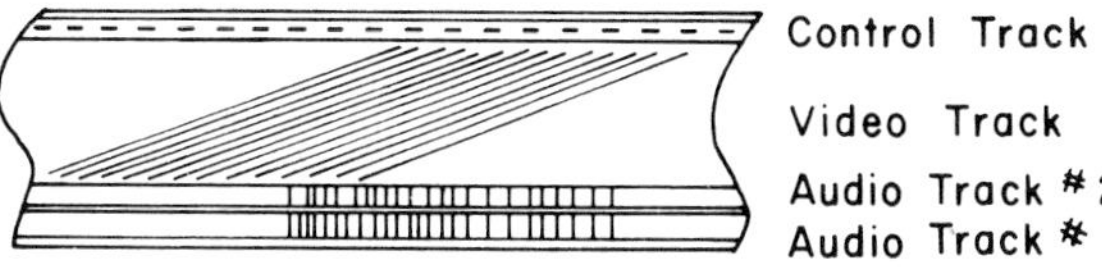

FIG. 15.5. Videotape track patterns. Pattern of recording on ¾-inch videotape. The control track and two audio tracks are applied in a linear manner similar to audio recording. The video track, however, is applied diagonally utilizing the helical scanning configuration, as described in the text, as a greatly increased amount of information must be recorded to produce a video picture. (From Charles Bensinger, The Video Guide, Video-Info Publications, 1977).

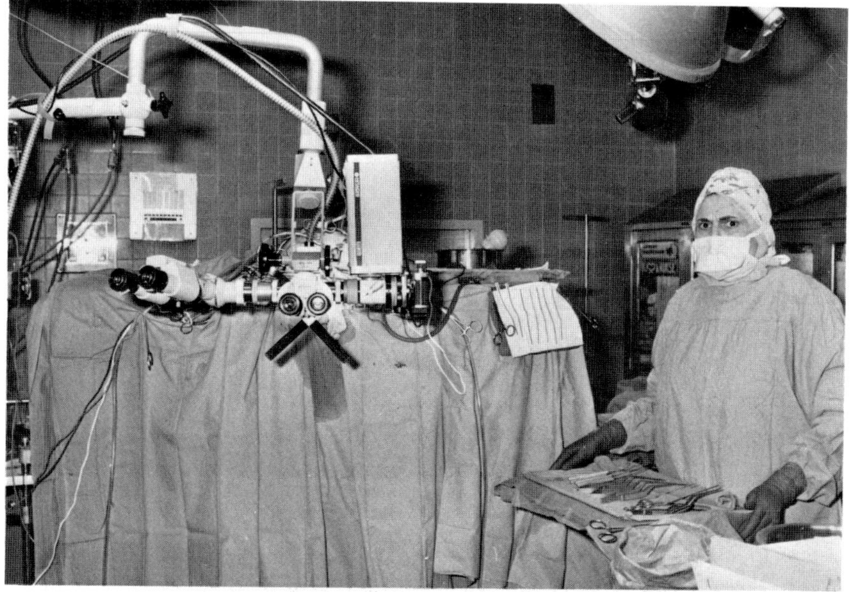

FIG. 15.6. View of microscope setup showing relationships of the video equipment and positioning of the equipment relative to the scrub nurse. In this case the patient is in the sitting position for a posterior fossa craniectomy.

by placing his assistant on the opposite side. The optical switch is placed on the microscope in such a manner as to rotate the video camera so that it is 90° from the axis of the surgeon's binocular objective. (Fig. 15.7) Placed in this manner, it will not compete for space with the surgeon's head nor will it impede his access to the nurse or operative field. A check is made at this point to be sure that the picture obtained on the monitor is correctly oriented. If it is not, the TV camera can be loosened from its mount and rotated to achieve proper orientation.

The interconnecting cable from the TV camera to its control unit is connected and if a microphone is desired to record a sound track, this too may be placed on the microscope adjacent to the camera or may be clipped to the surgeon's scrub suit (for those cameras which do not include an internal microphone) (Fig. 15.8). The output of the video

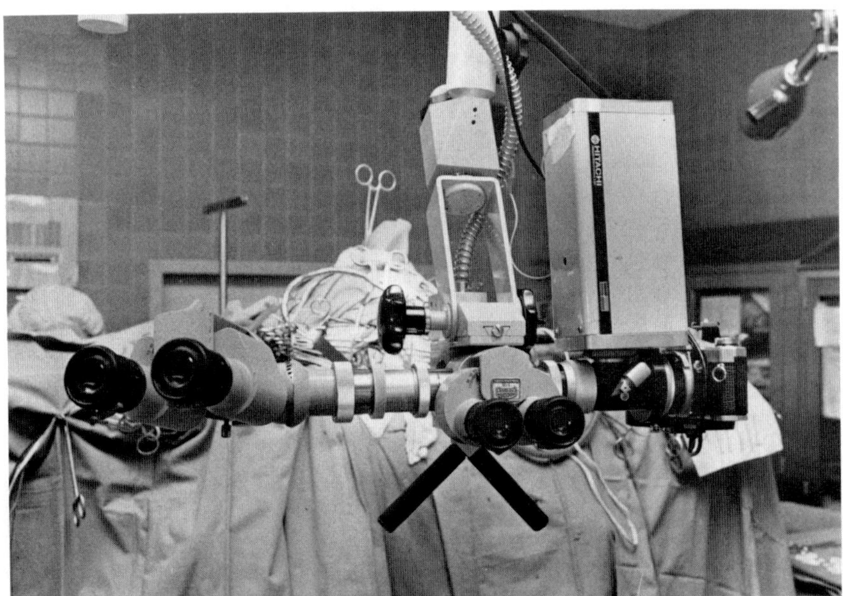

FIG. 15.7. Closeup view of the microscope with TV and still cameras mounted on the optical switch.

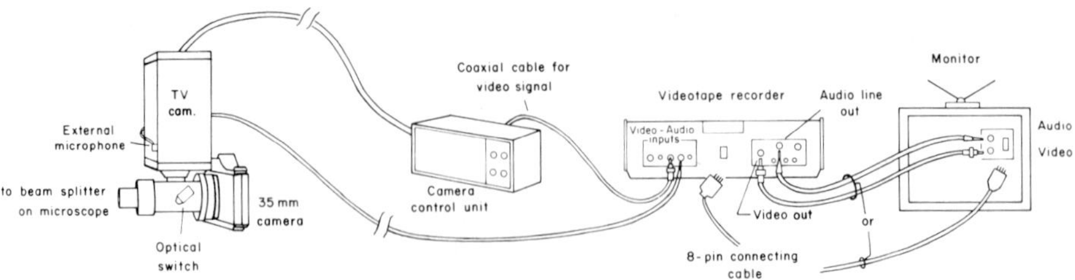

FIG. 15.8. Diagram of connections for use of video camera and videotape recorder.

control unit is connected to the input of the videotape recorder, and the output of the videotape recorder is connected to the television monitor. Most tape recorders and monitors are equipped with a standard 8 to 10 pin cable that allows their complete interconnection. Alternatively, a single coaxial cable can be connected from the video output of the recorder to the video input of the monitor. If several video monitors are used in the operating room, they can be connected in parallel as each video monitor will have two video inputs. In this manner, the signal is looped through each one. At the *last* video monitor in the chain, the switch marked 72 ohms, which is a terminator for the coaxial cable, should be placed in the *on* position. Obviously, if only one video monitor is used, then on that one the switch will be placed in the *on* position. Pressing the record button on the monitor will allow the video signal to be fed through the monitors even if the recorder is not in the play function, that is, even if the tape is not moving. However, a cassette tape must be inserted in the machine before this pass along of the video signal will occur.

The equipment is then ready to record any portions of the operation desired, but all of the operation will be visible to the staff in the operating room. To record, the recorder is placed in the play position and then returned to a stop or, if available, a pause mode when recording is no longer desired. We have found it useful to modify a tape recorder to include an external foot switch. This is a relatively simple modification that can usually be performed by your local TV service facility. This allows remote control of the pause function so that the surgical assistant can start and stop the recorder as desired during the operation.

Depending on the combination of ocular lenses and the focal length of the binocular tubes used, the diameter of the field seen by the camera may not be the same as that seen by the operator. We have found, for example, that it is useful to use 12.5× ocular lenses for the operator. This gives the operator a wider field with less magnification and encourages the use of a higher power setting on the magnification changer within the microscope. The picture seen by the TV camera and other photodocumentation devices is thus enlarged. The result, however, is that the field "seen" by the photodocumentation devices is smaller than that seen by the operator. He thus must be careful that he is not operating at the edge of his visual field and off the screen of the TV or still camera. The scrub nurse or assistants can be useful in advising him when he is operating off the center of the screen. A reticle can be inserted in the surgeon's ocular to define the field seen by the photodocumentation devices, but this has not been necessary in our experience. If 20× oculars are used, the field of the surgeon and photo devices is more nearly congruent.

It is important that the surgeon ascertain that the ocular lenses are properly focused prior to the start of the case. We have obtained our best results by having the surgeon wear his eyeglasses if he normally uses them and to use the appropriate highpoint ocular lenses. The individual adjustment of these eye pieces is then set at 0. In this manner, the surgeon's image will be in focus at the same time as the TV picture. The practice of correcting visual errors by adjusting the oculars can result in an out of focus video picture unless individual adjustments are made every time the magnification changer on the microscope is altered.

The f-stop on the photoadaptor or optical switch is adjusted to provide an adequate amount of illumination while viewing the video monitor. Over illumination is just as bad as inadequate illumination and will limit the ability to obtain true color fidelity. Illumination is generally not a problem while working on the cerebral surface but becomes more critical the deeper one proceeds. Reflections off bright objects such as cottonoid pledgets or shiny retractors in the operative field will significantly impair picture quality. This is because the video camera contains automatic circuitry to adjust the gain or brightness of the picture. A bright spot, therefore, might be interpreted as a bright overall picture and the gain accordingly reduced, throwing the area of interest into an inadequate exposure range. It has been our practice to record only small segments of an operation on videotape. While the use of a videotape recorder modified with a foot switch as mentioned above facilitates this, an acceptable alternative is to have personnel who are not scrubbed control the videotape recorder. Dr. Ted Kurze has made what seems like an excellent suggestion in this regard. Prior to the surgery, the case is discussed by the surgeon and the second assistant and keypoints in the operation pointed out. The second assistant is then assigned to capture these keypoints on the videotape. In this manner, this provides an additional educational function for this trainee.

A videotape can be erased and used over and over so that there should be no hesitancy about recording significant segments of the operation. Nevertheless, it is both time-consuming and boring to try to review a long procedure just to extract a few useful moments of information. With experience, however, selective recording techniques will be developed in which only desired portions of the procedures will be recorded.

Advanced Video Techniques

Once one acquires a basic video system and gains experience with it, the need for improvements will be readily seen. It is difficult and cumbersome to remove equipment from the operating room when it is desired to be used in a conference situation and for individual review. Thus, the next logical step is the purchase of additional equipment for use in one's office or conference facility. This will require a second videotape recorder and a second monitor.

Also, it is often desirable to edit out small segments of the material for a conference situation or to prepare a teaching videotape. Somewhat crude but generally satisfactory edits can be performed utilizing two recorders. However, superior machines are available with editing capabilities. Equipment such as this incorporates more accurate controling circuits allowing better editing. Among other things they perform the edit switchover, that is, the conversion from one machine to another during what is known as the vertical interval. This is the time when the picture is actually off the screen so that no breakup of the picture is seen and a clean edit results. To edit properly it is necessary that both machines be running at normal speed at the point that the edit is desired. To do this, both machines have to be backed up prior to the edit point an equal distance and then run forward to the edit point. To achieve this with precision, various editing consoles are available. Some of these are made by the individual videotape recorder manufacturers, while others are manufactured by independent companies. This equipment may use the control track pulses at the time of recording to effect an accurate edit, or even more accurate editing may employ a time code recorded on the audio channel.

Advanced editing techniques might also employ the use of character generators to add titles to the material and special effects generators to allow the insertion of additional material or the fading from one scene to another. This equipment is expensive but may be available in the audiovisual departments of larger teaching institutions or time may be rented on some of this equipment at local video production companies.

Summary

Video technology has advanced to the point that small lightweight cameras can be easily added to the operating microscope. This photodocumentation modality offers major advantages in the performance of the operation by facilitating the participation of the entire operating staff. In addition, it allows review and critical assessment of one's own performance which hopefully will lead to improvements. It has an outstanding educational value with many obvious areas of applicability. With the growth of the home video market, further improvement in equipment and further reductions in cost are likely.

ACKNOWLEDGMENTS

Most of the material in this chapter reflects the contributions and teachings of the many who have preceded the author in this area and are not original contributions. Especially helpful have been Dr. Leonard Malis, Dr. Theodore Kurze, Mr. Richard Feinbloom of the Designs for Vision Corporation, Mr. Peter Hoerenz of Carl Zeiss, and Mr. Bernard Munzelli of Hitachi Corporation. A useful source of basic nonmedical video information is *The Video Guide* by Charles Bensinger published by Video-Info Publications, P.O. Box 1507, Santa

Barbara, Calif. 93102. Portions of the material in this chapter are taken from a chapter entitled "Photodocumentation in Neurosurgery" by the author which is included in Volume II of *Cerebrovascular Surgery*, J. M. Fein and E. Flamm, Editors, 1981 (in press) and used with permission of the publisher, Springer Verlag, New York.

REFERENCE

1. Apfelbaum, R. I. An optical switch for improved photography through the operating microscope. Surg. Neurol. 6: 335–336, 1976.

ADDENDUM

Specific Information regarding Video Equipment

The material contained below is intended as a general guide and reflects the writer's personal opinion at the date of writing this (September 1980). Video technology is an extremely rapidly advancing field in which we see new and improved products being introduced often and significant improvements occurring frequently. The information below, therefore, should be used only as a general guide.

Video Cameras

The video camera must meet several requirements if it is to be used with the operating microscope. It must obviously be of a size and weight compatible with the microscope to avoid unbalancing or overloading it and to allow it to fit within the confines of the draping in the operative field. In addition, it must have adequate sensitivity to respond to the available light with good color fidelity. To achieve these goals most of the color camera systems on the market, which are applicable to microsurgery, consist of two units: The camera head itself which attaches to the operating microscope and the color processing unit to which it is connected by a control cable. The color processing unit contains the electronic wizardry which combines with the camera to produce the complete video signal. Some cameras have built in microphones as well. An excellent camera in our opinion is the Hitachi 9017. It has been designed for use on the operating microscope and weighs a mere 1.6 kg which is quite satisfactory. It has proven to be a reliable performer, giving consistently excellent results. It is priced in the neighborhood of $5,000 and has outperformed other cameras costing more than twice as much in side by side tests. While there are cameras on the market now which are smaller, the size of the Hitachi camera is quite adequate, and there seems to be little advantage to a smaller camera if it does not perform better or costs more.

There is a significant improvement anticipated in color cameras in the next decade when the vidicon tube is replaced by a semiconductor sensing system known as a charge coupled device (CCD). These are extremely small and will allow very tiny cameras to be perfected, while also reducing costs.

Videotape Recorders

The industry standard for small videotape recorders is the ¾-inch U-matic cassette recorder. The video cassette may be considered as similar to an audio cartridge, although it is much larger. With the use of video cassettes, individual threading and handling of tape is eliminated. This facilitates the use by nontechnically trained personnel and at the same time extends the life of the equipment, protecting it from misuse and damage as well as the wear and tear associated with handling. All ¾-inch U-matic cassette recorders use the same basic recording system patented by the Sony Corporation, and tapes prepared on any one may be played on any other (that is, as long as all are using the NTSC standard; see previous discussion about this in the text of the chapter). This system will produce a good quality videotape sufficient for editing and even, with proper electronic processing, for use on broadcast TV. Although Sony has been the pioneer in this area and is the industry leader, their competitors and imitators also produce excellent quality equipment.

The ½-inch videotape cassette systems have been recently heavily promoted for use in the home videotape market. There are, however, two competing formats. The so-called Beta format and the VHS format. These are *not* intercompatible with each other, and a tape recorded on one system cannot be played on the other. (In fact, they use different design cassettes.) While these machines are smaller and somewhat less costly than the ¾-inch machines, they are probably more appropriate for home use than for hospital-based medical use. Editing functions are not as readily available as with the ¾-inch format, and in addition, the lack of intercompatibility is a significant limiting factor. Also, picture quality deteriorates more rapidly with each succeeding generation (copy) than with the ¾-inch system. A basic ¾-inch videotape recorder can be obtained for about $2,000. More elaborate machines, having editing functions, cost two to three times as much.

Commercially recorded tapes may usually be obtainable in both the ¾-inch or either of the ½-inch formats. It is also possible to copy a tape from one machine to another in any format.

Video Monitors

A videotape monitor is also required. As mentioned before, this is basically a television set but takes its input directly from the video output of the recorder rather than from an RF signal over the air. Because monitors are a smaller proportion of any manufacturers market, they are priced significantly more than receivers alone.

A 19-inch or larger diagonal monitor should be purchased initially. It may be desirable to have several monitors depending on the geography of the operating theater. A single recorder and/or camera can supply a signal to drive several monitors without difficulty. The major manufacturers of video equipment are also good sources for monitors. Both the Sony and Sharp monitors, for example, are well regarded and either would be a good choice.

We have found it useful to assemble the operating room video equipment in a cabinet on wheels (Fig. 15.9). This allows placement of the monitor on the top shelf at eye level and the recorder below it. The lower section of the cabinet can then be used to house the camera control unit and provide storage for spare videotape as well as for microscope accessories which are not in use. If equipment is mounted on the cart, it may be removed from the operating theater and used in a conference setting as desired, although we have found it preferable to duplicate the equipment when practical and dedicate one recorder and monitor for operating room use only.

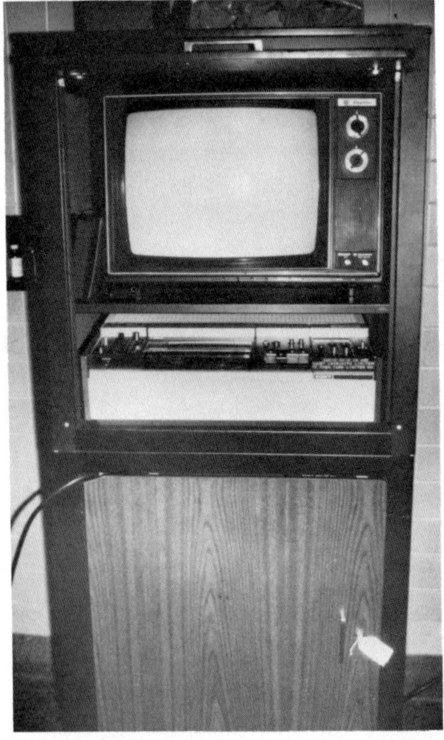

Fig. 15.9. Video equipment cabinet in operating room. The monitor and recorder are placed at convenient viewing and operating heights. Storage for videotapes and microscope accessories is provided in the lower compartment which also houses the camera control unit.

CHAPTER

16

Preparing Movies of Microsurgical Operations

ALBERT L. RHOTON, JR., M.D., AND CARLA J. LENKEY

The orientation of this paper is that of a "do it yourself" moviemaker. The surgical microscope has provided a marvelous opportunity to capture the delicate aspects of a neurosurgical operation using a camera that is easily attached to the microscope. The camera, because it is attached to the microscope, records the same detail seen by the surgeon while he is performing the operative task. Preparing operative movies without the surgical microscope involves a photographer coming to the operating room, filming over the surgeon's shoulder, and editing the film with the surgeon's help. This contrasts with the methods outlined here in which the surgeon fits the camera on the microscope, loads the film in the film magazine, selects the field for photography, and carries the developed film to a home study for viewing and editing during his spare time.

Colored movies provide a more accurate color reproduction and greater clarity of operative detail than tapes produced from a television camera and have the advantage of ease of display before large groups. A disadvantage of movie cameras is that they hold only enough film to record 3 minutes of the operation. Recording a 2-hour operation on film would involve a prohibitive cost, but could be done with a television monitor and tape deck for moderate cost. The fact that the movie cannot be run continuously upon initial consideration appears to be a disadvantage; however, by careful planning, one may on 100 to 300 feet of film capture most of the crucial aspects of a neurosurgical operation.

Film is easier to review and edit than television tapes. The film of several operations can be reviewed in only a few minutes. To edit movie film, one needs an inexpensive film editor, a splicer, and a few minutes of spare time. This contrasts with the condensation of a 2-hour television tape into a 15-minute tape which would take several hours, editing equipment often found only in a television studio, and personnel who are often available only during working hours. It is possible to transfer the information on movies to television tape. The quality of the TV image produced from film is excellent. The transfer from television tape to film, although possible, produces a less satisfactory image.

Preparing movies of microsurgical operations involves the selection of the following items: a movie camera that can be fitted on the operating microscope, a beam splitter, a cineadaptor, a reticule or micrometer disc that fits into one eyepiece on the binocular tube, and satisfactory lighting (Fig. 16.1) (3).

MOVIE CAMERA

Super 8- and 16-mm cameras have been fitted to the operating microscope (3–5). The 16-mm camera is preferred because 16-mm movies are more suitable for projection before groups. There are two 16-mm cameras which are commonly fitted to the surgical microscope: the Urban (Urban Engineering, Burbank, Calif.) and the Beaulieu (Carl Zeiss, Inc., New

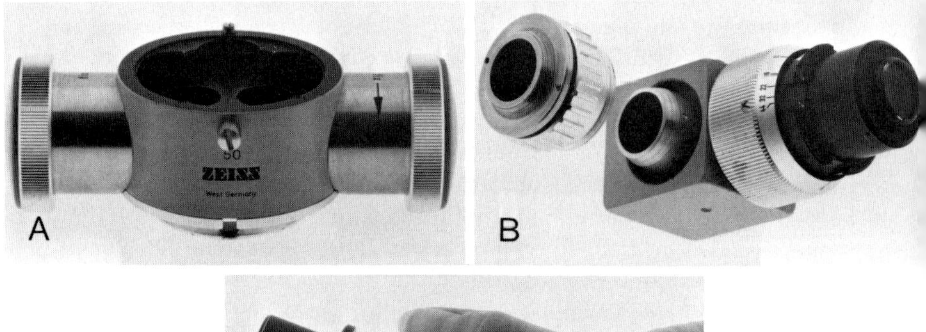

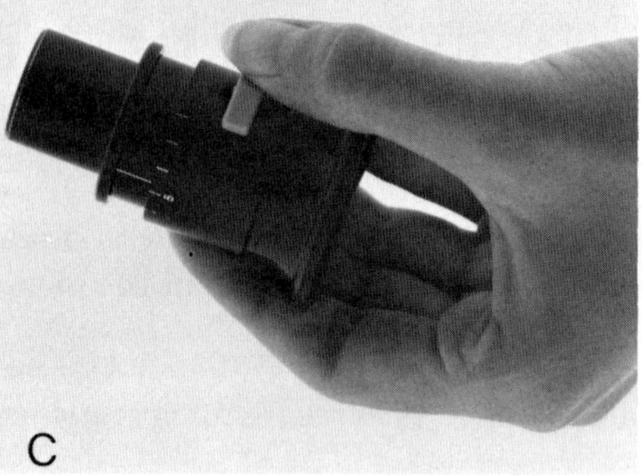

FIG. 16.1. (*A*) Zeiss beam splitter. The Zeiss beam splitter fits between the binocular tube and the body of the microscope. The rounded shafts on each side accept a photoadaptor to which the movie camera is attached. The number 50 on the beam splitter identifies the fact that one-half (50%) of the light reaches the surgeon's eye and one-half is directed into the accessory. (*B*) Cine adaptor to which the movie camera is attached. The metal ring to the left may be needed to fit some cameras to the adaptor. There are five f stops on the cine adaptor. Most applications require that the f stop be fully open. (*C*) Eyepiece which fits into the binocular tube. Satisfactory filming requires that the eyepiece setting be adjusted to correct for the surgeon's refractive errors if the surgeon does not wear his glasses and also for differences in the focus of the surgeon's eye and the camera.

York, N. Y.) (4, 5). The on-off switch for both is controlled by a foot pedal, and both hold 100 feet of film suitable for 3 minutes of filming. I prefer the Urban camera because of its light weight and ease of loading film and because the film magazines holding 100 feet of film can be changed without removing the camera from the microscope (Fig. 16.2) (4). The Beaulieu has the advantage of having a built-in light meter to control the exposure, but the camera must be removed from the microscope to load the film. The ease of changing film magazines is most important because this change is needed during the operation if one wishes to film for longer than 3 minutes. I prefer to load the film into the film magazine myself. This is a task which can be learned in a few minutes (Fig. 16.3).

BEAM SPLITTER

The beam splitter or divider consists of a semitransparent mirror which is placed in the path of the incident light beam and reflects the image

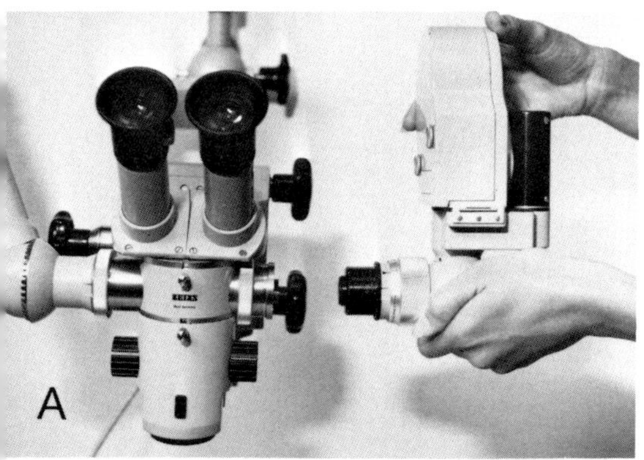

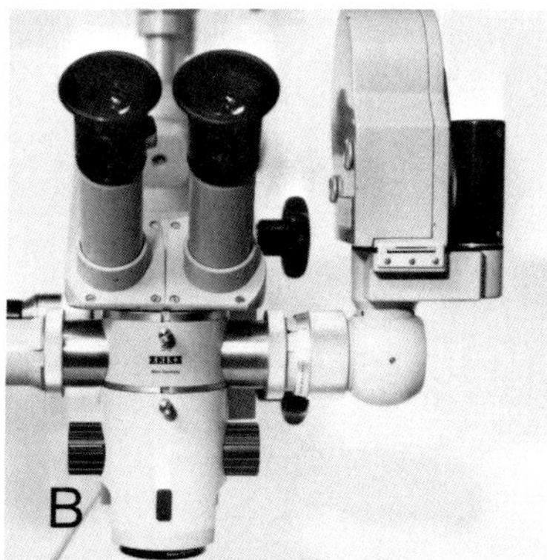

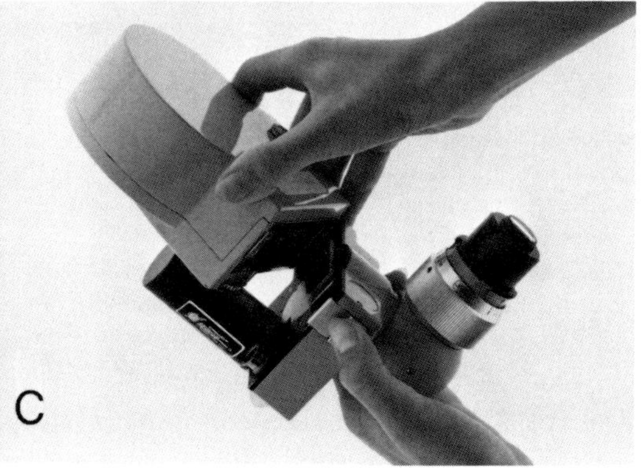

Fig. 16.2. (*A*) The Urban camera is held to the right of the beam splitter to which the camera attaches. (*B*) The cine adaptor attached to the camera has been fitted into the right side of the beam splitter. (*C*) The film magazines on the Urban camera clip easily onto the motor drive and cine adaptor. The motor drive and cine adaptor remain attached to the microscope during the changing of the film magazines. Several film magazines should be loaded before beginning the operation because each holds film for only 3 minutes of recording.

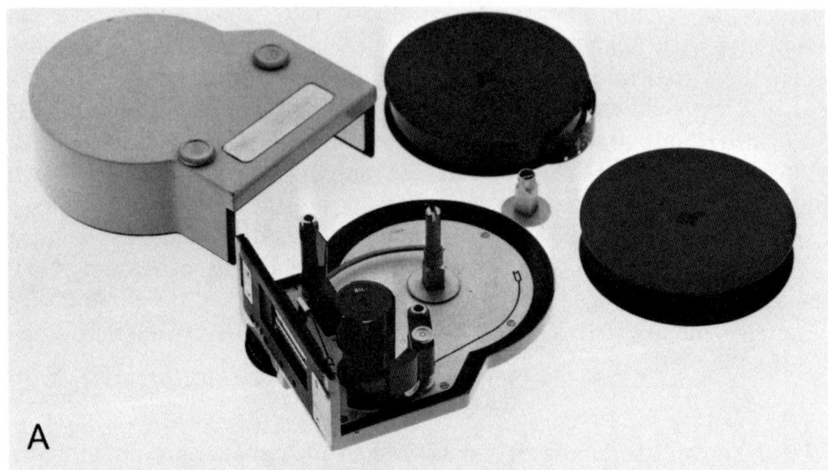

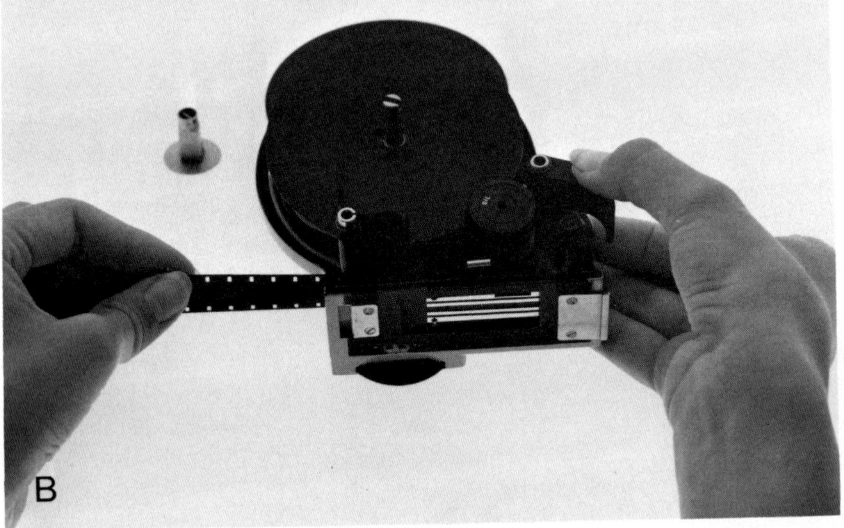

FIG. 16.3. (*A*) Urban camera opened and ready for loading film. The reel with the original film is above and the take-up reel with its adaptor are below. (*B*) The film is being loaded. (*C*) Film loaded. (*D*) Film magazine being closed.

into an accessory side tube. The beam divider is placed between the body of the microscope and the binocular tube. The Zeiss beam splitter directs the accessory images to the right and left side of the microscope (Carl Zeiss, Inc., New York, N. Y.). The most commonly used beam splitter (Zeiss, 50-50) directs one-half of the light into an accessory side tube. A "70-30" beam splitter (30% to the surgeon) allows more light for the accessories. The optical image seen by the surgeon is unaffected by the

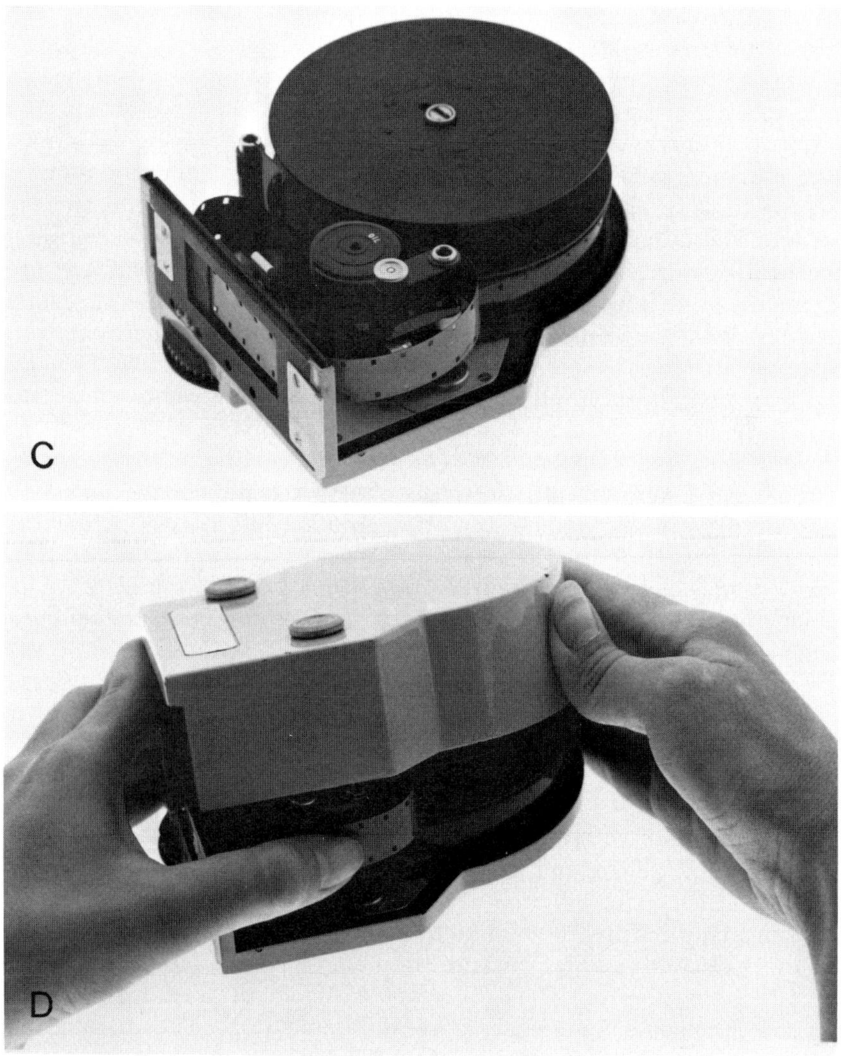

beam division except for the reduction in brightness of the image. The beam splitter 50 supplies the same amount of light to the observer tube and to the surgeon's eyepiece and is used primarily for an assistant's observer tube. The beam splitter 70 directs more light to the accessories than to the surgeon's eyepiece, an advantage when all the available light is needed by the movie or television camera. To minimize objectionable interference in the finished motion pictures caused by fingers and instruments obstructing the view, the camera is usually mounted on the left side of the beam splitter.

The number of accessories available has placed competing demands on the two ports of the beam splitter: there is a need for immediate viewing of the operation by nurses and anesthesiologists by displaying the output of a television camera on a monitor in the operating room; the need of the assistants to witness the operation through an observer tube; and the need of the surgeon to obtain still or cinephotography for teaching purposes. Two accessories, one on each side of the beam splitter, are commonly used; however, one may desire three or more accessories, such as a combination of a still 35-mm camera, television camera, and an observer tube, or another consisting of a movie camera, a still camera, and an observer tube, etc. Two means of attaching more than two accessories to the microscope are available. An optical switch, built to accommodate two accessories, may be attached to either of the two ports of the Zeiss beam splitter. Adjusting the switch directs the image to either, but not both, of the accessories. Another alternative, permitting the use of three or four accessories, is to place an Urban beam splitter in one or both sides of the binocular tube; thus two accessories may be attached to the Zeiss beam splitter between the binocular tube and the microscope body and another may be attached to each side of the binocular tube. Theoretically, six accessories could be used if optical switches were placed on each side of a conventional beam splitter or if beam dividers were placed in each side of the binocular tube.

CINE ADAPTORS

A photoadaptor with a light intensity control must be placed between the Zeiss beam splitter and the movie camera. The beam splitter accepts any one of three cine adaptors (Zeiss f-74, f-107 mm, and f-137). The f-107-mm adaptor is preferred for 16-mm movies of neurosurgery, although the magnification is lower because the field of view is larger than with the f-137-mm adaptor. The f-74 adaptor should be used for Super 8 cameras. Each cine adaptor offers five different f stops. The aperature is usually opened to the maximum during filming.

RETICULE

A micrometer disc or reticule is a small disc that fits into the eyepiece and has a focusing device and a rectangular frame on it. When filming, the camera is recording the monocular image seen by the eye on the side of the beam splitter to which the camera is attached. Thus, the disc is incorporated into the eyepiece on the side to which the camera is attached so that there is coincidence between the rectangular frame on the disc and the cine frame (Fig. 16.4).

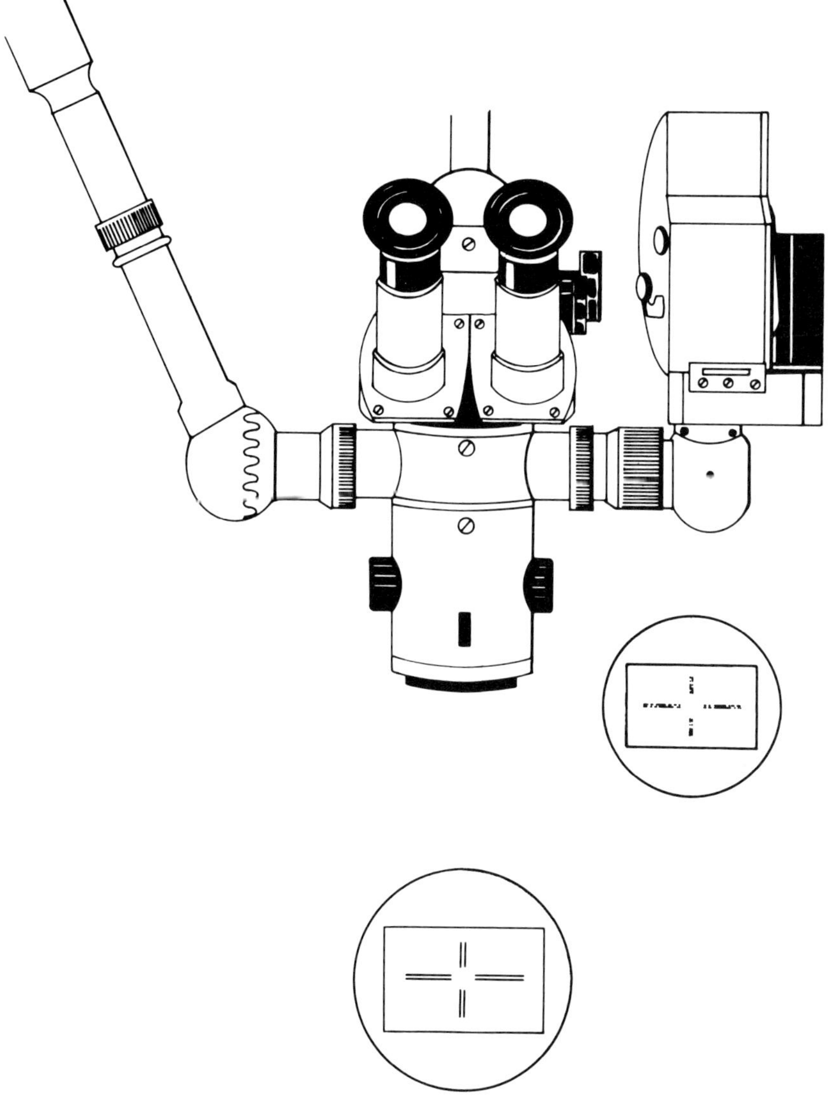

FIG. 16.4. Drawing of a Zeiss microscope. The Urban camera is attached to the right side of the beam splitter, and an observer tube is attached on the left side. Below the microscope is the image seen by the operator when a reticule or micrometer disc is fitted in one of the eyepieces. The reticule has a rectangular outline which outlines the approximate field seen by the camera and a series of four cross-hairs which, when properly adjusted to compensate for the surgeon's refractive error, are seen as four crossed pairs of parallel lines. The circular field to the right of the microscope shows the blurred image of the grid when the eyepiece with the reticule is improperly adjusted. The reticule should be fitted into the eyepiece on the same side as the camera.

The focusing device in the reticule provides an infinity correction setting for the eyepieces. It is improbable that satisfactory results will be obtained unless the reticule is used to select eyepiece settings that compensate for errors in the operator's vision. The reticule has four pairs of grid hairs which, when adjusted so as to correct for the surgeon's refractive error, will appear to be parallel. The movie camera attached to the beam splitter is in perfect focus only when a normal set of eyes has the field in focus with the eyepieces set at 0. If the surgeon has myopia or hyperopia, focusing the microscope up and down with the eyepiece on the zero setting until it is in good focus for the surgeon will throw the camera out of focus. The reticule has the advantage of selecting an eyepiece setting which corrects for the surgeon's refractive error and allows both the surgeon's and the camera's eye to be in focus at the same time. The surgeon should wear his glasses during the adjustment of the eyepieces using the reticule if he wears his glasses when operating with the microscope.

LIGHTING

The operating microscope is usually fitted with a lighting unit sufficient for operating, but not for photography. One common lighting unit insufficient for photography includes a 30-watt bulb and the transformer needed to illuminate it. For cinephotography a minimum of a 6-V, 50-watt lamp with a 100 va power supply is needed. Microscopes with a 30-watt bulb may be fitted with either a Zeiss or an Urban power booster and a 50-watt bulb which is automatically energized when the foot pedal switches the camera on. Even the 50-watt bulb may provide insufficient light for photography in some deep operative sites, such as the transsphenoidal exposure or when using 25- or 40-fold magnification. It is impossible to give optimal exposure data for all practical cases because of the different cameras, magnifications, lighting outfits, film speeds, and photographic situations. Some trial exposures are helpful in formulating exact exposure data. A recent trend has been to attach an accessory fiberoptic light to the microscope body directly adjacent to the objective lens, but this has the disadvantage that the accessory light is not coaxial. It was because of the need for increased light that the author developed a modification of the fiberoptic booster light (Applied Fiberoptics, Randolph, Mass.) (2). Recently we have started using the halogen light on the Zeiss 1H microscope and have found that this light is sufficient for our television and movie needs and, in some cases, it has been so bright that the light reaching the camera must be reduced by several f stops to prevent it from "brightening out" the image. Increasingly powerful fiberoptic light sources are also being developed and will replace the halogen and incandescent bulbs in the microscope body.

Fox (1) has summarized the methods for improving lighting for operating a camera as follows:

1. Use 50- instead of 30-watt bulbs
2. Keep bulbs and optical system clean
3. Discard bulbs with blue or dark spots in the light image
4. Use shorter focal length objective lens
5. Use eyepieces with greater magnification. They require less magnification (and hence less light loss) inside microscope unit
6. Avoid zoom lens system which absorbs more light
7. Use 30-70 beam splitter (70% to side arms) instead of 50-50 beam splitter
8. Open diaphragm to camera (but lose sharpness and depth of focus)
9. Select efficient film that requires less light
10. Make use of reflections in surgical wound
11. Remove black paint border around glass light deflector behind objective lens (some Zeiss microscopes)
12. Use add-on fiberoptic light sources (2)

FILM

There are many types of film that can be used in the camera. The two most common types of film used to make 16-mm movies of microsurgery are Kodak Ektachrome 7252 and Ektachrome 7242. The recommended film is Eastman Kodak commercial Ektachrome 7252 on 100-foot spools with doubly perforated edges. The original copy of Ektachrome 7252, when duplicated, results in the production of a better print for projection than does the 7242, but the original copy of the 7252 is less satisfactory for projection than the original copy of the 7242. Ektachrome 7242 is most commonly used when immediate projection of the original copy is desirable, as in newscasting. The ability to project the original copy is not a significant advantage in preparing movies of microsurgery because the original film should not be projected since the projector may scratch or damage it so that it is useless for making copies. One should select a film which, when edited, will produce the best copies, and that is Ektachrome 7252.

FILMING

The most common difficulties encountered are maintaining good focus, retaining the image within the reticule, insufficient light, reflections from the instruments, and attempts to film at too high a magnification.

One should select a magnification which will yield a large enough field that there is sufficient detail to orient a viewer to the site of the operation.

The camera films only a part of the field that is being seen by the surgeon. Thus, if your field becomes extremely restrictive, it is likely that there will not be sufficient orienting landmarks. Movies taken at 25- or 40-fold magnification are often of little value.

A common problem is that accurate focus is not maintained throughout the filming. It is common to find that novices do not fully appreciate the fine detail which they can see with the microscope. It is helpful to learn to expect the finest vessels on the neural surfaces to be crisply in focus. The image should be retained within the rectangle on the micrometer disc, and the eyepieces should be properly set to correct for refractive errors in both eyes and to correct for differences in the focus of the camera and the surgeon's eyes. The manual which accompanies the Urban camera provides a step-by-step description of how to focus the microscope for photography.

The surgical instruments should have a dull finish because the brilliant light from highly polished instruments reflected back through the surgical microscope can detract from the quality of the movies. Sharpness and sterilization are not affected by the dull finish.

DEVELOPING AND DUPLICATING THE FILMS

One needs to gain an appreciation of the various types of film in order to prepare movies for teaching purposes. The film used in the movie camera is called the original film. The original film should not be projected because it might be damaged and rendered useless for making copies. When I began filming operations, I had several originals of unique operations destroyed or badly scratched in a projector. When the original film is removed from the movie camera and sent for development, a work print is requested. The work print is the least expensive print. The work print may be projected while preserving the original film for making other prints. The other three types of copies of the original with which one needs to become acquainted are printing masters, answer prints, and projection prints. A printing master is a high quality reproduction of an original film suitable for serving as a template for reproducing copies for projection. Projection prints are high quality reproductions of a printing master or original suitable for projection. The original and printing master have the advantage of serving as a better template for producing copies for projection, but the projection print has the advantage of giving a better image on the screen than the original or master. When ordering a printing master or work print, it is advantageous to have edge numbers placed along the sides for editing. After you have completed your editing on your work print, you may use the numbers on the work print to edit the original or printing master. The edited original or printing master is sent to a studio for duplication of a first print, called the answer print.

The answer print is examined to check for needed corrections in lighting density, contrast, and color. After the corrections are made, the answer print is then duplicated into as many projection prints as needed. Projection prints released for showing are often referred to as release prints.

EDITING

When the original film is developed, one should order a work print. The work print is used for the initial viewing and editing. In my early filming, I found there was a tendency for the medical art studio to want to hold my original film and have me view it when a medical graphics person was available to project and edit the film with me. This was unproductive because coordinating my schedule with that of the art studio was almost impossible. Therefore, I began to store the film in my study, where I could view and edit it on an inexpensive film editor during evenings and weekends. Gloves may be worn, and great care taken not to scratch the original or master film. Splicing is done with a cold splicer which takes 10 to 15 seconds/splice. During the editing, light frames and blurred sequences are removed.

After a number of cases have been filmed, they are spliced together to yield a film of the desired length. Most films of individual microsurgical operations are only 5 to 6 minutes in length. The movies from individual operations may be combined one after the other to prepare movies of various lengths. It is rare that teaching conferences and, especially, presentations at scientific meetings allow the use of movies lasting longer than 15 to 20 minutes (3 or 4 cases). Original films cannot be repeatedly spliced into movies of different lengths; therefore, when asked to prepare a film of a different length than usual, a new printing master is ordered and edited to the desired length for making a projection print, rather than repeatedly editing the original film.

During editing, one needs to be aware of which side of the film the emulsion is on. Original film has the emulsion on the down side, that is, the emulsion is down when the film is run through a film editor from left to right. A copy, whether it be a printing master, work print, or projection print, reproduced from original film with the emulsion on the down side will have the emulsion on the up side. Thus, a work print ordered at the time the original is developed will have the emulsion on the up side. A copy produced from a master having the emulsion on the up side will have the emulsion on the down side, etc. When splicing film from different cases in sequence, the emulsion on the film from the different cases should be on the same side. It is difficult to splice film with the emulsion on different sides, and the focus shifts if it is projected. Turning film over (from emulsion down to emulsion up, or vice versa) will make an operation performed on one side look like it came from the opposite side; thus, a film from an operation in the left cerebellopontine angle, when turned, will appear to have come from the right cerebellopontine angle. Titles, on the other hand, cannot be rotated because that will make them appear backward on the screen.

TITLES

Titles are prepared by placing white press-on letters onto a sheet of clear acetate. The acetate sheets with the title are then laid over whatever colorful background you desire. The art studio then photographs the acetate sheet and background to provide a strip of film of sufficient length to be read easily. Each foot of film provides 2½ seconds of running at the time of projection. The titles are returned as a strip of original film which is spliced into the operative material. The titles should be produced so that they have the emulsion on the same side as the remainder of the film.

CONCLUSION

Cinematography offers an opportunity for self-study and improvement. Learning to maintain the accurate focus and the dry operative field needed for movies does much to improve one's operative skills, although the movies are often prepared for teaching others. I have learned a great deal by reviewing movies of past operations. Carefully prepared movies have repeatedly, upon reexamination, yielded new insights into operative anatomy and techniques. This is only one of many examples of the fact that the teacher learns more from his efforts than those being taught.

REFERENCES

1. Microsurgical treatment of neurovascular disease: A Report for the Joint Committee for Stroke Resources (Study Group on Microsurgical Treatment of Neurovascular Disease, John L. Fox, M.D., Chairman). Neurosurgery, *3:* 287–337, 1978.
2. Rhoton, A. L. Jr. Accessory light for the surgical microscope. Neurosurgery, *4:* 71–74, 1978.
3. Rhoton, A. L. Jr. Micro-operative techniques. *In Neurological Surgery*, edited by J. R. Youmans. W. B. Saunders, Philadelphia, in press, 1979.
4. Rand, R. W., and Urban, J. C. The surgical microscope: its use and care. *In Microneurosurgery*, edited by R. W. Rand, Ed. 2, pp. 7–19. C. V. Mosby, St. Louis, 1978.
5. Yasargil, M. G. *Microsurgery Applied to Neurosurgery.* Academic Press, New York, 1969.

III

Review of Current Adjuncts of Neurosurgery

CHAPTER

17

Posterior Fusions of the Cervical Spine

EBEN ALEXANDER, JR., M.D.

In the treatment of injuries of the cervical spine, first consideration must be given to protection of the neural elements. Relieving all pressure on the spinal cord and nerve roots and maintaining them in a neutral position affords the best opportunities for the return of neural function. To do that with certainty requires accurate reduction of bony elements followed by internal fixation, if necessary, for immediate stability and spinal fusion to prevent the late recurrence of malalignment.

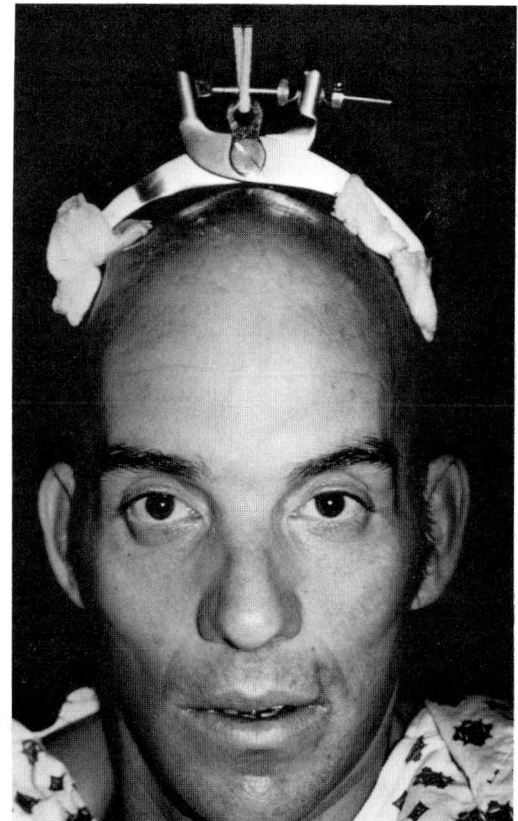

FIG. 17.1. Patient with Crutchfield tongs reducing and stabilizing cervical fracture.

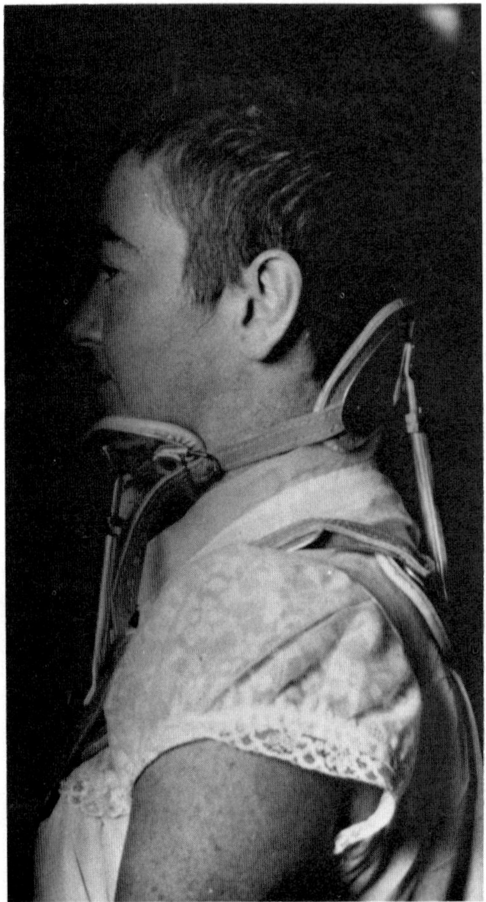

FIG. 17.2. Four-poster Zimmer brace, often used postoperatively if cervical spine is not fused.

As we reported in 1959, "The general routine of skeletal traction, internal fixation, and spinal fusion constitutes a method of treatment that needs to be varied but slightly in order to include a large percentage of all serious injuries of the cervical spine" (3). That there are options other than posterior fusion to stabilize the cervical spine after fracture is acknowledged. Reduction and prolonged traction through the use of Crutchfield tongs (Fig. 17.1), halo immobilization, brace immobilization (Fig. 17.2), anterior interbody fusion—all have their place. The concern of this presentation is to consider the patient who has been chosen for a posterior fusion, to indicate the most suitable methods of posterior fusion, and to review the evolution of those methods.

In 1939, Gallie (4) reported that fractures of the odontoid process were best treated with wire and bone fusion only of C1 and C2. Indeed, McLaurin et al. (6) and Salmon (8) more recently have published some cases satisfactorily treated by simple wiring at that level. However, some of our patients treated in that manner showed less than solid fusions on later flexion and extension roentgenograms. It seemed reasonable, for fractures of the odontoid, to incorporate C1, C2, and C3 into any fusion being performed (Fig. 17.3) since the heavy, well-formed spinous process and laminae of C2 forms a fulcrum over which the lever of a graft attached to C3 and to C1 can hold the C1 to C2 union solidly in place. At that level, therefore, we have fused C1, C2, and C3, wiring C1 to C2 and securing the graft to the laminae of C1, C2, and C3 with wire (Fig. 17.4).

At the lower levels, such as at C5 and C6, we have fused two vertebrae above and two vertebrae below the unstable area, wiring together the spinous processes of the two vertebrae involved in dislocation with No. 18 wire, and securing the graft to the laminae of all four vertebrae to provide adequate stability.

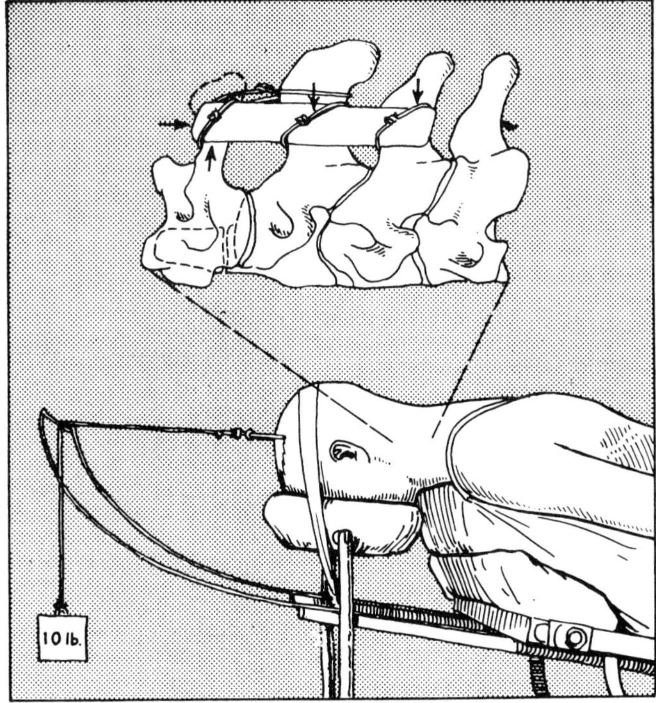

FIG. 17.3. Fusion across C1, C2, and C3 for fracture of the odontoid. (From E. Alexander *et al.* (2). Published with permission.)

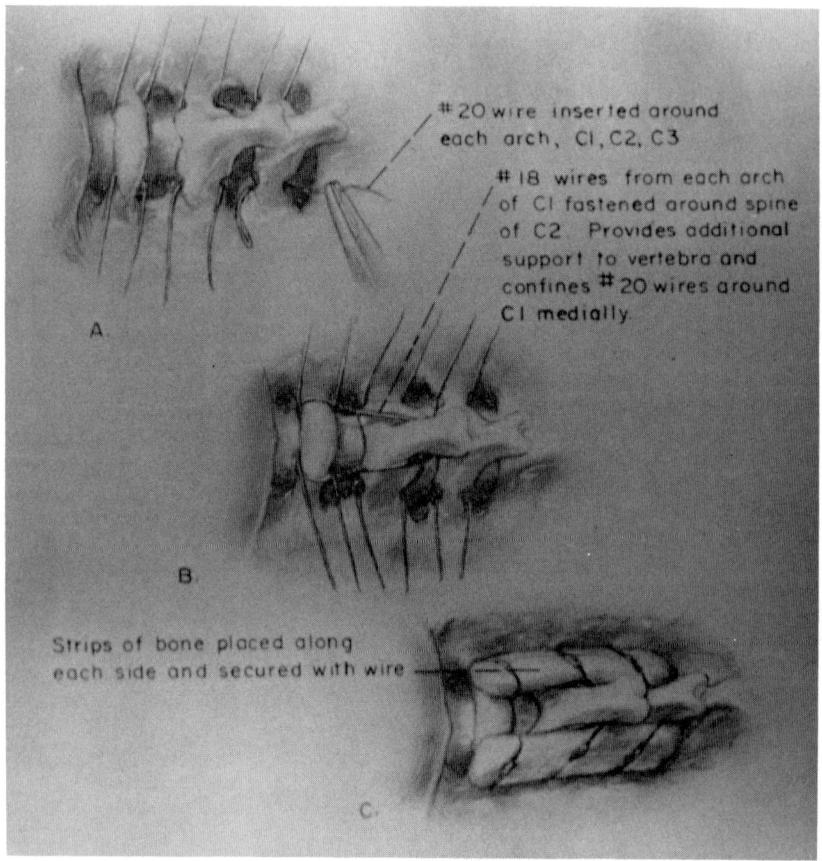

FIG. 17.4. (*A*) Portions of lamina have been removed to allow passage of No. 20 wires. (*B*) No. 18 wire is twisted around each side of C1 and tied behind spinous process of C2. (*C*) Wires are twisted around bone grafts. (From Kelly *et al.* (5). Published with permission.)

We first performed those fusions using autogenous iliac bone grafts (Fig. 17.5), and No. 20 or No. 22 stainless steel wire twisted or tied by the Harris wire tier. We soon learned, however, that while No. 20 wire was acceptable for securing the graft in place, No. 18 wire was needed for wiring the vertebral spinous processes together—anything less substantial would break. As our experience increased, we found that rib grafts (Figs. 17.6 to 17.8) fitted better and were easier to obtain than iliac crest grafts. However, in roentgenograms of some patients taken 6 to 12 months after operation, no bone was visible, although the fusions were stable.

It was with those patients in mind that, in 1961 and 1962, we did 5 fusions substituting acrylic for the bone (Fig. 17.9), wiring it in place just

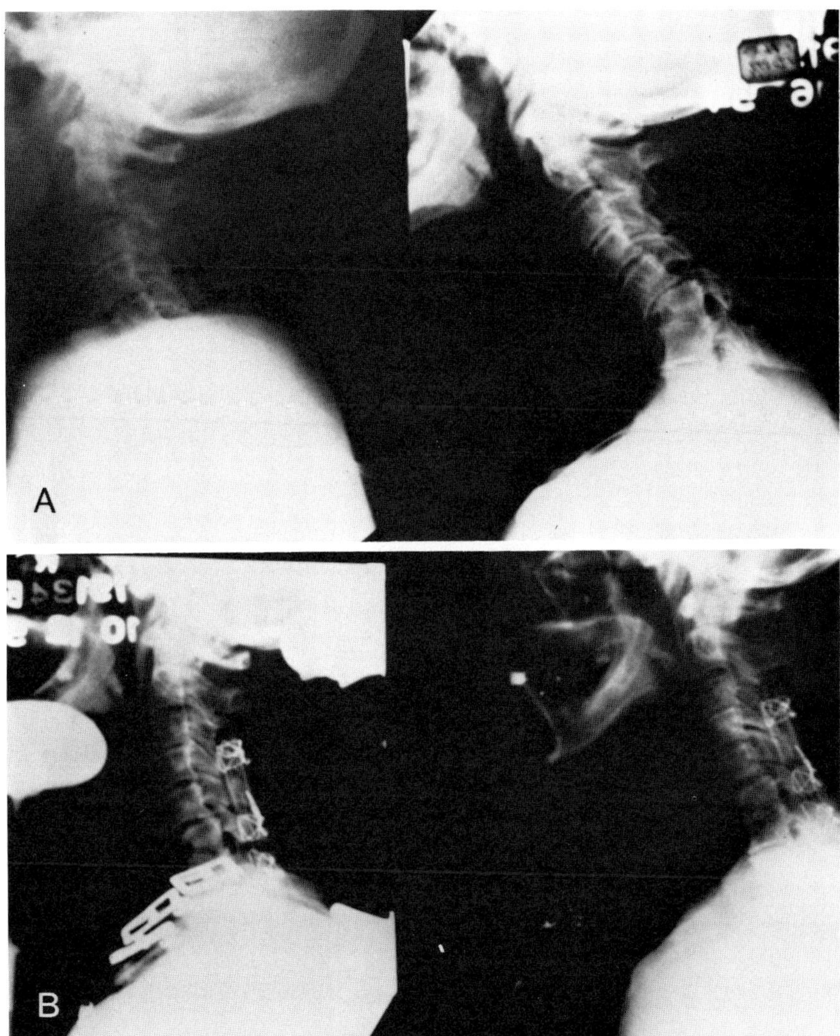

FIG. 17.5. (*A*) X-ray taken immediately after injury shows only top 5 vertebrae and no sign of fracture. *Top right*, x-ray taken 4 months later shows severe dislocation. Patient could not raise his arms. (*B*) Fracture was reduced, and bone grafts were wired into place.

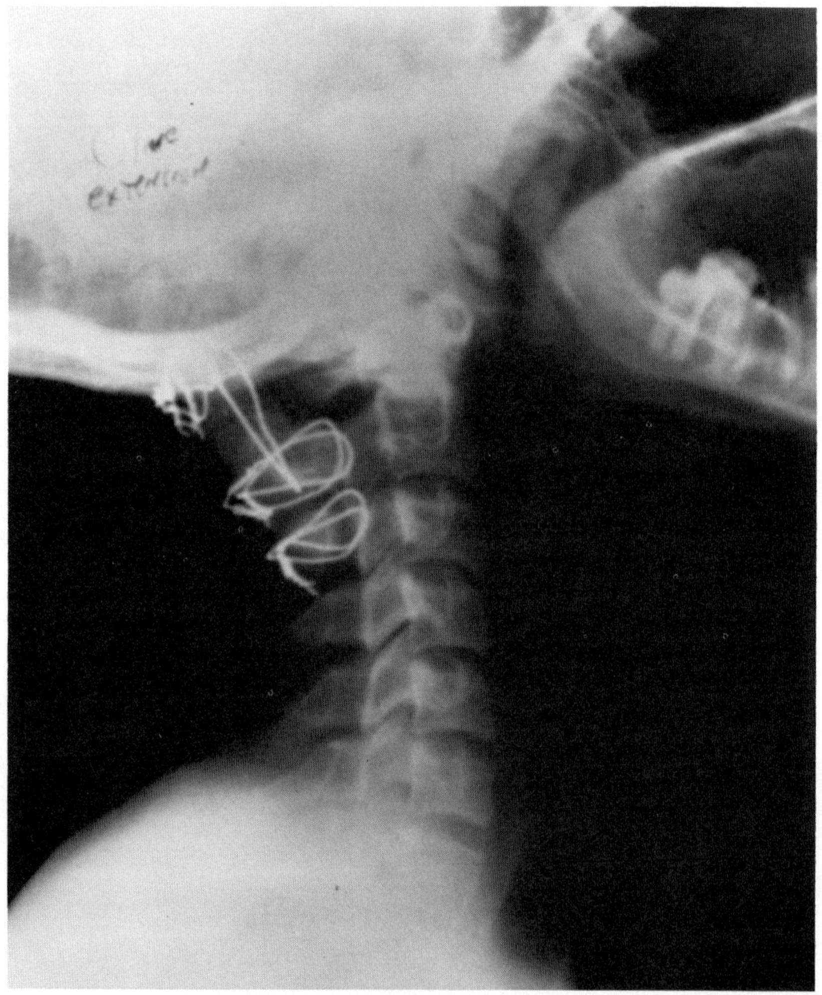

Fig. 17.6. Patient with congenital anomaly of the occipital-cervical area, requiring laminectomy of C1. Fusion between C2, C3, and occiput was done with rib graft.

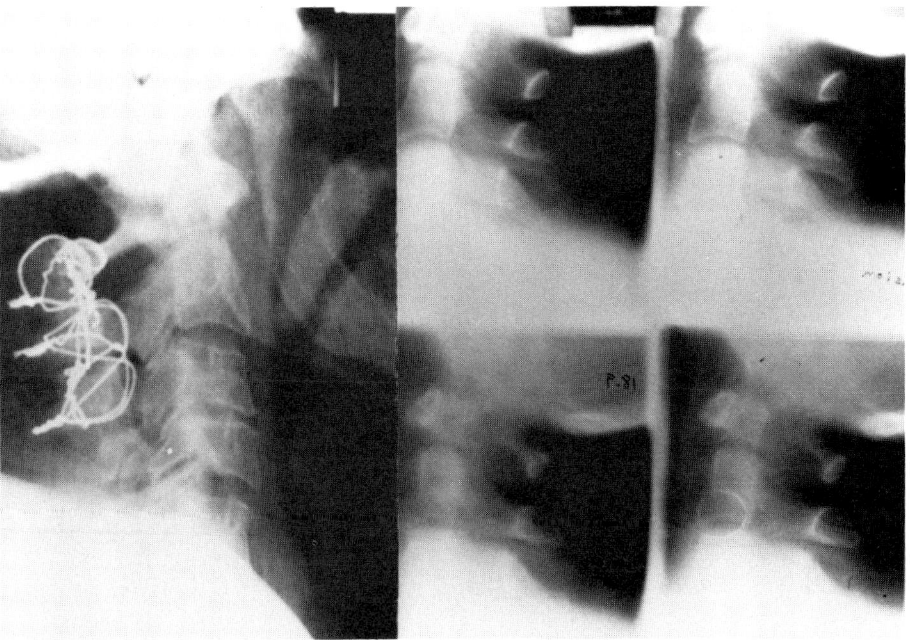

FIG. 17.7. Another patient with fracture of the odontoid (tomograms on *right*). Fusion with rib graft is shown on the *left*.

as we had the rib grafts. We shaped the acrylic in its bed, and when it began to harden and generate the heat of polymerization, we took it out until it was cool. We then put it back in and wired it in place with wires placed beneath the laminae. Thus, the acrylic was essentially tied to the laminae.

Those patients did well, and their fusions were stable (5), and since then we have continued to use acrylic more often than autogenous bone for posterior cervical spine fusion, except in growing children in whom we still use bone (7).

Parts of the early procedure using acrylic were tedious and parts were potentially dangerous, so we constantly sought alternative methods that would expedite the procedure, remove hazardous features, and make it more easily performed.

While attempting to remove an ill-seated acrylic graft, we found that acrylic adheres so strongly to stainless steel wire that, once it has set, it cannot be separated from the wire except with a drill. Utilizing that knowledge, we began to pass a No. 20 wire under each lamina, to twist the wire so that the ends protruded 1.0 to 1.5 cm above the lamina, and to cast the acrylic over the ends of the wire, thus incorporating the wire into the fusion (Figs. 17.10 to 17.13).

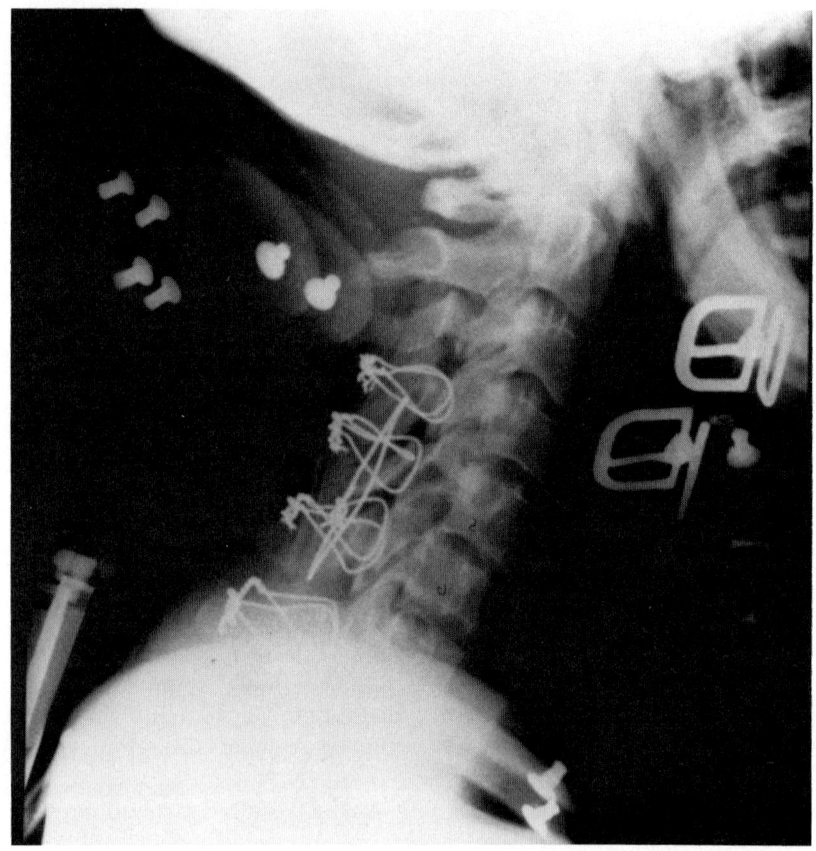

FIG. 17.8. Fracture of lower cervical spine treated with wiring and rib graft.

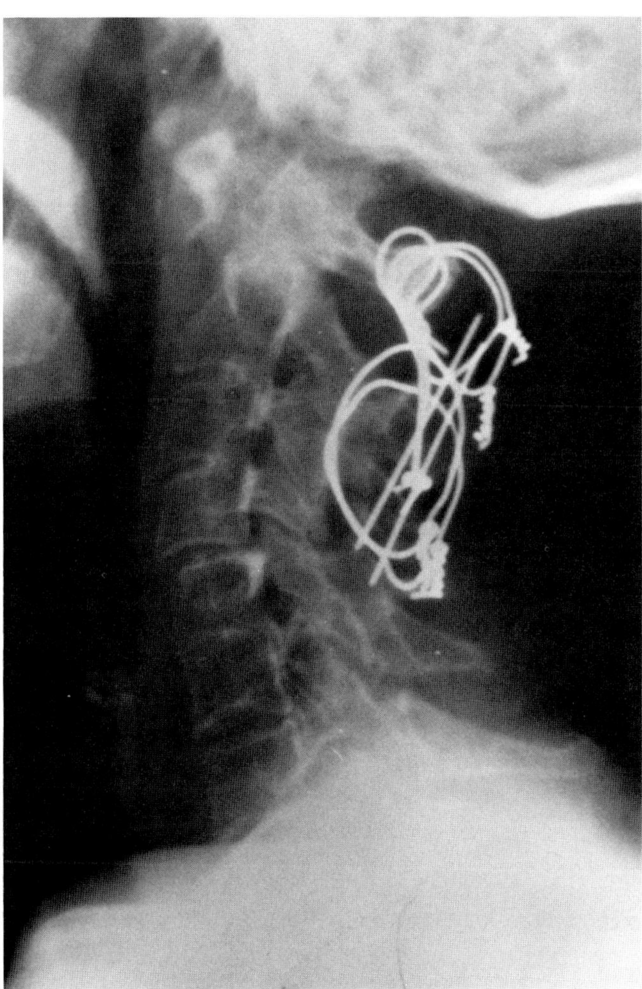

Fig. 17.9. C1 spinous process has been wired to C2 and C3. Acrylic has been cast and wired in place.

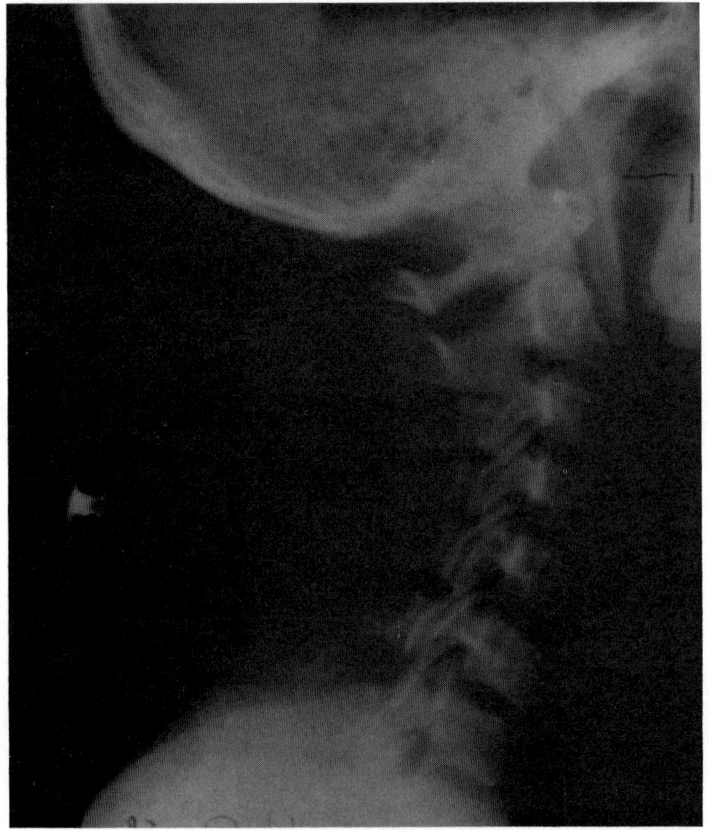

FIG. 17.10. Patient with fracture of C6 and C7; neck braced.

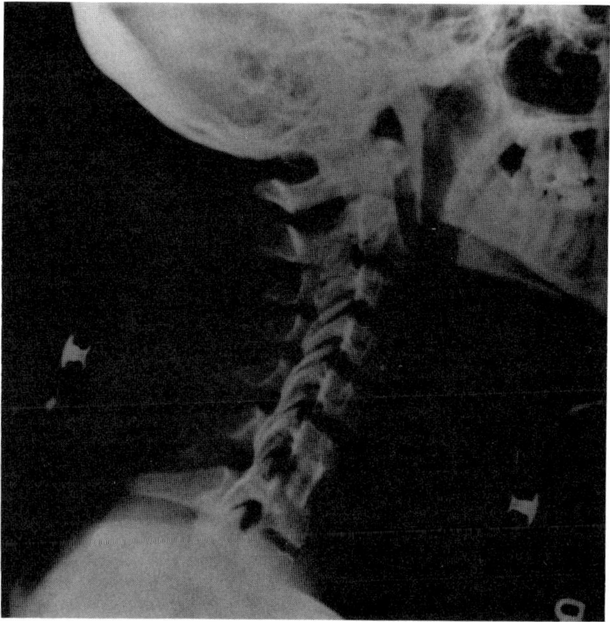

FIG. 17.11. Same patient having undergone anterior interbody fusion of C6, C7.

Whereas we had previously been concerned about the heat of polymerization of the acrylic as it fixed and had removed it for cooling, we found we could dissipate that heat by irrigating the acrylic with cold saline and let it fix in place.

These modifications worked well, but we were still left with the necessity of passing a No. 20 wire beneath each lamina before twisting it around the lamina, then to be incorporated in the acrylic. Two other recent modifications appear to be satisfactory answers to that problem: one, a modification of a small towel clip attached around (Fig. 17.14, *top*) the dorsal surface of each lamina or into small holes drilled into the lamina (Fig. 17.14, *bottom*); the other, devised by Dr. David Kelly, stainless steel Kirschner wires .062 inches in diameter placed through drill holes in the base of each spinous process. With both modifications, the reduction of any dislocation or subluxation, if not already effected by skeletal traction, is done as far as possible by open means (1) before final fusion is done. If necessary, an intraoperative cross-table lateral roentgenogram is taken to determine completeness of reduction.

No. 18 stainless steel wire is passed through an opening in the base of the spinous process (Fig. 17.15) above the dislocation and inferior to the posterior angulated spinous process below the dislocation. The wire is

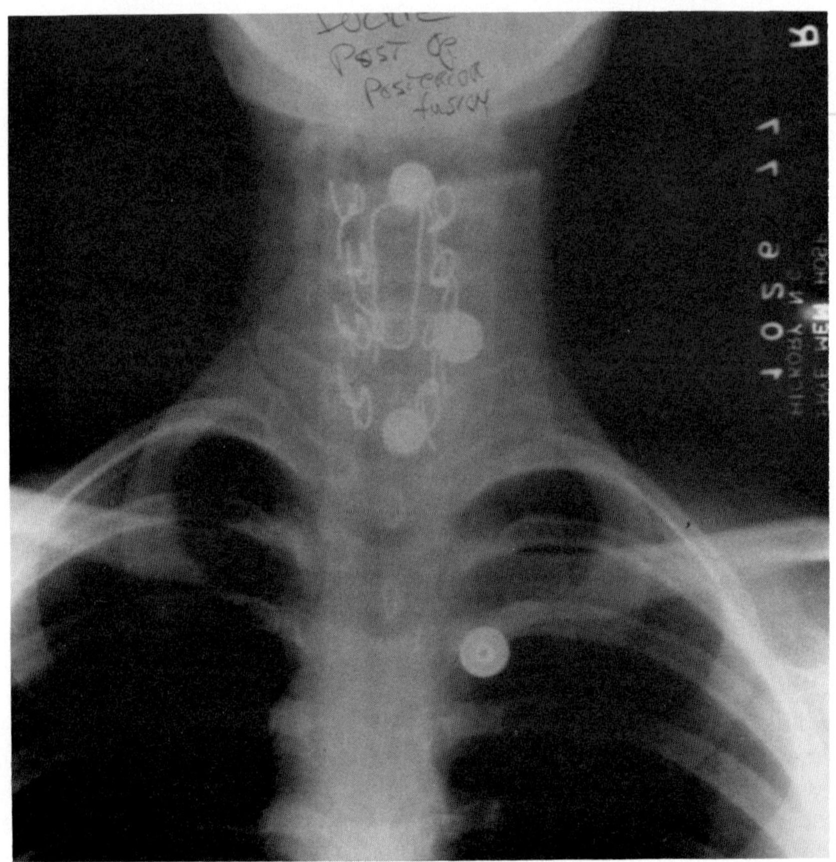

FIG. 17.12. Same patient. Anterior interbody fusion was absorbed; neck was redislocated. Anterior view of posterior fusion with acrylic wired in place.

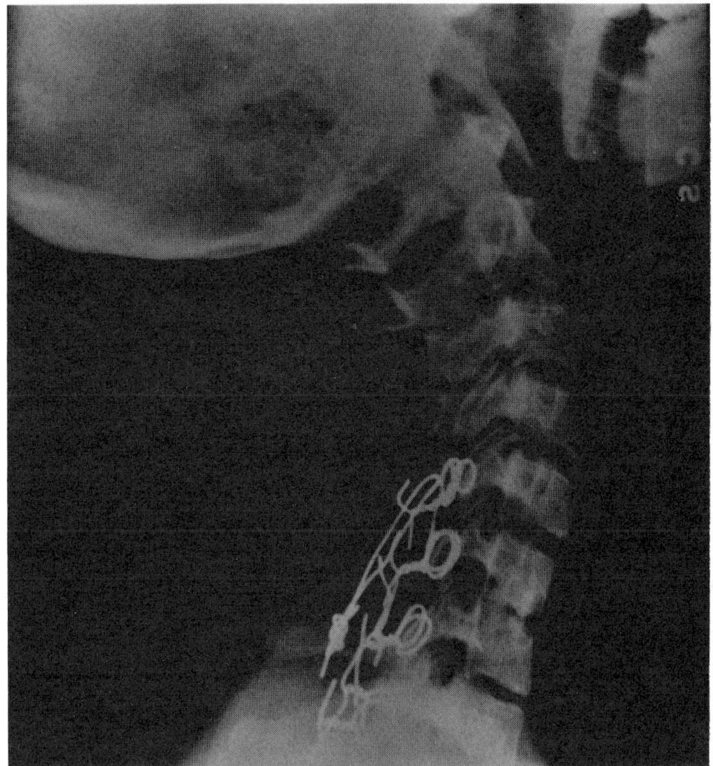

FIG. 17.13. Lateral view of same patient.

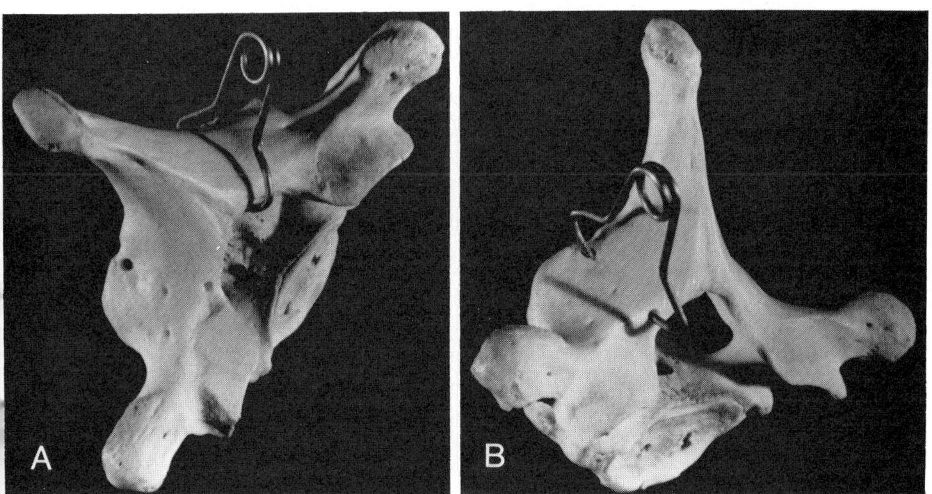

FIG. 17.14. Modified towel clip passed around lamina (*A*) or placed in holes in lamina (*B*).

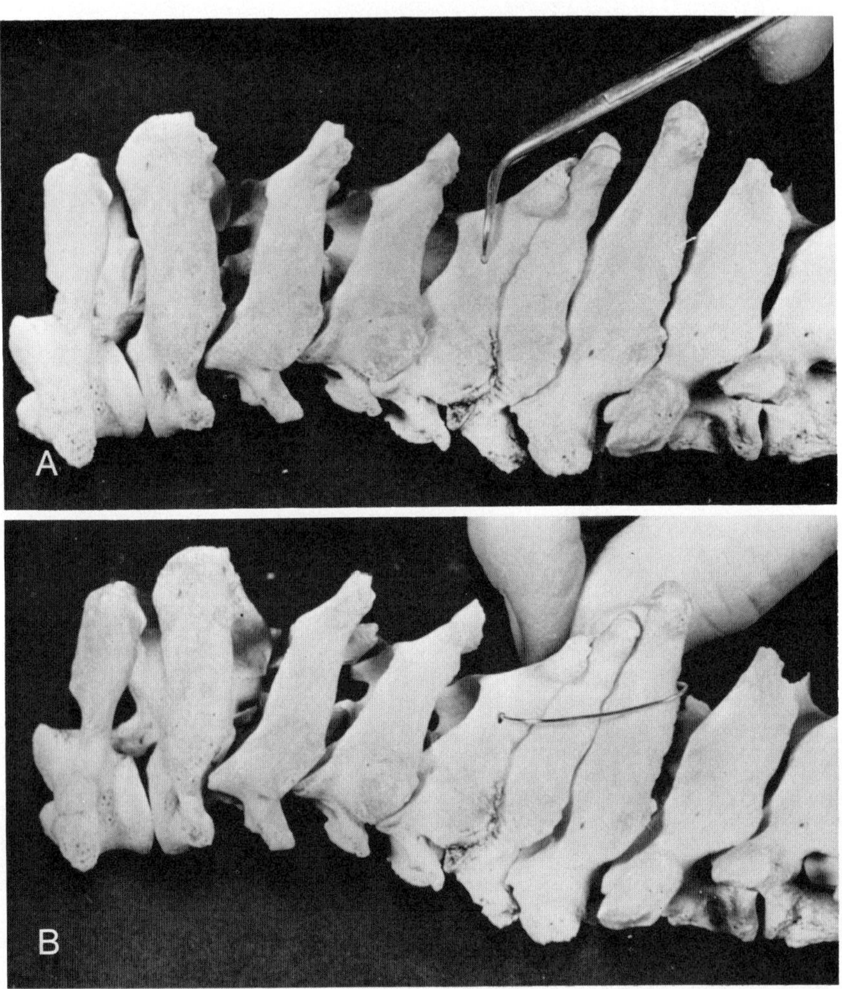

FIG. 17.15. (*A*) Towel clip used to make hole through spinous process of C5. (*B*) No. 18 wire passed through spinous process of C5 and beneath spinous process of C7.

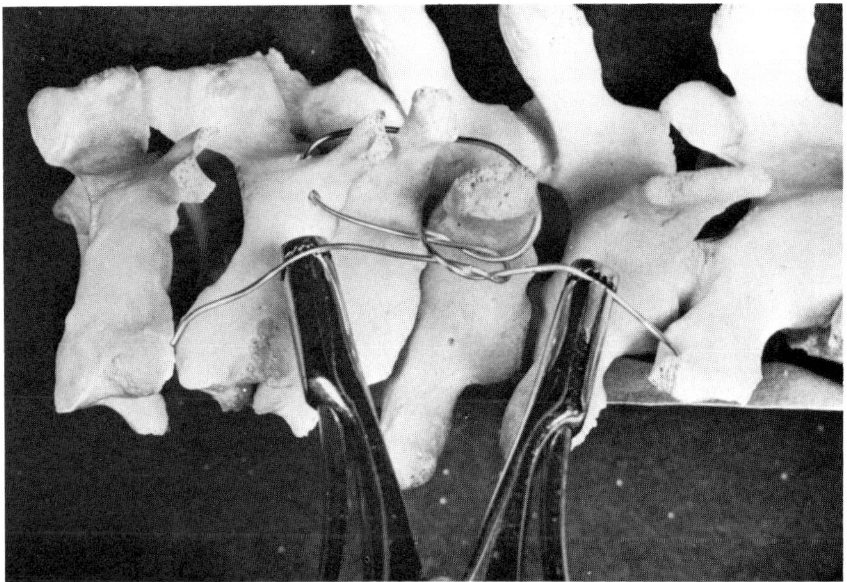

FIG. 17.16. Wire seen in Fig. 16.15 tied with Harris wire tier.

tied with a Harris wire tier (Fig. 17.16), the ends turned down ventrally toward the laminae.

Then, the special fusion clips are put in place, or with Dr. Kelly's method (Fig. 17.17), the Kirschner wires are driven through the holes made in the bases of the spinous processes. The pins or the clips, plus the No. 18 wire used to secure the spinous processes, are incorporated in a small, cigar-shaped piece of acrylic (Fig. 17.18) that has begun polymerizing so that it can be molded but is not so soft that it will flow or drop between the laminae to compress the dura. Roentgenographic appearance is shown in Fig. 17.19 (one patient), and in Fig. 17.20 (another patient).

In order to avoid passing a wire beneath the laminae of C1 when C1 is involved in the fusion, we have devised smooth stainless steel hooks that can be placed around the laminae and tied with No. 18 wire around the spinous process of C2 (Fig. 17.21).

In some instances, before the acrylic has hardened, a section of straight No. 20 stainless steel wire is buried in each cigar-shaped segment of acrylic to provide a radiographic tag (Fig. 17.22) in the acrylic, which is not radiopaque, should there be a future dislocation or fracture, and to provide further strength to the acrylic similar to that in reinforced concrete.

The wounds are readily closed with interrupted sutures in layers

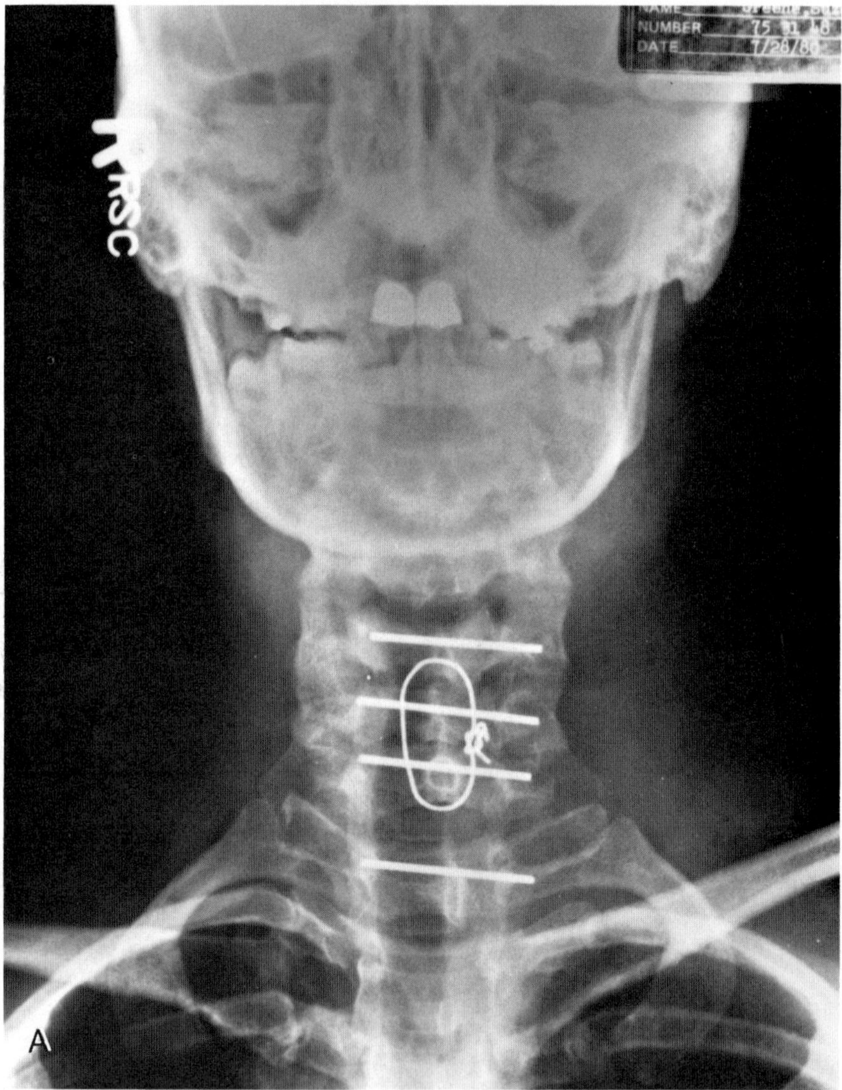

FIG. 17.17. Anteroposterior (*A*) and lateral (*B*) view of Kirschner wires through spinous processes and wiring of adjacent vertebrae.

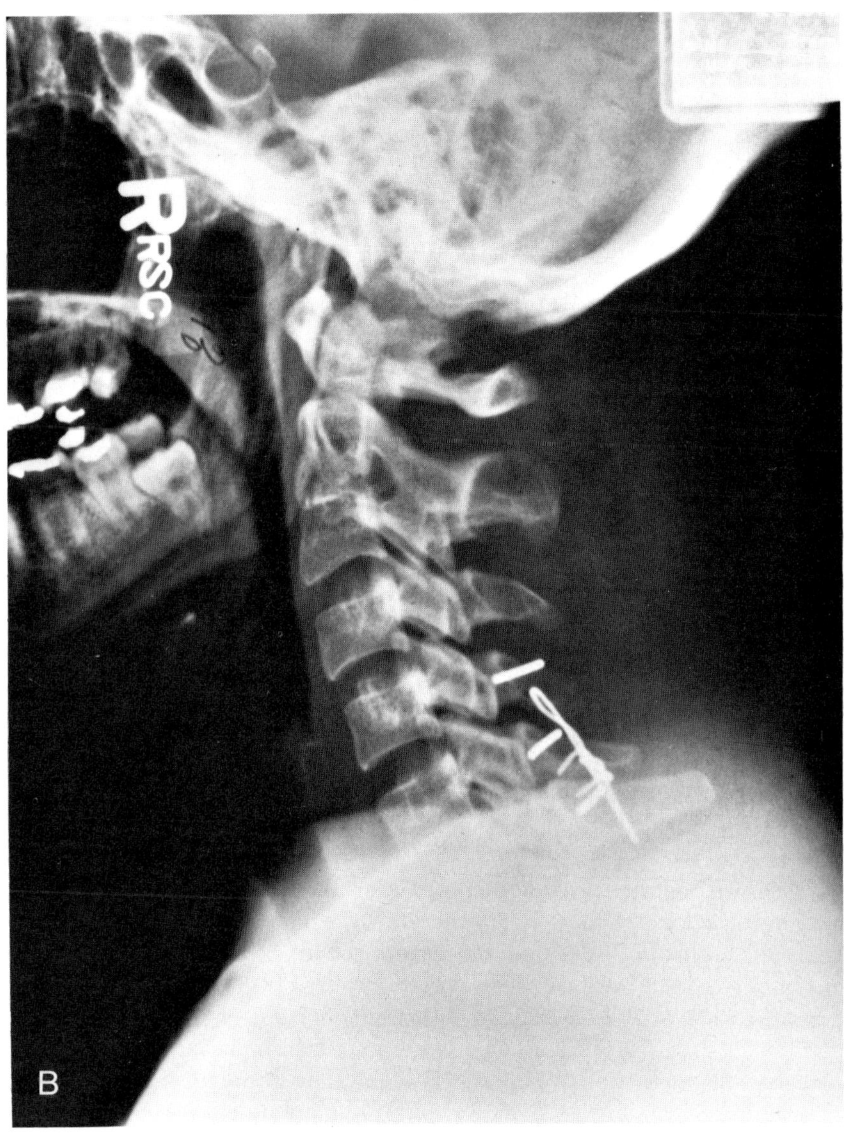
R
RSC
B

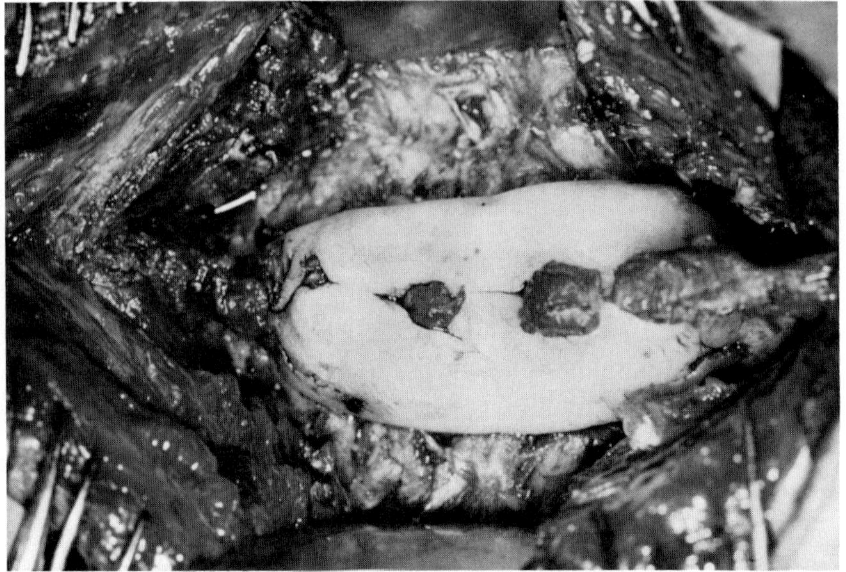

FIG. 17.18. Cigar-shaped pieces of acrylic are molded around clips and wires.

without drainage. The bulk of the acrylic implant is not so large that it presents as an additional mass.

The fusion at this stage is probably as solid as it will ever be except for the ligamentous healing requiring many weeks; so as soon as the patients are comfortable, they are allowed to begin ambulation, but are told to wear a Thomas collar when out of bed for the next 4 months. Obviously, if a patient has a serious neurologic deficit, his ambulation may be delayed. Some surgeons suggest using a 4-poster Zimmer brace or one of the other more sturdy braces, but we have not always found them to be necessary.

Roentgenograms are taken immediately after operation and about once a month during follow-up. At the end of 4 months, lateral films of the cervical spine, in flexion and extension, are taken to determine stability.

In one case of fracture of the superior facet of C4 with subluxation and compression of the C5 root, it was necessary to remove the facet. The spinous processes of C3 and C4 were not wired together, and postoperatively, although the subluxation is stable and the neurological function normal, the patient still has a slight malalignment of C3 on C4. In addition, at 4 months after operation he complained of neck pain again, and a lateral roentgenogram showed a collapse of the vertebra of C6, which we considered a pathological fracture. An anterior fusion, replacing the body of C6 with an autogenous iliac graft, was done, and the patient

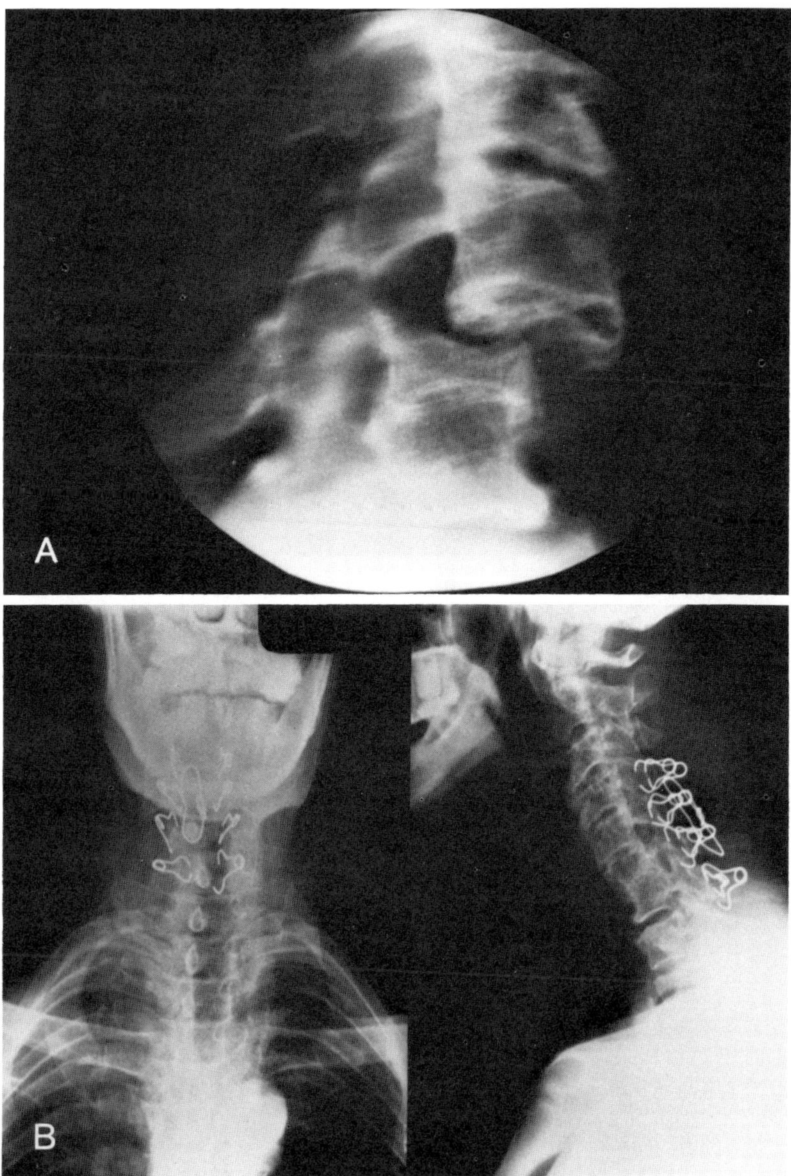

FIG. 17.19. (*A*) Tomogram showing severe dislocation of C5 on C6. (*B*) Fracture/dislocation reduced; C5 and C6 wired together; fusion clips, 2 above, 2 below, and 2 each in C5 and C6 are cast in acrylic.

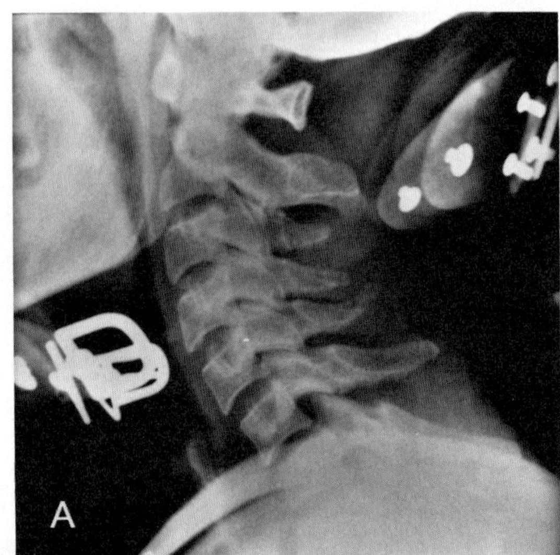

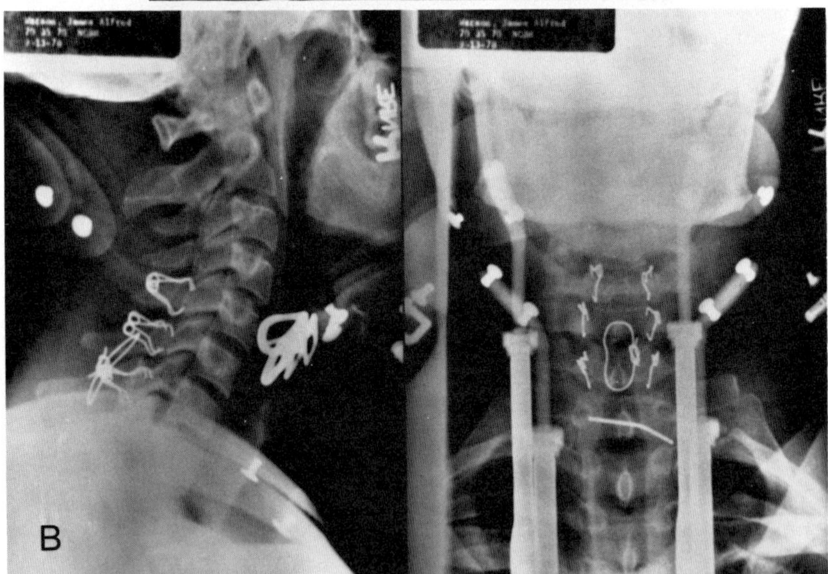

FIG. 17.20. (*A*) Dislocation of C7 on T1 was reduced and brace applied, but dislocation has recurred. (*B*) Anteroposterior and lateral X-rays after fusion with acrylic cast over clips at C5 and C6 and Kirschner wire through C7.

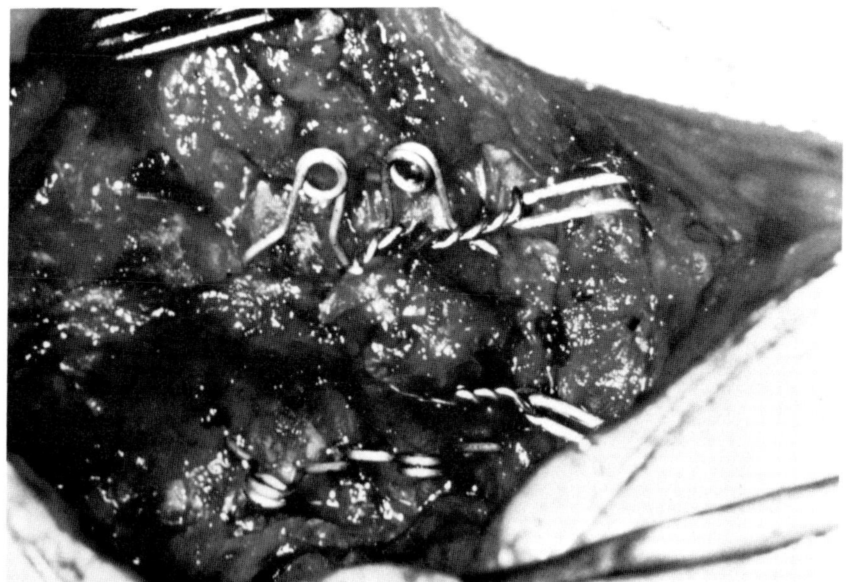

FIG. 17.21. Clips in place and stainless steel hooks have been placed over laminae of C1.

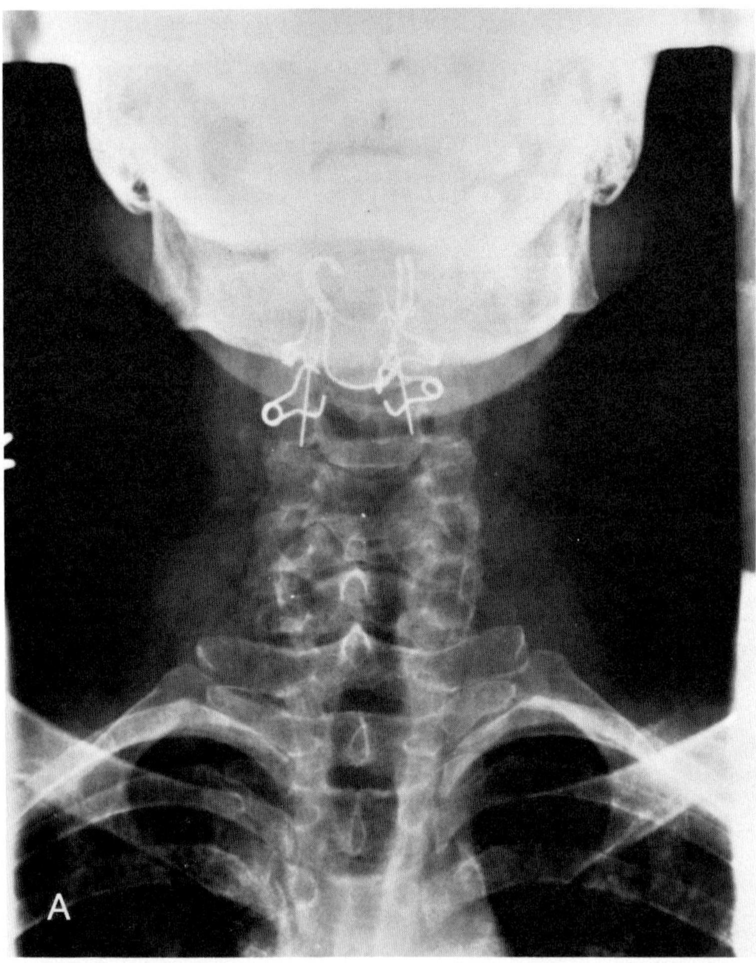

FIG. 17.22. Anteroposterior (*A*) and lateral (*B*) X-rays showing hooks over laminae of C1, clips through laminae of C2 and C3, and 2 straight wires placed longitudinally in the acrylic.

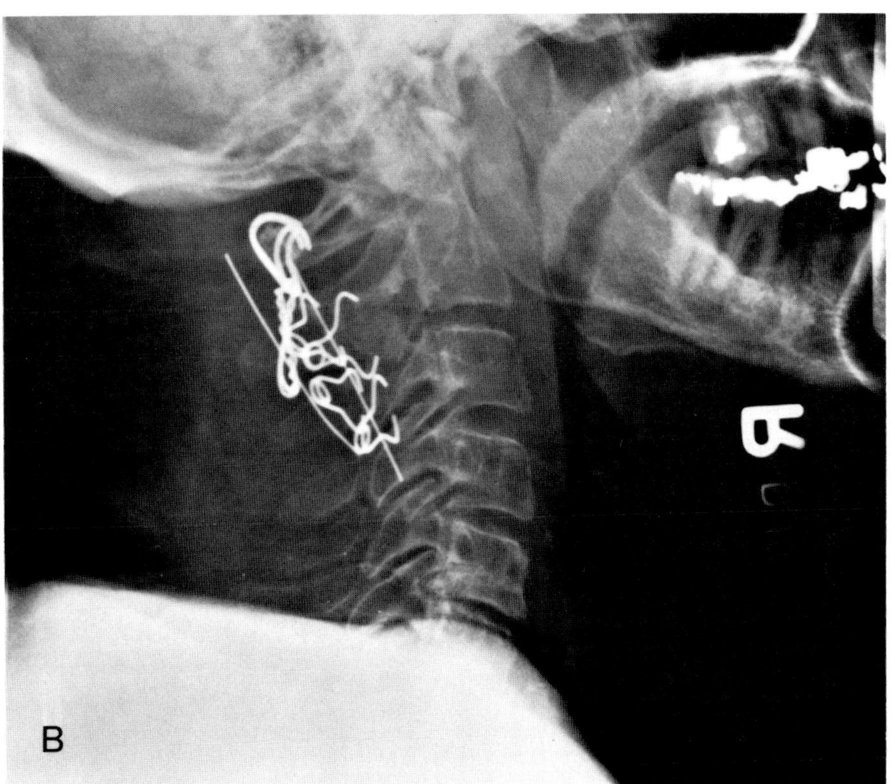
B

has since done well. The bone that was removed showed no abnormality and the cause of the collapse of C6, not apparent roentgenographically even 2 months after the original injury, remains unknown.

About 15 cases that have been done with one or the other of these last modifications have all been stable.

The overall method has proved to be expeditious, safe, and satisfactory for the treatment of cervical spine injuries.

REFERENCES

1. Alexander, E., Jr., Davis, C. H., Jr., and Forsyth, H. F. Reduction and fusion of fracture dislocations of the cervical spine. J. Neurosurg., *27:* 587–591, 1967.
2. Alexander, E., Jr., Forsyth, H. F., Davis, C. H., Jr., and Nashold, B. S., Jr. Dislocation of the atlas on the axis. The value of early fusion of C1, C2, and C3. J. Neurosurg., *15:* 353–371, 1958.
3. Forsyth, H. F., Alexander, E., Jr., Davis, C. H., Jr., and Underdal, R. The advantages of early spine fusion in the treatment of fracture-dislocation of the cervical spine. J. Bone Joint Surg., *41A:* 17–36, 1959.
4. Gallie, W. E. Fractures and dislocations of the cervical spine. Am. J. Surg., *46:* 495–499, 1939.
5. Kelly, D. L., Jr., Alexander, E., Jr., Davis, C. H., Jr., and Smith, J. M. Acrylic fixation of atlanto-axial dislocations. Technical note. J. Neurosurg., *36:* 366–367, 1972.
6. McLaurin, R. L., Vernal, R., and Salmon, J. H. Treatment of fractures of the atlas and axis by wiring without fusion. J. Neurosurg., *36:* 773–780, 1972.
7. McWhorter, J. M., Alexander, E., Jr., Davis, C. H., Jr., and Kelly, D. L., Jr. Posterior cervical fusion in children. J. Neurosurg., *45:* 211–215, 1976.
8. Salmon, J. H. Fractures of the second cervical vertebra: internal fixation by interlaminar wiring. Neurosurgery, *1:* 125–127, 1977.

CHAPTER

18

The Ideal Shunt for Hydrocephalus

EBEN ALEXANDER, JR., M.D.

When shunting for hydrocephalus with polyethylene tubing was instituted in the early 1950's, it was first ventriculoureteral (4), then primarily ventriculoperitoneal. However, without a valve to prevent retrograde flow, there was frequent blockage of the tubing and a high incidence of infection, which necessitated multiple revisions in sick children with increased pressure (6). Use of the ventriculoatrial shunt (2, 3, 5) added

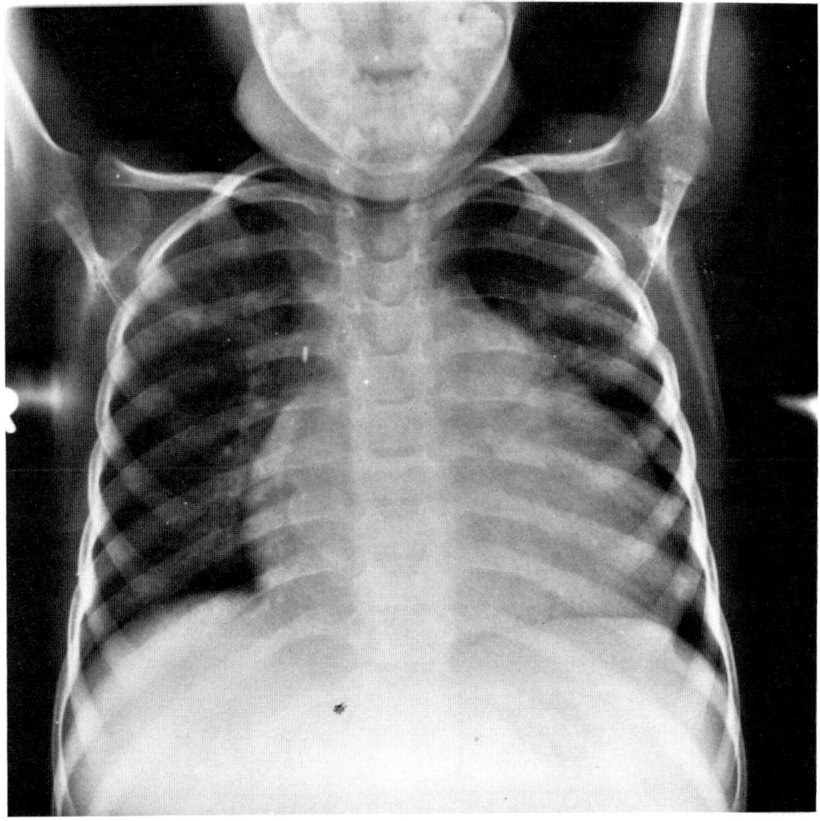

FIG. 18.1. Cor pulmonale as complication of ventriculoatrial shunt.

occasional blood stream infections, several pulmonary complications including cor pulmonale (Fig. 18.1), and occasional venal caval obstruction; if the distal shunt tube became disconnected, it sometimes lodged in the heart (Fig. 18.2).

With the development of the Holter valve (1), Shillito was one of those who led the return to the use of the ventriculoperitoneal shunt. David Kelly spent a year with Matson and Shillito, and he reintroduced the ventriculoperitoneal shunt to our service at the North Carolina Baptist Hospital. That shunt worked so well in combination with the valve that

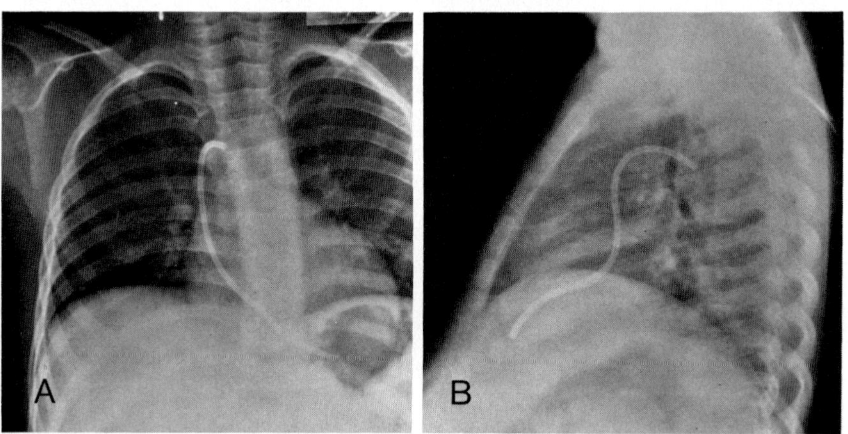

FIG. 18.2. Anteroposterior (*A*) and lateral (*B*) views of disconnected distal tubing from ventriculoatrial shunt lodged in heart.

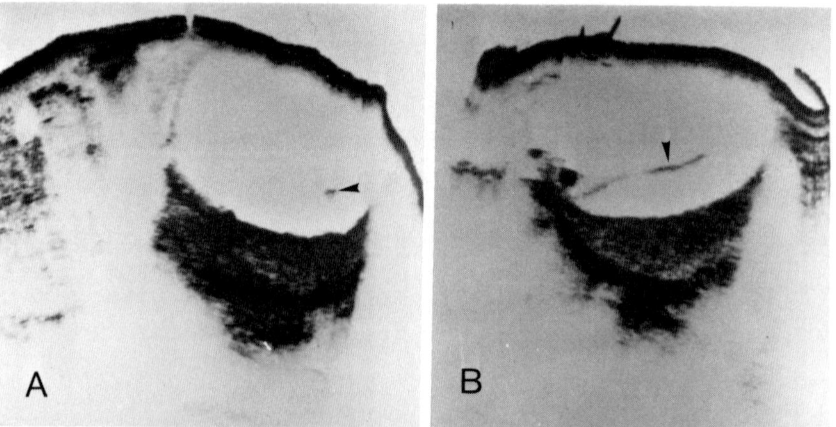

FIG. 18.3. Ultrasonic scans of left upper quadrant ((*A*) *transverse scan*; (*B*) *longitudinal scan*) showing pseudocyst around distal tubing (*arrowhead*). Cyst is evidence of inability of peritoneum to absorb fluid shunted from the ventricles.

all of our shunts are now placed in the peritoneum initially. Revisions are done electively when necessary. Only in the rare patient, who for some reason cannot absorb fluid in the peritoneum (Fig. 18.3), have we had to turn to a ventriculoatrial shunt. If a long-term successful ventriculoatrial

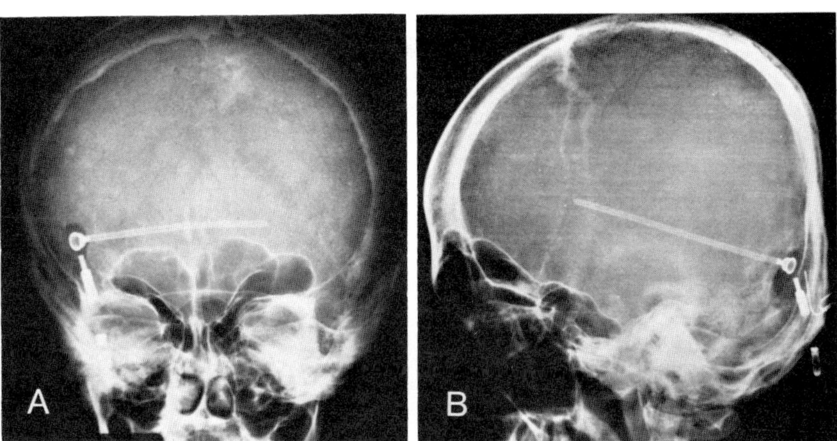

FIG. 18.4. Anteroposterior (*A*) and lateral (*B*) views show proximal tube of Rickham reservoir lying across midline.

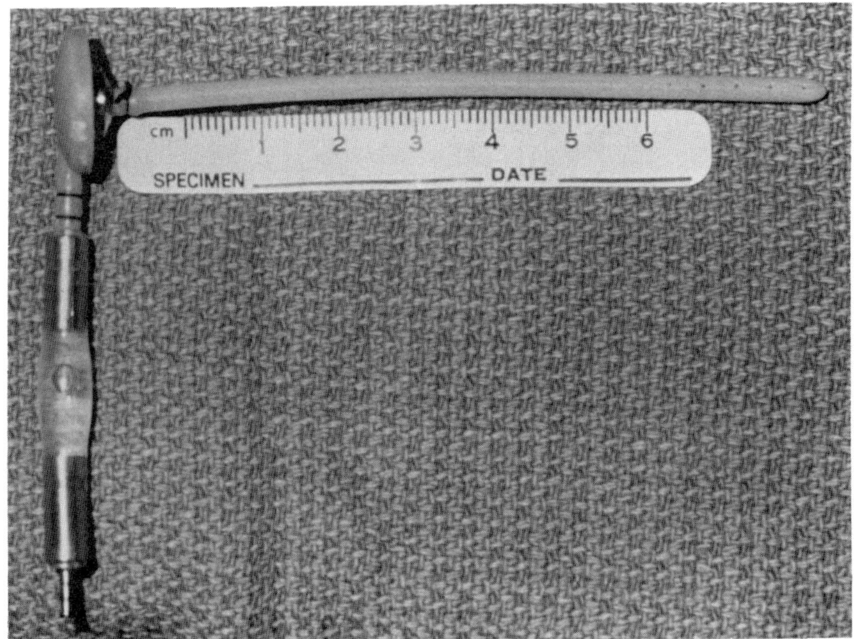

FIG. 18.5. Rickham reservoir connected directly to Holter valve, a connection that frequently separates when the Holter valve is pumped.

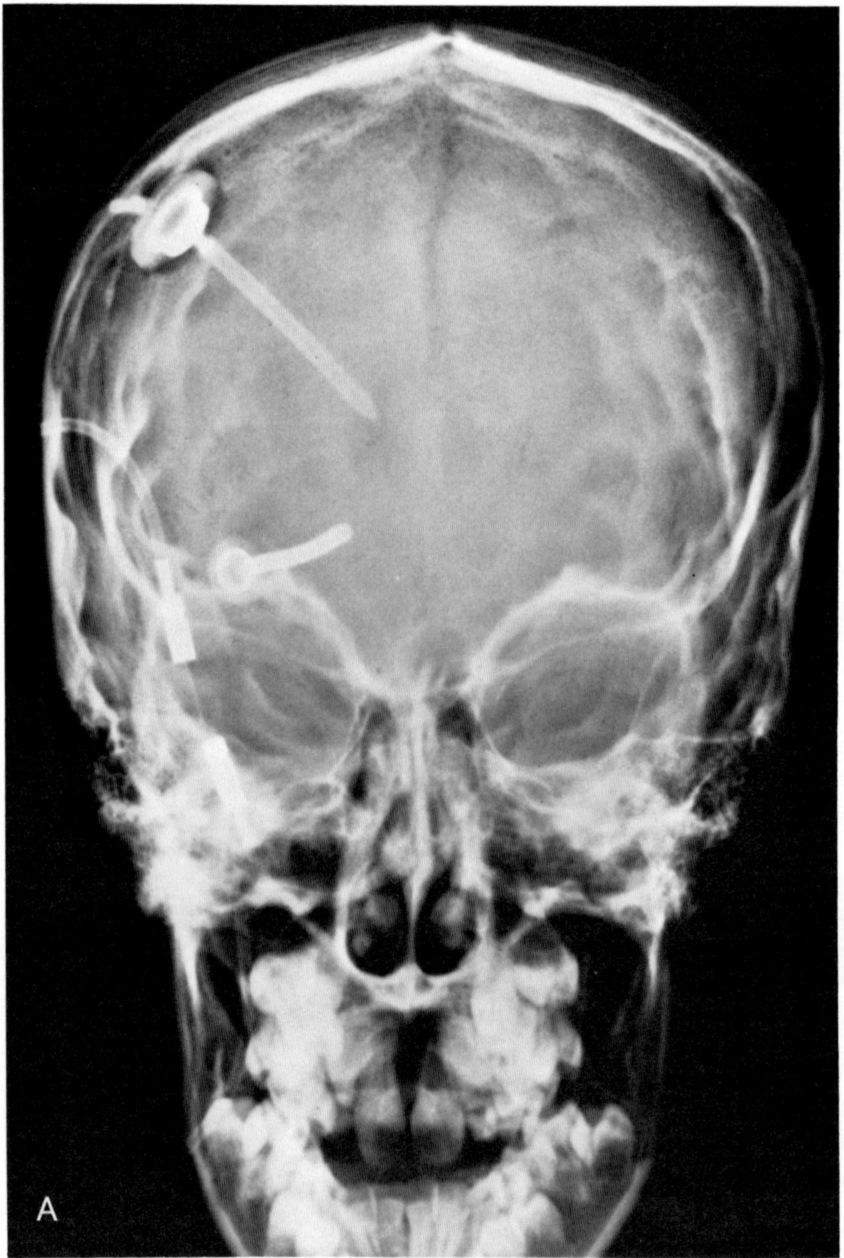

FIG. 18.6. Anteroposterior (*A*) and lateral (*B*) views showing separation of Holter valve from Rickham reservoir. Old parietal Rickham reservoir had been left in place.

shunt requires revision and lengthening, we replace it in the right atrium; if that is not possible, we again try to use the peritoneum as the absorptive surface.

COMPLICATIONS

Despite the overall improvement in shunting procedures, there exist many factors that can prevent their proper functioning. The rationale for illustrating these so dramatically is not to indicate the large number of problems, but to study the ways in which the majority of complications can be avoided. They are primarily complications of technique.

Improper Positioning of the Proximal Shunt

By CT scanning, we now know that the lateral ventricles in most children in whom a low-pressure Holter valve shunt is functioning

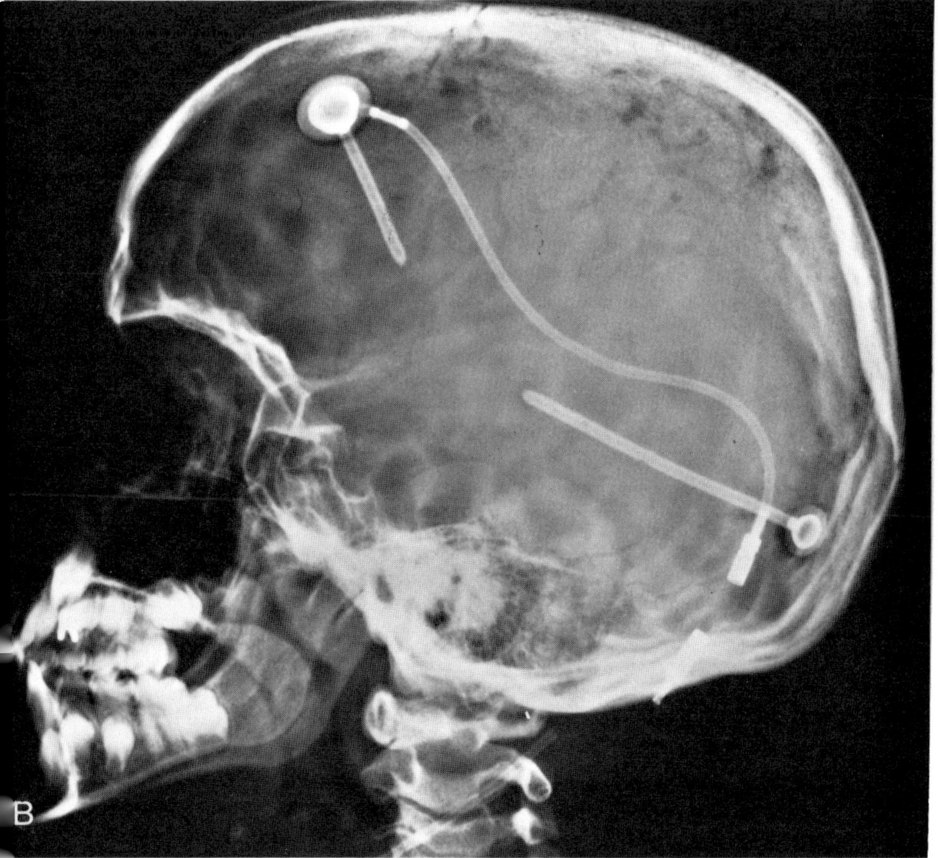

Fig. 18.6. (*B*)

properly become small—sometimes slit-like; if the proximal catheter is in the posterior or midportion of the second part of the lateral ventricle, its lumen may become occluded by the choroid plexus or brain, unless its tip is far forward, cephalad to the foramen of Monro. If a proximal tube—whether it is an angled tube, a Rickham reservoir, or a Leroy reservoir—is put into the ventricle by the posterior parietal route, it will be directed at right angles to the surface of the skull at the point where it enters the skull. Unless the tubing can be put in within 3 to 4 cm of the midline posteriorly, it does not lie in the direction of the ventricle, but most often will be seen lying across the midline (Fig. 18.4).

Disruption

Figs. 18.4 and 18.5 illustrate direct connection of the side arm of the Rickham reservoir to the Holter valve. When the Holter valve has to be pumped for any reason, that connection is put under excessive strain and it may disconnect. The insertion of a 3-cm piece of silicone tubing between the side arm of the Rickham reservoir and the Holter valve will prevent that complication.

On occasion, the distal tube may become separated from the Holter valve (Fig. 18.6), particularly in active young children. Care must be taken in tying these tubes together, using nothing smaller than no. 3 braided silk and tying it firmly but not so tightly that it cuts the tubing. Smaller silk will cut the tubing even more easily.

When connecting new tubing during a revision, the largest connector available should be used. Some of the metal connectors have a small neck and can be pulled apart; the tube can then be lost in the abdomen (Fig. 18.7).

If a patient develops a subdural hematoma while he has a shunt, it may be necessary to occlude the shunt temporarily in order to reexpand the brain after the subdural hematoma has been drained. A tantalum clip placed across the tubing to occlude it may cut (Figs. 18.8 and 18.9) or puncture (Fig. 18.10) the tube.

Migration of the Shunt

The importance of suturing the Holter valve to the skull, particularly in a growing child, is emphasized by Fig. 18.11, which shows the tube in the ventricle, well forward and near the foramen of Monro, and Fig. 18.12, taken just 2 weeks later, which shows the valve outside the skull, the tubing outside the cranial cavity. The shunt is not working, as can be seen by the separation of the sutures. The proper technique for securing the proximal end of the Holter valve in the parietal region of the skull is illustrated in Fig. 18.13. In the adult skull, two drill holes are made at angles meeting at the inner table or medullary cavity of the skull, and

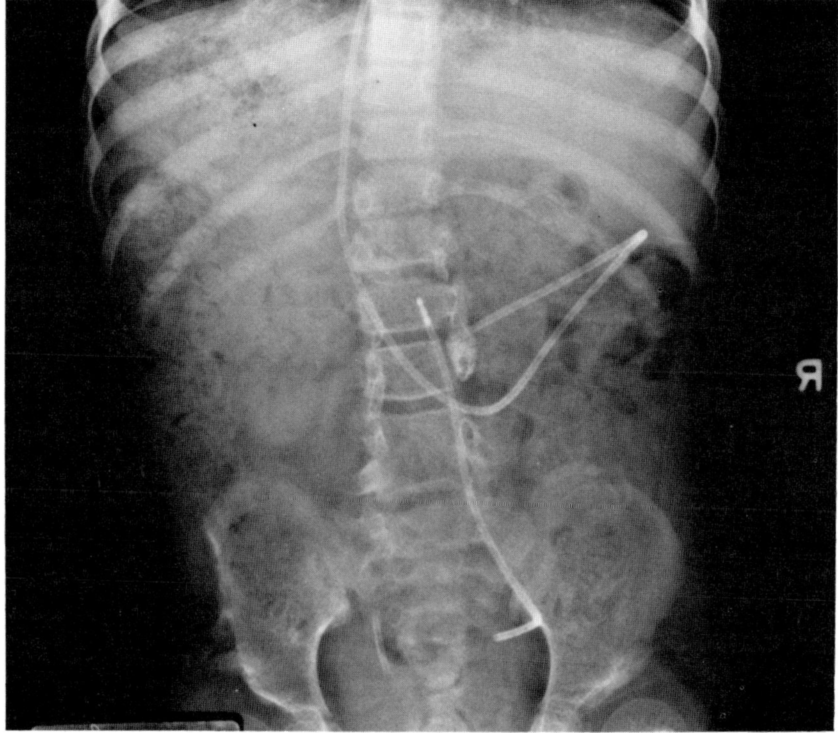

FIG. 18.7. Two disconnected distal shunts lie in the peritoneum. The smaller of the two has been present for 4 years.

two no. 3 silk sutures are passed through these holes. The Holter valve is then tied tightly to the skull, the silk being wrapped around the Holter valve twice so that it will not slip. In the infant, whose skull is thin, it is relatively easy to pass a needle extradurally through the skull, or, if necessary, a small drill hole can be made to facilitate that passage.

Infection

Note in Fig. 18.13 that the valve is placed away from the incision, and only a flap will lie over any elevated part of the shunt apparatus. That is particularly important in small infants, but is important in all other patients as well. No part of the Holter valve or of the Rickham reservoir should be directly under a skin incision. Furthermore, when silk sutures are tied onto the connectors, the knots should be tied on the "down" side of the connectors so that the "profile" of the knots will not exert a force to threaten the integrity of the incision.

Wounds should be closed in two layers with absorbable 4-0 suture

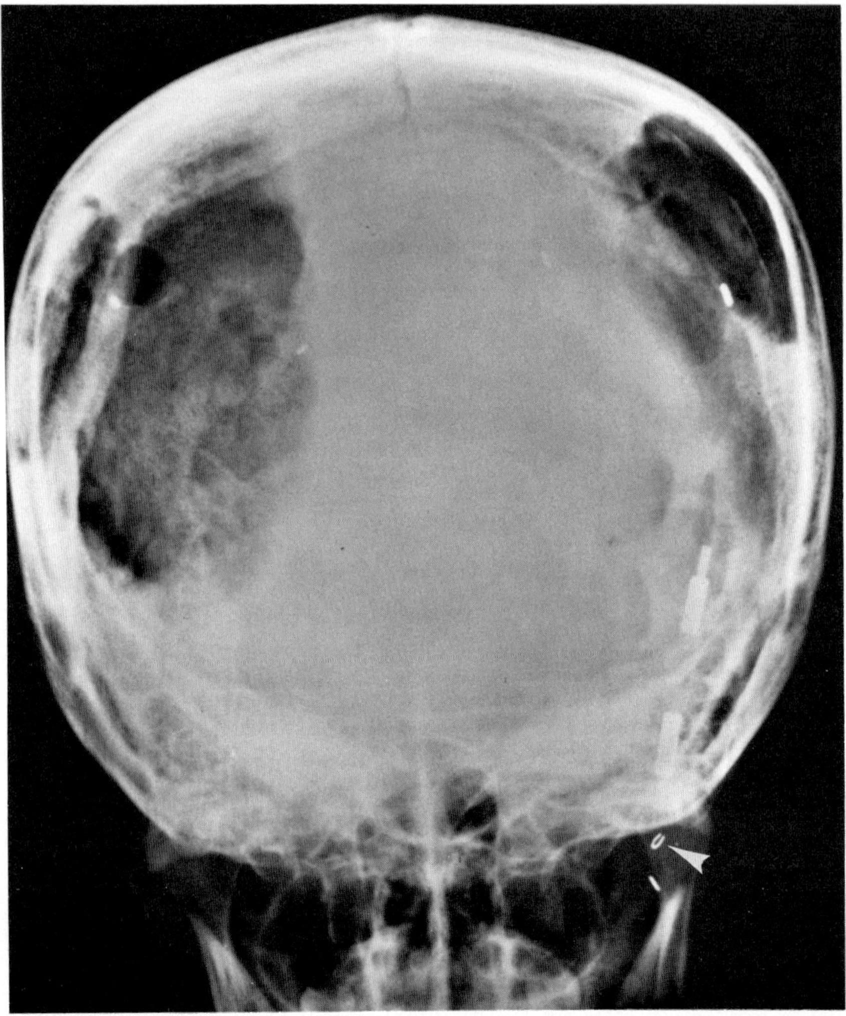

FIG. 18.8. Anteroposterior view shows large subdural hematomas (outlined by clips on inner membranes) and tantalum clip (*arrowhead*) just below Holter valve. Distal tubing cut by the clip has slipped down into the neck and out of view.

material for the galeal layer (or, in infants, for the subcutaneous layer). Two-layer closure should be done as well on all of the wounds in the neck or chest wall that are made so that the tubing from the Holter valve can be guided to the peritoneum. The failure of one wound, even a small wound, can lead to uncontrollable infection in the whole shunt system (Fig. 18.14).

In passing the tubing into the peritoneum, we believe that the length

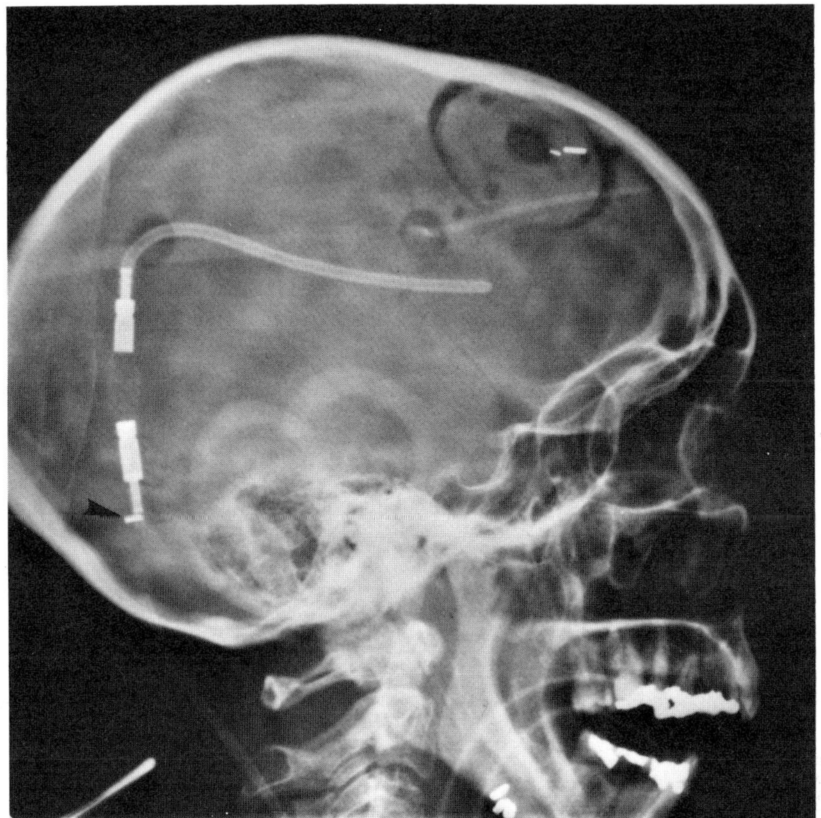

FIG. 18.9. Tantalum clip (*arrowhead*) has cut distal tubing.

of tubing to put in is a length sufficient to reach the symphysis pubis but not beyond it. We try to place the tube in the midline over the liver, but frequently it slips down into the peritoneal cavity and, on occasion, can become obstructed (Fig. 18.15). In one patient in our series, an overly long tube was used and it entered the small bowel (Fig. 18.16). An uncontrolled infection developed, and the entire shunt had to be removed. That would also be the course if a tube entered—as tubes have been known to do—the large bowel, the bladder, the lower rectum, the vagina, an inguinal hernia, or the scrotum.

Obstruction

Two or three small holes cut in the side of the distal tubing within 3 cm of its end facilitate continued drainage and functioning of the tube. However, those openings must never be larger than one-fourth the

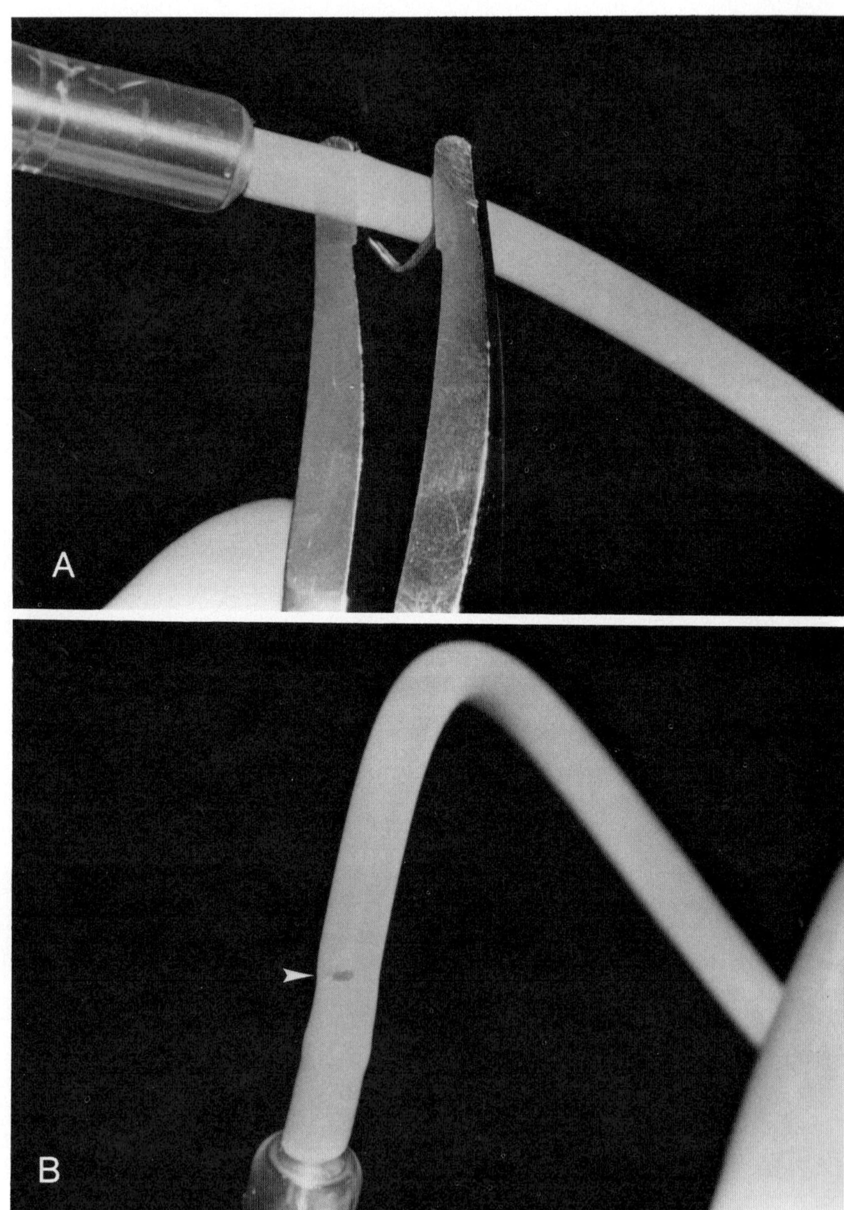

FIG. 18.10. (*A*) Weck tantalum clip being placed on silicone tubing at distal end of Holter valve. (*B*) Puncture (*arrowhead*) caused by clip.

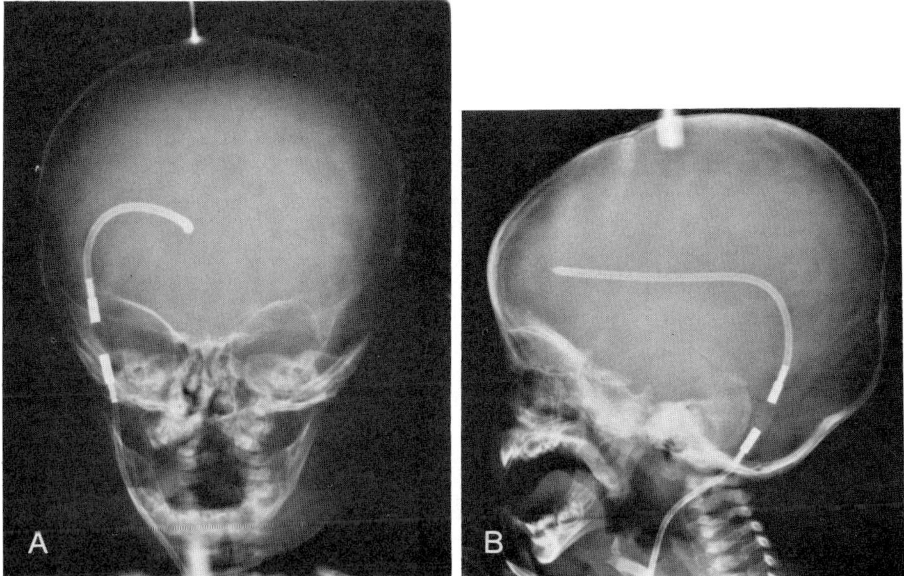

FIG. 18.11. Anteroposterior (*A*) and lateral (*B*) views showing proximal catheter lying well forward in ventricle near the foramen of Monro.

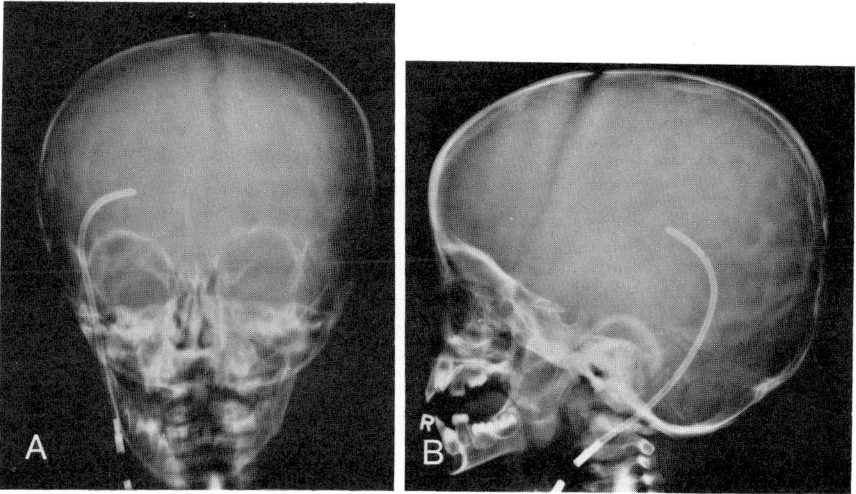

FIG. 18.12. Anteroposterior (*A*) and lateral (*B*) views taken 2 weeks later. Holter valve had not been sutured to the skull and had slipped down, pulling the proximal catheter out of the ventricle. Separated sutures indicate shunt malfunction.

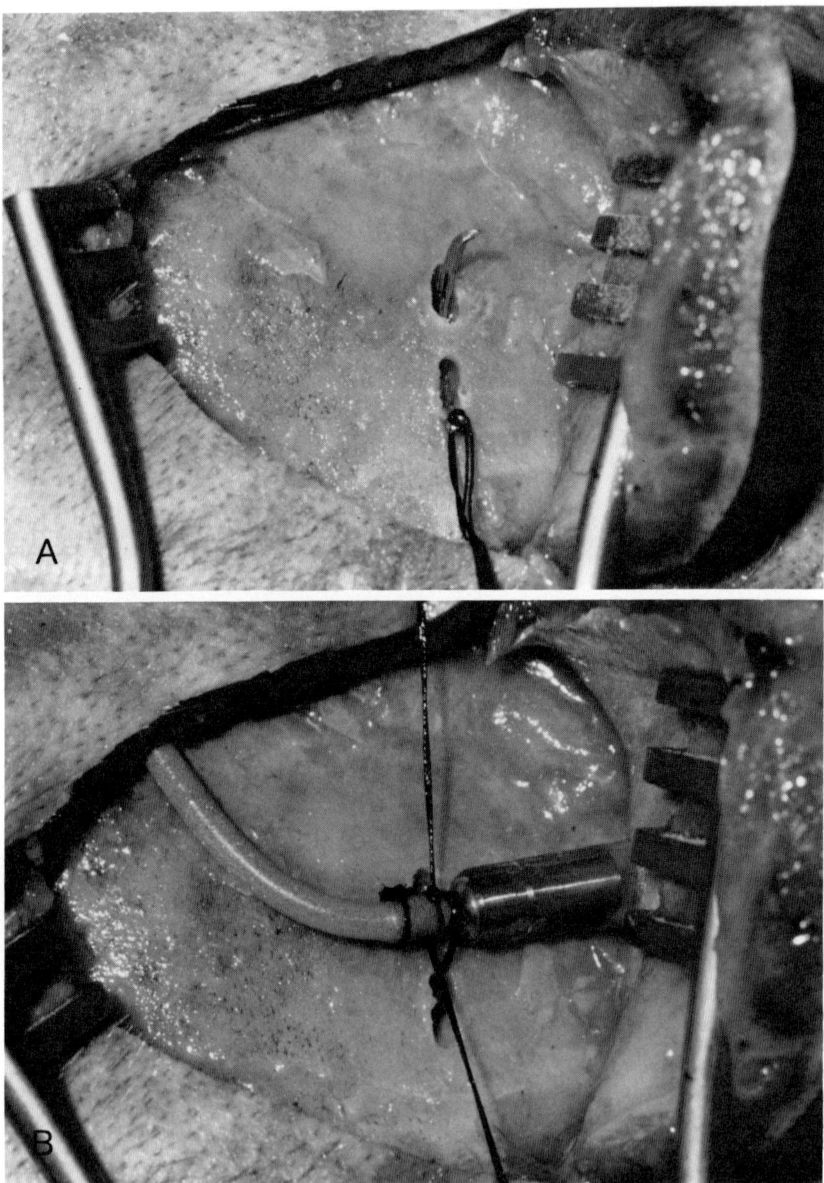

FIG. 18.13. Cadaver study. Technique for securing Holter valve to skull. (*A*) Flap is retracted, drill holes have been made in skull well away from the incision line, and 3-0 silk suture is being pulled through. (*B*) Holter valve is tied securely to skull.

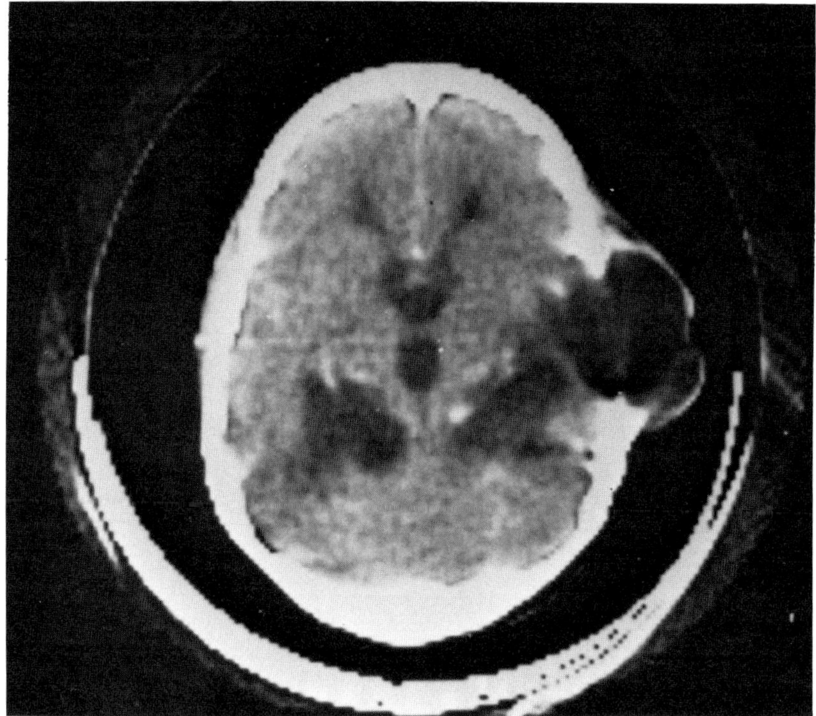

FIG. 18.14. Recurrence of hydrocephalus after removal of grossly infected shunt.

circumference of the tube or they will allow the tube to bend back on itself so that flow is completely obstructed (Figs. 18.17 and 18.18).

THE HOLTER VALVE

Here at the Bowman Gray School of Medicine-Baptist Hospital (BGSM-BH) complex, we have used the Holter valve system for our ventriculoperitoneal shunts almost since the valve's introduction in 1957. Since that year, the equipment has been greatly improved. The newer silver-impregnated tube causes so little reaction in the tissue that only a very thin pseudomembrane forms around the tube, making it an easy process to remove and replace tubing during elective revisions. The entire system is now radiopaque. The valves are highly dependable, and only very rarely can some complication in a shunt be attributed to the valves or the tubes themselves. The Holter valve, particularly the newer, elliptical Holter valve, has a positive pumping action. If it pumps easily when pressed upon in the parietal region, one can be reasonably certain that the distal end of the shunt is open; if it collapses when pumped and then

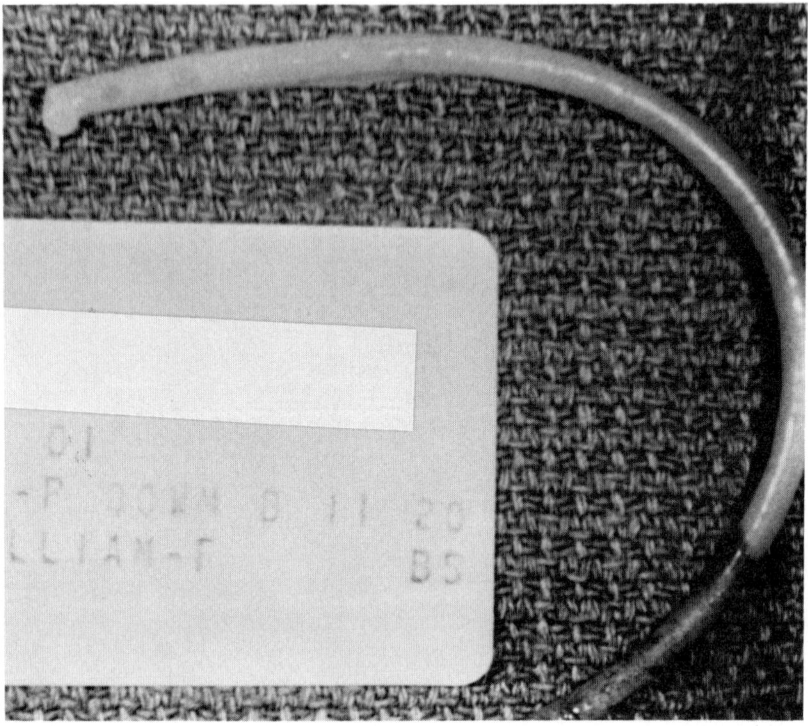

FIG. 18.15. Obstructed distal tubing.

gradually fills over the course of 30 to 60 seconds, then the proximal end in the slit-like ventricles is patent; if it pumps, but does not refill readily, the proximal end is probably blocked.

THE PROCEDURE AT BGSM-BH

When we establish a ventriculoperitoneal shunt, we give all of our patients prophylactic antibiotic therapy immediately before the first incision is made, and continue the dose for 48 hours thereafter. Usually, we give cephalothin to older patients; nafcillin to infants. We prepare the skin extensively, first with PhisoHex wiped off with alcohol, then with 3.5% iodine applied twice and wiped off with 70% ethyl alcohol until no evidence of the iodine remains. We use Steridrapes, and, as I have already mentioned, close the wounds in layers, including the small incisions made as needed along the track of the peritoneal tube. We use no nonabsorbable suture material beneath the skin, since silk may erode through the thin skin of a baby's scalp or chest wall to cause serious infection.

To reduce the number of occlusions of the proximal tubing, such as the one illustrated in Fig. 18.19, we have devised the following system.

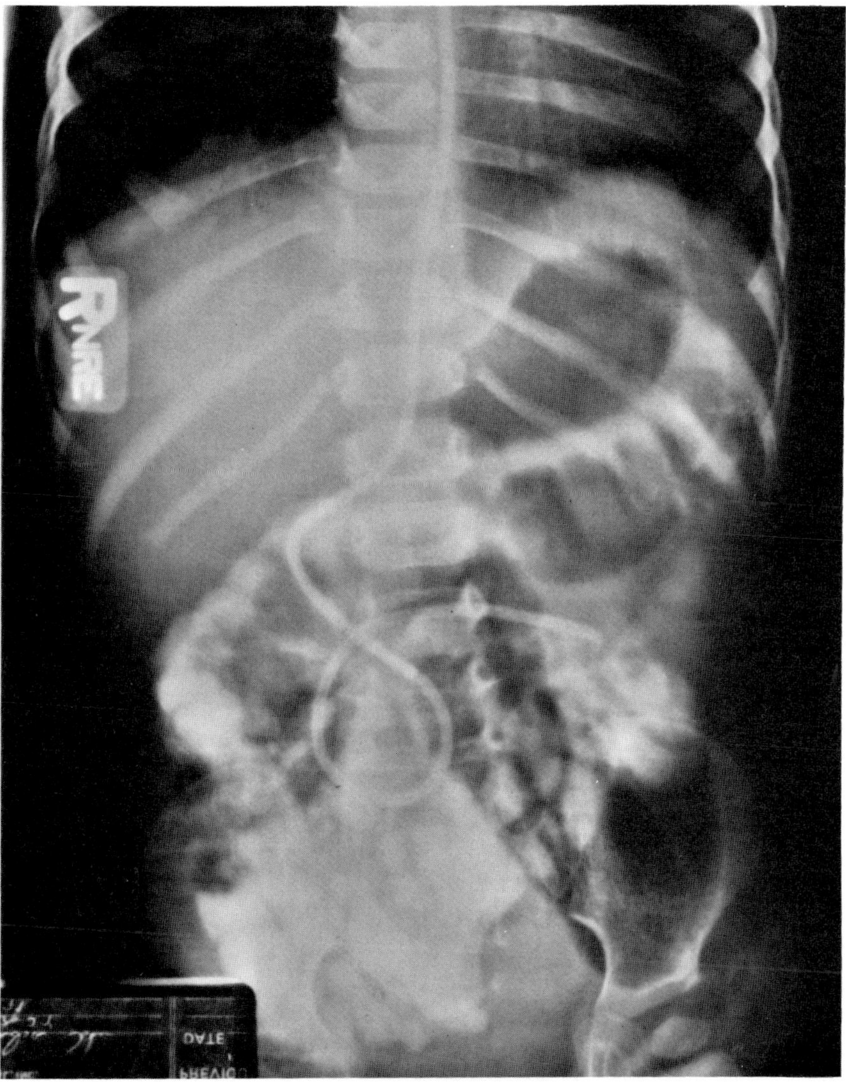

FIG. 18.16. Too long distal catheter has penetrated small bowel.

Since even the best of shunts may become obstructed, particularly as the ventricles shrink and become slit-like, we use a large Rickham reservoir (7) recessed through a large burr hole into the skull so that the profile of the reservoir is rarely higher than that of the scalp itself. This large burr hole in the frontal region is centered 4 cm from the midline at the coronal suture, as can be seen in Fig. 18.20*A*. The outline of the

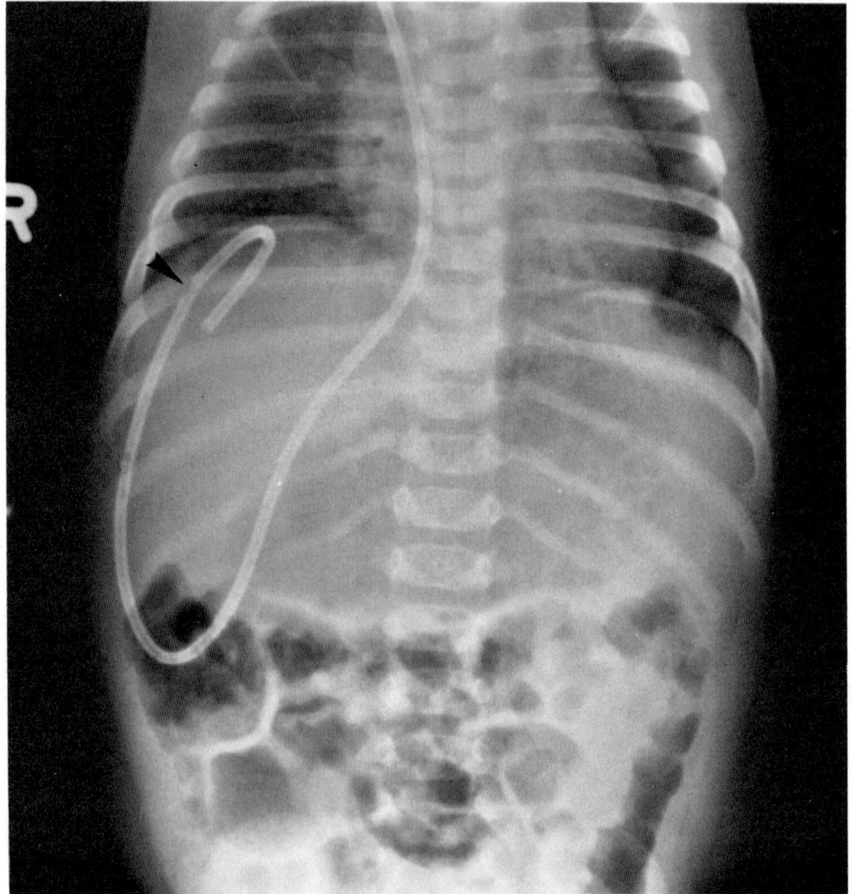

FIG. 18.17. Hole in side of tubing (*arrowhead*) is too large and catheter will bend.

coronal suture can be seen; the ruler shows the distance from the midline. A small hole is then drilled out on the posterior side toward the Holter valve in the parietal region to accommodate the side arm of the Rickham reservoir so that the reservoir can be truly seated without a high profile (Fig. 18.20*B*).

In adult patients, 5 cm of ventricular tubing is the maximum needed (Fig. 18.21*A*) and if the opening in the skull is 4 cm from the midline and if the Rickham reservoir is inserted directly at right angles to the skull (Fig. 18.21*B*), the distal end of the catheter should be directly into the anterior horn of the ventricle just anterior to the foramen of Monro and away from the choroid plexus. A small opening is made in the dura mater, small enough that the catheter attached to the Rickham reservoir must

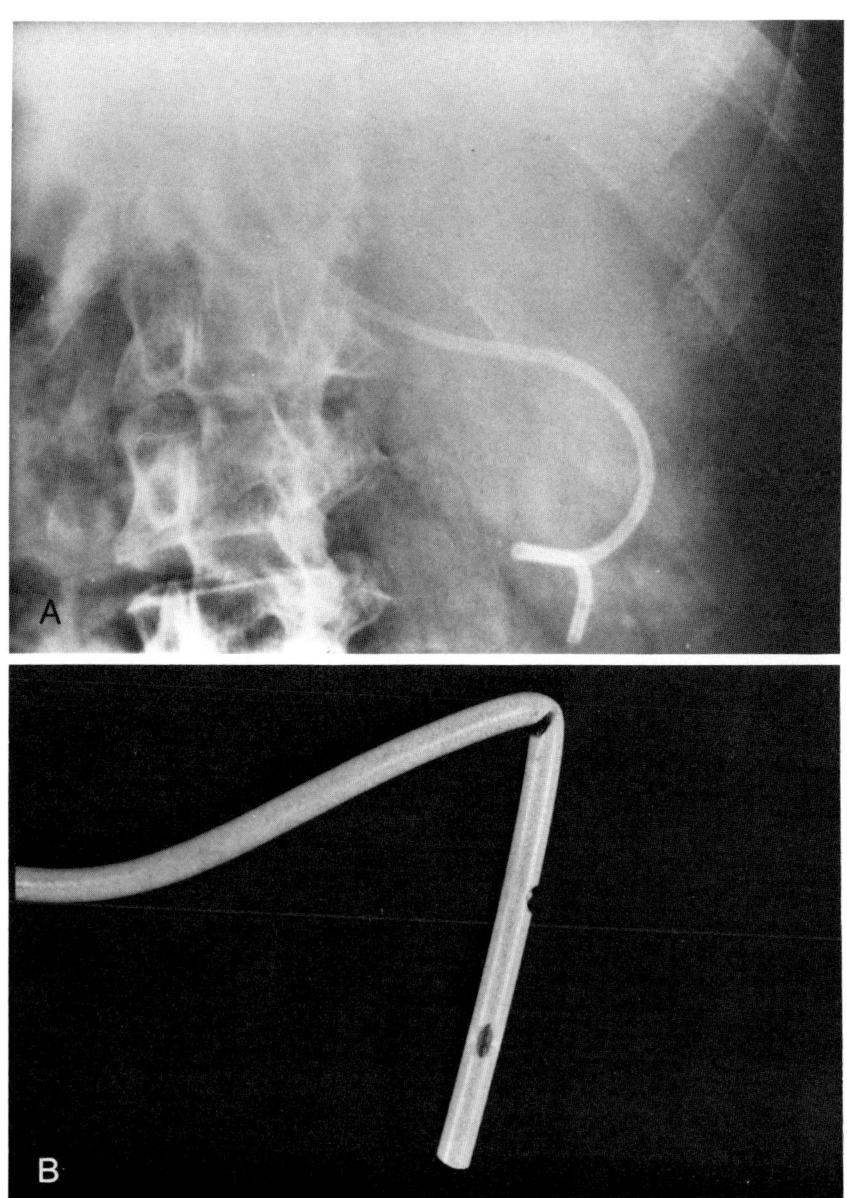

FIG. 18.18. (*A*) Tubing has bent back on itself at site of side hole. (*B*) Tubing after it was removed from patient.

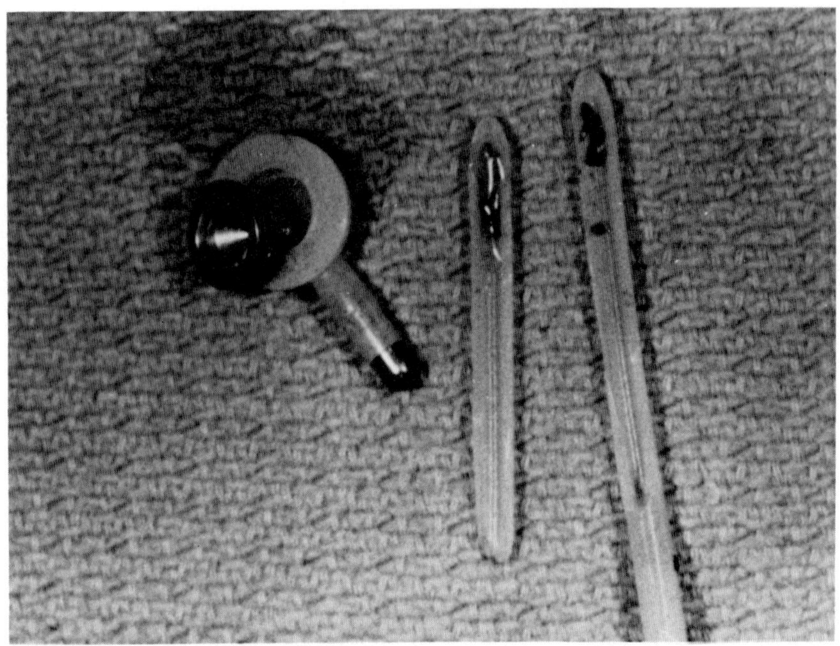

FIG. 18.19. Rickham reservoir with tube removed and split open to show clot in distal end.

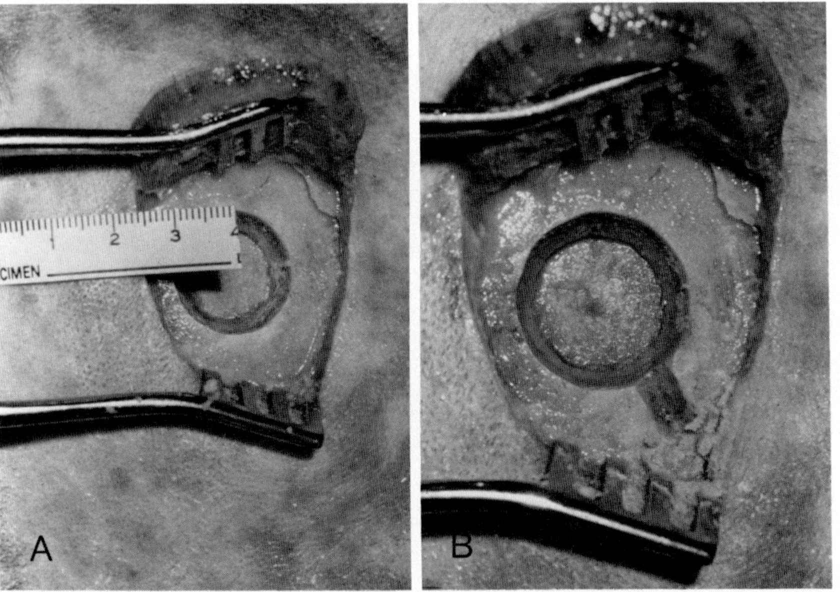

FIG. 18.20. Cadaver study. (*A*) Burr hole for Rickham reservoir is made 4 cm from midline just anterior to coronal suture. (*B*) Channel has been drilled out for side arm of reservoir.

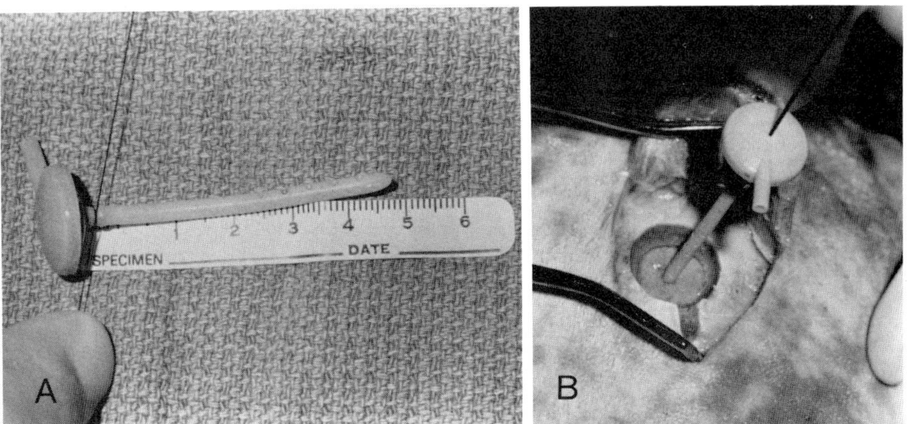

FIG. 18.21. Cadaver study. (*A*) Rickham reservoir for adult; tie is 3-0 silk. (*B*) Stylette passes directly through center of cap to guide reservoir stem at right angles to skull.

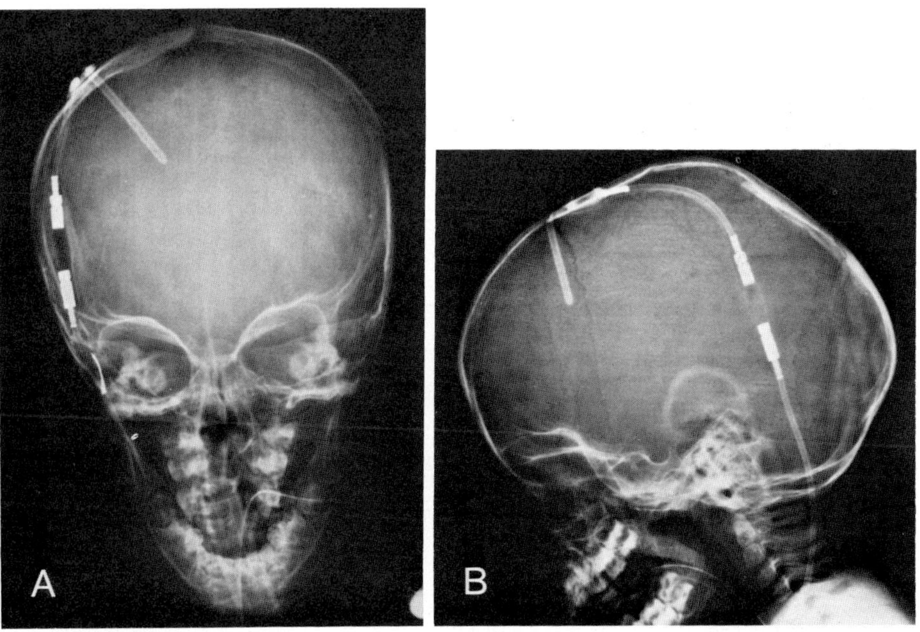

FIG. 18.22. Anteroposterior (*A*) and lateral (*B*) views showing poor placement of Leroy reservoir in infant.

be forced through the dura to prevent leakage around the catheter, and possibly to prevent the formation of subdural hematomas.

We pass the tube attached to the side arm of the Rickham reservoir beneath the scalp to the Holter valve in the posterior parietal region; in

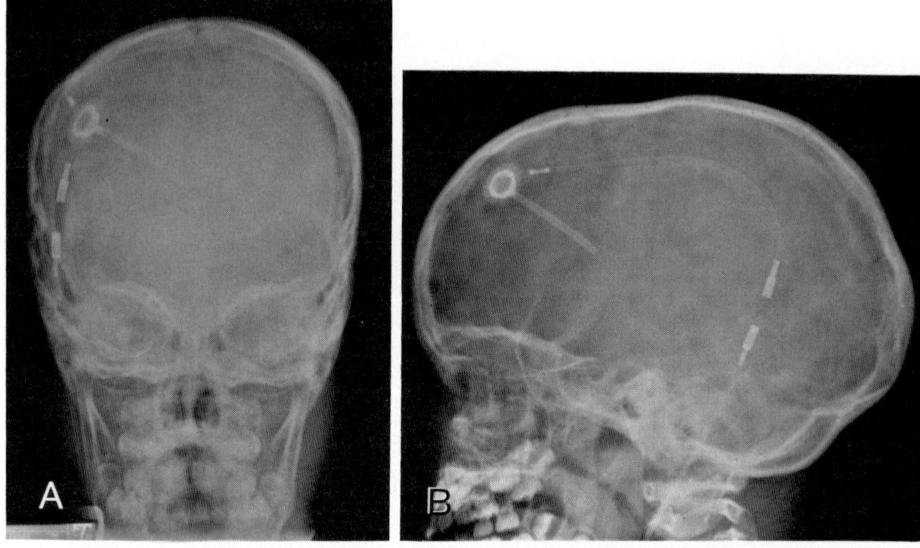

FIG. 18.23. Anteroposterior (*A*) and lateral (*B*) views showing that Rickham reservoir has been placed too far forward and too far lateral.

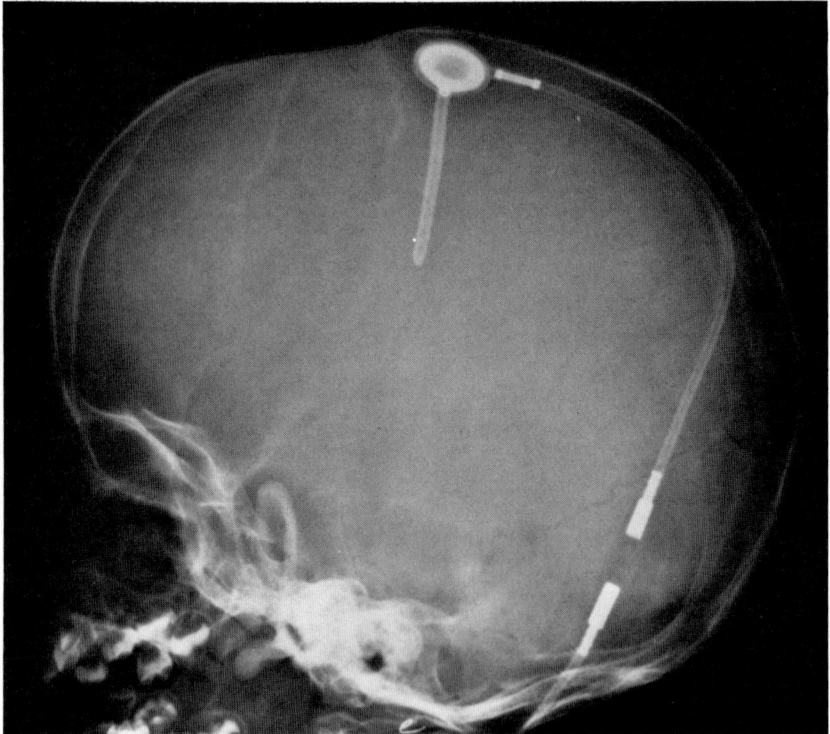

FIG. 18.24. Rickham reservoir has been placed too far back, behind coronal suture.

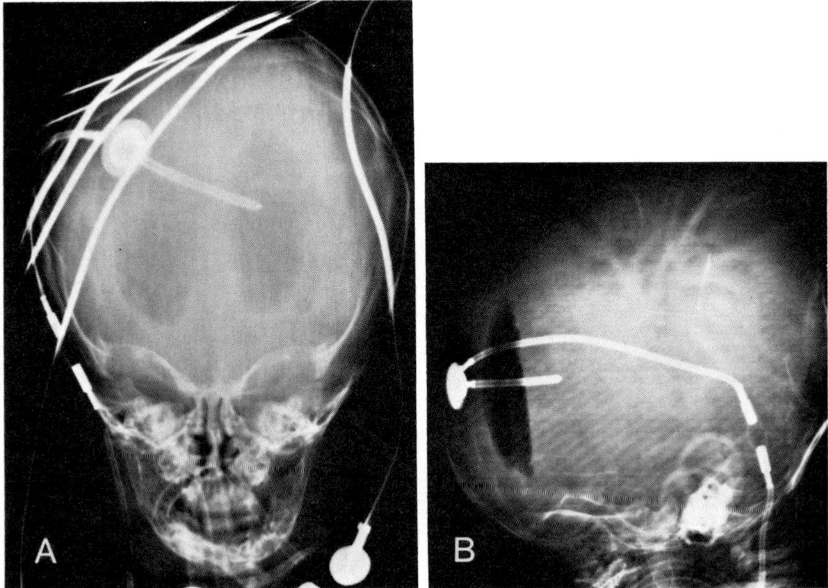

FIG. 18.25. Anteroposterior (*A*) and lateral (*B*) views show that frontal Rickham reservoir is too far forward, too far lateral, and, for this position, too long, since it has crossed the midline.

all cases, we place this tube rather high, suturing the proximal end of the Holter valve to the skull.

If the patient returns with apparent shunt obstruction, it is a simple matter for the physician to shave the hair over the Rickham reservoir and to put a small no. 23 needle into the reservoir. He can obtain spinal fluid, measure pressure, or attach a manometer filled with fluid to the needle, and if the Holter valve is working properly, he can use it to pump down the column of fluid. That ability to pump the Holter valve is reassuring for the physician examining a child with signs and symptoms suggestive of shunt obstruction. Some obstructions of the proximal end can be relieved by irrigating the proximal tube with a no. 19 needle passed down to the distal end of the proximal tube.

By studying roentgenograms taken immediately postoperatively to demonstrate the position of the shunt, we know, in cases with successful results, that we have used the measurements I have given you. Failure to use those exact measurements produces unsatisfactory results, as is illustrated in Figs. 18.22 through 18.25.

Fig. 18.22 shows poor placement of a Leroy shunt in a small baby. The shunt is not deep enough, and when the ventricles became slit-like, the shunt did not work. We did not recognize the problem in time, and despite our efforts, the baby died because of shunt obstruction.

In many instances, we have placed the Rickham reservoir too far forward or too far from the midline. In Fig. 18.23, the distal end of the proximal shunt is carried too far back into the ventricle behind the foramen of Monro and is not deep enough in the anterior horn of the ventricle.

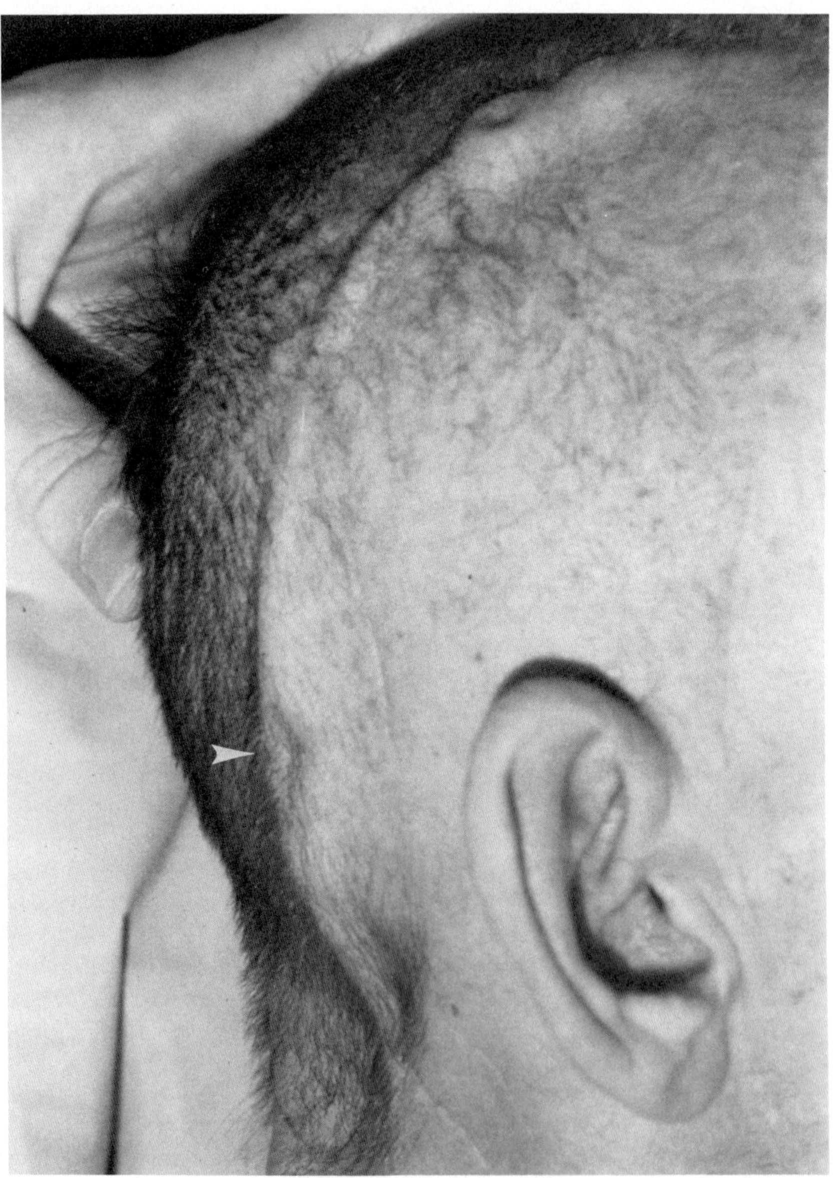

FIG. 18.26. Closed Portnoy On/Off device can be seen beneath scalp at top of picture. Holter valve (*arrowhead*) has collapsed.

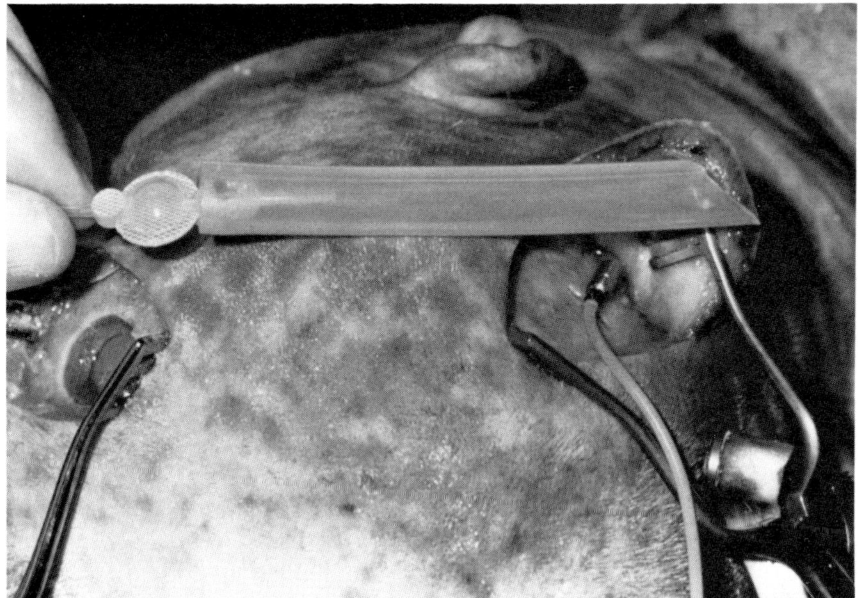

FIG. 18.27. Cadaver study. Chest drainage tube will be used to pass Portnoy On/Off device under scalp from burr hole on left to Holter valve on right.

In other instances, the catheter is placed behind the coronal suture (Fig. 18.24) so that the distal tube is lying in part 2 of the ventricle, not away from the choroid plexus in the anterior horn, and the catheter is too close to the motor cortex, a part of the brain that must be avoided. In Fig. 18.25, the catheter is much too far forward and too far lateral, and for that position, much too long, so that it has crossed the midline.

In small infants, it is difficult to judge exactly how long the catheter attached to the Rickham reservoir should be. In an adult, 5 cm is exactly the right length; in a 2-week-old child, 3.5 to 3.8 cm is about the right length, but may still be too long. It is best to determine the length for each individual case.

No matter what shunt system is used and no matter what type of pressure valve is used, subdural hematomas secondary to mild trauma will form in these patients. In the last 2 or 3 years, we have been experimenting with the Portnoy On/Off device to help alleviate that problem. We drain the hematoma (both in children and adults), put in the Portnoy On/Off device at the same operation, close the system, and leave it closed until the subdural hematoma is evacuated and the brain has reexpanded. In Fig. 18.26, the Portnoy On/Off device high in the parietal region can be seen through the scalp. The valve is obviously closed, since pumping the Holter valve behind the right ear has left the valve collapsed.

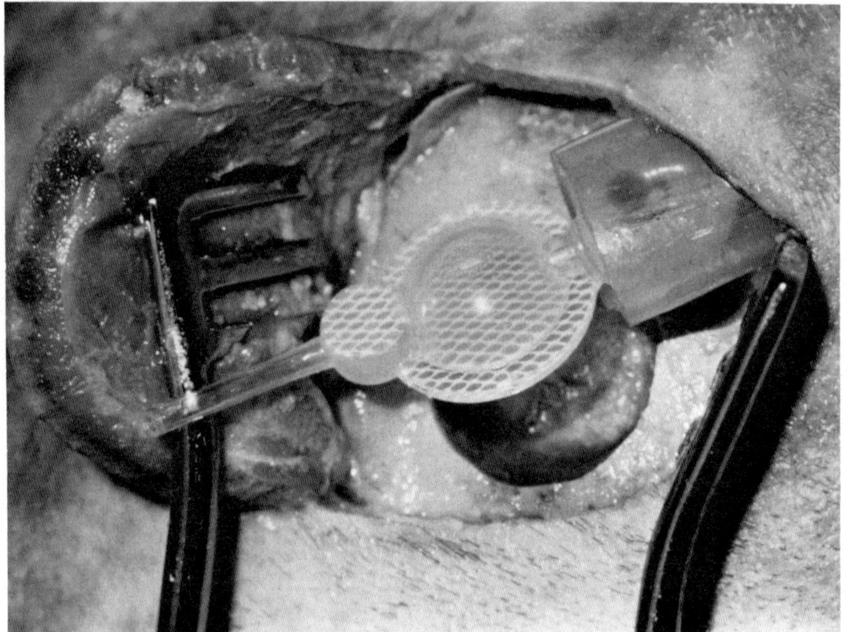

FIG. 18.28. Portnoy On/Off device is being passed beneath scalp.

In some older patients with cortical atrophy, we have inserted the Portnoy On/Off device between the Rickham reservoir and the Holter valve at the time the shunt is inserted.

Figs. 18.27 through 18.29 illustrate one method of passing the Portnoy On/Off device between the Rickham reservoir and the Holter valve. The more distal part of the Portnoy On/Off device is placed into a piece of plastic chest drainage tube which carries it through to the incision where the Holter valve is tied in place. That places the device well under the scalp and away from the incision. Disadvantages of using this method are:

1. More hair, one half of the head, must be shaved.
2. An additional incision must be made in the scalp.
3. More "hardware" must be buried under the skin.
4. More connections must be made, so that
5. Slightly more time is required to insert the shunt.

Some have expressed a preference for other valve systems when the CSF protein is elevated, since a high concentration of CSF protein tends to prevent any kind of shunt from functioning satisfactorily. However, we have not found any other shunt system to be clearly superior to the Holter system. The positive pumping action of the Holter valve, which

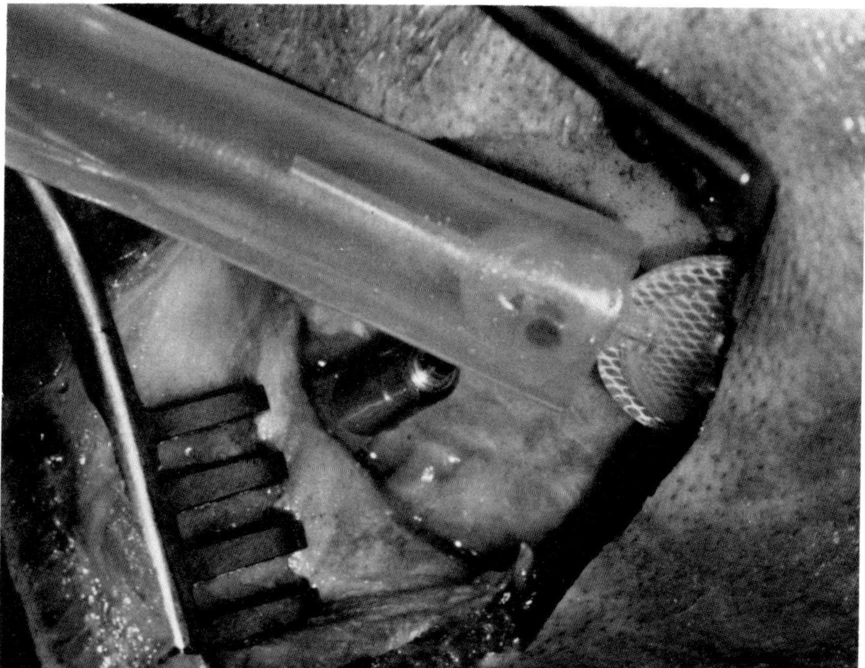

FIG. 18.29. Portnoy On/Off device is being pulled under scalp for attachment to Holter valve.

enables us to test the system—particularly if a Portnoy On/Off device is inserted so that we can selectively flush either the proximal or the distal end by pressure through the scalp on the Portnoy device—provides us with as much information about the functioning of a shunt as we have ever had. That capability, combined with the complete radiopacity of the shunt system, allows us to determine whether the shunt is functioning, whether it is completely connected, and, in some instances, whether it is defective.

All shunt systems for hydrocephalus have inherent disadvantages. The ventriculoperitoneal shunt system, combined with a Holter valve and a Rickham reservoir, has been chosen for use at BGSM-BH because our evaluation of the complications of it and other systems has shown that it is the most satisfactory shunt system for our use.

REFERENCES

1. Hlavinka, D. J. Treatment of hydrocephalus. Res. Rev., Bowman Gray School of Med. *1*: 35–42, 1961.
2. Jackson, J. D. Ventriculo-atrial shunt in the management of hydrocephalus. South. Med. J., *58*: 405–408, 1965.

3. Mark, V. H., and Sweet, W. H. Ventriculo-atriostomy; a technical note: the accurate placement of the distal end of the shunt into the right atrium without x-ray control. Neurochirurgia (Stuttg), *3*: 115–120, 1960.
4. Matson, D. D. A new operation for the treatment of communicating hydrocephalus. Report of a case secondary to generalized meningitis. J. Neurosurg., *6*: 238–247, 1949.
5. Nulsen, F. E., and Becker, D. P. Control of hydrocephalus by valve-regulated shunt. J. Neurosurg., *26*: 362–374, 1967.
6. Raimondi, A. J., Robinson, J. S., and Kuwamura, K. Complications of ventriculo-peritoneal shunting and a critical comparison of the three-piece and one-piece systems. Child's Brain, *3*: 321–342, 1977.
7. Rickham, P. P., and Penn, I. A. The place of the ventriculostomy reservoir in the treatment of myelomeningoceles and hydrocephalus. Dev. Med. Child Neurol., *7*: 296–301, 1965.

CHAPTER

19

Archaeology: The Big Neurosurgical Dig

EBEN ALEXANDER, JR., M.D.

As a member of the editorial board of the *Journal of Neurosurgery* and as a sometime contributor to the medical literature, I have long been interested in the neurological and neurosurgical procedures that were done with good reason in the past but are no longer being done. Just as archaeological explorations at sites of ancient cities give clues to how past civilizations developed and changed, so would a similar "dig" into our neurosurgical past give an indication of how the procedures we do today developed and why earlier procedures were abandoned.

I have three reasons for presenting some of those abandoned tools and procedures to you now:

1) I think you will find some of them amusing.
2) I think you will share with me a sense of humility when you are reminded of the very desperate circumstances under which some of the early workers performed their surgical procedures, and how important their early efforts were, in the sense that they led in time to procedures that have proved to be helpful.
3) I think you will be stunned to realize how recent it was that some of these techniques and procedures were the only ones available.

I have found it impossible to maintain any chronological pattern here, so I'll just take you on a tour through a pile of diagnostic artifacts and then for a look at some of the operative procedures of the past.

Myelography

The start of contrast myelography in this country is known to most of you—Mixter and Barr (45), by injecting lipidol into the spinal canal, were able to recognize a ruptured disc as the cause of certain radiographic and clinical findings that had been attributed by Stookey (62), Dandy (19), and others to the presence of a chondroma. However, lipidol, the only contrast material then readily available, caused a fairly severe reaction within the nervous system and was difficult to inject because of its density. So, some turned to thoratrast, which was not much better, because it was radioactive and easily deposited throughout the ependyma, or to diodrast, which was extremely irritating to the nervous system.

The development of Pantopaque was, therefore, heralded as a breakthrough, and a test that obviously had great diagnostic potentials became safer and easier to perform.

Angiography

Once contrast agents became safer, angiography became more popular. It began to replace air studies, and became the primary means of diagnosing subdural hematomas: no longer were unconscious patients taken to the operating room for the making of 3 burr holes on each side of the head. Cerebral angiography was expanded to help us diagnose intracerebral as well as extracerebral lesions, and is still a useful tool, even in this era of computed tomography (CT).

However, the development of contrast agents that were safe to use in the blood stream and of safer techniques for injecting those agents without a very high incidence of complications was a long, slow process. Thoratrast was much less irritating to the brain than lipidol and gave excellent contrast, but if it spilled into the neck around the carotid artery it caused intense scarring and, in some cases, later malignancy. Furthermore, it was deposited in the liver and spleen and other parts of the reticuloendothelial system where there, too, it was the cause of later malignant tumors.

Initially, most cerebral arteriograms were done by the percutaneous carotid route—later, by retrograde injection through the brachial artery. Only when Conray, Renografin, and similar materials were introduced and the femoral approach by catheterization was used did these procedures become safe. The neurosurgical literature in the early 1950s is replete with reports concerning the complications of angiography, some authors reporting complications, some reporting no complications, and others reporting how to avoid them.

Diagnosis of Brain Abscesses with Opaque Dyes

With the advent of the CT scan, many diagnostic contributions of the past have fallen by the wayside. Ventriculography and pneumoencephalography, with their risks and profound patient discomfort, are becoming increasingly rare. Courtland Davis and I (3) reported the use of micropaque barium in suspension for injection into intracranial cysts and abscesses (Fig. 19.1). It was an elegant method, which helped us follow abscesses until they either disappeared or enlarged to the point that it was obvious that they must be further treated surgically, but it is a method that is no longer necessary.

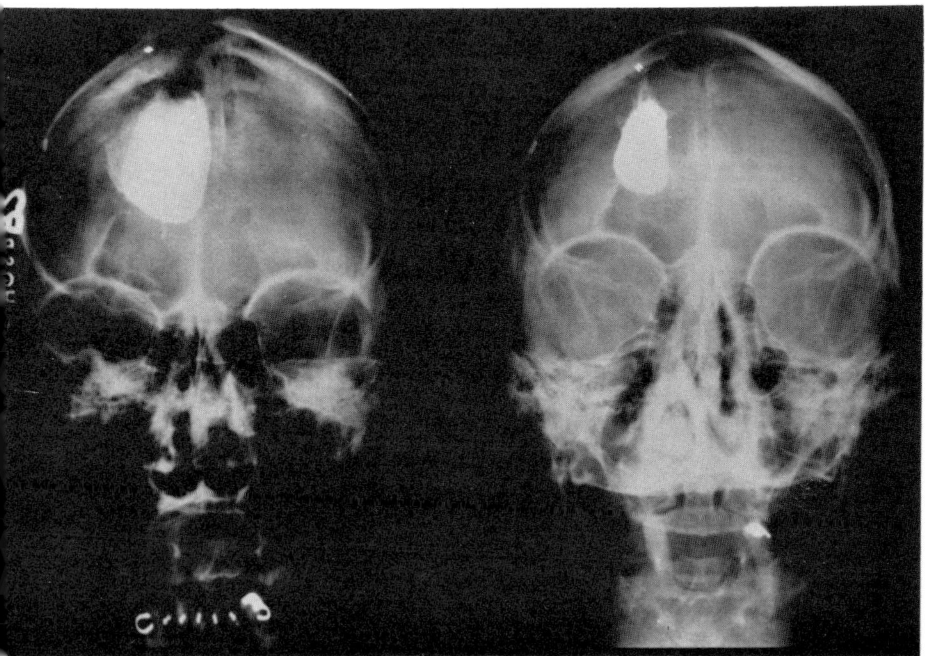

FIG. 19.1. Micropaque barium in brain abscess before (*left*) and after (*right*) aspiration of abscess, showing shrinkage of abscess cavity. (From E. Alexander and C. H. Davis, Jr. (3). Published with permission.)

Roentgen Stereoscopy

The ability to see films in 3 dimensions was developed by radiologists more than 4 decades ago (44) (Fig. 19.2). It was an essential part of reading chest and skull radiographs. It is still in use in most radiology departments but is fast losing its value in competition with tomograms and CT scans. Last month, one of our residents, only 2 years out of medical school, had never heard of the procedure.

SURGICAL PROCEDURES

Increasing Blood Supply to the Brain

In 1949, an article was published by Claude Beck (9), then a professor of surgery at Western Reserve University, and others, entitled "Revascularization of the Brain through Establishment of a Cervical Arteriovenous Fistula" (Figs. 19.3 to 19.5). Their rationale was that if a patient had a poorly developed or smaller than normal brain, with accompanying mental retardation and seizures, an increase in the cerebral blood flow might help increase the size of the brain and improve its function. They

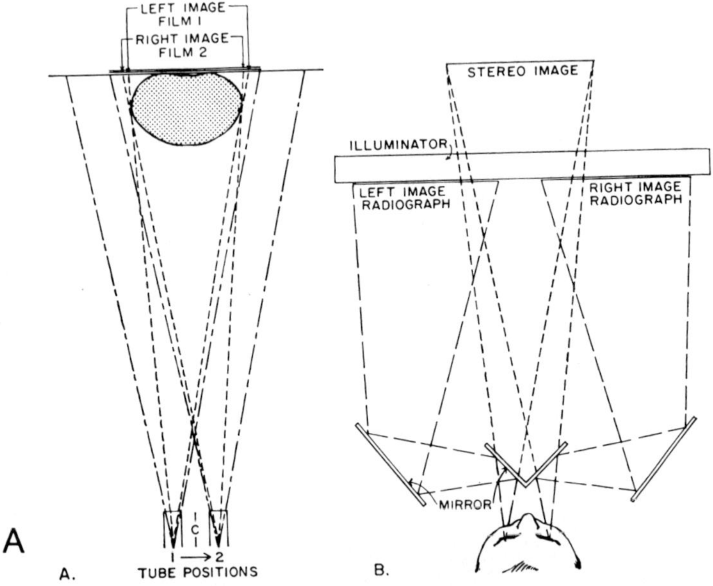

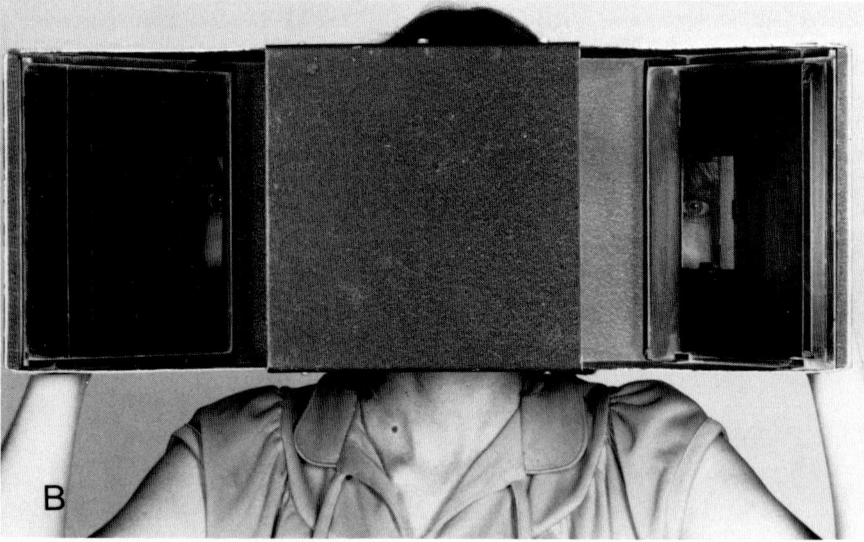

FIG. 19.2. (*A*) Principles of roentgen stereoscopy. (From I. Meschan (44). Published with permission.) (*B*) Technician using stereoscopic viewer as in *top B*.

based their hypothesis on the analogy of an arteriovenous fistula in an extremity, which does increase the blood supply to the whole extremity with resultant growth of that extremity. Their experimental work had shown that if the carotid artery was anastomosed to the jugular vein on

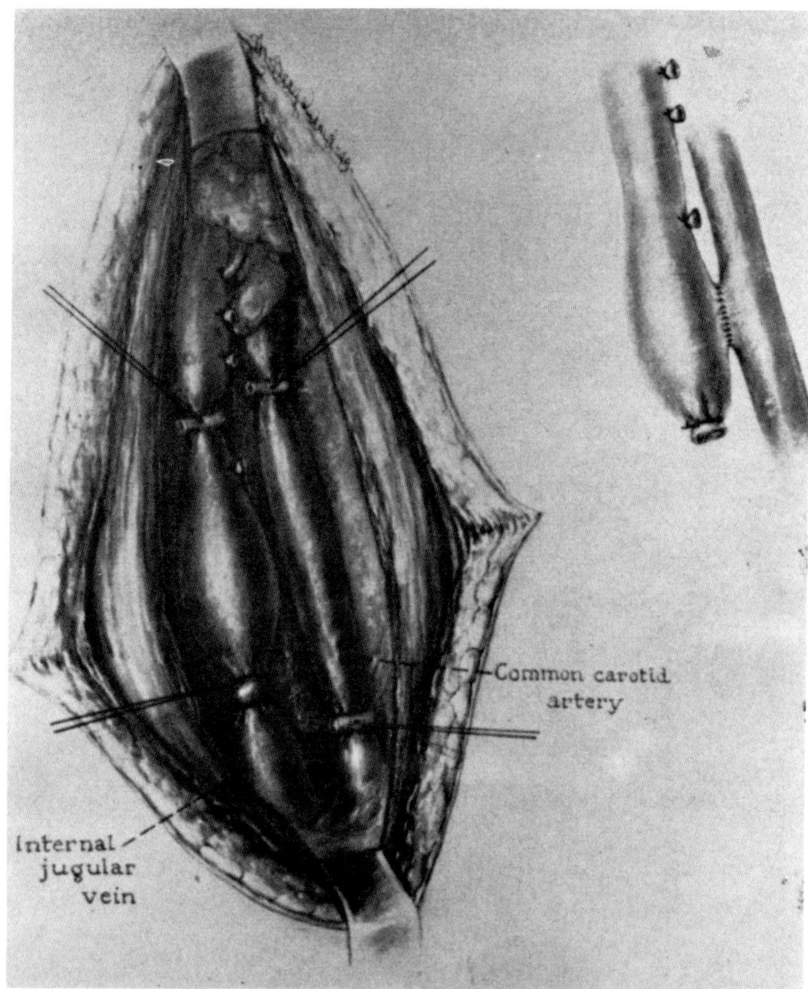

FIG. 19.3. Attempted revascularization of brain by anastomosing carotid artery and jugular vein. (From C. S. Beck *et al.* (9). Published with permission.)

one side of the neck, the blood flow to the head would be greatly increased, the pressure of the spinal fluid would increase, and presumably the brain would be more adequately vascularized. They reported one case of a microcephalic child in whom the head circumference grew from 42 to 45 cm in a short time after the operation and was accompanied by separation of the sutures. Two or three other microcephalic children had fewer seizures and seemed to move their hemiplegic extremities better after a carotid artery-jugular vein fistula had been established, so Beck and his colleagues hoped that the children would continue to improve.

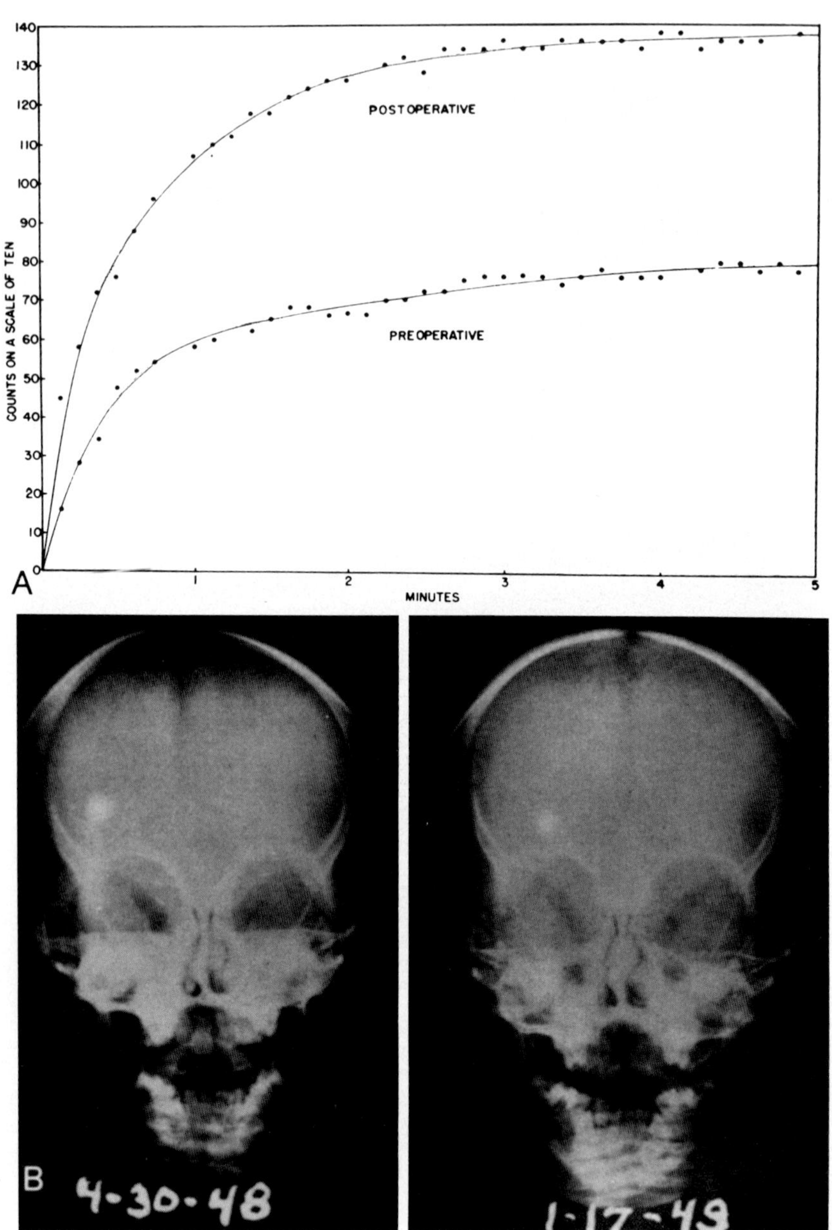

FIG. 19.4. (*A*) Increase in cerebral blood flow and (*B*) separation of sutures indicating increase in size of intracranial contents following carotid artery-jugular vein anastomosis. (From C. S. Beck *et al.* (9). Published with permission.)

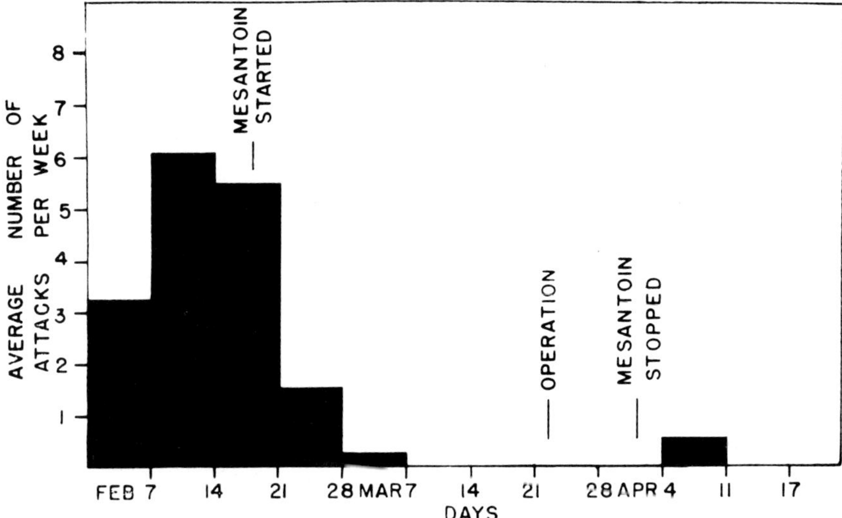

FIG. 19.5. Decrease in seizures following carotid artery-jugular vein anastomosis. (From C. S. Beck et al. (9). Published with permission.)

However, in time, Gurdjian *et al.* (32) did a follow-up of that study in 38 monkeys, anastomosing the carotid artery to the jugular vein. They did not find that this procedure improved the oxygenation of the brain; rather, in general, it resulted in the blood's being shunted back to the heart through the jugular vein on the other side of the neck. There was stagnation of the blood and a lowered oxygen value in the sagittal sinus, even though the oxygen content in the neck veins was elevated. Thus, a procedure that looked promising was sidelined after further study.

Approaching Aneurysms

Perhaps you don't know that Soma Weiss, Hersey Professor of Medicine at the Harvard Medical School, had a middle cerebral artery aneurysm diagnosed in the early 1940s. The diagnosis was made clinically; it was predicted that he would die of recurrent hemorrhage; and he did. Although the cream of the crop of neurosurgeons saw him, none at that time considered his aneurysm a matter for surgical treatment.

A bit later, when there was a start to approaching intracranial aneurysms surgically, many, many methods were tried to improve the mortality of the procedure. Today, some of those seem a little farfetched, but they are "shards" of our past, and many predict present procedures.

Hypotension during exposure of the aneurysm was felt to be an advantage, and it was initiated in many ways, all without the drugs and many of the anesthetic procedures that are available today. Endotracheal tubes were rarely used, and blocking agents were unavailable.

Gillies (30) and Griffiths (31) described total spinal anesthesia below T1 as a method of reducing blood pressure and intracranial blood flow (Figs. 19.6 and 19.7). This was done in a logical way, and their papers were excellent papers. The anesthesia could be carried higher if an endotracheal tube was put in place, and the blood pressure depended entirely on the tilt of the table—the higher the head, the lower the pressure. We operated on 2 patients with anterior communicating aneurysms by this method.

Soon after, the blocking agent trimethaphan camsylate was developed. When given systemically, trimethaphan camsylate reduced the blood pressure, the effect again depending entirely on the raising of the head of the table and the pooling of blood in the lower extremities. Bucy (54) was one of the authors of an excellent article on that subject.

From New Zealand, Hodder (33) reported lower limb negative pressure equipment for the reduction of cerebral blood flow during neurosurgical procedures. This was an intriguing apparatus comprising 2 cylinders

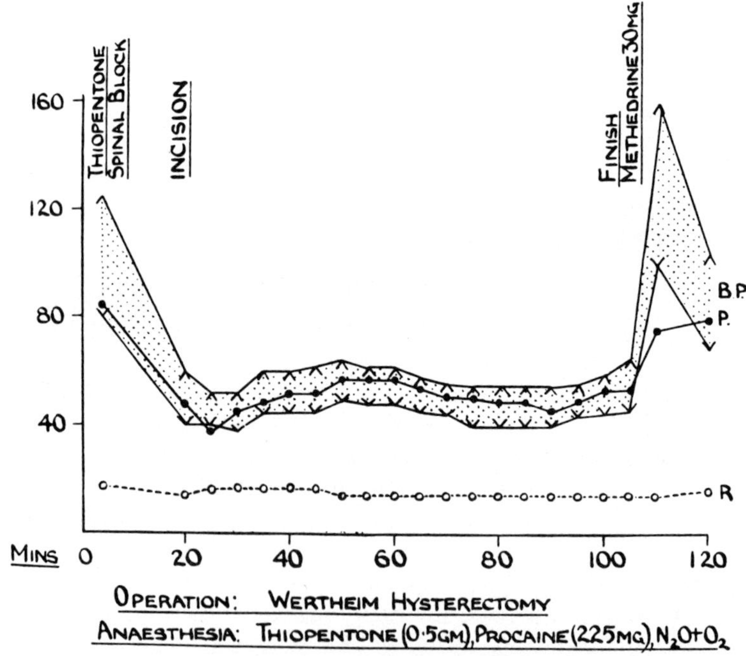

FIG. 19.6. Decrease in blood pressure caused by total spinal anesthesia. Also used for intracranial operations. (From J. Gillies (30). Published with permission.)

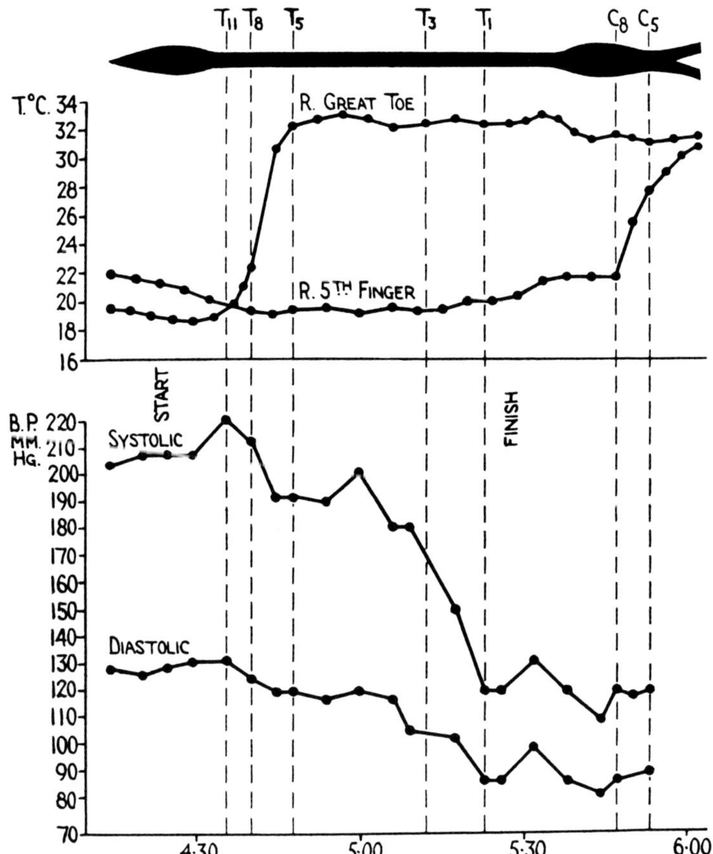

(AFTER SARNOFF AND ARROWOOD, 1947). SUBARACHNOID INJECTION OF 0·2% PROCAINE HYD. AT LEVEL OF 3RD L.V. AS SOLUTION REACHES HIGHER SEGMENTS, SYMPATHETIC PREGANGLIONIC FIBRES ARE BLOCKED AND PROGRESSIVE CHANGES IN BLOOD PRESSURE AND SKIN TEMPERATURE OCCUR.

FIG. 19.7. Decrease in blood pressure caused by total spinal anesthesia up to T1. (From J. Gillies (30). Published with permission.)

which, in effect, sucked blood into the lower extremities so that the blood pressure in the head would be reduced (Fig. 19.8).

Then there developed an enthusiasm for providing **hypothermia** during the operative treatment of intracerebral aneurysms (Fig. 19.9). This came after the introduction of chlorpromazine and the recognition that the brain surrounding the aneurysm should be as avascular as possible (22).

One of the geniuses of neurosurgery, Temple Fay (24), was one of those

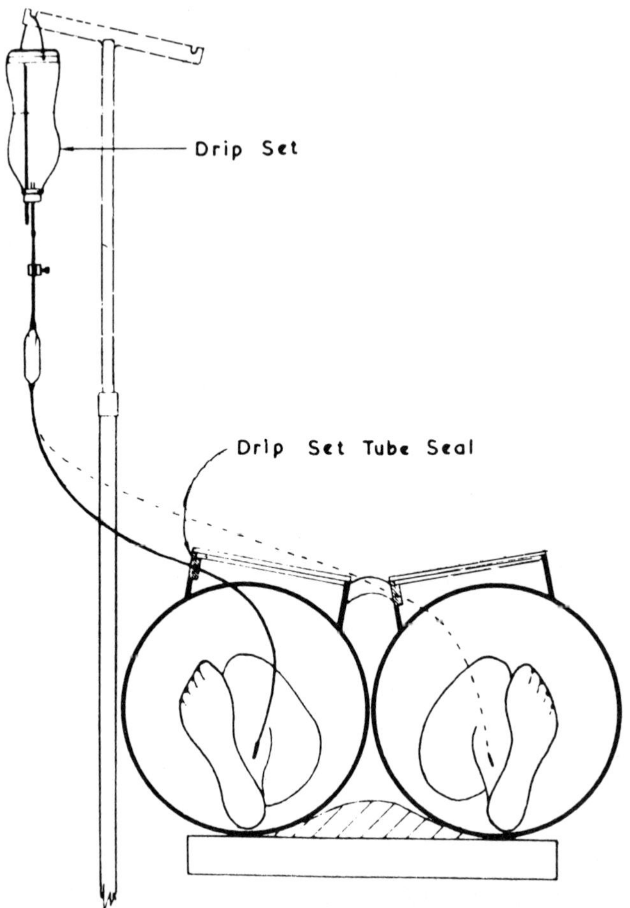

FIG. 19.8. Apparatus for lowering blood pressure in the head by drawing blood into the lower extremities. (From B. H. Hodder (33). Published with permission.)

who worked extensively with hypothermia, his interest being to refrigerate the brain for the treatment of brain tumors, rather than for the removal of cerebral aneurysms. Fig. 19.10 shows some of the instruments he used, and some of those instruments in the tumor bed.

Curing Headache

For a while, **cervical sympathectomy** appeared to be promising for the treatment of some types of headache. It was frequently used unilaterally for that purpose, creating a Horner's syndrome which was supposed to increase the circulation to the brain. Some patients with bilateral headaches had bilateral sympathectomies, and some of those, I am told, had prefrontal lobotomies when their headaches failed to improve.

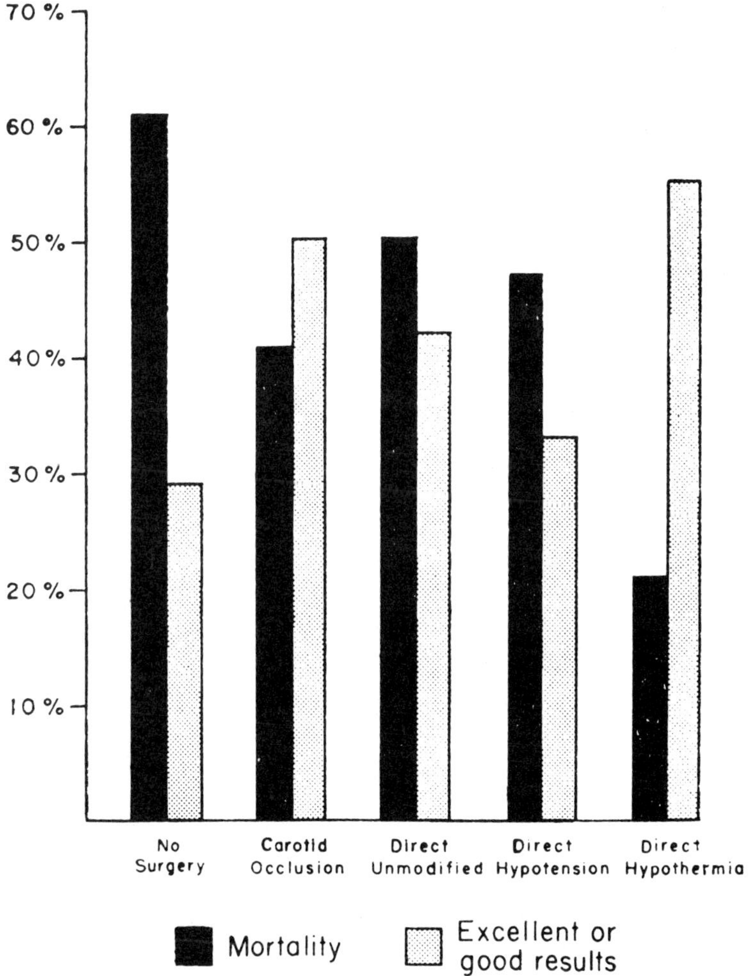

FIG. 19.9. Summary of results from various methods of managing intracerebral aneurysms. (From C. H. Davis, Jr. and E. Alexander, Jr. (22). Published with permission.)

Shunting for Hydrocephalus

Hydrocephalus has been a problem as long as any of us have any memory of neurosurgery, and the effectiveness of the forms of treatment today make it difficult for one to become too agitated over the small number of problems that remain.

For aqueduct stenosis, the old PSP test (phenolsulfonphthalein test) was used to try to localize the site of blockage (10, 56) (Fig. 19.11). Dandy (18) and later Leksell (40) developed methods for opening the aqueduct (Fig. 19.12) and Torkildsen (66) developed his much safer procedure of bypassing the obstruction (Fig. 19.13). It is amazing to see how far we

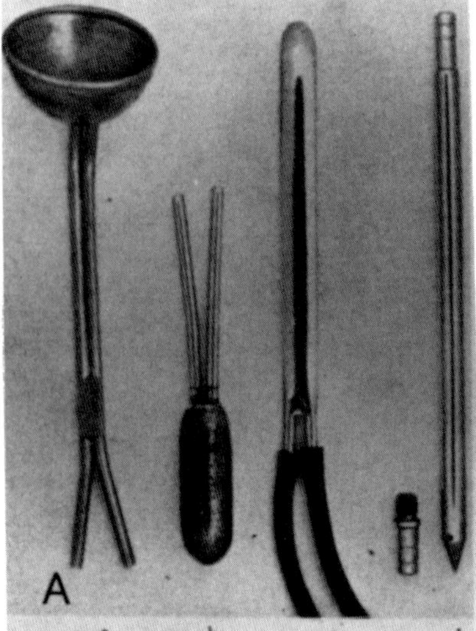

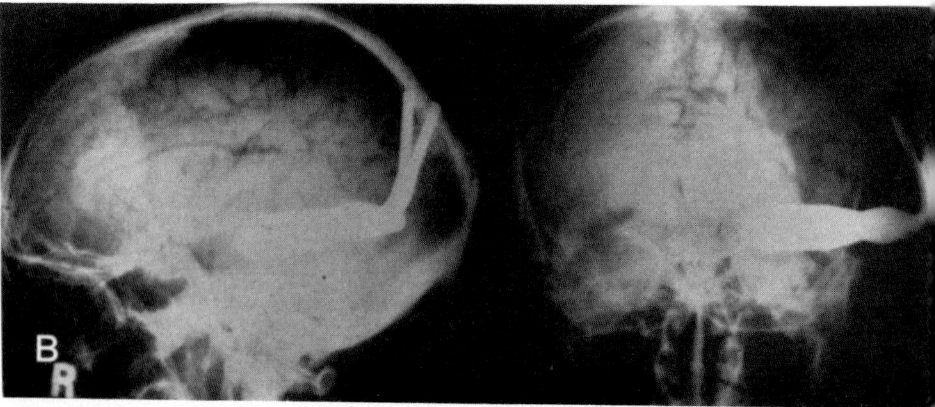

Fig. 19.10. Method for refrigerating brain for the management of brain tumors. (*A*) Instruments required; (*B*) instruments in place. (From T. Fay (24). Published with permission.)

have come and to recognize the importance of the contributions Matson (43) made during his residency at Duke University—the introduction of the ventriculoureteral and lumbar-subarachnoid-ureteral shunts (Fig. 19.14). These shunts worked well on a short-term basis, but a child who developed fever and vomiting or diarrhea quickly became dehydrated, and there was a high incidence of recurrent ascending infection. I might mention, however, that one of our patients has had a functioning lumbar-subarachnoid-ureteral shunt for over 20 years.

When Courtland Davis and I (2) placed a shunt in one patient with the

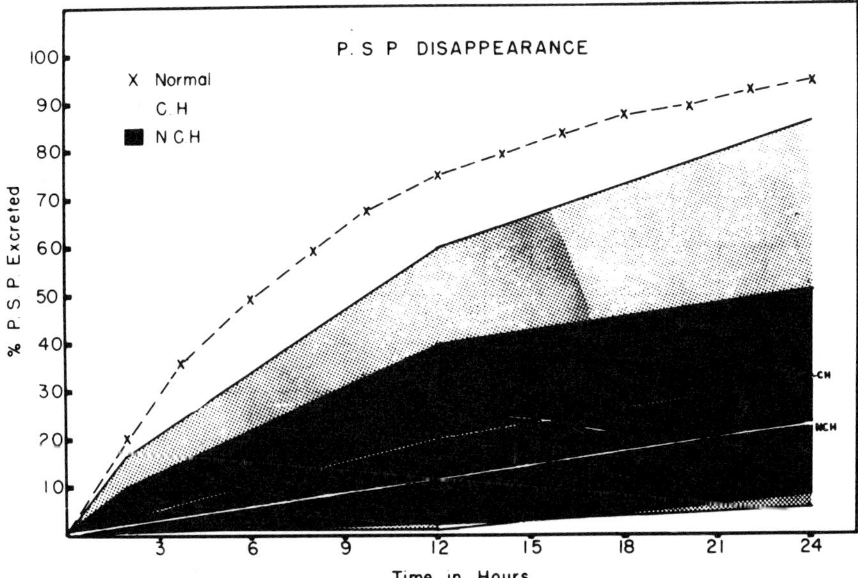

FIG. 19.11. Phenolsulfonphthalein (*P.S.P*) dye test used to localize site of block of cerebrospinal fluid causing hydrocephalus. (From W. M. Craig and H. W. Dodge, Jr. (14). Published with permission.)

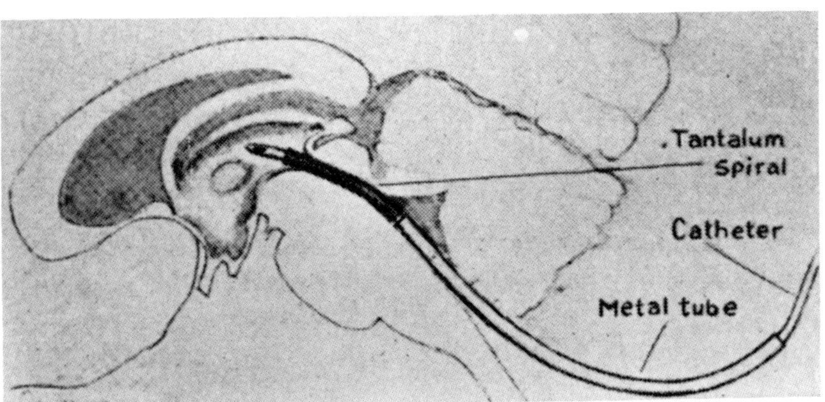

FIG. 19.12. Early technique to shunt cerebrospinal fluid from aqueduct. (From J. E. Scarff (56). Published with permission.)

congenital absence of one kidney, we placed the distal end of the tube in the peritoneum and found that the shunt worked as well as did those placed in the ureter. Soon, we began to use ventriculoperitoneal shunts with frequency (Fig. 19.15).

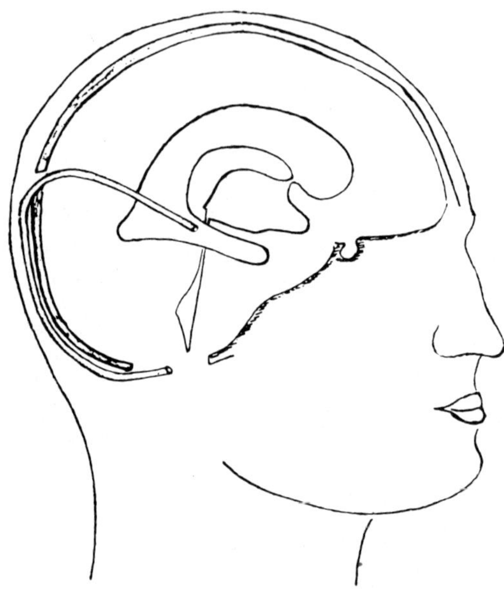

FIG. 19.13. Torkildsen shunt. (From A. Torkildsen (66). Published with permission.)

About that time, Nosik (48) (Fig. 19.16*A*) introduced the ventriculomastoid shunt, and Svien and his colleagues (63) modified and improved it (Fig. 19.16*B*). It was an easy shunt to establish, but had only short-term beneficial effects and almost always led to recurrent meningitis.

Neurosurgeons became biased against the ventriculoperitoneal shunts because they occluded so frequently, and soon ventriculoatrial shunts became the rage. During that period, and it was before the days of good x-ray equipment in the operating room, Robertson and his colleagues (53) described the use of the electrocardiogram in the placement of the atrial catheter as demonstrated in Fig. 19.17. However, ventriculoatrial shunts also led to a good deal of trouble—I remember one patient who had 22 operations over a 2- to 3-year period before something began to work well on a long-term basis. Some of the lumbar-subarachnoid-peritoneal shunts had at least as many revisions and repositionings over a similar period of time. The solution to many of the problems of occlusion proved to be the valve (49) (Fig. 19.18).

Polyethylene (Fig. 19.19), the brand name of a plastic that had been introduced in World War II in England as a light-weight insulation material for the wire used in the Mosquito bomber, proved to be almost nonreactive in the human body (35). Matson and I worked for over a year trying to develop a valve from that material, but we never made a satisfactory one. It was only when silicone became available that Spitz

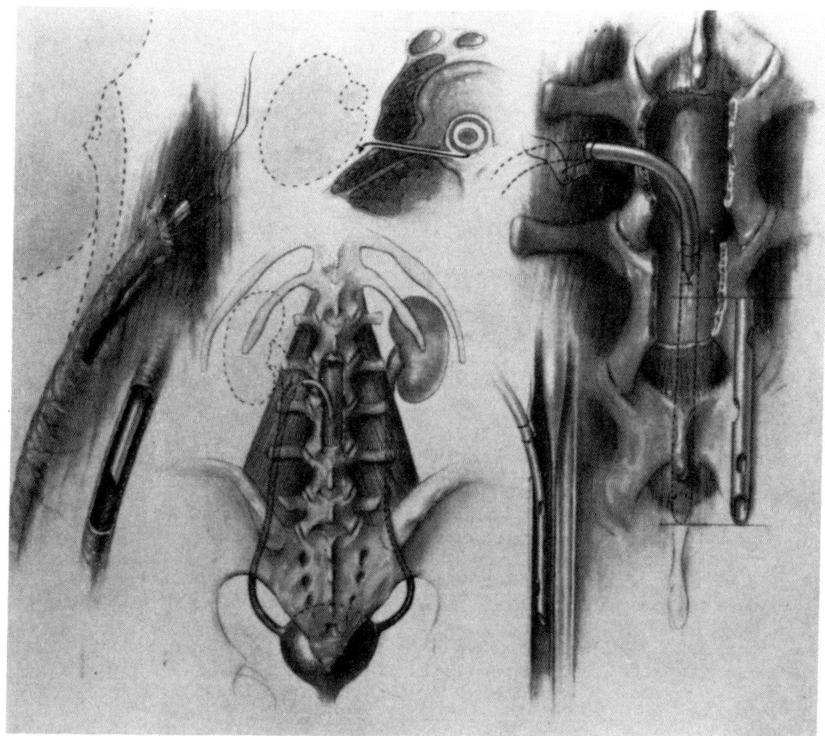

FIG. 19.14. Lumbar-subarachnoid-ureteral shunt. (From D. D. Matson (43). Published with permission.)

and Holter were able to develop the Holter valve, which has proved the most satisfactory of all valve systems. With the valve in place, the shunts could be placed in the peritoneum again where they have worked very well.

Peripheral Nerve Procedures

During World War II the repair of peripheral nerves was a large part of the work of neurosurgeons. Many efforts were made to improve on the anastomoses and the results. The use of homogenous nerve grafts was reported on by Spurling and associates (60) (Fig. 19.20), who found that this simply led to severe fibrosis and was not effective. That has remained the case today, except in transplants of small purely sensory or motor nerves, such as digital nerves and the facial nerve.

For a while, there was great enthusiasm for demonstrating the effects of nerve lesions by measuring sweating on the extremities, *i.e.*, by detecting decreased electrical resistance (52) (Fig. 19.21).

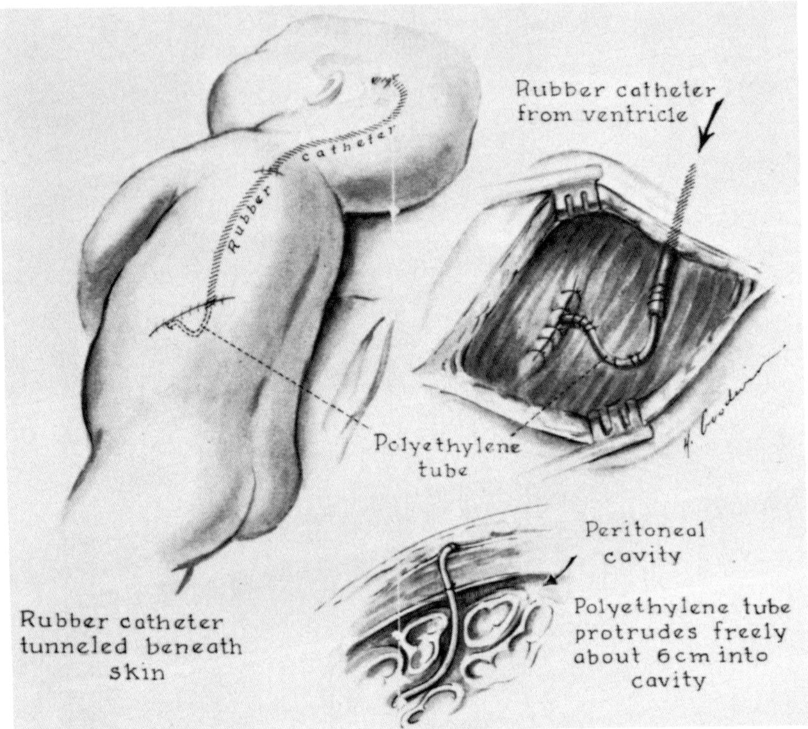

FIG. 19.15. Ventriculoperitoneal shunt. (From E. Alexander, Jr. and C. H. Davis, Jr. (2). Published with permission.)

Tantalum, an element refined at great cost, was made into extremely fine wire and swedged onto needles with which to effect nerve anastomoses, and it is still used for that purpose. It was also cast into fine foil that could be annealed into a strip or made into more solid plates (69). Since it was so nonreactive in the body, it seemed to be an ideal substance to wrap around a nerve anastomosis to prevent scar tissue from growing in. It looked beautiful at the end of the operation (Fig. 19.22), and we could hardly believe that it wouldn't work, but it wouldn't. Complications developed: in addition to our old bugaboo, scarring, there was slipping and multiple fragmentation of the tantalum sheaths, almost all of which had to be removed.

Much of the repair of peripheral nerves remains an enigma, but the foundations have been laid on which future techniques for repair can be erected.

Correcting Cranial Defects

Cranial defects, too, were common during World War II, and progress in their correction was made during that period. Previously, silver plates,

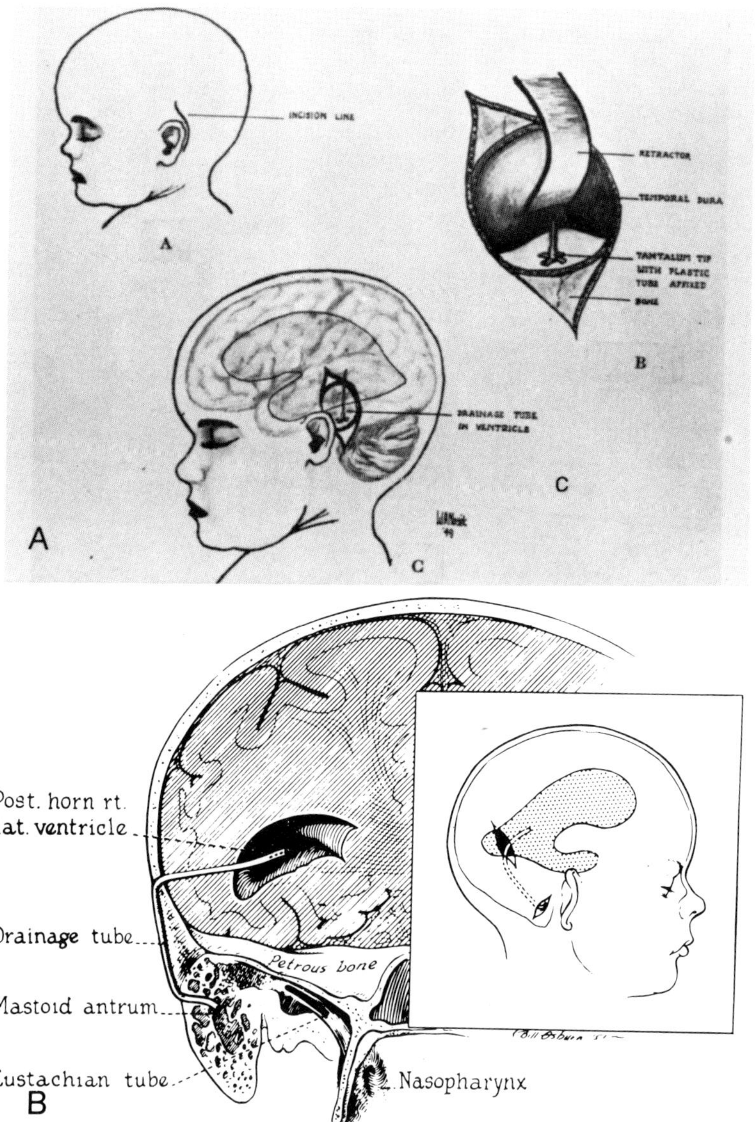

FIG. 19.16. (*A*) Ventriculomastoid shunt. (From W. A. Nosik (48). Published with permission.) (*B*) Modification. (From H. J. Svien *et al.* (63). Published with permission.)

cellophane plates, and plates of other foreign materials had been used, but the enthusiasm was primarily for vitallium, a very hard metal used primarily in orthopedic surgery. Vitallium had to be fashioned and fitted, and required a 2- or 3-stage operation with a lot of screws and hardware. Unfortunately, even then, many vitallium plates had to be removed.

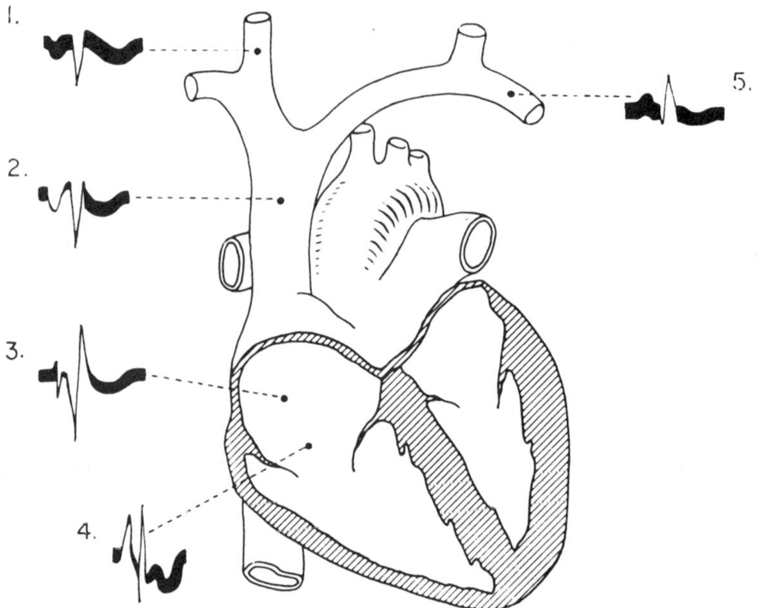

Fig. 19.17. Use of electrocardiogram to guide placement of distal end of ventriculoatrial shunt into right atrium. (From J. T. Robertson *et al.* (53). Published with permission.)

Tantalum proved much easier to work with because it was softer and more malleable, but again, it usually had to be fixed in place with screws or wedges, and many of those worked out, with resulting infection (Figs. 19.23 and 19.24). Preparing the defect for the plate was an involved procedure, and it often opened up sinuses and other areas that were prone to develop infection (41).

The use of polyethylene was a step in the right direction (5). The material could be heated and shaped into whatever form one needed (Figs. 19.25 and 19.26); it perhaps would still be popular today if acrylic had not proved to be so effective. Acrylic could be cast and polymerized and molded (Fig. 19.27) so that it would fit exactly to the skull defect without any protrusion through the scalp (23). It has stood the test of time and has effectively replaced all other methods of closing skull defects.

Tic Douloureux

Tic douloureux has been approached by so many forms of treatment and that it is difficult to keep them all straight. Davidoff and Feiring (21) studied the method originally described by Hutchinson (34) of giving large doses of ferrous carbonate, but found it not to be effective. Woodhall

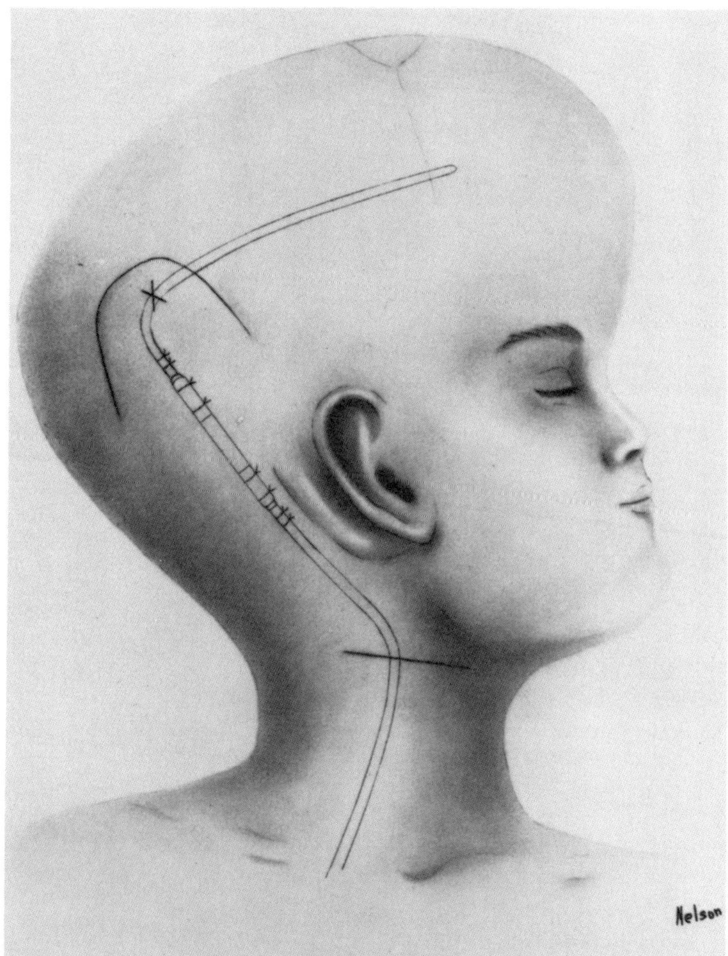

FIG. 19.18. Incision needed for securing Holter valve. (From F. E. Nulsen and D. P. Becker (49). Published with permission.)

and Odom (71) used stilbamidine, which produced a relative numbness of the extremities (including the head) and was effective to some extent. Courtland Davis and I (4) reported the use of huge doses of vitamin B_{12}, 1000 mg given 3 times a day for 3 days, and then given in decreasing amounts. This had been a means of treating severely painful tabetic crises; it had been helpful (13), and it seemed to us a sensible means of treating trigeminal neuralgia. Unfortunately, it was largely unsuccessful over the long term.

The early surgical approaches to the treatment of tic douloureux were

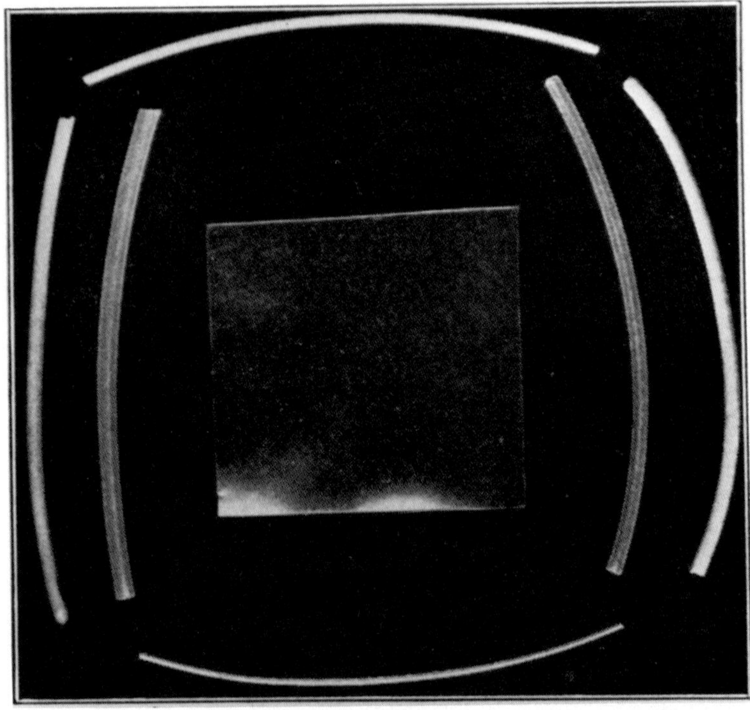

FIG. 19.19. Polyethylene tubes and plate for use in surgical procedure. (From F. D. Ingraham *et al.* (35). Published with permission.)

by Krause (39), Cushing (17), and others who removed the trigeminal ganglion (Fig. 19.28). Soon, Frazier (27) reported cutting the retroganglion fibers, which proved to be a permanent and much less mutilating procedure.

In 1938, Sjöqvist (58, 59) described division of the descending tract of the Vth cranial nerve in the medulla (Figs. 19.29 and 19.30), a procedure we all used a few times.

Some of you can recall the concern that many of the senior neurosurgeons had in the early 1960s over the belief that all neurosurgery residents should learn the standard operation of subtemporal division of the Vth cranial nerve. There just were not enough of those cases to go around. As a matter of fact, the procedure is rarely used today, and relatively few neurosurgeons know how to do it. Now, patients with tic douloureux are first treated with phenytoin sodium and carbamazepine, and if their pain is not relieved, posterior fossa decompression as described by Jannetta (36–38) or retroganglion neurolysis as described by Sweet and Wepsic (64) and Tew (65) is used; one or the other of these is almost always effective.

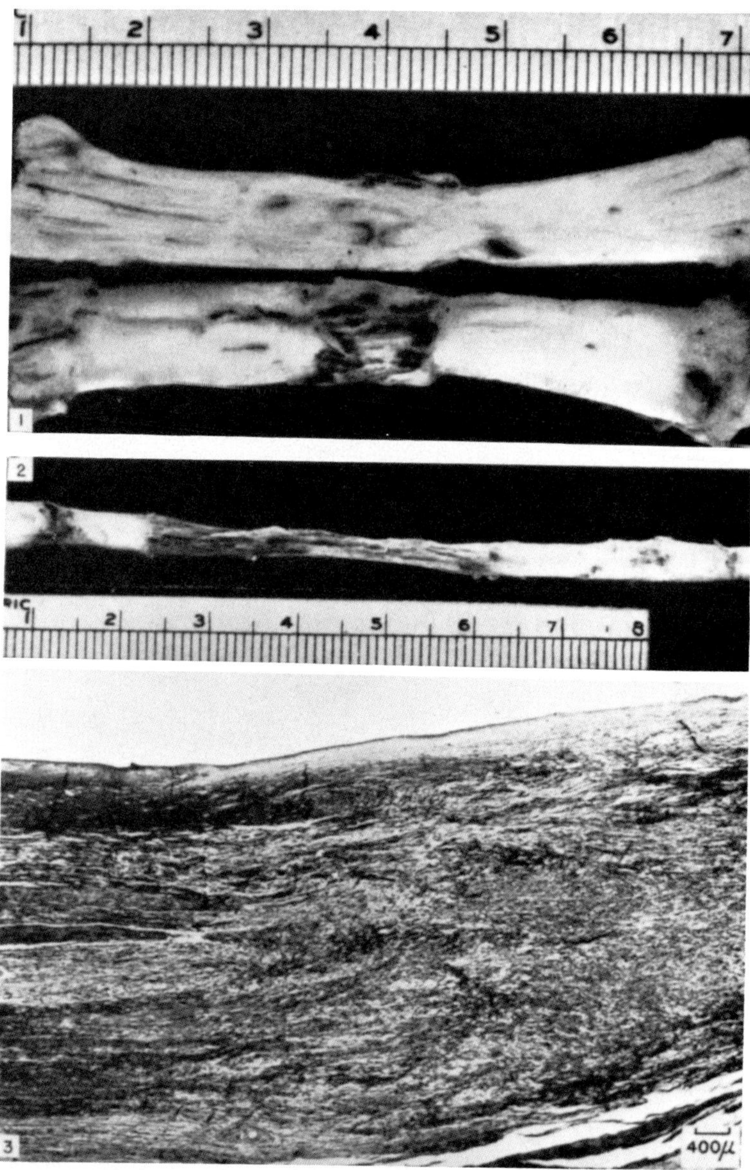

FIG. 19.20. Failure of homogenous nerve grafts in large nerves of the arm. (From R. G. Spurling *et al.* (60). Published with permission.)

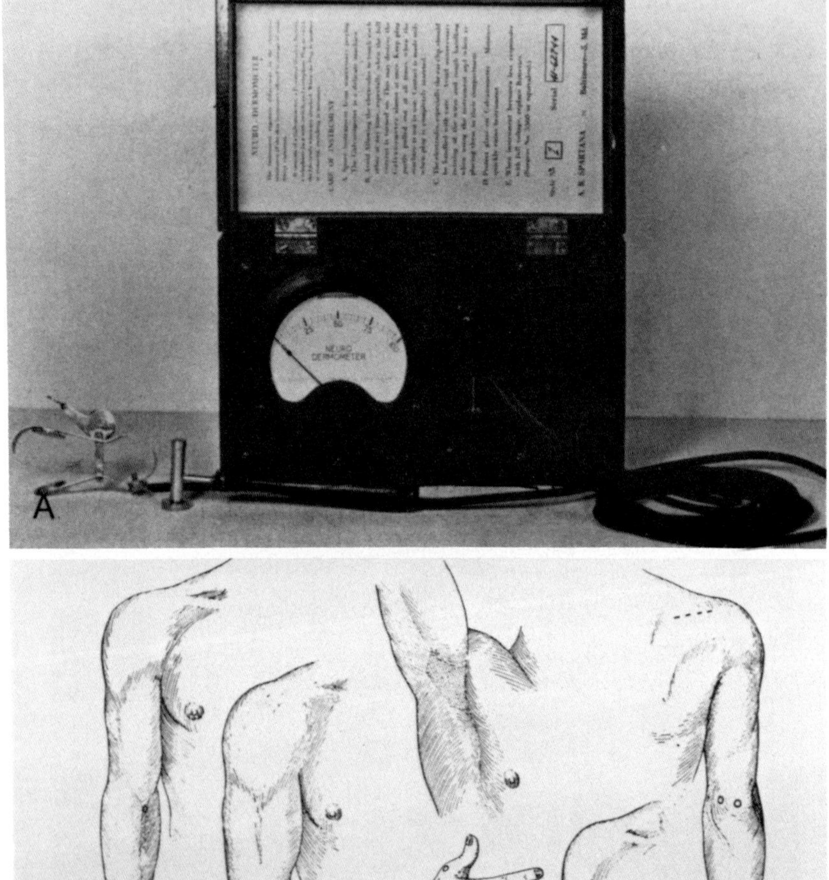

FIG. 19.21. (*A*) Dermometer used to measure sweating, a technique for charting peripheral nerve lesions. (*B*) Denervated areas produced by lesion of ulnar nerve at the elbow. (From C. P. Richter (52). Published with permission.)

Vertigo

There was also a good deal of enthusiasm for unilateral sectioning of the VIIIth cranial nerve for the treatment of vertigo (20) (Fig. 19.31), and many such procedures were done. The result, of course, was deafness on that side. This procedure is rarely, if ever, needed at the present time.

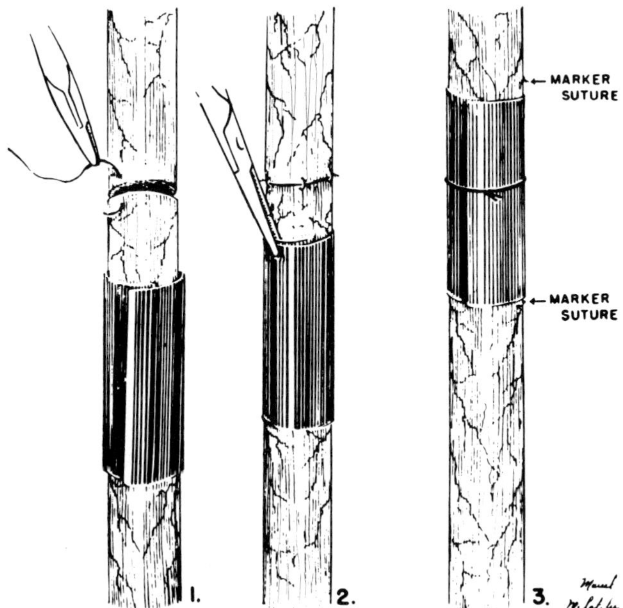

FIG. 19.22. Application of tantalum sleeve to protect area of nerve anastomosis. (From J. C. White and H. Hamlin (69). Published with permission.)

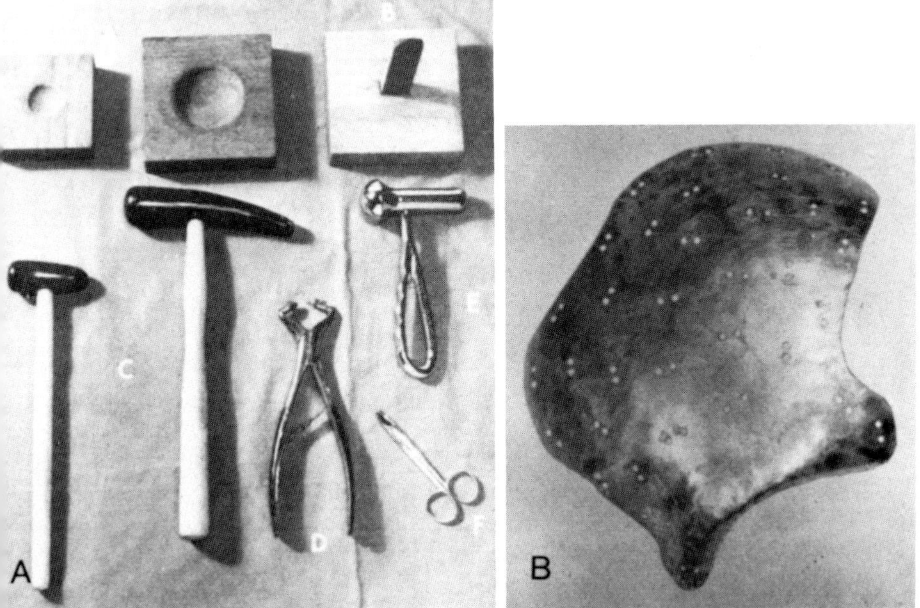

FIG. 19.23. (*A*) Tools for plating a cranial defect with tantalum. (*B*) Tantalum plate ready for attachment to cranium. (From W. Lewin *et al.* (41). Published with permission.)

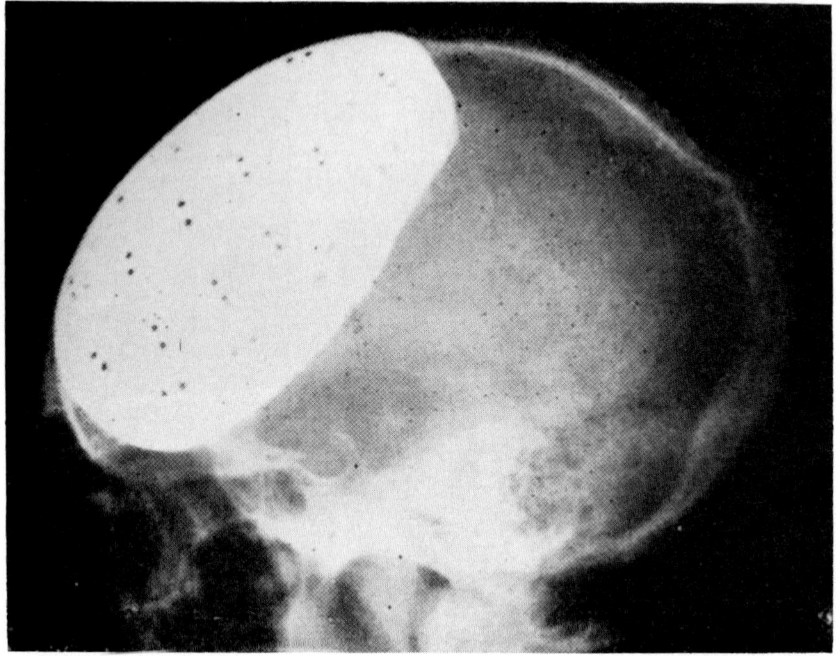

FIG. 19.24. Tantalum plate in place. (From W. Lewin *et al.* (41). Published with permission.)

Hemifacial Spasm

Not so far back, and not so archaic, was the method of partial section (Fig. 19.32) of the facial nerve for hemifacial spasm as described by Scoville (57). That was, in fact, a very effective procedure that produced a discrete lesion, but the facial paralysis almost always recurred. The present methods of posterior fossa exploration are probably much more effective in the long run.

Operating for Exophthalmos

A problem for neurosurgeons was malignant exophthalmos associated with hyperthyroidism (Fig. 19.33). Surgical methods were devised to remove the lateral, superior, and inferior walls of the orbit (14) (Fig. 19.34)—all aimed at relieving the progressive vision-threatening pressure on the eyeball. Ophthalmologists and otolaryngologists as well as neurosurgeons made contributions to the procedures. Surgical treatment for malignant exophthalmos is rare today, since the endocrine/medical care of these patients has become so satisfactory.

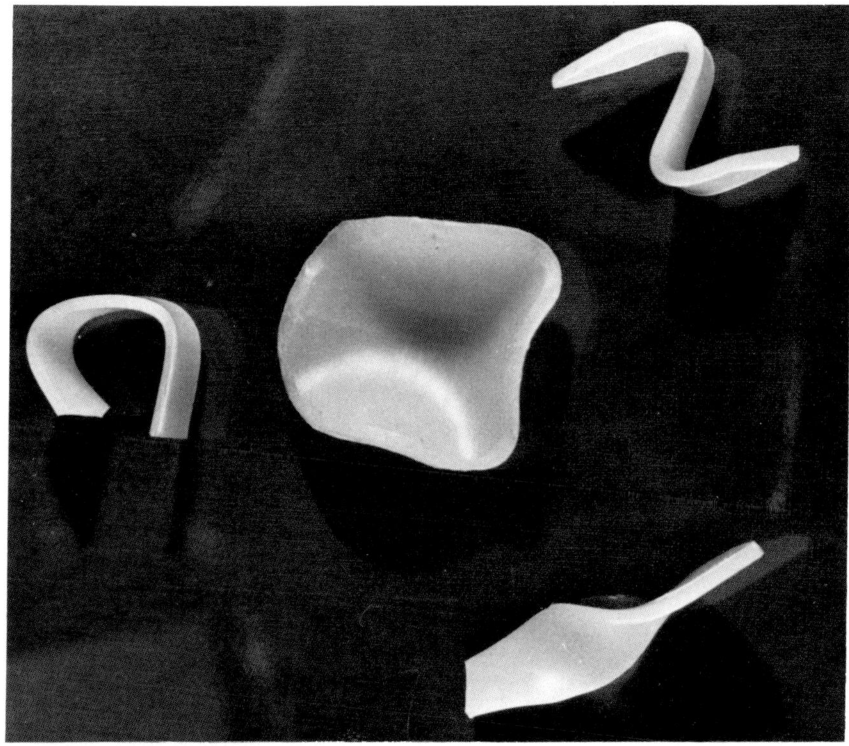

FIG. 19.25. Polyethylene shaped in hot water. (From E. Alexander, Jr. and P. H. Dillard (5). Published with permission.)

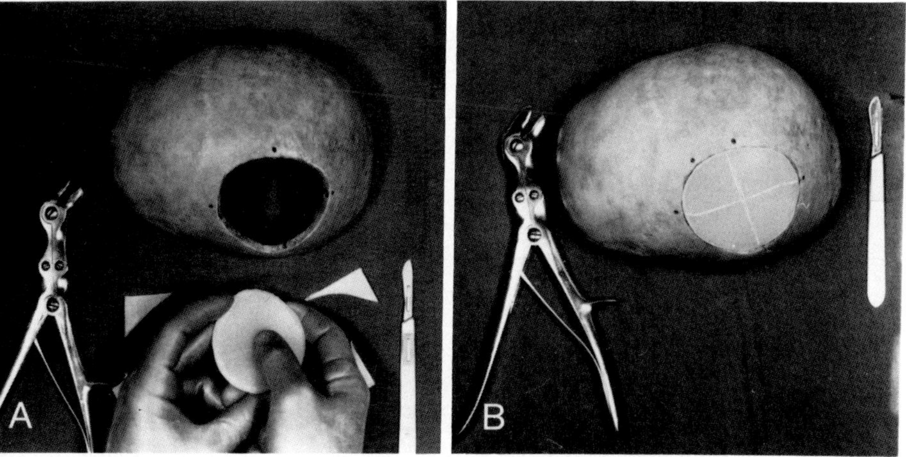

FIG. 19.26. (*A*) Polyethylene plate being fashioned to fit cranial defect. (*B*) Plate in defect. (From E. Alexander, Jr. and P. H. Dillard (5). Published with permission.)

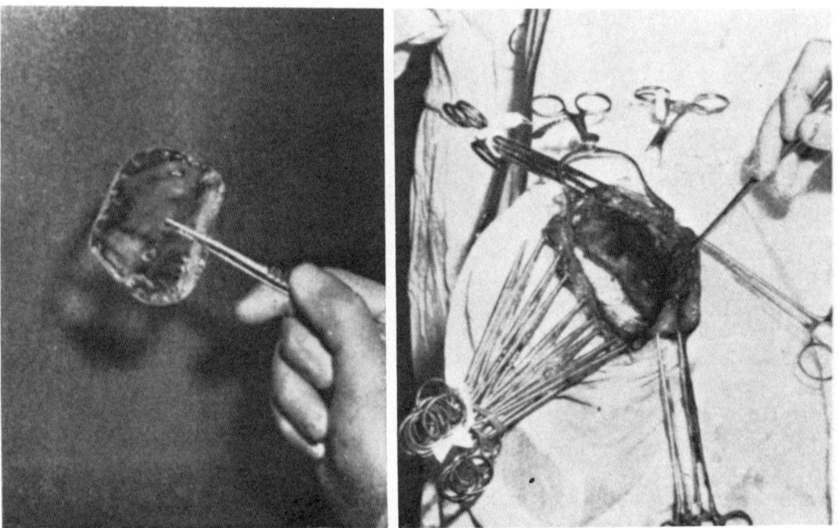

FIG. 19.27. Acrylic plating of cranial defect. (From C. W. Elkins and J. E. Cameron (23). Published with permission.)

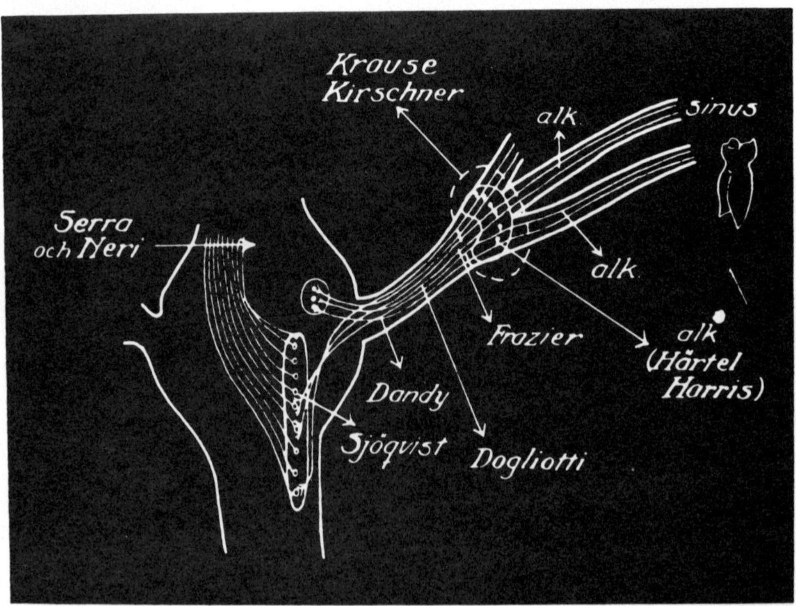

FIG. 19.28. Early surgical treatment of trigeminal neuralgia. (From O. Sjöqvist (59). Published with permission.)

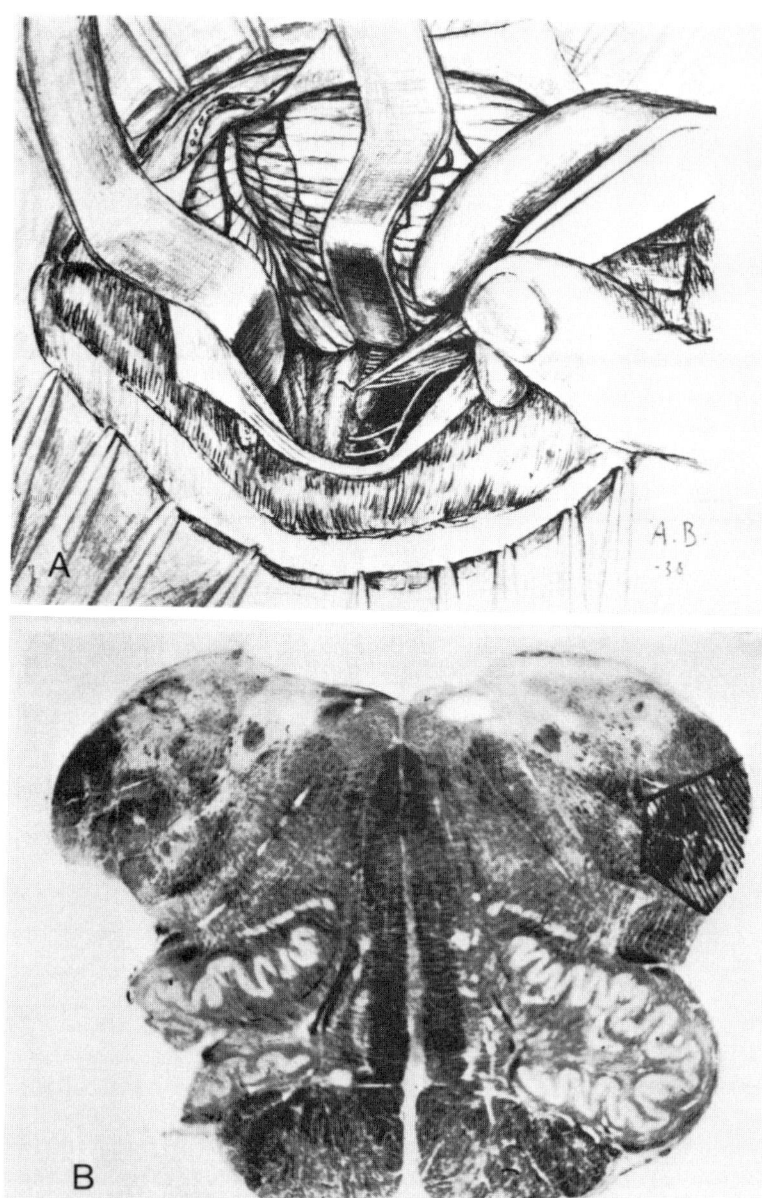

FIG. 19.29. (*A*) Approach for division of spinal trigeminal tract for tic douloureux. (*B*) Postoperative lesion. (From O. Sjöqvist (58). Published with permission.)

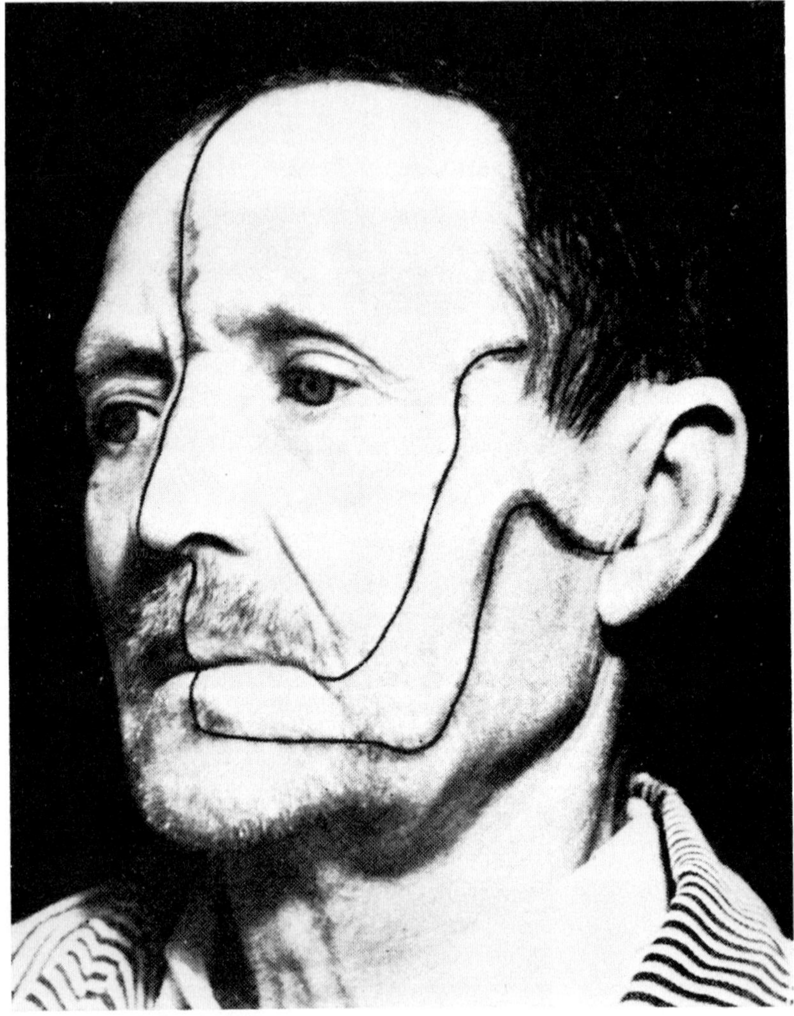

FIG. 19.30. Sensory loss following division of spinal trigeminal tract. (From O. Sjöqvist (58). Published with permission.)

Cervical Spine Traction

The introduction of traction for the handling of cervical spine injuries was primarily by Crutchfield (16), but many others had devised tongs for that purpose. For some patients, mobility seemed advisable. Fig. 19.35 shows one of our patients, an elderly man with a fractured odontoid that was stabilized with 2 sets of Crutchfield tongs and a strong piece of rubber attached to a halo apparatus above his head. A similar procedure was reported by Abbott and Hale in 1953 (1) (Figs. 19.36 and 19.37).

While we are looking at gadgets, I must show you a means we had of treating facial fractures. Our colleagues in otolaryngology were seeking a better way to place traction on the face than immobilizing the patient in bed, so we put together this device using 2 sets of Crutchfield tongs placed in the skull almost at right angles to each other, heavy wires, and plaster (Fig. 19.38). It worked very satisfactorily, and we published our results in *Surgery, Gynecology, and Obstetrics* (6). The device was much cheaper than the more complex devices that have come along since.

Early Approaches to Hemostasis and Dural Substitutes

The early methods of hemostasis and for covering the exposed brain should be exhibited as artifacts. They lead us back to Bailey and his colleagues (7), who used fibrin foam, which was developed from the early fractionation of blood by Cohn. Fibrin foam proved to be an effective hemostatic method used by the neurosurgeons at Harvard, but was replaced by the much more readily manufactured and cheaper Gelfoam of a later period. Fibrin could also be made into a film (Fig. 19.39) to cover the cortex and other exposed areas of the brain; it was absorbable, but it was difficult to suture and it, too, fell into disuse with the development of materials such as homologous frozen dura and silicone grafts.

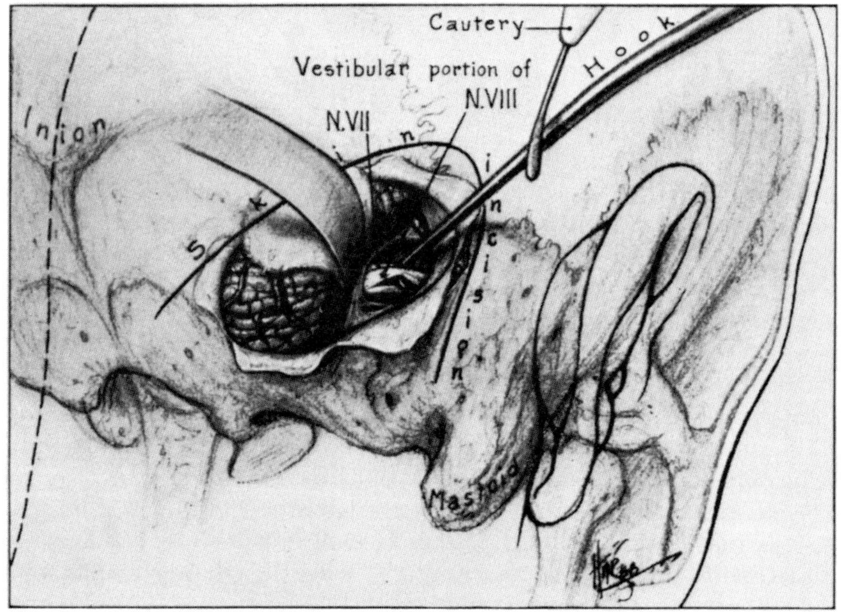

FIG. 19.31. Section of cranial nerve VIII for treatment of vertigo. (From W. Dandy (20). Published with permission.)

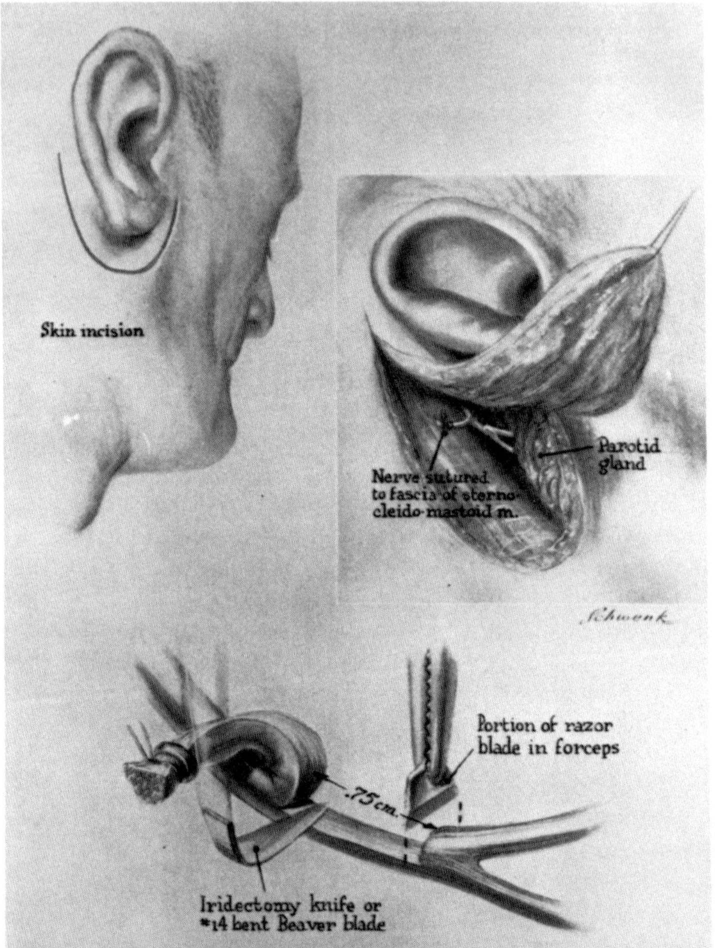

FIG. 19.32. Partial section of cranial nerve VII for hemifacial spasm. (From W. B. Scoville (57). Published with permission.)

Challenging Parkinsonism

In the 1940s, the treatment of that most debilitating of diseases, parkinsonism, was done largely by the neurologists, who had scopolamine, belladonna, trihexyphenidyl, and related drugs at their command.

Some early surgical approaches were attempted, but the most intriguing was that devised by Earl Walker in 1949 (67)—cerebral pedunculotomy (Fig. 19.40). Many surgeons used it, and although the patients were severely paralyzed on the contralateral side for a period of time, it did, in fact, help a number of patients to recover function.

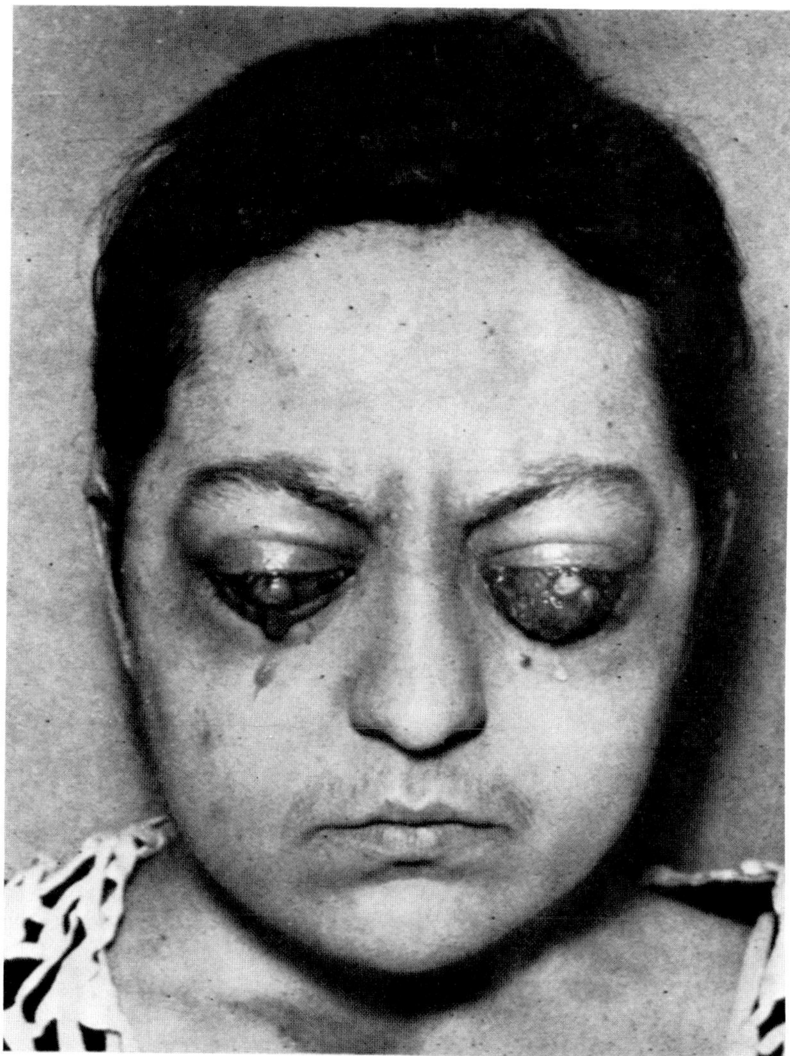

FIG. 19.33. Malignant exophthalmos. (From W. M. Craig and H. W. Dodge, Jr. (14). Published with permission.)

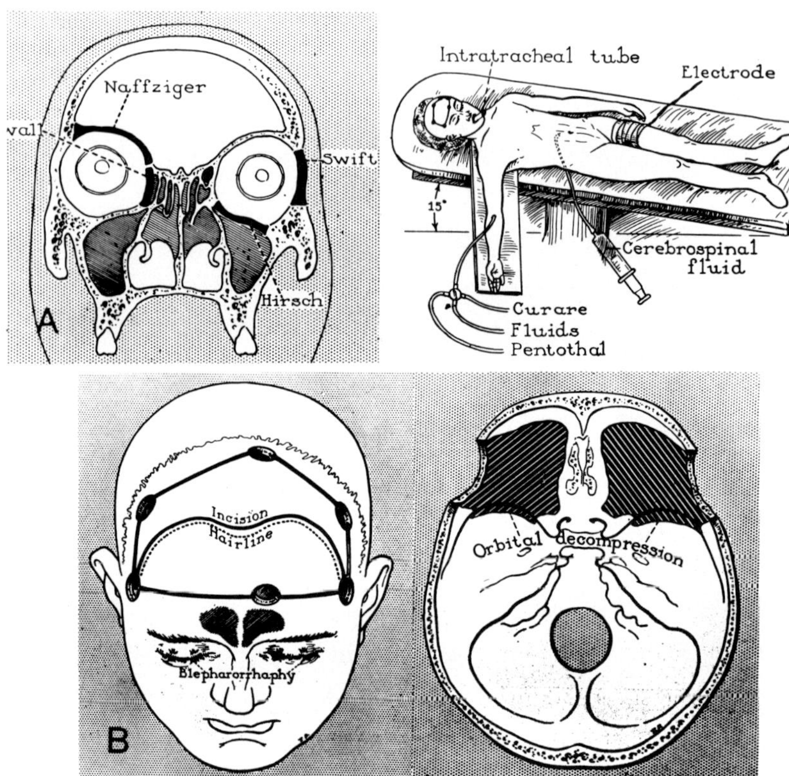

FIG. 19.34. Semidiagrammatic representation of various operative methods for relieving orbital pressure in patients with malignant exophthalmos. (From W. M. Craig and H. W. Dodge, Jr. (14). Published with permission.)

Irving Cooper, attempting to do a cerebral pedunculotomy, found marked arachnoid adhesions around the peduncle and encountered severe bleeding. He controlled the bleeding with a clip, but assumed that he had severely damaged the patient. However, to his gratification, the patient was much improved, and to his credit, Cooper (11) investigated this further and found that he had occluded the anterior choroidal artery. On the basis of vascular studies, he concluded that this vessel primarily supplied the globus pallidus (Fig. 19.41), and it was with that conclusion in mind that he devised the procedure for chemopallidectomy (12, 50) (Fig. 19.42). As time went on, of course, the lesions proved to be more effective if made in the ventrolateral nucleus of the thalamus, and soon, a number of surgeons were making discrete and exact lesions located by stimulation and intraoperative monitoring. The procedure of thalamotomy for parkinsonism was an elegant, effective procedure, and would probably still be widely used if levodopa and similar agents had not been developed. Today, thalamotomy is done at only a few medical centers. It is interesting, however, that some of the patients who had thalamotomies as long ago as 15 years still show marked improvement on the side affected by the operation, and they have never developed dystonia on that side, in contrast to those patients who develop dystonia as a result of large doses of levodopa.

Prefrontal Lobotomy

In the 1940s, psychiatric disease was common—as it is now—but there were no good drugs for the control of patients with psychiatric disorders, and the hospitals were full to overflowing. It was for that reason prefrontal lobotomy was developed. Crawford and Fulton and their coworkers (15) performed ablations of the frontal lobes in two soon-to-be-famous chimpanzees named Becky and Lucy (Fig. 19.43). They had tested these animals preoperatively and then retested them postoperatively and noted any changes in behavior. Fulton presented their findings in Spain, where

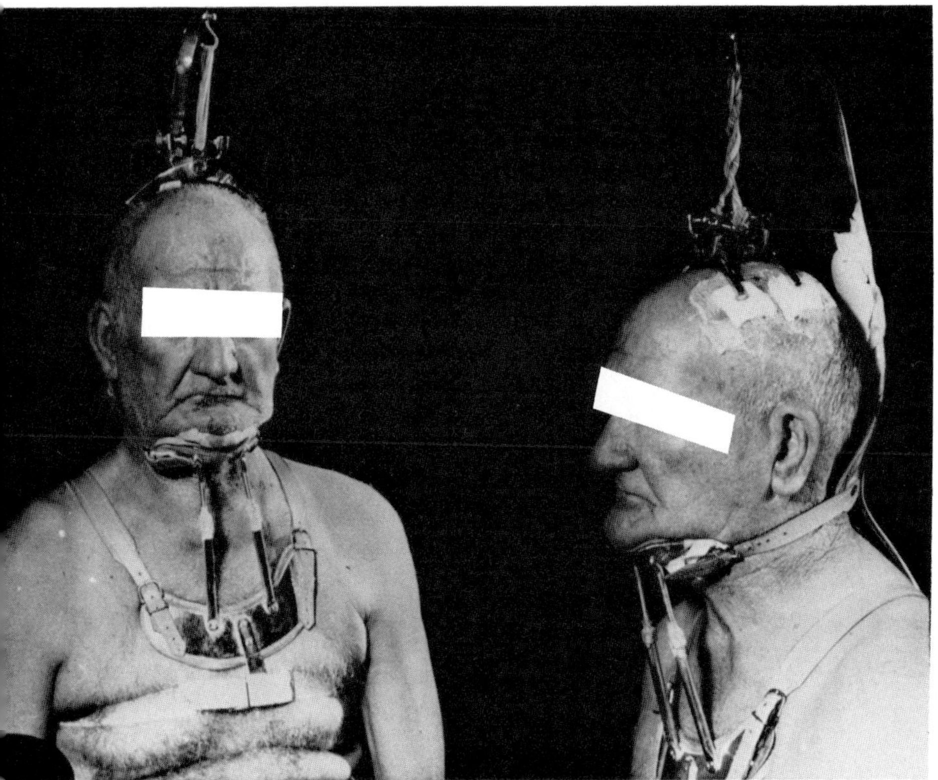

FIG. 19.35. Use of Crutchfield tongs and halo frame for stabilization of odontoid fracture.

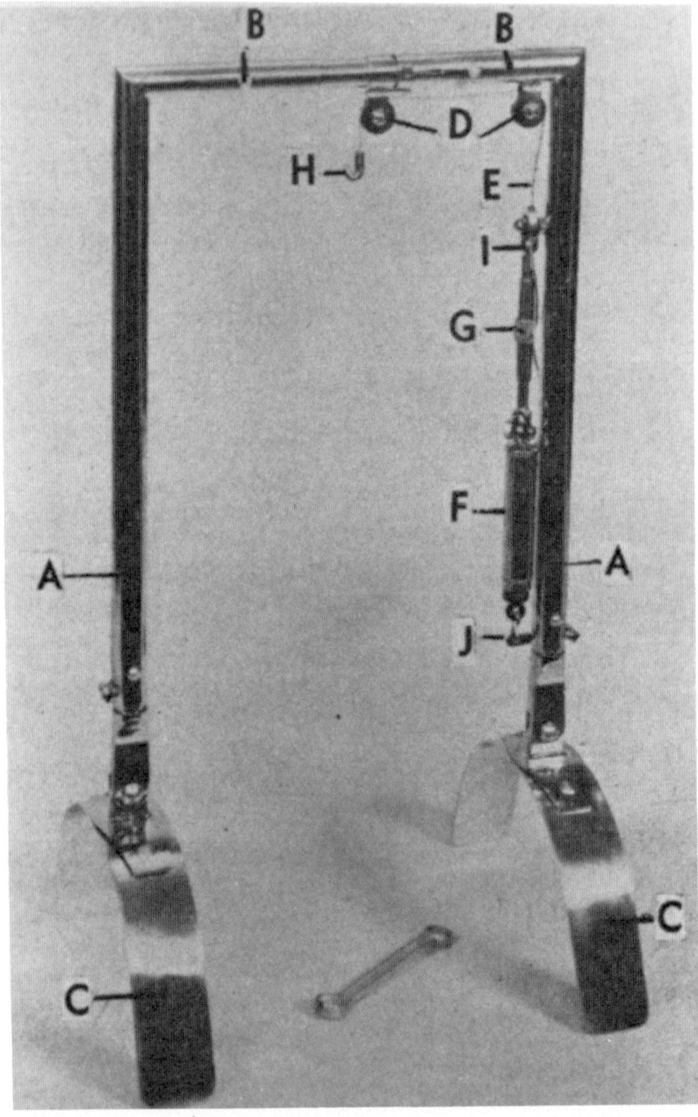

Fig. 19.36. Precursor of halo frame. (From K. H. Abbott and N. Hale (1). Published with permission.)

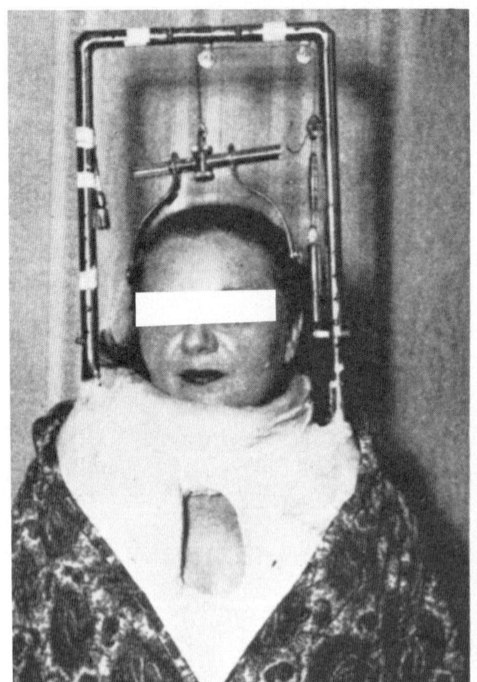
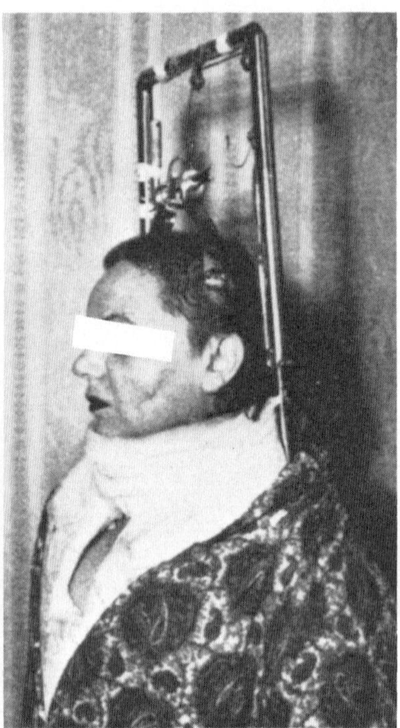

FIG. 19.37. Patient in cervical trapeze for stabilization of dislocation of C4 over C5. (From K. H. Abbott and N. Hale (1). Published with permission.)

he was heard by Moniz (46), who soon was doing prefrontal lobotomies on patients (Fig. 19.44). Ironically, it was Moniz, rather than Fulton and his coworkers, who received the Nobel Prize in 1949 "for his discovery of the therapeutic value of prefrontal leucotomy in certain psychoses" (61).

Soon, prefrontal lobotomies were being done across the world (Fig. 19.45), and they were accepted as providing both psychiatric and economic advantages. In England, for example, papers were published showing the economic benefit of doing prefrontal lobotomies in patients who required much supervision and attention by the staff of the hospital. Postoperatively, such patients were almost invariably improved to the extent that they could move to less "acute" parts of the hospital, with a saving to the state.

The psychiatric benefits of prefrontal lobotomy were marked in many cases, particularly when the more conservative selective lobotomies were done. I would like to quote one of my discussions of prefrontal lobotomy in 1951, "It may be true, as some predict, that this procedure is only a temporary expedient, a valuable and most instructive one in the therapy of mental disorders; and it may be that chemical and hormonal therapy

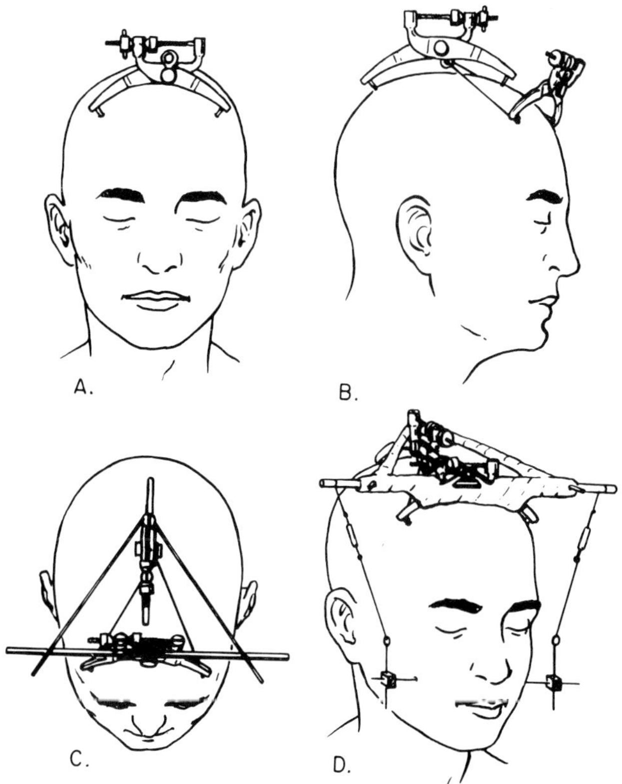

FIG. 19.38. Stabilization of facial fracture with Crutchfield tongs. (From E. Alexander, Jr. *et al.* (6). Published with permission.)

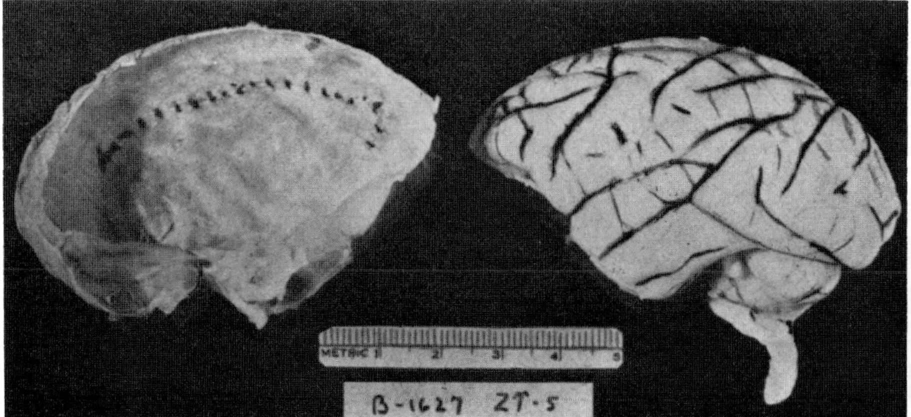

FIG. 19.39. Use of fibrin film to cover cerebral hemispheres in absence of dura. (From O. T. Bailey *et al.* (7). Published with permission.)

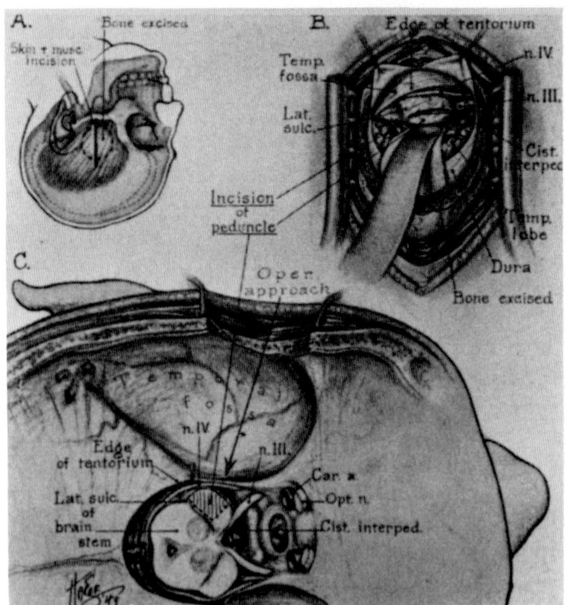

FIG. 19.40. Cerebral pedunculotomy for relief of parkinsonism. (From A. E. Walker (67). Published with permission.)

will, in time, bring far greater improvements, but whatever the future development, prefrontal lobotomy has proved itself useful in certain cases of mental disease, both from the individual patient's point of view, and from the point of view of the broad socio-economic problems found in the state mental hospitals."

The procedure was even done as an outpatient procedure by Fiamberti (25) in 1937 and later by Freeman (28) (Fig. 19.46), who used a transorbital approach—the so-called "ice pick operation."

About the only part of this procedure that has remained viable is bilateral cingulotomy, first described by Eldon Foltz (26) (Fig. 19.47) and still being done by a number of surgeons, including Ballantine *et al.*(8).

Display of Miscellaneous Artifacts

There are a number of interesting developments of past years that we've largely lost sight of, but I simply mention them briefly to call your attention to them.

Love and Erb (42) described "transplantation" of the spinal cord in cases of severe kyphoscoliosis (Fig. 19.48) in the days before the circulation of the spinal cord was clearly understood and before the development of the Harrington rods.

The treatment of closed head injuries has always been difficult, but

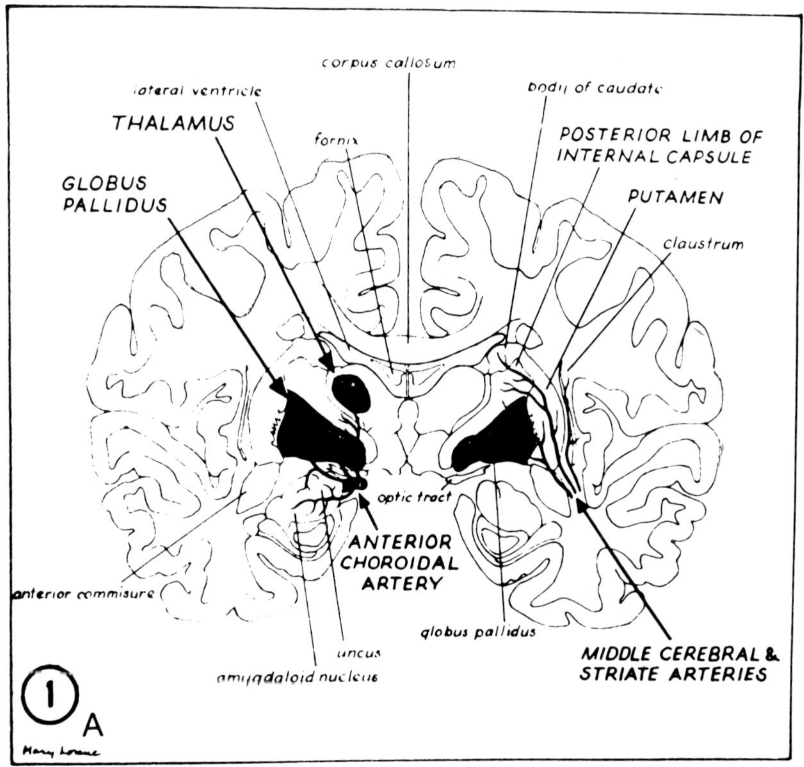

FIG. 19.41. (*A*) Vascularization of globus pallidus. (From I. Cooper and J. B. Gonzalo (12). Published with permission.)

was even more difficult before we had aids such as intracranial pressure monitoring, mannitol, barbiturates, and tilt tables. In 1950, Arthur Ward (68) suggested that huge doses of atropine, 1/10 of a grain, used twice a day, would be of help in counteracting the effects of acetylcholine in the nervous system.

The evolution of the treatment of paraplegia has covered a number of eras, but the days of tidal drainage as devised by Munro (47) (Fig. 19.49) are long remembered by those who were in neurosurgery at that time. Tidal drainage was an ingenious method: it irrigated the bladder automatically and kept it clean, but there was a truism, possibly expressed by Matson, "It takes one resident full-time to keep one Munro tidal drainage apparatus going satisfactorily."

At one time, poliomyelitis was the scourge of the young and of many older persons as well. The iron lung (Fig. 19.50) was the only thing that kept many severely afflicted polio victims alive. The development of polio

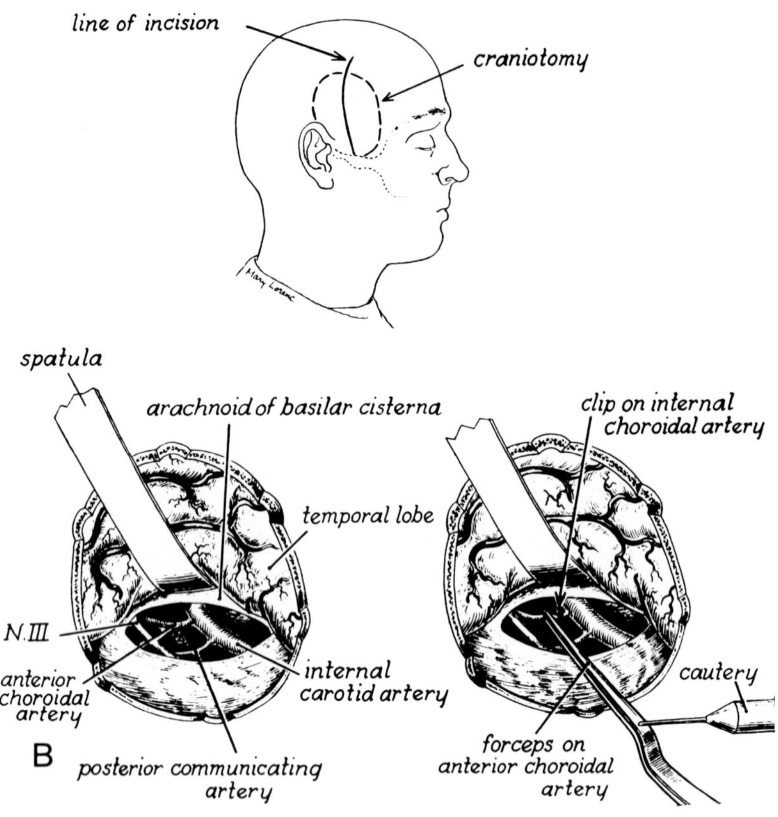

Fig. 19.41(*B*)

vaccines has made the disease one of the forgotten horrors of medicine in the Western world, and for patients with other causes of spinal paralysis, the modern bedside respirators attached to a tube in the patient's trachea are far less cumbersome and allow easier patient care.

The treatment of epilepsy was a long and difficult one, and really there have been no breakthroughs since Penfield and Erickson published their book, *Epilepsy and Cerebral Localization*, in 1941 (51). However, the procedure of hemispherectomy for the patient with unilateral seizures and an atrophic brain on one side was best exemplified by the work of Lyle French *et al.* (29). He and his coworkers performed a number of those procedures (Fig. 19.51), and they were very effective. The experience of many of the rest of us has also been gratifying. With the introduction of a number of anticonvulsants, and with the ability to easily determine levels of anticonvulsant agents in the blood so that there is

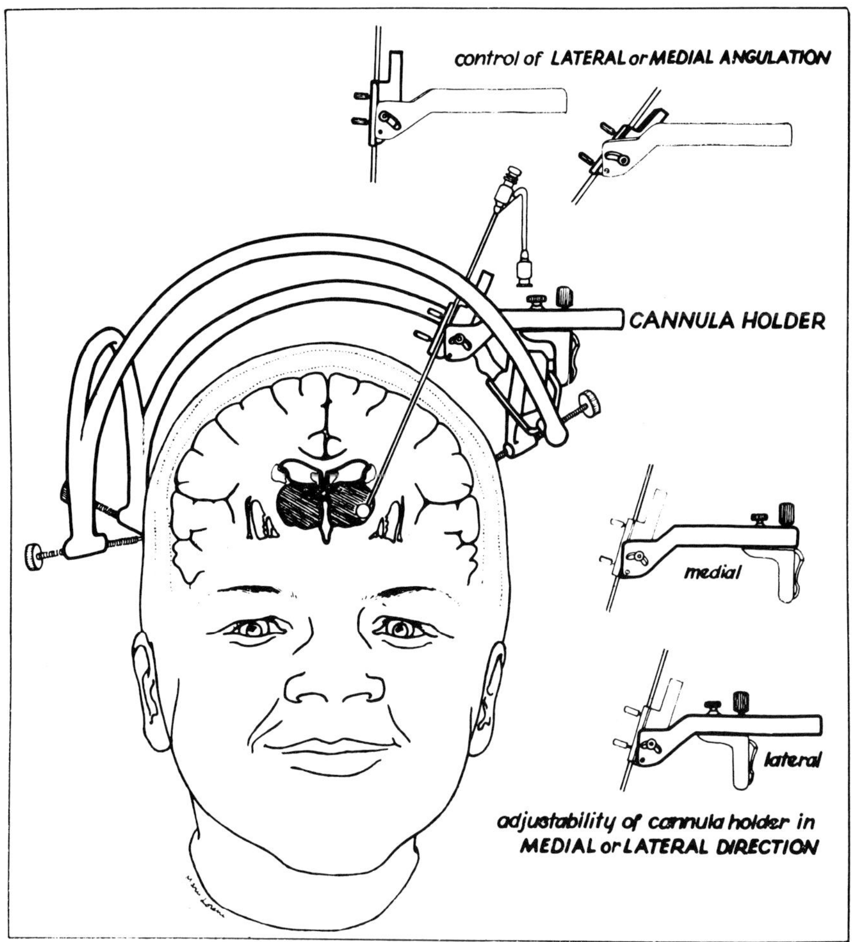

FIG. 19.42. Chemopallidectomy for parkinsonism. (From C. Parera and I. S. Cooper (50). Published with permission.)

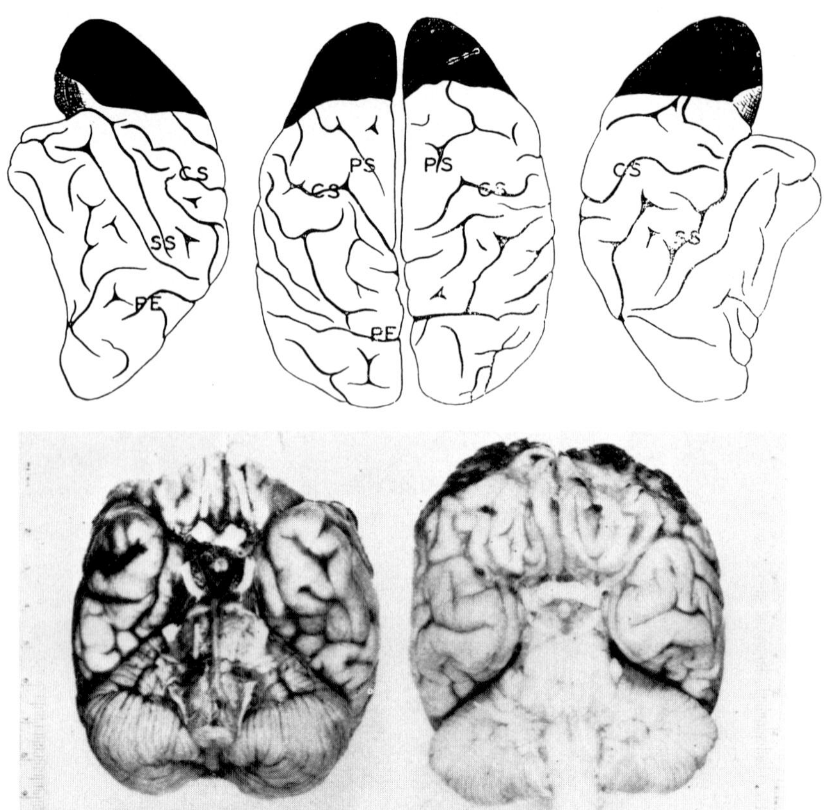

FIG. 19.43. Cortical ablations in chimpanzees Lucy and Becky. (From M. P. Crawford *et al.* (15). Published with permission.)

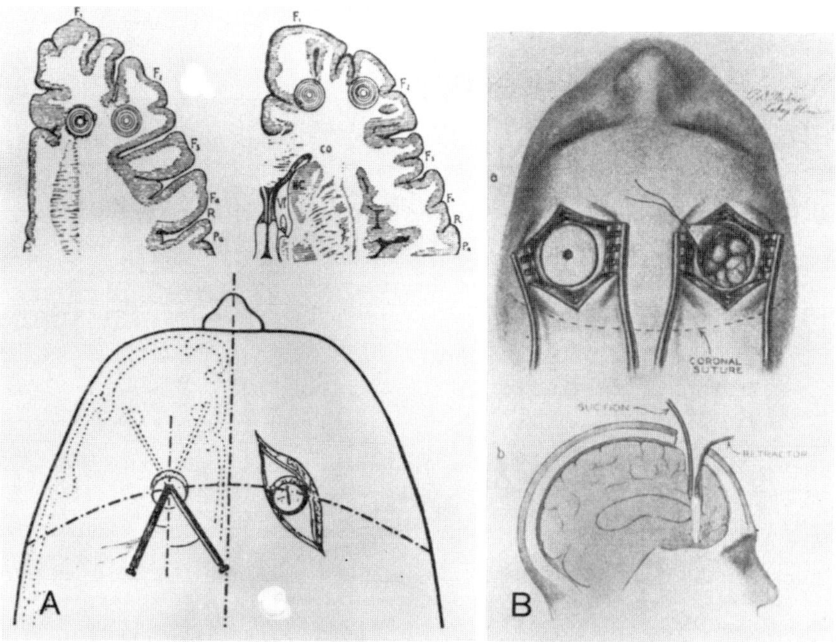

FIG. 19.44. Prefrontal lobotomy. (From J. E. Scarff (55). Published with permission.)

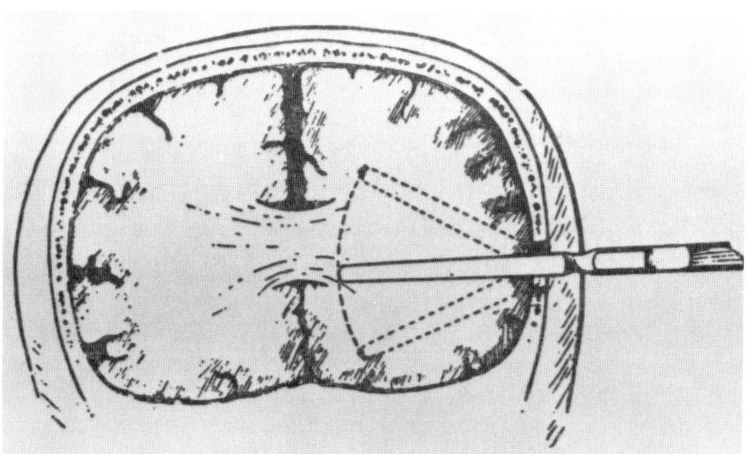

FIG. 19.45. Precursor to standard technique of prefrontal lobotomy. (From J. E. Scarff (55). Published with permission.)

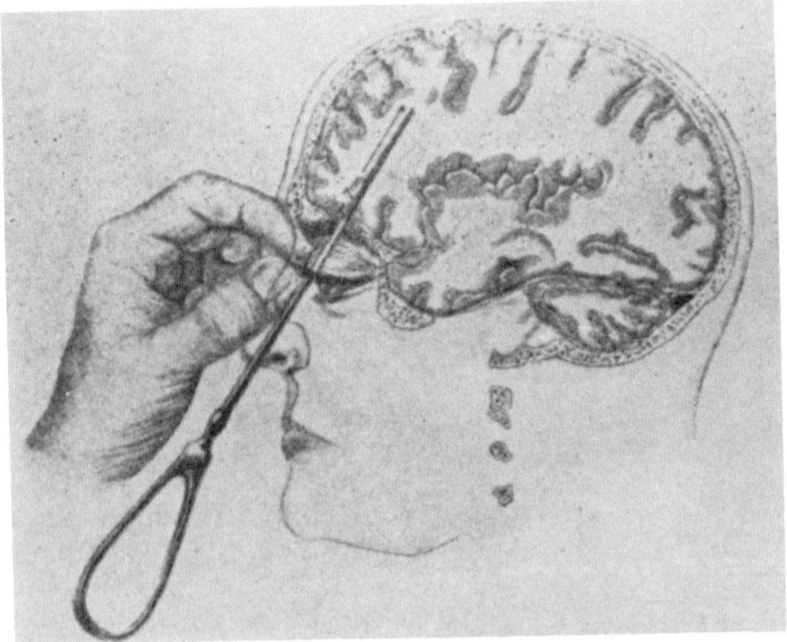

FIG. 19.46. "Ice pick" lobotomy. (From J. E. Scarff (55). Published with permission.)

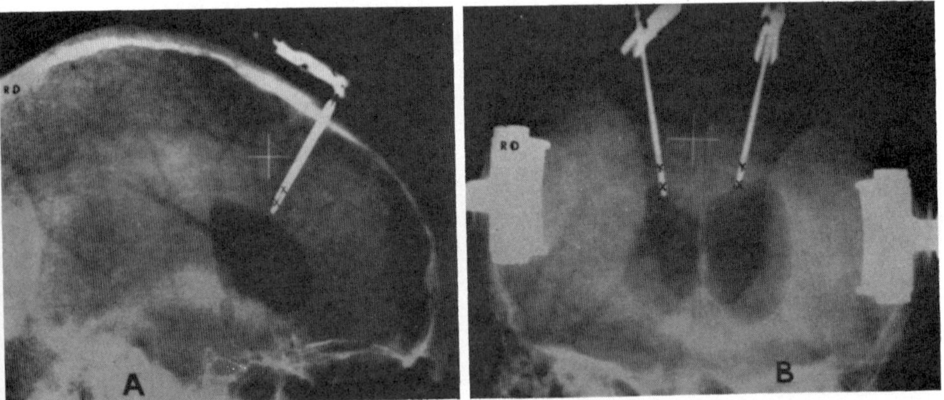

FIG. 19.47. Bilateral cingulotomy. (From E. L. Foltz (26). Published with permission.)

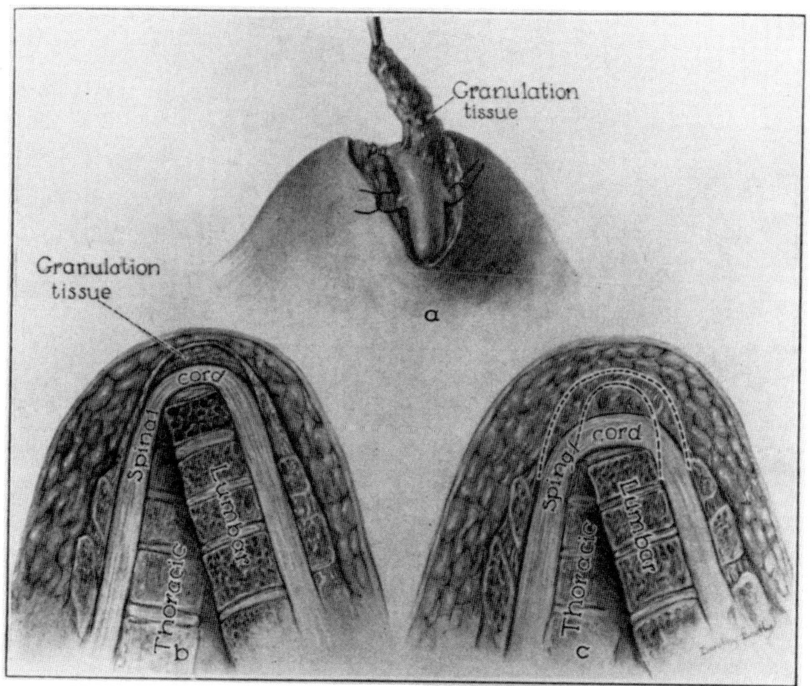

FIG. 19.48. Transplantation of spinal cord to relieve compression caused by severe kyphosis. (From J. G. Love and H. R. Erb (42). Published with permission.)

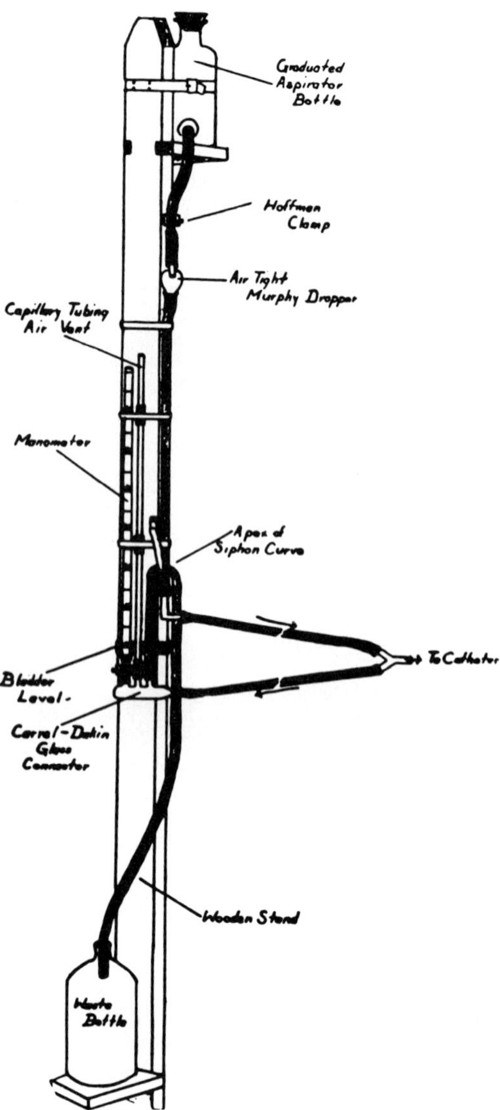

FIG. 19.49. Tidal drainage for management of patients with paraplegia. (From D. Munro (47). Published with permission.)

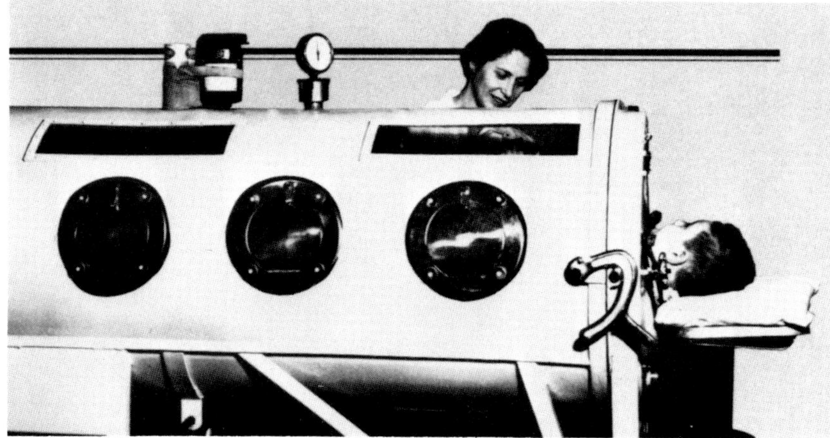

FIG. 19.50. Iron lung.

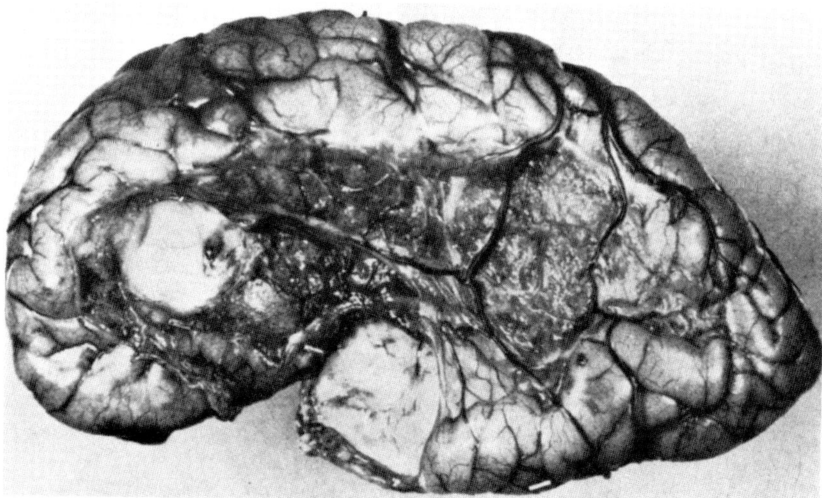

FIG. 19.51. Specimen of brain removed at time of hemispherectomy. (From L. A. French *et al.* (29). Published with permission.)

better control of seizures, hemispherectomy is rarely done now, but it still is a very effective procedure in isolated cases.

Neurosurgeons as well as general surgeons were deeply involved in the 1940s and 1950s in the surgical control of severe hypertension by extensive thoracolumbar sympathectomy (70) (Fig. 19.52). Some of the results of the studies were excellent, but the development of effective drug therapy for hypertension made that operation obsolete.

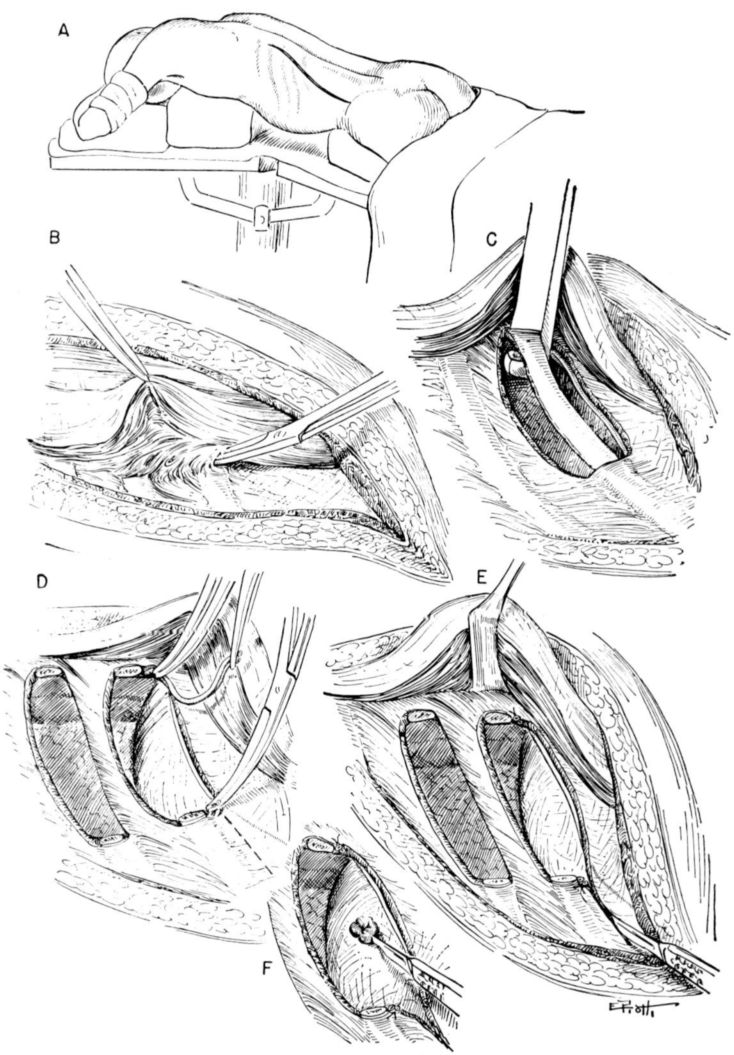

Fig. 19.52. Thoracolumbar sympathectomy for control of essential hypertension. (From J. C. White and H. Hamlin (70). Published with permission.)

Conclusions

This has been a "dig" into old neurosurgery, into an era when most of this audience, if actually on hand, were still in knickers or in bloomers, as the case may be. In recent years, neurosurgery has become so much easier, so much more enjoyable, and of so much more lasting benefit to the patients that one can scarcely help but be enthusiastic about the future. The use of steroids to reduce cerebral edema, the use of antibiotics to control or prevent infection, good anesthesia, selective angiography, embolization of tumors and vascular malformations, balloon techniques for the treatment of aneurysms, and the CT scan—all have come into being as a result of contributions from the basic and medical sciences. These tools all serve to make our efforts easier and to extend our capabilities.

As a matter of fact, as the ordinary types of neurosurgery become easier, new fields of endeavor open, and some of the areas that seem discouraging to us now may yet fall to the advances that are coming our way. By the same token, many of the seemingly ideal procedures that we use today may also succumb to superior procedures and become part of our past. In time, our present procedures may only be important in their ability to move, amuse, and entertain neurosurgeons of the future.

REFERENCES

1. Abbott, K. H., and Hale, N. Cervical trapeze. An apparatus for ambulatory treatment of fractures of the cervical spine. J. Neurosurg., *10:* 436–437, 1953.
2. Alexander, E., Jr., and Davis, C. H., Jr. Recent advances in the treatment of infantile hydrocephalus. N.C. Med. J., *14:* 610–613, 1953.
3. Alexander, E., Jr., and Davis, C. H., Jr. The radiographic demonstration of cysts and abscesses of the brain. Use of micropaque barium in suspension. J. Neurosurg., *21:* 288–291, 1964.
4. Alexander, E., Jr., and Davis, C. H., Jr. Trigeminal neuralgia: conservative management with massive vitamin B_{12} therapy. N.C. Med. J., *14:* 1–4, 1953.
5. Alexander, E., Jr., and Dillard, P. H. The use of pure polyethylene plate for cranioplasty. J. Neurosurg., *7:* 492–498, 1950.
6. Alexander, E., Jr., Harrill, J. A., and Satterwhite, W. M., Jr. Skeletal traction for facial fractures. Surg. Gynecol. Obstet., *119:* 1326–1327, 1964.
7. Bailey, O. T., Ingraham, F. D., Neuhauser, B. D., and Cobb, C. A., Jr. Fibrin film in neurosurgery, further studies. The insertion of fibrin film between the sutured dura and the intact leptomeninges: the effect of roentgen therapy on tissue reactions to fibrin film. J. Neurosurg., *4:* 465–471, 1947.
8. Ballantine, H. T., Jr., Levy, B. S., Dagi, T. F., and Giriunas, I. B. Cingulotomy for psychiatric illness: report of 13 years' experience. *In* Neurosurgical Treatment in Psychiatry, Pain, and Epilepsy, edited by W. H. Sweet, S. Obrador, and J. G. Martin-Rodriguez, pp. 333–353. University Park Press, Baltimore, 1977.
9. Beck, C. S., McKhann, C. F., and Belnap, W. D. Revascularization of the brain through establishment of a cervical arteriovenous fistula. Effects in children with mental retardation and convulsive disorders. J. Pediatr., *35:* 317–329, 1949.

10. Bering, E. A. The use of phenolsulphonphthalein in the clinical evaluation of hydrocephalus. J. Neurosurg., *13:* 587–595, 1956.
11. Cooper, I. Surgical occlusion of the anterior choroidal artery in parkinsonism. Surg. Gynecol. Obstet., *99:* 207–219, 1954.
12. Cooper, I., and Gonzalo, J. B. Implications of a five-year study of 700 basal ganglia operations. Neurology (Minneap.), *8:* 701–707, 1958.
13. Costello, R. T. A new treatment for the "lightning pains" of tabes dorsalis. Urol. Cutan. Rev., *51:* 260–263, 1947.
14. Craig, W. McK., and Dodge, H. W., Jr. Surgical treatment of progressive exophthalmos. Ann. Surg., *136:* 366–374, 1952.
15. Crawford, M. P., Fulton, M. D., Jacobsen, C. F., and Wolfe, J. B. Frontal lobe ablation in chimpanzee: a resume of "Becky" and "Lucy." Pub. Assoc. Res. Nerv. Ment. Dis., *27:* 3–58, 1948.
16. Crutchfield, W. G. Skeletal traction for dislocation of the cervical spine. Report of a case. South. Surg., *2:* 156–159, 1933.
17. Cushing, H. A method of total extirpation of the Gasserian ganglion for trigeminal neuralgia: By a route through the temporal fossa and beneath the middle meningeal artery. J.A.M.A., *34:* 1035–1041, 1900.
18. Dandy, W. E. The diagnosis and treatment of hydrocephalus due to occlusion of the foramina of Magendie and Luschka. Surg. Gynecol. Obstet., *32:* 112–124, 1921.
19. Dandy, W. E. Loose cartilage from intervertebral disk simulating tumor of the spinal cord. Arch. Surg., *19:* 660–672, 1929.
20. Dandy, W. Surgery of the brain. *In* Lewis' Practice of Surgery, Vol. 12, p. 196. W. F. Prior Company, Inc., Hagerstown, Md., 1945.
21. Davidoff, L. M., and Feiring, E. H. Ferrous carbonate in the treatment of tic douloureux. Acta Psychiatr. Neurol., *24:* 403–410, 1949.
22. Davis, C. H., Jr., and Alexander, E., Jr. Intracranial aneurysms: an evaluation of methods of treatment. South. Med. J., *52:* 357–360, 1959.
23. Elkins, C. W., and Cameron, J. E. Cranioplasty with acrylic plates. J. Neurosurg., *3:* 199–205, 1946.
24. Fay, T. Early experiences with local and generalized refrigeration of the human brain. J. Neurosurg., *16:* 239–260, 1959.
25. Fiamberti, A. M. Proposto di una tecnica operatoria modificata e semplificata per gli interventi alla Moniz sui lobi prefrontali in malati di mente. Rass. Studi Psichiat., *26:* 797–805, 1937.
26. Foltz, E. L. Current status and use of rostral cingulumotomy. South. Med. J., *61:* 899–908, 1968.
27. Frazier, C. H. The division of the sensory root of the trigeminus for the relief of tic douloureux; an experimental, pathological and clinical study, with a preliminary report of one surgically successful case. Part II. Phila. Med. J., *8:* 1039–1049, 1901.
28. Freeman, W. Transorbital lobotomy. Preliminary report of ten cases. Med. Ann. Dist. Columbia, *17:* 257–261, 1948.
29. French, L. A., Johnson, D. R., Brown, I. A., and Bergen, F. B. Cerebral hemispherectomy for control of intractable convulsive seizures. J. Neurosurg., *12:* 154–164, 1955.
30. Gillies, J. Anaesthetic factors in the causation and prevention of excessive bleeding during surgical operations. Ann. R. Coll. Surg. Engl., *7:* 204–221, 1950.
31. Griffiths, H. W. C., and Gillies, J. Thoraco-lumbar splanchnicectomy and sympathectomy. Anaesthesia, *3:* 134–146, 1948.
32. Gurdjian, E. S., Webster, J. E., and Martin, F. A. Carotid-internal jugular anastomosis in the rhesus monkey. J. Neurosurg., *7:* 467–472, 1950.
33. Hodder, B. H. Improved lower-limb negative-pressure equipment for the reduction of

cerebral blood pressure in neurosurgery. J. Neurosurg., *14:* 695–699, 1957.
34. Hutchinson, B. Cases of Neuralgia Spasmodica, Commonly Termed Tic Douloureux, Successfully Treated, Ed. 2. Longman, London, 1822.
35. Ingraham, F. D., Alexander, E., Jr., and Matson, D. D. Polyethylene, a new synthetic plastic for use in surgery. Experimental applications in neurosurgery. J.A.M.A., *135:* 82–87, 1947.
36. Jannetta, P. J. Arterial compression of the trigeminal nerve in patients with trigeminal neuralgia. J. Neurosurg., *26:* 159–162, 1967.
37. Jannetta, P. J. Observations on the etiology of trigeminal neuralgia, hemifacial spasm, acoustic nerve dysfunction and glossopharyngeal neuralgia. Definitive microsurgical treatment and results in 117 patients. Neurochirurgia, *20:* 145–154, 1977.
38. Jannetta, P. J. The cause of hemifacial spasm: definitive microsurgical treatment at the brainstem of 31 patients. Otorhinolaryngology, *80:* 319–322, 1975.
39. Krause, F. Entfernung des ganglion gasseri und des central davon gelegenen trigeminusstames. Dtsch. Med. Wochenschr., *19:* 341–344, 1893.
40. Leksell, L. A surgical procedure for atresia of the aqueduct of Sylvius. Acta Psychiatr. Neurol. Scand., *24:* 559–568, 1949.
41. Lewin, W., Graham, M. P., and Northcroft, G. B. Tantalum in the repair of traumatic skull defects. Br. J. Surg., *36:* 26–41, 1948.
42. Love, J. G., and Erb, H. R. Transplantation of the spinal cord for paraplegia secondary to Pott's disease of the spinal column. Arch. Surg., *59:* 409–421, 1949.
43. Matson, D. D. A new operation for the treatment of communicating hydrocephalus: report of a case secondary to generalized meningitis. J. Neurosurg., *6:* 238–247, 1949.
44. Meschan, I. Roentgen signs in clinical practice, Vol. 1. In Basic Principles and Radiology of the Skeletal System, p. 40. W. B. Saunders, Philadelphia, 1969.
45. Mixter, W. J., and Barr, J. S. Rupture of the intervertebral disc with involvement of the spinal canal. N. Engl. J. Med., *211:* 210–214, 1934.
46. Moniz, E. Essai d'un traitement chirurgical des certaines psychoses. Bull. Acad. Med. (Paris), *115:* 385–392, 1936.
47. Munro, D. The Treatment of Injuries to the Nervous System, p. 85. W. B. Saunders, Philadelphia, 1952.
48. Nosik, W. A. Ventriculomastoidostomy. Technique and observations. J. Neurosurg., *7:* 236–239, 1950.
49. Nulsen, F. E., and Becker, D. P. Control of hydrocephalus by valve-regulated shunt. J. Neurosurg., *26:* 362–374, 1967.
50. Parera, C., and Cooper, I. S. A modification of the chemopallidectomy guide. J. Neurosurg., *17:* 547–550, 1960.
51. Penfield, W., and Erickson, T. C. Epilepsy and Cerebral Localization. Charles C Thomas, Springfield, Ill., 1941.
52. Richter, C. P. Instructions for using the cutaneous resistance recorder, or "dermometer" on peripheral nerve injuries, sympathectomies, and paravertebral blocks. J. Neurosurg., *3:* 181–191, 1946.
53. Robertson, J. T., Schick, R. W., Morgan, F., and Matson, D. D. Accurate placement of ventriculo-atrial shunt for hydrocephalus under electrocardiographic control. J. Neurosurg., *18:* 255–257, 1961.
54. Sadov, M. S., Wyant, G. M., Gleave, G., and Bucy, P. C. Controlled hypotension. II. A preliminary report on "Arfonad" (RO 2-2222). J. Neurosurg., *11:* 143–150, 1954.
55. Scarff, J. E. Fifty years of neurosurgery, 1905–1955, reprinted from Surgery, Gynecology, and Obstetrics. *In* Fifty Years of Surgical Progress, edited by L. Davis, pp. 303–399. Franklin H. Martin Memorial Foundation, Chicago, 1955.
56. Scarff, J. E. Treatment of hydrocephalus: an historical and critical review of methods and results. J. Neurol. Neurosurg. Psychiatry, *26:* 1–26, 1963.

57. Scoville, W. B. Partial section of proximal seventh nerve trunk for facial spasm. Surg. Gynecol. Obstet., *101:* 494–497, 1955.
58. Sjöqvist, O. Studies on pain conduction in the trigeminal nerve. A contribution to the surgical treatment of facial pain. Acta Psychiatr. Neurol. (Suppl.), *17:* 1–139, 1938.
59. Sjöqvist, O. Trigeminal neuralgia. A review of its surgical treatment and some aspects of its etiology. Acta Chir. Scand., *82:* 201–217, 1939.
60. Spurling, R. G., Lyons, W. R., Whitcomb, B. B., and Woodhall, B. The failure of whole fresh homogenous nerve grafts in man. J. Neurosurg., *2:* 79–101, 1945.
61. Stevenson, L. G. Nobel Prize Winners in Medicine and Physiology, 1901–1940, pp. 264–271. H. Schuman, New York, 1953.
62. Stookey, B. Compression of the spinal cord due to ventral extradural cervical chondromas. Arch. Neurol. Psychiatry, *20:* 275–290, 1928.
63. Svien, H. J., Dodge, H. W., Jr., and Lake, C. F. Ventriculomastoid shunt in the management of obstruction to the aqueduct of Sylvius in the adult: report of case. Staff Meetings Mayo Clin., *17:* 215–218, 1952.
64. Sweet, W. H., and Wepsic, J. G. Controlled thermocoagulation of trigeminal ganglion and rootlets for differential destruction of pain fibers. Part 1. Trigeminal neuralgia. J. Neurosurg., *39:* 143–156, 1974.
65. Tew, J. M. Radionics Procedure Technique Series. Radionics, Inc., Burlington, Mass., 1974.
66. Torkildsen, A. A new palliative operation in cases of inoperable occlusion of the Sylvian aqueduct. Acta Chir. Scand., *82:* 117–124, 1939.
67. Walker, A. E. Cerebral pedunculotomy for the relief of involuntary movements. I. Hemiballismus. Acta. Psychiatr. Neurol., *24:* 723–729, 1949.
68. Ward, A., Jr. Atropine in the treatment of closed head injury. J. Neurosurg., *7:* 398–402, 1950.
69. White, J. C., and Hamlin, H. New uses of tantalum in nerve suture, control of neuroma formation, and prevention of regeneration after thoracic sympathectomy. Illustration of technical procedures. J. Neurosurg., *2:* 402–413, 1945.
70. White, J. C., Smithwick, R. H., and Simeone, F. A. The Autonomic Nervous System. Anatomy, Physiology, and Surgical Application, Ed. 3, p. 424. Macmillan, New York, 1952.
71. Woodhall, B., and Odom, G. L. Stilbamidine isethionate therapy of tic douloureux. J. Neurosurg., *12:* 495–500, 1955.

CHAPTER

20

Medical and Surgical Management of Functional Pituitary Tumors

MARTIN H. WEISS, M.D.

The remarkable progress of the past decade in the surgical treatment of both intra- and suprasellar functional pituitary tumors has been paralleled if not stimulated by the evolution of a neuropharmacologic armamentarium which presently provides effective replacement therapy for many neuroendocrine deficiencies. Parallel advances in neurochemistry have begun to provide us with agents whose actions are directed at the therapy of functional pituitary tumors and therein complement our surgical capacity to eradicate these lesions.

Pituitary tumors occur with significant frequency; recent studies report an incidence of pituitary adenomas of 13 to 16% in the general population (10). Clearly, such lesions most commonly constitute incidental findings which have little or no impact upon a patient's well-being. The majority of *symptomatic* pituitary tumors secrete excess amounts of adenohypophyseal hormones resulting in varied functional disorders. Our interest, as neurosurgeons, focuses upon two aspects of pituitary tumors; first, the decompression of parasellar structures rendered compromised by extrasellar extension of such lesions, and secondly, the eradication of excess adenohypophyseal hormonal secretion in order to alter the systemic consequences of such aberrant endocrine function. Several drugs have recently become available which appear effective in reducing hormone secretion in tumors producing prolactin, growth hormone, or ACTH. This neuropharmacological addition to our therapeutic armamentarium is beginning to play a significant role in the treatment of patients with functional pituitary tumors.

Application of these therapeutic medical modalities, however, appears to be limited at the present time. Experience to date seems to indicate that the available agents do not consistently reduce tumor size and that the effects of these agents on hormone secretion disappear upon withdrawal of the drug. In this review, we will discuss the mechanism of action, clinical application, and therapeutic results of the varied modalities, pharmacological and surgical, available for treatment respectively of prolactin, growth hormone, and ACTH secreting pituitary tumors.

PROLACTIN-SECRETING TUMORS

Prolactin is the only pituitary hormone whose secretion is predominantly under tonic inhibition by the hypothalamus mediated by an as yet undefined transmitter termed "prolactin-inhibiting factor" (PIF) (Fig. 20.1). The neurotransmitter dopamine is believed to regulate PIF secretion in the hypothalamus and dopamine receptors have been detected on prolactin-secreting cells within the pituitary. Administration of dopamine or dopamine agonists will block prolactin release by an apparent direct action on pituitary lactotrophs. Although dopamine is thus well established as a physiologic inhibitor of prolactin release, numerous studies suggest the presence of additional hypothalamic factors that also inhibit prolactin secretion. On the other hand, evidence indicates that serotonin and serotonin-like agents may have a stimulatory effect on prolactin secretion; thyrotropin releasing hormone (TRH), the natural stimulator of TSH release, also stimulates the secretion of prolactin from pituitary lactotrophs both *in vitro* and *in vivo*. Serotonin antagonists are capable of blocking the stimulation of prolactin release induced by suckling, TRH, and sleep. The inhibition of prolactin release by dopaminergic agents, however, constitutes the present basis for the pharmacological treatment of prolactin-secreting pituitary tumors.

Two groups of drugs have been used: dopamine precursors and ergotamine derivatives. *l*-Dopa, a precursor of dopamine that crosses the blood-brain barrier, effectively lower serum prolactin levels and restores menses in patients harboring prolactinomas. The relatively short half-life and undesirable side effects of L-dopa, however, have mitigated against wide clinical application of this drug in this setting. Ergot derivatives have also proved effective in suppressing prolactin release in patients with prolactin-secreting pituitary tumors. In particular, the compound 2 bromo-α-ergocryptine (bromocryptine) demonstrates marked potency in inhibiting prolactin secretion with relative absence of major side effects. This drug is a long-lasting dopamine agonist and, like dopamine, has both

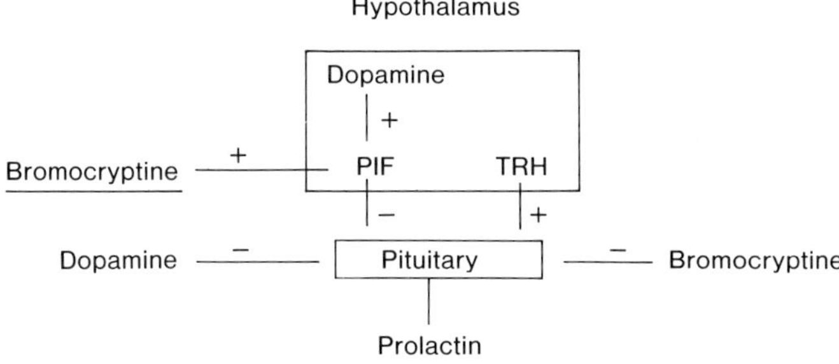

FIG. 20.1. Prolactin's secretion is under tonic inhibition by the hypothalamus mediated by PIF.

hypothalamic and pituitary sites of action. Evidence from our laboratories and others indicates that bromocryptine will inhibit prolactin secretion from lactotrophs grown in tissue culture (10). The inhibitory effects of bromocryptine, therefore, do not require the presence of an intact hypothalamic pituitary axis.

Primary bromocryptine treatment of patients harboring prolactin-secreting tumors is presently controversial (8). Utilization of this agent in the presence of a known pituitary tumor has not been approved by the FDA. However, a number of clinics in the United States and throughout the world have accumulated a sizeable experience with the utilization of bromocryptine in the presence of prolactin-secreting tumors (3, 5, 7, 9, 10, 15).

A common circumstance in which such treatment is proposed arises in the management of a female patient harboring an intrasellar prolactin-secreting tumor who desires restoration of fertility in the hope of becoming pregnant. Our experience has shown that 90% of patients treated with bromocryptine, 5 to 10 mg/day, will undergo resolution of hyperprolactinemia and restoration of menses (7). By comparison our surgical experience with over 150 patients harboring prolactin-secreting pituitary tumors reveals a restoration of normal prolactin levels postoperatively in approximately 70% of cases, a *chemical* cure rate approximating virtually every major clinical series of prolactinomas reported to date (13). It is apparent, therefore, that the medication is at least equally effective to surgical efforts at restoring normal levels of serum prolactin. Bromocryptine appears to be well tolerated when properly prescribed. A starting dose of 1.25 or 2.5 mg orally once daily is followed by progressive increases to 5 to 10 mg daily in divided doses; this increase in dosage is usually carried out over a period of 2 to 3 weeks; as yet, no serious contraindications to prolonged administration of this drug have been reported.

The side effects of bromocryptine are the consequences of its dopaminergic activity. Postural hypotension will be the most frequent side effect reported acutely; if the drug is given in small amounts initially and slowly increased thereafter, hypotension is usually not a chronic problem. Nausea, vomiting, and intestinal discomfort are also frequent complaints; but, if the drug is taken with meals, these symptoms are generally reduced if not totally eliminated. At high dosages, cold-induced digital spasms (Raynaud's syndrome) and cardiac irregularities with frequent extrasystoles have been reported. As such, any evidence of severe cardiovascular or vascular disease are a relative contraindication to the administration of any ergot alkaloid, including bromocryptine.

Should a woman with a prolactin-secreting tumor become pregnant subsequent to taking bromocryptine, one must be concerned about three potential risks as a consequence of this sequence. First, such tumors may undergo rapid enlargement during pregnancy. Reports of such occurrences indicate that between 3 and 15% of such patients will undergo symptomatic enlargement of their tumors (3, 5, 9, 15); the risk of such an event appears to be in direct proportion to the size of the tumor at the time of conception (10). A number of studies have reported that the signs and symptoms of tumor enlargement occurring during pregnancy have regressed following successful delivery of the child (3, 8). Because of this risk, however, our policy has been to recommend surgery for any patient harboring a tumor of dimensions 1 cm or greater as defined by high resolution computerized tomography prior to any attempt at induction of fertility. If postoperative prolactin values are reduced to normal and fertility ensues, no further pharmacologic therapy need be utilized. However, if hyperprolactinemia should persist postoperatively, one may then utilize bromocryptine to induce fertility while obviating concern about excessive tumor growth during pregnancy. In the event that inordinate tumor growth should occur in the absence of previous surgical therapy, one may elect to proceed with surgical intervention during the pregnancy; we have found, on the other hand, satisfactory results with reinstitution of bromocryptine which has reversed the symptoms sufficiently to allow completion of pregnancy and postpartum resection of tumor.

A second potential risk is the possible teratogenic effect of bromocryptine on the fetus. The incidence of congenital defects recorded in clinics throughout the world who have used bromocryptine induction of pregnancy, ranges between .05% and 1% of live births (10). This low incidence of birth defects falls within the range seen in the normal population. It appears, therefore, that there is no existing evidence to indicate any increased risk of teratogenic effect from the use of bromocryptine.

There is a significantly higher incidence of spontaneous abortion in patients who become pregnant subsequent to bromocryptine therapy; approximately 30% of these patients will undergo spontaneous abortion (10). However, this is not higher than the generally known increased frequency of spontaneous abortion in patients who have had difficulty conceiving and who require some form of neuropharmacologic manipulation to induce fertility.

Surgery of prolactin-secreting tumors showing no evidence of major extrasellar extension is directed at removing all grossly visible tumor while retaining normal functional adenohypophysis so as to avoid postoperative hypopituitarism. The availability of adjuvant neuropharmacological aids to ensure postoperative restoration of normal prolactin levels where necessary emphasizes the need for preservation of adenohypophyseal function. The existence of high resolution computed tomography should virtually eliminate negative explorations for such lesions; preservation or improvement of adenohypophyseal function postoperatively must be a major objective of any surgical venture.

Treatment of prolactin-secreting tumors with significant extrasellar extension poses a somewhat different problem. Surgery appears to be the most favorable primary mode of therapy for such lesions. Once again, preservation of adenohypophyseal function, where present preoperatively, is to be sought. There are scattered reports of decreasing size of prolactin-secreting tumors treated with significant amounts of bromocryptine (up to 20 mg/day) (8, 12), but our experience with this as a primary form of therapy has been totally inconsistent. There is evidence that bromocryptine may prove synergistic to postoperative radiotherapy utilized after resection of large prolactin-secreting pituitary tumors, a claim which will require careful scrutiny and confirmation as provided in a controlled clinical trial (12).

At the present time, it appears that bromocryptine is an excellent agent that may be utilized with a high degree of success to induce fertility in the presence of small prolactin-secreting tumors. Such patients who become pregnant require careful follow-up during the course of pregnancy with respect to clinical evaluation along with repeated visual field and visual evoked response assessments. Evidence proporting a cytotoxic effect of the agent and/or prolonged effectiveness following withdrawal of bromocryptine is as yet forthcoming.

TUMORS SECRETING GROWTH HORMONE

Regulation of growth hormone secretion by somatotrophs in the adenohypophysis appears to be under a balanced influence of growth hormone-releasing factor (GRF) as well as growth hormone-inhibiting hormone (somatostatin) synthesized and/or released by hypothalamic neurons (Fig. 20.2). Hypothalamic release of GRF appears to be regulated by three neural centers; the ventromedial and arcuate nuclei of the hypothalamus and the limbic system. Specific neurotransmitters appear to stimulate GRF release from specific areas; α-adrenergic catecholamines induce release by the ventromedial nucleus of the hypothalamus, dopamine induces release from the arcuate nucleus of the hypothalamus, and serotonin mediates release of GRF from the limbic system. Interestingly enough, in a high percentage of growth hormone-secreting tumors, an aberrant response to neurotransmitters is observed in that TRH will paradoxically stimulate the release of growth hormone and dopamine will suppress release of growth hormone, whereas it normally stimulates its release (14) (Fig. 20.3).

Primary therapy of growth hormone-secreting tumors in the vast majority of cases at the present time calls for surgical enucleation of the

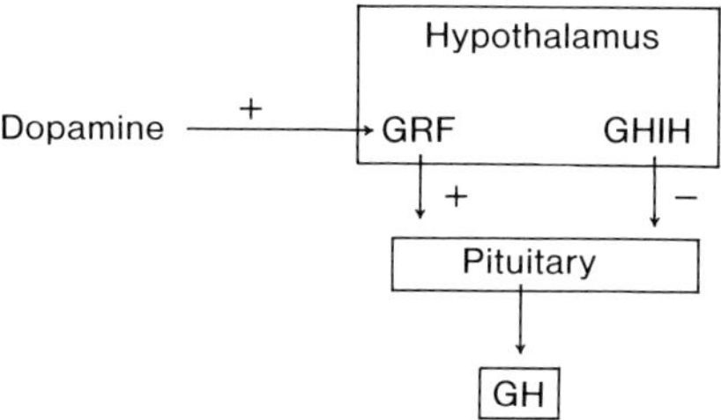

FIG. 20.2. Regulation of GH secretion is under a balanced influence of GRF as well as GHIH.

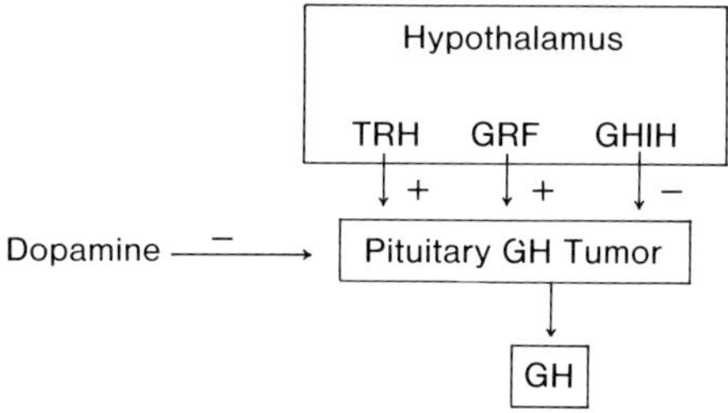

FIG. 20.3. TRH stimulates the release of GH and dopamine suppresses release of GH, whereas it normally stimulates its release.

tumor. Surgery affords the opportunity for selective removal of the tumor while preserving normal adenohypophyseal function; no pharmacological therapy available to date offers this desirable potential outcome. Even the use of high energy particle radiation results in a significant incidence of posttherapy hypopituitarism which increases in incidence over time due to the ongoing effects of such therapy.

The pharmacological attempt at management of growth hormone-secreting tumors focuses upon two disimilar groups of agents; the chemically synthesized inhibitory hormone somatostatin and a variety of dopaminergic drugs. Somatostatin, a polypeptide synthesized in the hypothalamus along with other endocrine sites markedly inhibits the release of growth hormone. This agent acts directly upon the pituitary, and administration of somatostatin to acromegalic patients leads to a profound fall in growth hormone levels. However, the agent must be administered parenterally, has an extremely short half-life, diminishes the secretion of other essential hormones, such as glucagon and insulin, and may be inherently toxic. As such, it is unacceptable for clinical use. Analogues of somatostatin which are relatively specific for growth hormone-secreting cells are being developed; such agents hold promise for future clinical therapy.

It was previously noted that the administration of L-dopa paradoxically suppresses growth hormone levels in acromegalic patients; this action is presumably at the level of the pituitary. It is now known that a number of dopaminergic drugs will also acutely lower growth hormone levels. Due to its long-acting dopaminergic activity, bromocryptine has been found to effect a sustained reduction of growth hormone levels in acromegalic patients. Studies to date indicate that this drug will generate a fall of approximately 50% in growth hormone secretion in a high percentage of patients (10, 14). Achievement of this effect has generally required utilization of significantly higher doses of bromocryptine than required for the treatment of hyperprolactinemia (20 to 60 mg/day), resulting in a significantly higher percentage of patients who experience untoward side effects from the medication (10). In addition, although physical features of acromegaly may be significantly improved with a 50% fall in growth hormone levels, this reduction in hypersomatotropinemia may be insufficient to reverse the malignant systemic endocrine consequences of prolonged elevation of serum growth hormone. At our institution, we have formulated a protocol to treat patients who have mild acromegaly (growth hormone levels generally less than 20 mg/ml), are over age 55, and who are without clinical signs of malignant endocrinopathy (clinical diabetes and/or significant hypertension) with a trial of bromocryptine therapy. This group does not appear to be at major risk from the mildly elevated serum growth hormone and may be satisfactorily maintained on a medical regimen without need for additional therapy. It must be recognized that such therapy is costly since this expensive medication must be taken for a prolonged period, and patients complain of chronic GI distress. In addition, this represents a small fraction of patients who present with acromegaly. For the vast majority of patients, surgery offers the best opportunity to eradicate the disease, preserving existing adenohypophyseal function with minimal side effects.

The objective of surgical therapy in acromegaly (14) calls for eradication of abnormal growth hormone dynamics with preservation of adenohypophyseal function where that is possible. The malignant nature of the systemic complications of untreated acromegaly call for radical exenteration of the sella turcica if such is necessary to assure resolution of the hypersomatotropinemia.

ACTH-SECRETING PITUITARY TUMORS

Recent evidence indicates that at least 80% of cases of Cushing's disease are caused by ACTH-secreting pituitary tumors, in women the frequency may be greater than 95% (10). Regulation of ACTH secretion by the adenohypophysis has not, as yet, been well defined. It is known that monamines, acetylcholine, melatonin, and γ-aminobenzoic acid appear to play a role in regulation of ACTH secretion (10). The exact nature of these effects and the sites of action are certainly not well understood. Considerable data exists, however, implicating the significant role of

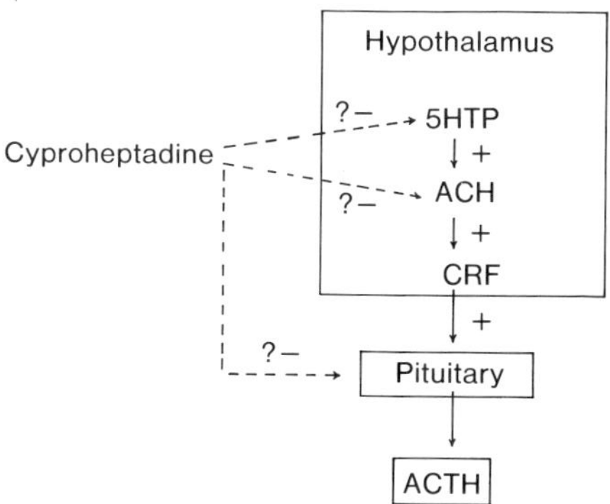

FIG. 20.4. Serotonin stimulates the release of CRF from the hypothalamus by direct effect upon cholinergic neurons.

serotonin in the regulation of the pituitary adrenal axis (Fig. 20.4). Apparently serotonin stimulates the release of corticotropin-releasing factor (CRF) from the hypothalamus by direct effect upon cholinergic neurons. It is also possible that melatonin inhibits corticotropin-releasing factor by a pathway that is as yet unknown.

The knowledge that serotonin appears to stimulate the release of ACTH led Krieger and her group to utilize the serotonergic antagonist cyproheptadine for the treatment of Cushing's disease (6). In addition to an antiserotonergic effect, cyproheptadine has been reported to have anticholinergic, antidopaminergic, and antihistaminergic effects. After an initial report of three patients with Cushing's disease found to be responsive to cyproheptadine, subsequent studies have revealed that as many as 50% of patients with Cushing's disease will have a clinical and biochemical response when treated with this drug (1, 4, 6, 10). The agent is administered at a dose of 25 mg/day in divided doses. A biochemical depression in serum cortisol levels appears in approximately 1 to 3 months after full doses of the drug are established. Clinical remission, however, lags somewhat behind the biochemical response, becoming apparent within 4 to 6 months after initiating treatment. Several patients with elevated ACTH levels due to Nelson's syndrome have also been reported to have a significant suppression of these ACTH levels along with decrease in skin pigmentation (1, 4). Patients have been demonstrated, at 6 to 12 months after initiation of treatment, to have normal suppressibility of ACTH by dexamethasone along with a restoration of normal cortisol circadian rhythm (1). A recent report by Aronin and Krieger details a patient with Nelson's syndrome who maintained clinical and laboratory remission for some 18 months after withdrawal of cyproheptadine therapy (1); however, patients have generally undergone an exacerbation of the basic disease process once therapy has been discontinued.

Patients with Cushing's disease and those with Nelson's syndrome are eligible for drug treatment only if local tumor extension does not require surgical decompression. There is, unfortunately, no way of predicting which patients will respond to drug treatment; effectiveness of treatment has not correlated with either the extent of clinical symptomatology nor size of the tumor mass. Several patients have been reported in whom an initial failure to respond to cyproheptadine therapy was followed by a positive response of the drug after surgical extirpation of tumor mass which has not resulted in chemical cure (10). In addition, patients harboring serious systemic consequences of Cushing's disease may require reduction of hypercortisolemia at a more rapid rate than can be anticipated with cyproheptadine therapy. In this case, it has been found desirable to proceed directly with surgical treatment, since the mortality and morbidity of transsphenoidal surgery is so minimal.

Somnolence and hyperphagia constitute the major side effects experienced with chronic ingestion of cyproheptadine. The somnolence usually disappears spontaneously. Hyperphagia, however, can prove to be of major concern, particularly in children being so treated. Prolonged administration of the drug for up to 16 months has been reported with no undue side effects, there appears to be no contraindication to prolonged administration of this agent (10).

Surgery of patients with Cushing's disease has taken on the most interesting dimension of all of our functional pituitary tumors. In those patients with abnormal sella turcicas and measurable ACTH, we have not failed to find a definitive lesion which has enabled extirpation of the tumor with preservation of adenohypophyseal function. However, we have also seen a number of patients who have normal sella turcicas by tomographic appearance along with high resolution computerized tomographic scans. In these patients, we have found that cure of the disease has required a total extracapsular enucleation of the gland, should one not find a tiny tumor after extensively filleting the gland. It is our feeling that symptomatic Cushing's disease is such a malignant entity that postoperative panhypopituitarism is a more desirable state than persistent unremitting hypercortisolemia.

The past 10 years has witnessed the emergence of sophisticated technical approaches to surgery of functional pituitary tumors which has been paralleled by an enhanced understanding of the physiology and biochemistry of hormone interactions at the hypophyseal-pituitary level. Such understanding has yielded the development of a still infantile group of pharmacological agents which hold promise as a significant addition to our therapeutic armamentarium. This delightful marriage between surgery and medicine in providing a comprehensive approach to the therapy of these intriguing disorders remains an exciting and stimulating prospect for all of us in the future.

REFERENCES

1. Aronin, N., Krieger, D. T. Sustained remission of Nelson's syndrome after stopping cyproheptadine treatment. N. Engl. J. Med. *302:* 453–455, 1980.
2. Hagen, C., Lindholm, J., Suenson, E., Riishede, J., Hummer, L., and Jacobson, H. H. Relationship between plasma prolactin concentration and pituitary function in patients with a pituitary adenoma. Clin. Endocrinol. *11:* 671–679, 1979.
3. Jewelewicz, R., and Vande Wiele, R. L. Clinical course and outcome of pregnancy in 25 patients with pituitary microadenomas. Am. J. Obstet. Gynecol., *136:* 339–343, 1980.
4. Jialal, I., and Pillay, N. L. Cyproheptadine therapy in Cushing's disease and Nelson's syndrome. So. African Med. J. *57*(9): 305, 1980.
5. Kelly, W. F., Doyle, F. H., Mashiter, K., Banks, L. M., and Gordon, H. Pregnancies in women with hyperprolactinemia: Clinical course and obstetric complications of 41 pregnancies in 27 women. Br. J. Obstet. Gynaecol., *86:* 698–705, 1979.
6. Krieger, D. T., Amorosa, L., and Linick, F. Cyproheptadine-induced remission of Cushing's disease. N. Engl. J. Med., *293:* 893–896, 1975.
7. March, C. M., Kletsky, O. A., and Davajan, V. Clinical response to CB-154 and the pituitary response to thyrotropin releasing hormone gonadotropin releasing hormone in patients with galactorrhea-amenorrhea. Fertil. Steril., *28*(5): 521–525, 1977.
8. McGregor, A. M., Scanlon, M. F., Hall, R., and Hall, K. Effects of bromocryptine on pituitary tumor size. Br. Med. J., *2:* 700–703, 1979.
9. Shewchuk, A. B., Adamson, G. D., Lessard, P., adn Ezrin, C. The effect of pregnancy on suspected pituitary adenomas after conservative management of ovulation defects associated with galactorrhea. Am. J. Obstet. Gynecol., *136:* 659–666, 1980.
10. Vigneri, R., and Goldfine, I. D. Pharmacologic therapy of patients with pituitary tumors secreting prolactin, growth hormone, and adrenocorticotropin. Adv. Intern. Med., *25:* 69–89, 1980.
11. Wajchenberg, B. L., Silveria, A. A., Goldman, J., Cesar, F. P., Marino, R., Jr., and Lima, S. S. Evaluation of resection of pituitary microadenoma for the treatment of Cushing's disease in patients with radiologically normal sella turcica. Clin. Endocrinol. *11:* 323–331, 1979.
12. Wass, J. A. H., Thorner, M. O., Charlesworth, M., Moult, P. J. A., Dacie, J. E., Jones, A. E., and Besser, G. M. Reduction of pituitary tumor size in patients with prolactinomas and acromegaly treated with bromocryptine with or without radiotherapy. Lancet, *2:* 66–69, 1979.
13. Weiss, M. H. Surgery of the pituitary gland. Bull. Los Angeles Neurol. Soc., *42*(3–4): 190–200, 1977.
14. Weiss, M. H. Acromegaly: Selection parameters and operative results. Clin. Neurosurg., in press 1981.
15. Zarate, A., Canales, E., Alger, M., and Forspach, G. The effect of pregnancy and lactation on pituitary prolactin-secreting tumors. Acta Endocrinol. (Hbh), *92:* 407–412, 1979.

CHAPTER

21

Neurological Manifestations of External Carotid Artery Disease

RICHARD M. HODOSH, M.D., and STEPHEN C. BOONE, M.D.

INTRODUCTION

Communications between the external carotid artery (ECA) and internal carotid artery (ICA) have been recognized since the time of Galen when the first descriptions of the normal anatomic features in lower mammals was recorded. Subsequent investigations by Elsching (10) in 1893 revealed that dye injected into the external carotid artery and external maxillary artery of cadavers could be traced into the ophthalmic arteries of both the ipsilateral and contralateral side. Marx (18) in 1949 provided the initial angiographic evidence, in human subjects, of the existence of collateral function.

More recently, rapid advances in radiographic imaging, cerebrovascular physiology, and surgical techniques have made the practicing neurologist and neurosurgeon even more aware of the potentially important contribution of the external circulation to the maintenance of a normal homeostatic state. Significant collateral contributions of external carotid pathways (4, 12, 17, 20) are frequently demonstrated in patients who survive an internal carotid artery occlusion without a major neurological deficit (20, 26). It has become evident that obstructions to flow in some external carotid arteries ipsilateral to a completely occluded internal carotid artery may result in serious neurological consequences. When associated with occlusion of other extracranial vessels in the cerebrovascular circuit, external carotid obstructions have been reported to cause facial pain (13), amaurosis fugax (3, 4, 16), painful ocular ischemia, and transient ischemic attacks in the carotid as well as the vertebrobasilar systems. Intermittent hypoperfusion through the external carotid artery has frequently been incriminated as a cause of these recurrent ischemic symptoms. A convincing argument for an embolic phenomena through the external carotid artery has also been made by the observation of retinal emboli distal to previously documented internal carotid occlusions (1–3). Ulcerative lesions at the origin of the external carotid, the common carotid, or thrombus within the "stump" of the occluded internal carotid artery are thought by many to be the source of this embolic material (1, 2).

Considerable controversy exists concerning the relative functional significance of the alternative external pathways to the cerebral and retinal circulation, and the role that various modes of surgical treatment may play in augmenting the normal circulation (5, 6, 8, 10, 15, 19, 23, 25, 27). Countee (7) emphasizes the position that surgical procedures on the external carotid artery can be expected to relieve symptoms of transient cerebral ischemia only when preoperative arteriograms demonstrate that the involved external carotid artery is a major source of blood supply to the symptomatic hemisphere distal to the occluded internal carotid artery. Dietrich *et al.* (8) have stated that angiographic visualization of these collateral connections is not a prerequisite for external carotid artery surgery.

With the increasing number of patients who are now being referred to neurosurgical units for consideration of extracranial-intracranial (EC/IC) bypass procedures it is becoming more important that detailed evaluation of the anatomic variations in collateral circulation be taken into account in planning the appropriate mode of therapy, whether it ultimately be conservative medical treatment or more intricate bypass procedures.

ANATOMICAL CONSIDERATIONS

Anatomical studies by Szapiro and Pakula (26) have demonstrated the significant communications which exist between the external and internal circulation when one common carotid artery is experimentally injected with the ipsilateral internal carotid artery being simultaneously occluded. Fig. 21.1 demonstrates these anastomatic channels which exist between the ECA and ICA as well as the vertebral system (12).

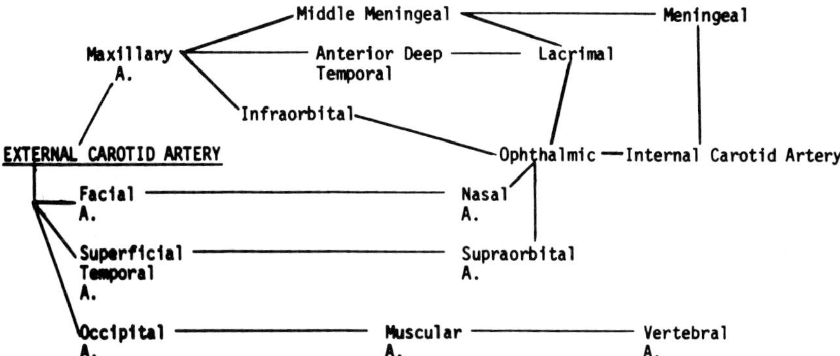

FIG. 21.1. Anastomotic channels between the external carotid artery and the internal carotid artery.

The second important collateral system which is responsible for maintaining cerebral perfusion in altered anatomic situations is the corticoleptomeningeal anastomoses which form a network over the surface of the brain, mostly in the depths of the gyri. More specifically there are three types of "candelabra" anastomoses in this system:

1. Medial frontal branches of the callosomarginal artery which anastomose with the ascending frontal, insular, and posterior parietal branches of the middle cerebral artery.
2. Communications with the parietooccipital and temporal branches of the posterior cerebral artery and the angular and temporal branches of the middle cerebral artery.
3. Finally, there are anastomoses which exist between vessels of the posterior clivus, pericallosal arteries, and the parietooccipital and posterior callosal branches of the posterior cerebral artery.

The third major collateral pathway between the external and internal system is the so called "Rete Mirable" (20) which is the result of anastomoses between corticoleptomeningeal and dural meningeal arteries.

SURGICAL CONSIDERATIONS

Various management decisions are involved in the choice of appropriate surgical therapy for patients with internal carotid artery occlusion and associated involvement of the external carotid artery system. Over the last several years we have attempted to develop a general scheme which has been useful in guiding our approach in the treatment of these patients. During the previous 4 years 145 patients with cerebrovascular disease have undergone varying surgical procedures. The surgery has consisted of 65 carotid endarterectomies and 98 extracranial-intracranial arterial anastomoses. Twelve of these patients were found to have an ipsilateral internal carotid artery occlusion and external carotid artery stenosis.

This group of 145 patients presented either with transient ischemic attacks (TIAs), strokes in evolution, or nondevastating cerebral infarction. All patients underwent routine laboratory testing to include CBC, blood sugar, uric acid, and lipid profile. Complete cardiovascular histories and examinations were performed by a cardiologist to determine if: (a) the heart was the source of emboli; (b) cardiac arrhythmias were present which might produce hypotension and subsequent TIAs; (c) the cardiac status was stable enough to permit cerebrovascular surgery. Static and dynamic brain scans with intravenous technetium-99 were performed as well as CT scans of the head with and without contrast enhancement. Most patients underwent noninvasive vascular evaluation either employing one or a combination of the following tests: Carotid phonoangiography, directional doppler, Gee OPG, and Kartchner OPG. Finally, all patients underwent complete angiography of the aortic arch, the cervical and intracranial carotid arteries, and vertebral arteries. When an occlusion of the internal carotid artery was suspected, prolonged injections with increased volumes were performed as has been suggested by Countee (7).

All surgery was completed under general anesthesia using nitrous oxide and narcotics. Intraoperative shunting was employed in those situations in which stump pressures were 50 mm Hg or less or when EEG recordings demonstrated slowing or decreased amplitude. The main objective of the first operation was to perform an external carotid endarterectomy. This was performed in the usual manner through a slanting arteriotomy from the common carotid toward the internal carotid side of the common carotid artery to facilitate the completion of possible endarterectomy of the internal carotid artery (Fig. 21.2).

If the prolonged injection angiogram suggested patency either by anastomotic filling of the intracranial artery down past the siphon or by a wisp of dye seen in the internal carotid in the neck, an internal carotid endarterectomy was attempted. A 1-cm arteriotomy in the distal internal carotid artery was initially performed in these situations. If back bleeding was obtained, then the incision was extended proximally and a routine endarterectomy was performed (Fig. 21.2). If minimal or no back bleeding was obtained, then a no. 3 Fogarty catheter was threaded up the internal carotid artery for a distance of about 7 cm—the balloon was inflated and the catheter was extracted. If no back bleeding was obtained and there was a known stump of the internal carotid artery, then a large hemoclip

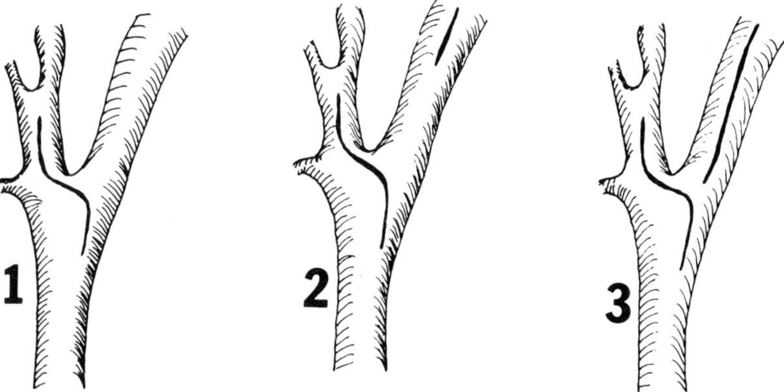

FIG. 21.2. Diagram of arteriotomy of the internal and external carotid arteries.

was used to occlude its origin (Fig. 21.3). The stump of a known occluded internal carotid artery was also hemoclipped in the same manner even if an endarterectomy was not attempted.

If the internal carotid artery was successfully opened, then no further surgery was contemplated. If the internal carotid artery was not opened, and the patients remained symptomatic after their ECA endarterectomy, an extracranial-intracranial arterial anastomosis was performed. An algorithm of this sequence is shown in Fig. 21.4 for review. Table 21.1 illustrates a breakdown of the operative procedures performed. Two patients had an external carotid TEA as the only procedure while three patients also had an attempted internal carotid TEA. Two patients had internal carotid stump ligation. Six patients eventually had an EC-IC bypass.

A review of the 12 patients is presented in Table 21.2. The mean age of the patients was 65 (range from 56 to 79). Nine of the patients were males. Eleven of the 12 patients had significant contralateral carotid artery disease with seven of them requiring contralateral carotid artery surgery. Nine patients revealed evidence of coronary artery disease. Eleven of 12 were at one time heavy smokers. Two patients demonstrated a type IV hyperlipidemia, and one had diabetes mellitus.

In the immediate postoperative period all patients were monitored in an intensive care unit. Ischemic symptoms were treated with volume expansion and pressors. Sodium nitroprusside was the agent employed to treat undesired blood pressure elevations. Postoperative angiography was performed in all patients included in this series.

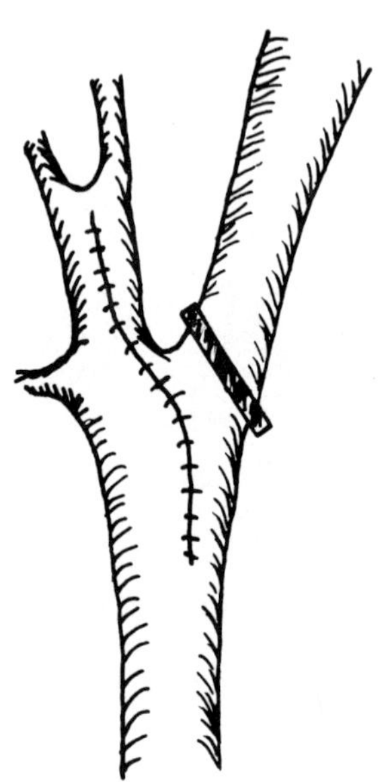

Fig. 21.3. Hemoclip ligation of the internal carotid artery stump.

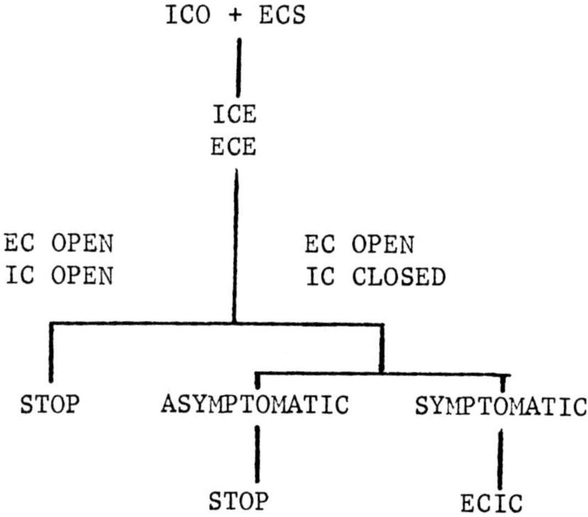

FIG. 21.1. Algorithm for surgical management of ipsilateral internal carotid occlusion and external carotid stenosis. ICO, internal carotid occlusion; ECS, external carotid stenosis; ICE, internal carotid endarterectomy; ECE, external carotid endarterectomy; EC, external carotid; IC, internal carotid; ECIC, extracranial, intracranial anastomisis.

TABLE 21.1

Operative Procedures: A Summary of Operations Used to Manage Ipsilateral Internal Carotid Occlusion and External Carotid Artery Stenosis

PROCEDURE	NUMBER
EXTERNAL CAROTID ENDARTERECTOMY	2
ECA-TEA AND ICA-TEA	3
ICA STUMP LIGATION	2
ECA-TEA AND EC/IC BYPASS	6

RESULTS

The technical results are presented in Table 21.3. Only one of the three internal carotids remained patent as judged by postoperative angiography. One of six patients undergoing an EC-IC bypass was not a technically successful result in terms of patency. This patient was the only person to have his superficial temporal artery decrease in size following the external carotid endarterectomy.

The clinical results proved to be more rewarding (Table 21.4). There were no deaths and no added morbidity. Patients were considered improved if their neurological deficit improved and/or if there was a cessation or reduction in their TIA frequency. The only patient who failed to demonstrate evidence of clinical improvement was one of the two patients in whom internal carotid endarterectomy was unsuccessful.

TABLE 21.2

Review of 12 Patients with Internal Carotid Occlusion and External Carotid Stenosis

MEAN AGE	65 (56-79)
SEX	9 MALES; 3 FEMALES
CONTRALATERAL CAROTID DISEASE	11
CONTRALATERAL SURGERY	7
HEART DISEASE	9
SMOKER	11
HYPERLIPIDEMIA	2
DIABETES MELLITUS	1

TABLE 21.3

*Technical Results**

PROCEDURE	SUCCESSFUL	NOT SUCCESSFUL
ECA-TEA	2	0
ECA AND ICA TEA	1	2
ECA-TEA AND ICA STUMP LIGATION	2	0
ECA-TEA AND EC/IC	5	1

* Operative procedure classified as successful if angiogram demonstrated patent endarterectomy or EC/IC bypass.

TABLE 21.4

Clinical Results

PROCEDURE	IMPROVED	NO CHANGE	WORSE
ECA-TEA	2	0	0
ECA AND ICA TEA	2	1	0
ECA-TEA AND ICA STUMP LIGATION	2	0	0
ECA-TEA AND EC/IC	6	0	0
TOTAL	12	1	0

CASE MATERIAL

The following cases are presented to offer a sampling of the categories of cases of internal carotid occlusion with symptoms referrable to combined external carotid artery involvement.

Case 1: Bilateral Internal Carotid Occlusion

W.A. is a 56-year-old white male who presented with a right hemiparesis and global aphasia 6 months prior to surgery. His initial angiographic evaluation revealed bilateral ICA occlusions, occlusion of the left vertebral, and filling of the right vertebral via muscular branches of the

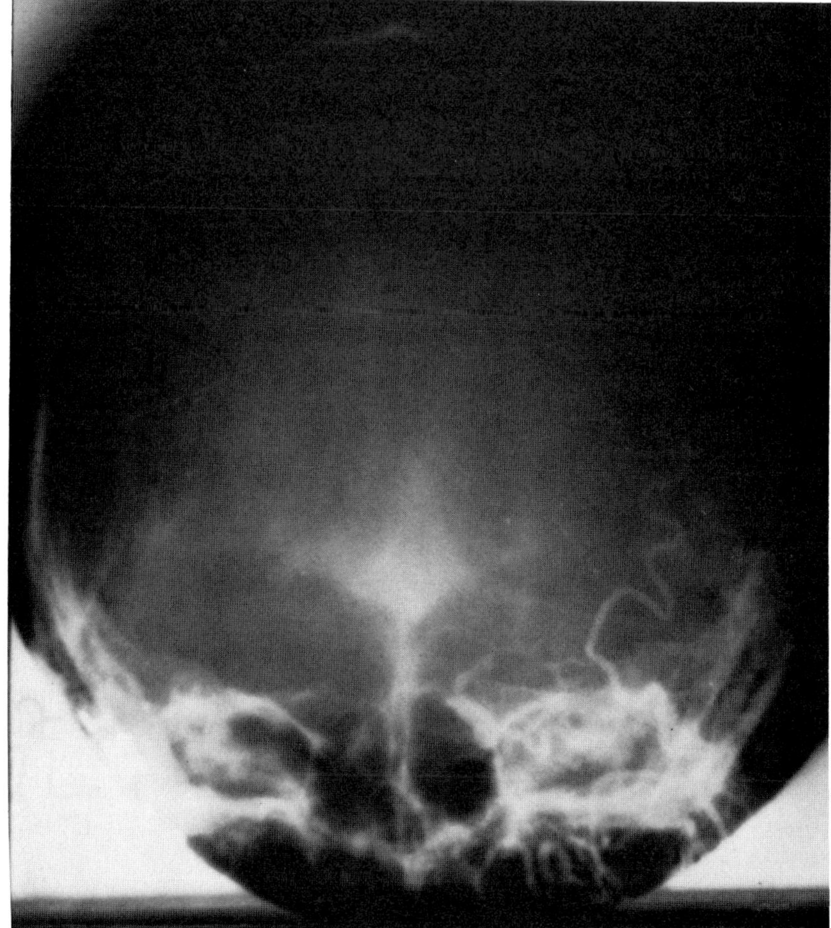

FIG. 21.5. Case 1. Preoperative left AP carotid angiogram demonstrating complete occlusion.

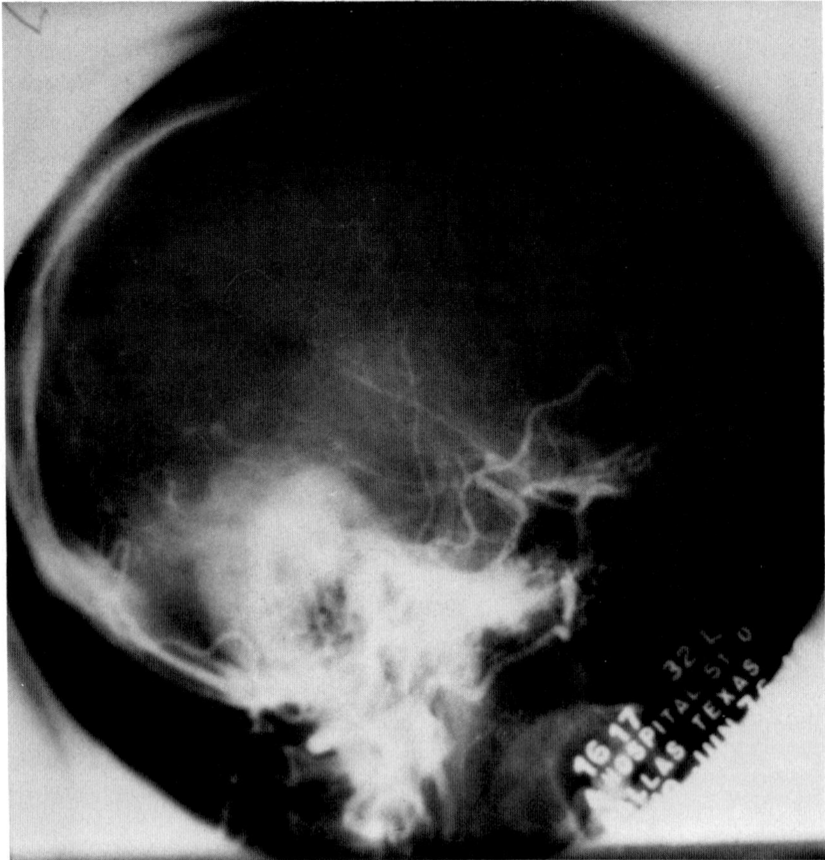

FIG. 21.6. Case 1. Preoperative left lateral carotid angiogram demonstrating complete occlusion.

external carotid artery (Figs. 21.5 and 21.6). His aphasia persisted over the next several months; however, there was gradual improvement in his right hemiparesis to the point where his weakness was barely detectable on clinical examination. CT scanning revealed evidence of multiple bilateral hemispheric infarcts. For the 6 to 8 weeks prior to surgery the patient experienced episodes of increased right sided weakness three to four times per week and lasting 30 to 120 minutes on each occurrence.

Because of the occurrence of these superimposed TIAs the patient underwent a left EC/IC bypass followed 2 weeks later by a right EC/IC bypass. There has been no recurrence of his TIAs for 3½ years, and interestingly his aphasia improved significantly after his second operation. Figs. 21.7 and 21.8 demonstrate the radiographic findings in this patient 1½ years after bypass.

COMMENT

This case demonstrates the extreme situation in which internal carotid circulation has been totally lost and the external circulation was burdened with providing cerebral blood flow (CBF) for both hemispheres. We feel that the occurrence of his TIAs occurred secondary to a hypoperfusion syndrome which was relieved by the bypass procedures. It is of note that there was an immediate and significant improvement in his aphasia after shunting, thus lending clinical support to the concept of "idling neurons."

Case 2

H.H. is a 74-year-old right handed white male who presented with several episodes of TIAs consisting of transient right hemiparesis and aphasia. His neurological examination was normal except for a slight right upper extremity pronator drift. Diagnostic evaluation revealed a

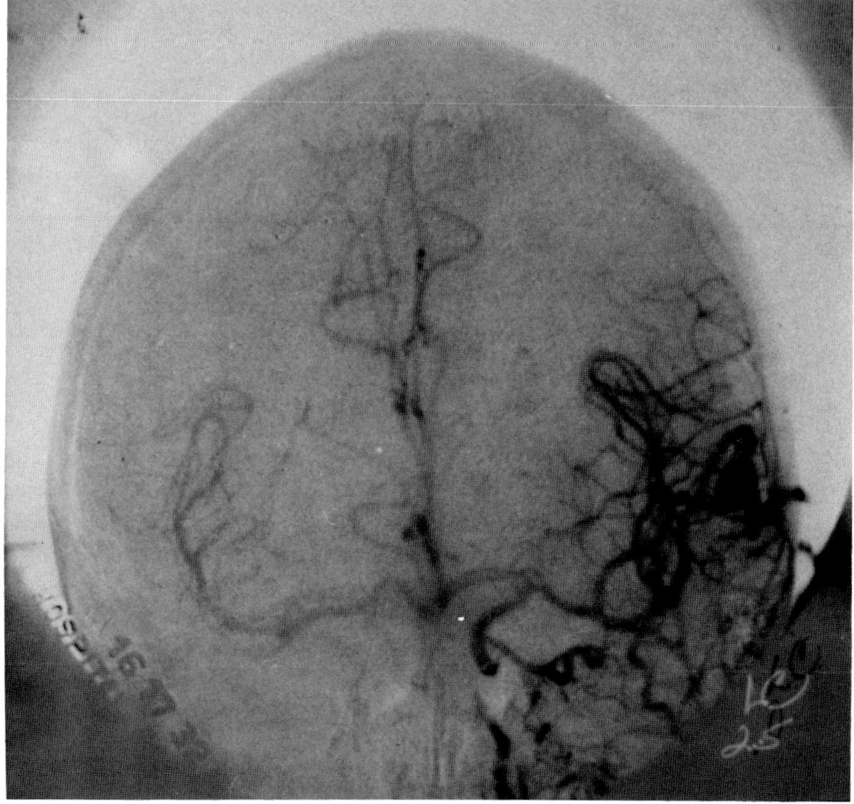

FIG. 21.7. Case 1. Postoperative left AP carotid angiogram 1½ years after surgery demonstrating patent EC-IC bypass with filling of both hemispheres. Note significant dilation of the superficial temporal artery.

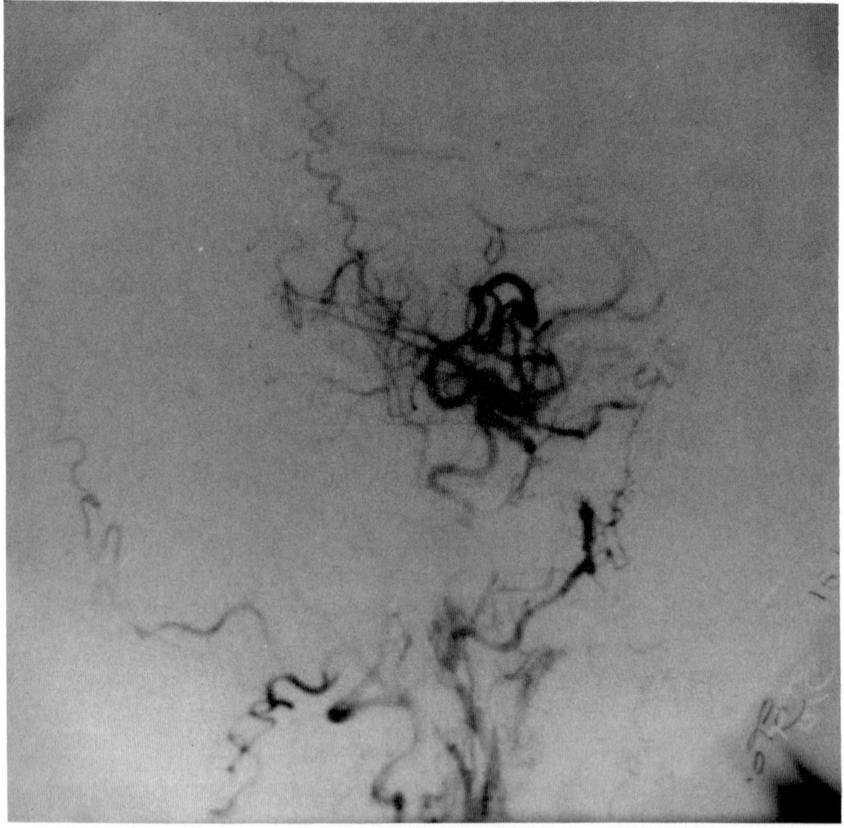

FIG. 21.8. Case 1. Postop left lateral carotid angiogram.

normal static brain scan with diminished flow to the left carotid artery. CT examination showed cortical atrophy that was symmetrical and compatible with his age. Noninvasive peripheral vascular studies demonstrated a hemodynamically significant lesion in the left internal carotid artery. Cerebral angiography revealed a complete occlusion of the left internal carotid artery (Fig. 21.9) as well as a stenosis of the proximal left external carotid and the right external carotid artery. A left external carotid endarterectomy was performed, and he has remained asymptomatic for more than 1 year.

COMMENT

This case illustrates the situation in which external carotid endarterectomy may alter the collateral supply enough to prevent TIAs and even possible stroke.

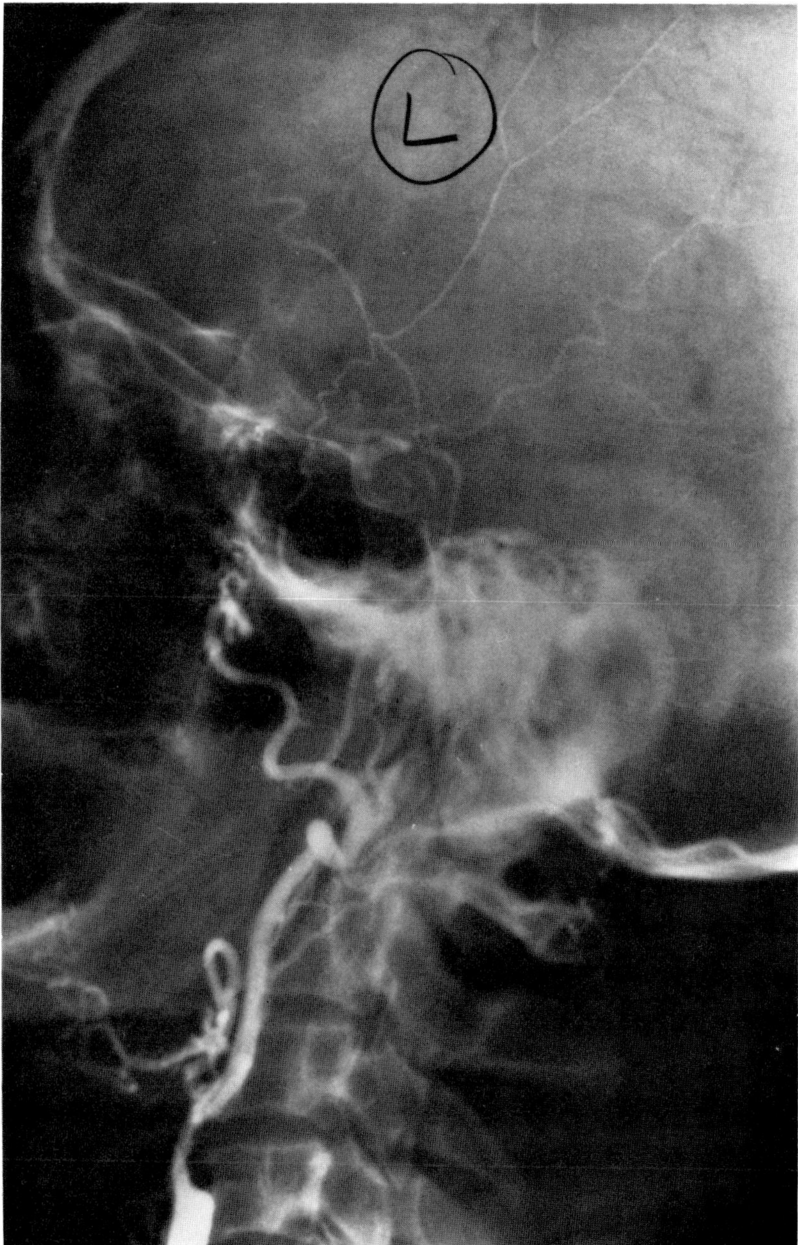

FIG. 21.9. Left common carotid angiogram, case 2. The internal carotid artery is occluded, and the external carotid artery which is supplying collateral flow to the intracranial internal carotid artery is significantly stenotic.

Case 3

P.H. is a 62-year-old left handed male who developed the sudden onset of a left hemiparesis and dysphasia which resolved over a 24-hour period. His neurological examination at that time was normal. A brain scan showed decreased flow through the right carotid with a normal static scan. A CT scan, performed 3 weeks after the initial symptoms, demonstrated a small right temporal lobe infarct. Noninvasive evaluation was positive for a lesion in both carotid arteries. A prolonged injection of the right carotid artery demonstrated a high grade stenosis or occlusion of the right internal carotid artery with an associated high grade stenosis of the external carotid artery (Fig. 21.10). A right external and internal carotid endarterectomy was successfully completed with patency documented by postoperative angiography (Fig. 21.11). His postoperative course has been totally free of any neurological symptoms.

COMMENT

This case nicely illustrates the radiographic technique of prolonged arterial injection to demonstrate the patency of a seemingly occluded internal carotid artery. Once again the collateral circulation can be implicated in helping to maintain the patency of the internal carotid via anastomoses through collateral branches.

Case 4

D.B. is a 46-year-old right handed white male with several episodes of dysphasia and right sided weakness which were occurring two to three times per week for the 6 weeks prior to admission, despite aspirin therapy. His diagnostic work was unremarkable with the exception of OPG evidence of diminished flow through the left internal carotid artery and an angiogram which revealed marked stenosis of the left external carotid artery and total occlusion of the left internal carotid artery with an irregular proximal stump (Fig. 21.12). A left external carotid endarterectomy was performed. Also a hemoclip was applied to the internal carotid stump to prevent the stump from serving as a source of emboli (Fig. 21.13).

Postoperatively the patient has remained asymptomatic for more than 10 months.

COMMENT

This case supports the earlier observations of Barnett and Peerless (1, 2) which suggest that the external system can function as a conduit to the intracranial circulation for emboli from an occluded internal carotid stump. Furthermore, this case demonstrates that hemoclip application is

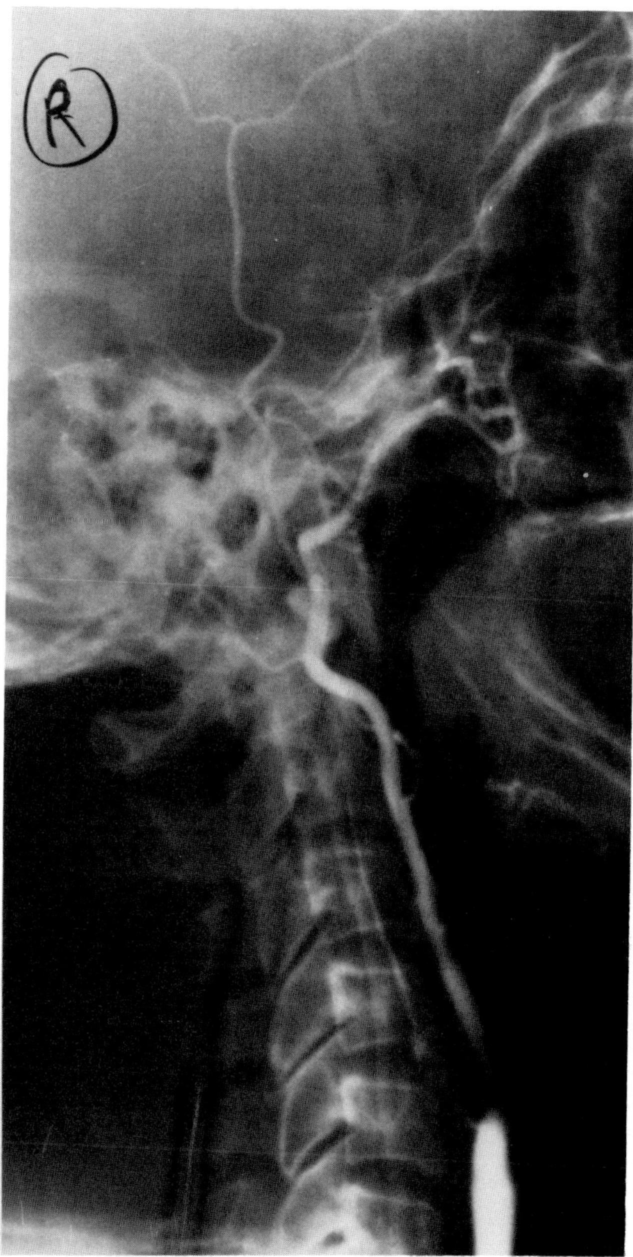

FIG. 21.10. Prolonged injection right common carotid angiogram on case 3. Note a severe stenosis of the external carotid artery and a wisp of dye in the internal carotid artery.

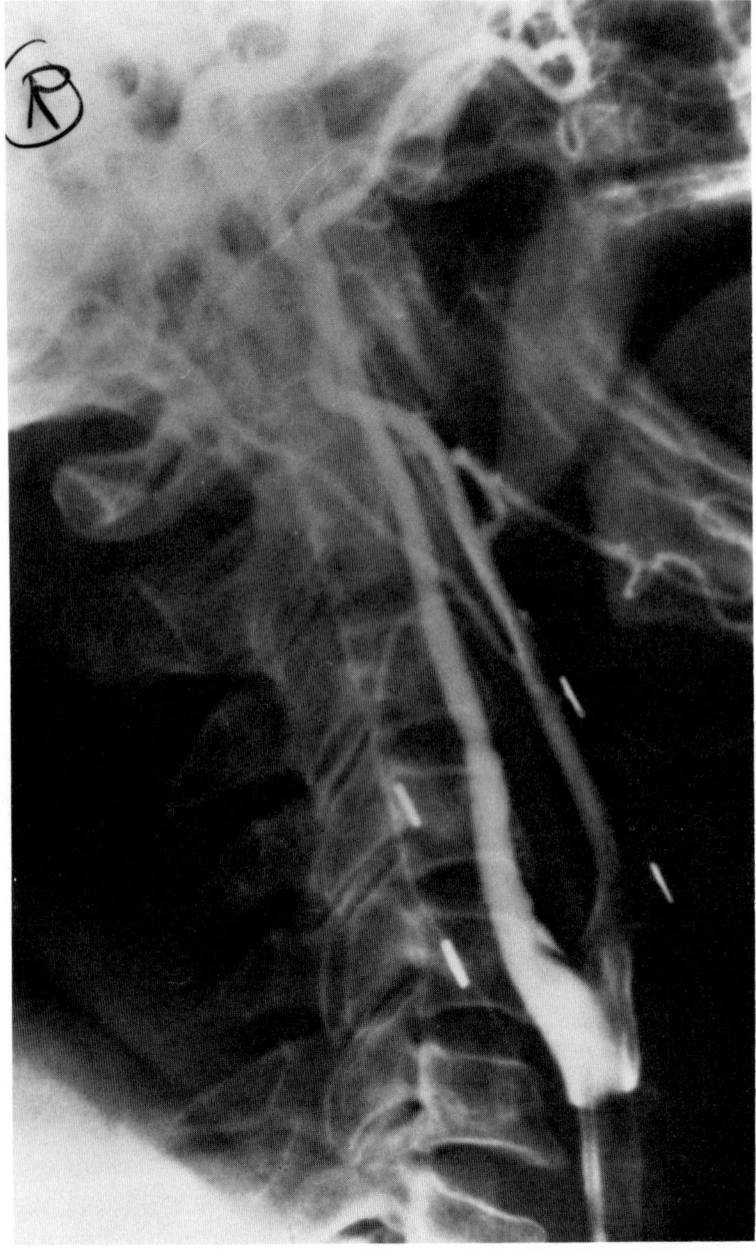

FIG. 21.11. Postoperative right common carotid angiogram on case 3.

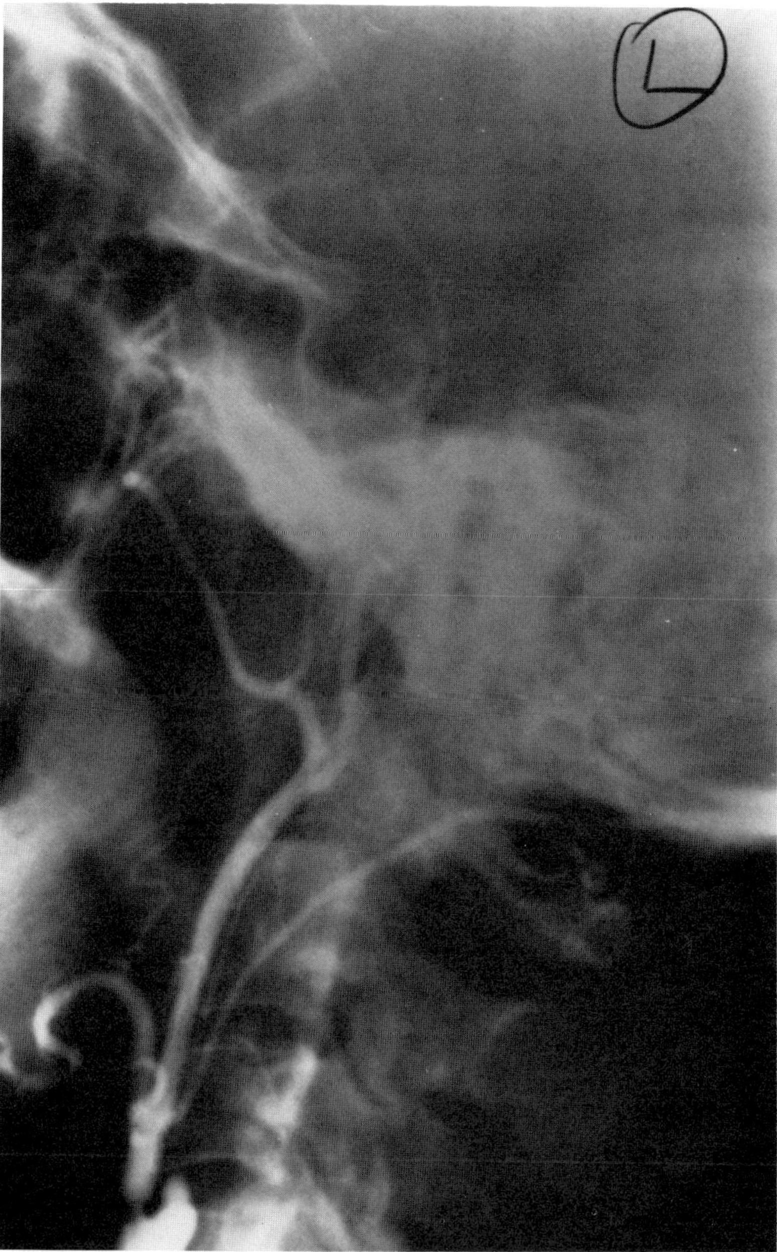

FIG. 21.12. Preop left common carotid angiogram on case 4. Note the high grade stenosis of the external carotid artery and the internal carotid stump.

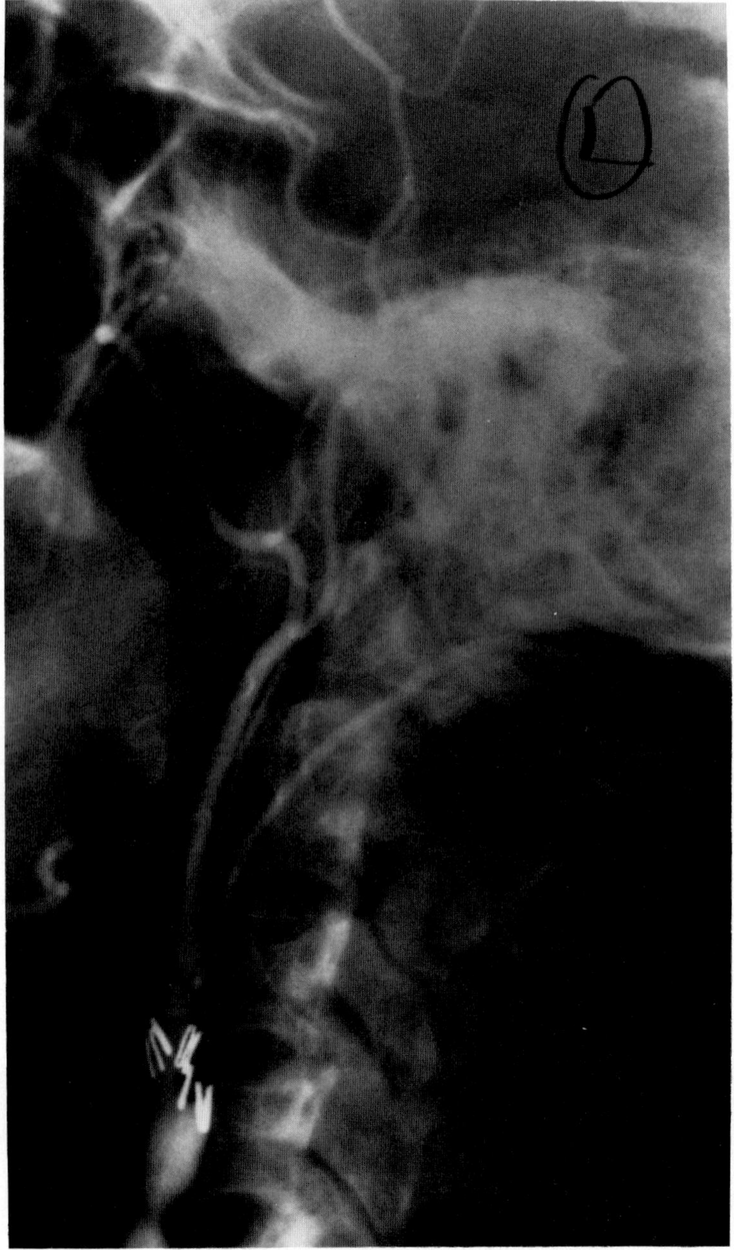

FIG. 21.13. Postoperative angiogram on case 3. This illustrates the hemoclip occlusion of the internal carotid artery stump.

a simple and effective means to obliterate the stump and create a smooth vascular margin.

Case 5

R.H. is a 59-year-old right handed male who had a transient episode of dysphasia and three episodes described as a loss of consciousness. His

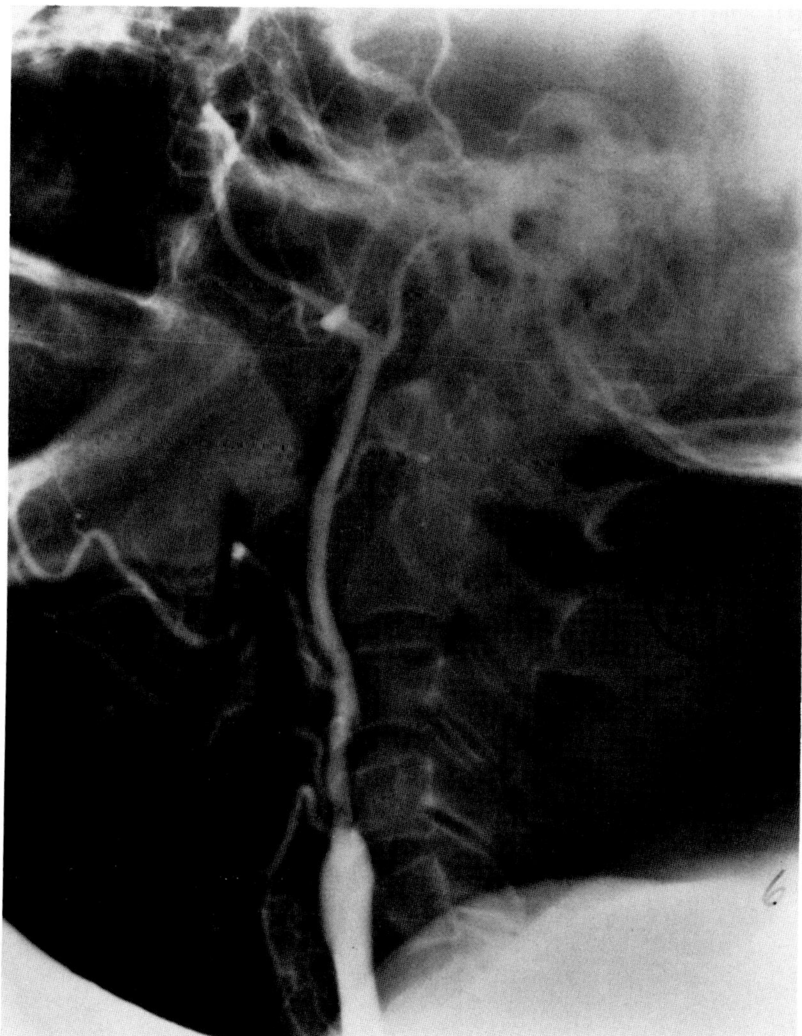

FIG. 21.14. Left common carotid angiogram on case 5. Note the internal carotid occlusion and the external carotid stenosis.

neurological exam was normal. Lipid profile and glucose levels were normal. Flow studies revealed diminished flow on the left side. Cerebral angiography revealed an occluded left internal carotid artery and a 50% stenosis of the left external carotid artery (Fig. 21.14). Because his symptoms were felt to be left hemisphere-related it was elected to proceed with an EC/IC bypass on the left. However, it was elected to perform an external carotid endarterectomy prior to the bypass in order to allow the superficial temporal artery (STA) to increase in size from its 0.7 mm

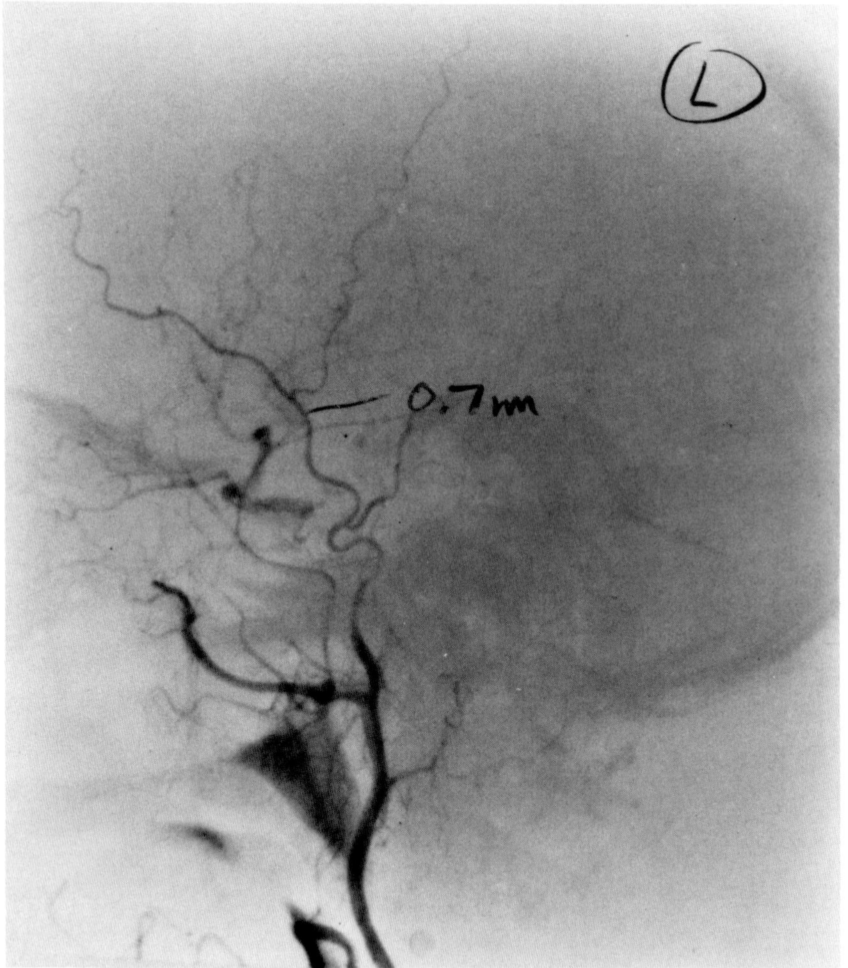

FIG. 21.15. Left common carotid angiogram on case 5. The superficial temporal artery (STA) measures 0.7 mm in diameter.

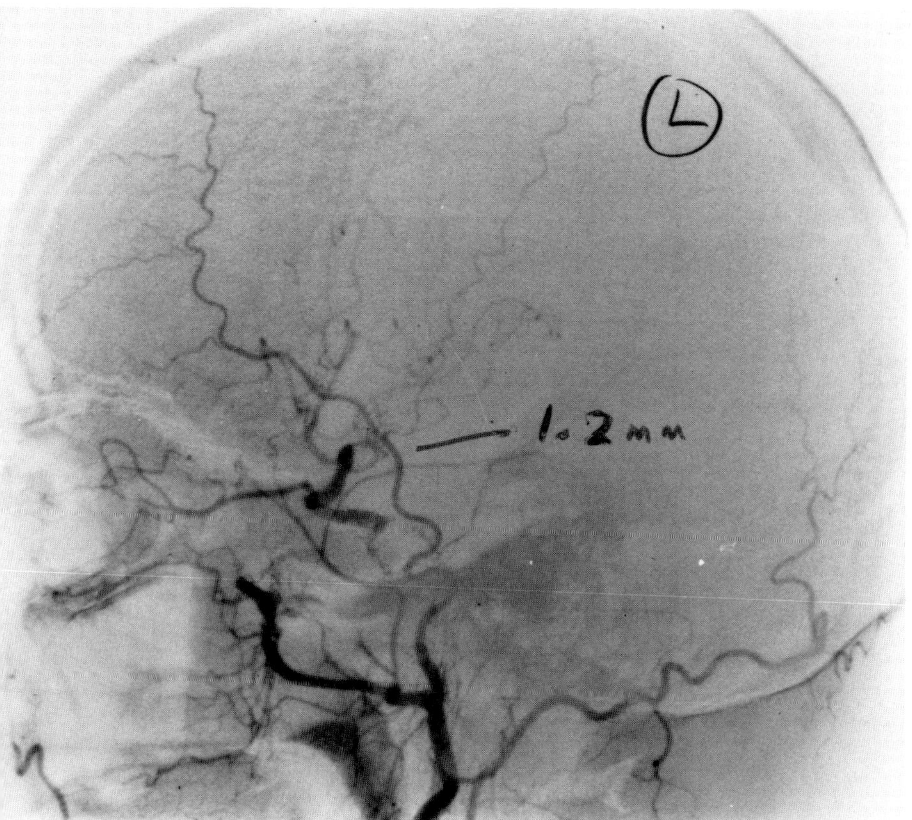

FIG. 21.16. Left common carotid angiogram on case 5, 3 weeks after a left external carotid endarterectomy. The superficial temporal artery has enlarged to 1.2 mm in diameter.

diameter (Fig. 21.15). Fig. 21.16 demonstrates that the STA subsequently increased to 1.2 mm 3 weeks after the endarterectomy of the external carotid. A successful STA-MCA bypass was ultimately achieved with the STA eventually increasing in size to 2.4 mm in diameter (Fig. 21.17). The patient has remained symptom-free for more than 15 months.

COMMENT

This case vividly documents the possible enlargement of the superficial temporal artery following an ipsilateral external carotid endarterectomy. Furthermore, it also demonstrates the STA enlargement that has been reported to occur after successful bypass procedures from a high pressured external system to a lower pressured internal circulation.

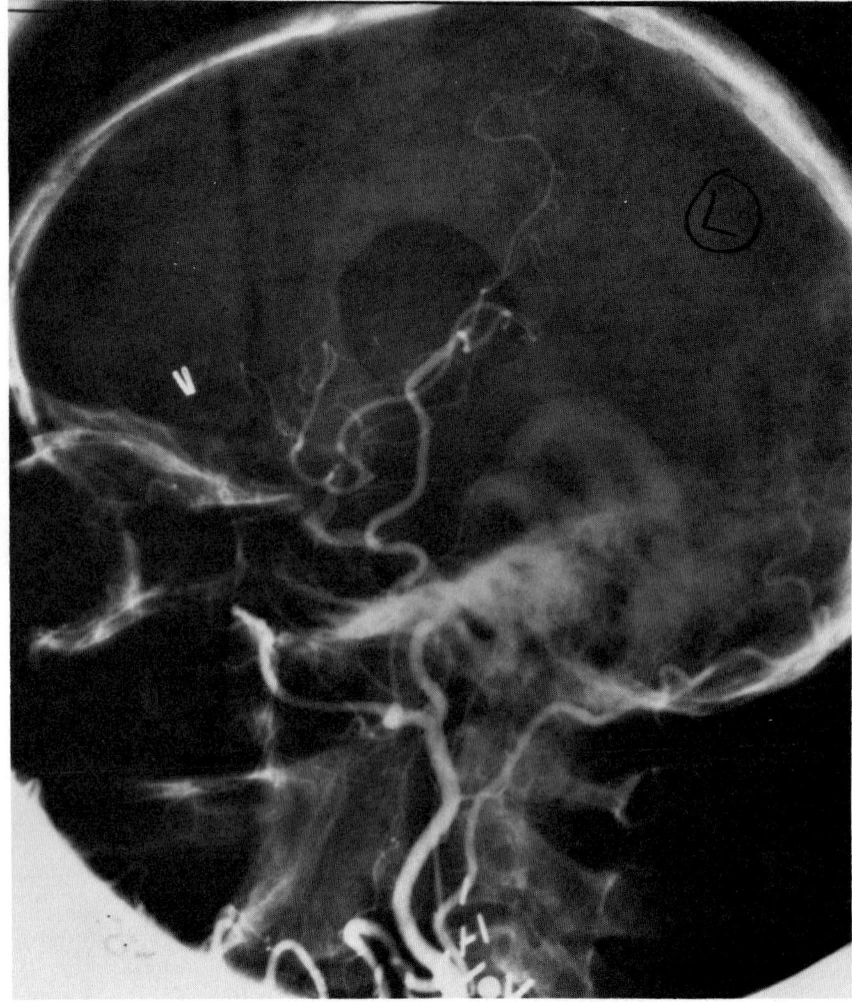

FIG. 21.17. Left common carotid angiogram on case 5 following a left STA-MCA bypass. The superficial temporal artery has enlarged to 2.4 mm in diameter.

SUMMARY

The management of patients with neurological signs and symptoms related to disease of the external carotid artery requires appreciation of the anatomical variations of its contributions to the intracranial circulation. Neurological signs may be produced by inadequate flow, thrombus, or distal embolization in the external carotid artery when there is associated disease of the ipsilateral internal carotid artery. The surgical management cannot be generalized in simple terms and must be individualized for each patient so as to provide him with the best results with the lowest possible morbidity and mortality. The cases presented in this section are offered only to demonstrate examples of the numerous therapeutic alternatives that exist for these patients with potential life-threatening and crippling disease.

REFERENCES

1. Barnett, H. J. M., Peerless, S. J., and Wei, M. The "stump" of the internal carotid artery: A source of further cerebroembolic ischemia (abstr.). Stroke, *8:* 14–15, 1977.
2. Barnett, H. J. M., Peerless, S. J., and Kaufmann, J. C. E. "Stump" of internal carotid artery—a source of further cerebroembolic ischemia. Stroke, *9:* 448–456, 1978.
3. Burnbaum, M. D., Selhorst, J. B., Harbison, J. W., and Brush, J. J. Amaurosis fugax from disease of the external carotid artery. Arch. Neurol., *34:* 532–535, 1977.
4. Caplan, H. A. Collateral circulation of the brain. Neurology, *11:* 9–15, 1961.
5. Clayson, K. R., and Edwards, W. H. Importance of external carotid artery in extracranial cerebral vascular occlusive disease. South. Med. J., *70:* 904–909, 1977.
6. Connoly, J. E., and Steimer, E. A. Endarterectomy of the external carotid artery. Arch. Surg., *106:* 799–802, 1973.
7. Countee, R. W., and Vijayanathan, T. External carotid artery and internal carotid artery occlusion: angiographic, therapeutic, and prognostic consideration. Stroke, *10:* 450–460, 1979.
8. Dietrich, E. B., Liddicoat, J. E., McCutchen, J. J., and DeBakey, M. E. Surgical significance of the external carotid artery in the treatment of cerebrovascular insufficiency. J. Cardiovasc. Surg., *9:* 213–223, 1968.
9. Ehrenfeld, W. K., and Lord, R. S. Transient monocular blindness through collateral pathways. Surgery, *65:* 911–915, 1969.
10. Elsching, G. Arch. Ophthalmol., *39:* 151, 1893.
11. Fields, W. S. Selection of stroke patients for arterial reconstructive surgery, Editorial. Am. J. Surg., *125:* 527–529, 1973.
12. Hawkins, T. D. Collateral anastomoses in cerebral vascular occlusion. Clin. Radiol., *17:* 203–219, 1966.
13. Herishanu, Y., Bendheim, P., and Dolberg, M. External carotid occlusive disease as a cause of facial pain. J. Neurol., Neurosurg. Psychiatry, *37:* 1963–1965, 1974.
14. Jackson, B. B. The external carotid artery as a brain collateral. Ann. Surg., *113:* 375–378, 1967.
15. Jacques, S. S., Garner, J. T., Tager, R., Rosenstock, J., and Field, T. Improved cognition after external carotid endarterectomy. Surg. Neurol., *10:* 223–225, 1978.
16. Lord, R. S. Monocular transient ischemic attacks in the external carotid artery. Med. J. Aust., *1:* 742–745, 1973.
17. Margolis, M. T., and Newton, T. H. Lateral pathways between the cavernous portion of the internal carotid and external carotid arteries. Radiology, *93:* 834–836, 1969.
18. Marx, F. An arteriographic demonstration of collaterals between internal and external carotid arteries. Acta. Radiol., **31:** 155–160, 1949.
19. Moran, J. M., Reichman, O. H., and Baker, W. H. Staged intracranial and extracranial revascularization. Arch. Surg., *12:* 1424–1428, 1927.
20. Mount, L. A., and Taveras, J. M. Arteriographic demonstration of the collateral circulation of the cerebral hemisphere. Arch. Neurol. Psychiatry, *78:* 235–253, 1957.
21. Padget, D. F. The development of the cranial arteries in the human embryo. Contrib. Embryol. Carnegie Inst., *32:* 205–261, 1948.
22. Richter, H. Collaterals between the external carotid artery and the vertebral artery in

cases of thrombosis of the internal carotid artery. Acta. Radiol., *40:* 108–112, 1953.

23. Samson, D. S., Hodosh, R. M., and Clark, K. Microsurgical treatment of transient cerebral ischemia. J.A.M.A., *241:* 376–378, 1979.
24. Samson, D. S., Watts, C., and Clark, K. Cerebral vascularization for transient ischemic attacks. Neurology, *27:* 767–771, 1977.
25. Sundt, T. M., Jr., Siekert, R. G., Piepgrass, D. G., Sharbrough, F. W., and Houser, O. W. Bypass surgery for vascular disease of the carotid system. Mayo Clin. Proc., *51:* 677–692, 1976.
26. Szapiro, J., and Pakula, H. Anatomical studies of the collateral blood supply to the brain and retina. J. Neurol. Neurosurg. Psychiatry, *26:* 414–417, 1963.
27. Taveras, J. M., Mount, L. A., and Friedenberg, R. N. Angiographic demonstration of the external-internal carotid anastomoses through the ophthalmic artery. Radiology, *63:* 525–530, 1964.
28. Thompson, J. E., and Talkington, C. M. Carotid endarterectomy. Ann. Surg., *184:* 1–15, 1976.
29. Yasargil, M. G. (ed.). Microsurgery Applied to Neurosurgery, pp. 105–114. George Thieme Verlag Stuttgart, 1969.

CHAPTER

22

Use of Transplantable Tissue in Neurosurgery*

DONALD J. PROLO, M.D., F.A.C.S.

A frontier largely overlooked by the community of neurosurgeons is transplantation biology. Courted often by surgeons involved in organ transplantation, a busy neurosurgeon interprets these entreaties with resignation in the presence of an irretrievably impaired brain-injured patient. A prevalent misconception, therefore, is that the neurosurgeon's role is solely that of a provider rather than user of salvageable portions of the decedent. Although organ transplantation will likely forever exceed the presumptive moral and technological limits of our specialty, the implantation of cadaveric tissues has flourished and will continue to expand as they become more plentiful, safe, and effective in the management of patients.

Neurosurgeons are in fact conspicuous practitioners of the art of transplantation. In a real sense every craniotomy represents a form of fresh autogeneic (autologous) orthotopic skull grafting (30). Lumbar and cervical fusions with fresh iliac crest donor bone extend the application of fresh autografts in clinical neurosurgery. Fascia lata grafting of dural defects augments further the use of fresh autografts. Autogeneic peripheral sensory nerves are commonly utilized for interfascicular nerve grafting where defects in functionally important nerves cannot otherwise be bridged without tension (2, 24, 37, 41). Whereas in these procedures the genome of donor and recipient is identical, an expanding role for processed cadaveric implants of bone, dura mater, and fascia lata fulfills goals of anatomical reconstruction without burdening the individual with the creation of painful defects elsewhere in the body. The underlying principles of transplantation biology and their surgical implications are therefore highly germane to practicing neurosurgeons.

Terminology

Despite the frequency with which grafting of bone, dura, and nerve are done in neurosurgery, our literature has largely overlooked progress in

* This investigation was supported in part by Office of Naval Research Contract N00014-76-C-0621.

transplantation and its apposite contributions to our specialty. An understanding of the biology of transplantation presupposes knowledge of operant terms used to define types of grafts. This terminology is based on the genome of the donor and the immunologic reactions of the recipient to viable grafts and nonviable implants (36, 43). Whereas autograft refers to a tissue or an organ from the same individual, the preferred associated adjective is now autogeneic rather than autologous or autogenous. In an analogous fashion isograft is allied with the adjective isogeneic for grafts from an identical twin or between members of an inbred strain. An allograft (previously homograft) represents a living tissue or organ whose genetic constitution differs from the recipient of the same species. The corresponding adjective allogeneic substitutes for the older term homogenous. Similarly xenograft and xenogeneic have replaced the former heterograft and heterogenous for transplantation across species lines. Dead processed tissue from the same species is an alloimplant and from another species a xenoimplant.

Principles of Transplantation

Changes which occur in tissue after transplantation are of two broad types: degenerative and proliferative. The superiority of fresh autografts of bone and nerve are well recognized (6, 13, 14, 26, 37). Transplantation of a fresh autograft conveys viable cells along with an immunologically identical matrix for the reconstitution of the recipient tissue. The antigenic exclusiveness of an individual lies predominantly on cell membranes, but also on structural proteins, enzymes, and other components of the interstitium (45). Processing techniques which eliminate cells through autodigestion and extract lipoproteins reduce immunogenicity and thereby enhance acceptance by the unrelated recipient (43). Hence alloimplants of devitalized tissue which selectively retain inductive proteins are advantageous over fresh allografts which contain significant antigenic markers. In general the transplantation of fresh unprocessed tissues and organs among unrelated members of a species is contraindicated, except where the tissue is immunologically privileged (such as the cornea) or matched for tissue type (such as the kidney). All of the considerations relevant to allografts apply even more strongly to xenogeneic transplantation.

The four biological mechanisms which subserve the transplantation of tissue are: (a) immunological; (b) vascular and cellular invasions (for example, neuro- or osteoconduction); (c) induction of identical tissue formation (neuro- or osteoinduction); and (d) remodelling (6, 18). An optimal implant would restore the anatomical integrity of the part and by the processes stipulated above become viable. By contrast alloplastic substances, such as plastics and metals, are variably inert, subject to encapsulation through an inflammatory foreign body reaction, and are susceptible to infection. The search for suitable tissue grafts and implants is predicated upon the superiority of actual or potential living tissue over foreign materials which at best would remain metabolically isolated from physiological processes.

Methodology

Autografts and allografts must be processed with observance of techniques which facilitate the successful restitution of the recipient tissue. Because one advantage of fresh autografts is cell survival, the aseptic harvesting of bone, peripheral nerve, or fascia must immediately precede their transplantation to a well-prepared, vascular recipient bed. The handling of fresh autografts must be gentle. Imminent dehydration from warm operating room lights and air exposure must be avoided along with contact with cytotoxic chemicals (saline, antibiotics, bone wax, rust inhibitors on scalpel blades, etc.) (1, 45). Any storage of the fresh autograft will likely result in cell death and some autodigestion of matrix proteins through enzymatic action (43).

By contrast the banking of devitalized alloimplants necessitates compliance with rigorous standards for donorship, harvesting of tissues, sterilization or confirmation of sterility, processing, storage, and distribution. Allogeneic tissues must preferentially be rendered sterile, acellular, and depleted of other potentially antigenic substrates. Aseptic procurement of tissue from cadavers does not ensure sterility. Proof of sterility from culture of the graft (or portion of it) would likely chemically injure it, compromise its structural integrity, or through handling secondarily contaminate it. Furthermore the pool of potential donors of tissue vastly expands when processing techniques include direct sterilization of the implant. The method of sterilization must effectively rid the tissue of surface and interstitial bacteria, fungi, and viruses without altering the biochemical and biomechanical character of the implant. Potential toxic residues must be eliminated to avoid injury to the recipient (7, 31).

Preservation techniques such as freezing and freeze-drying reduce antigenicity, temporarily arrest degradation of the matrix, maintain its structure, and allow thereby safe storage and distribution (11, 27, 43). Processing methods which selectively leave undisturbed the inductive protein(s) and promote the extraction or degradation of other immunogenic substances are favored (43, 45).

Sterilization of tissues through the years has included the use of boiling, autoclaving, chemicals (including antibiotics), and irradiation. Boiling is inefficient and like autoclaving causes denaturation of proteins in bone which leads to impaired remodelling and resorption of the implant (7). Benzalkonium chloride, β-propiolactone, and various antibiotics inhibit the inductive capacity of bone (45). The minimal bacteriocidal level of gamma irradiation is over 2 Mrads, and the virucidal level is in excess of 4 Mrads. These levels of irradiation cause biomechanical alterations in the tissue, increase the solubility of collagen and glycosaminoglycans, interfere with the covalent bonds of the collagen and its molecular helical structure, destroy the fibrillar network of the matrix observed by ultrastructural studies, and totally eradicate the inductive capacity of bone (5, 42, 45). Furthermore unusually stable free radicals are induced in the apatite which are potentially mutagenic and oncogenic (7, 17). The use of irradiation as a sterilant of tissue is to be deplored.

In contrast to the other agents, gaseous ethylene oxide has proven to be an effective and safe sterilant of bone, dura mater, and fascia lata. Through a series of experiments in our laboratory, we have demonstrated the penetration of this agent into wet bone, the desorption of ethylene oxide and its toxic reaction products in tissue, and the eradication of even the most highly resistant sporogenous *Bacillus subtilis* from bone (31).

Though Inclán reawakened interest in cadaver bone banking in 1942, Cloward since 1946 has successfully been using his own banked allogeneic bone for lumbar and cervical arthrodeses. Recently he has also been sterilizing his bone with ethylene oxide (9).

Guidelines for the banking of transplantable tissues and organs have been formulated by the American Association of Tissue Banks. In time this organization will certify laboratories whose methods for the procurement, processing, storage, and distribution of organs and tissues are scientifically appropriate and freely evaluable. Neurosurgeons now may safely procure bone, dura, and fascia from the United States Navy Tissue Bank, National Naval Medical Center, Bethesda, Maryland, the University of Miami Tissue Bank in Miami, Florida, and the Neuroskeletal Transplantation Laboratory at the Institute for Medical Research, 751 South Bascom Avenue, San Jose, California.

Applications

CENTRAL NERVOUS SYSTEM

Functional restitution after central nervous system injury at present is a chimerical enterprise, but nevertheless a focus of intense investigation. Of special interest are the experiments of Kao *et al.* (16) and Richardson *et al.* (32), wherein the gaps between ends of spinal cord were bridged with autogeneic and allogeneic peripheral nerves. Though no functional recovery occurred, there was a population of central neurons which grew into the grafts. At present these inchoate studies have no practical application.

PERIPHERAL NERVES

Fresh autografts of peripheral sensory nerves are widely used in microscopic interfascicular nerve repair (2, 13, 37). Millesi (24) found connective tissue proliferation occurred with tension, that the major source of connective tissue was the epineurium, and that connective tissue invasion and intraneural scarring took place only in the presence of tension. Even delayed tension consequent on extension of a nearby joint caused a traction lesion at the suture line. Hence for lesions greater than 2 cm, interfascicular nerve grafting is recommended (41).

Allografts ideally would compensate for defects in peripheral nerve without the need to sacrifice the patient's sensory nerve. Unfortunately, frozen irradiated and lyophilized allografts have had success ranging from no recovery to 50% restitution of function (8, 12, 22, 39). The immune response causes this failure with ultrastructural studies showing rejection of Schwann cells and subsequent rupture and collapse of their neurilemmal tubes (28). Marmor (21) and Pollard and Fitzpatrick (29) have demonstrated a reduced immune response in irradiated allogeneic nerves with lessened numbers of lymphocytes and plasma cells, but there is still a very dense deposition of collagen between neurilemmal tubes that impairs neurotization. The histoincompatibility between donor and recipient animal is reduced with immunosuppressant agents (40, 46), but only variable success in humans has been achieved with this method (12, 22). Peripheral nerve allografts have not achieved a state of clinical usefulness.

BONE

Fresh autografts of cancellous and cortical bone have consistently been found superior to any alternative graft or implant (4, 6, 14, 26). Without the imposition of immunological barriers and with the probability of some cell survival (especially in cancellous bone), the graft serves as an additional source of osteogenesis and further acts as a trellis or scaffold for the ingrowth of vessels (6, 43). The cell population that survives consists of osteoprogenitor cells and very few osteocytes within 0.3 mm from the cortical surface. Revascularization proceeds within the cancellous grafts within 1 to 3 weeks and into cortical grafts much more slowly over months (43). Incorporation is the process of envelopment and interdigitation of the donor old bone with new bone deposited by the recipient. The quantity of donor cortical bone may be 90% of its original volume years after grafting in contrast to the more rapid resorption and accretion (remodelling) occurring in cancellous autografts. Through osteoconduction the original structure of the graft provides a scaffold for the ingrowth of capillaries and perivascular tissue. Through osteoinduction pleuripotential migratory mesenchymal cells are converted into osteoprogenitor cells (43). This process is regulated by a hypothetical morphogenetic insoluble noncollagenous polypeptide, specific enzymes, and enzyme inhibitors. The failure rate of autografts ranges between 13% and 30, but depends much upon the particular application (7, 43).

Fresh allografts convey cells and other substrates which are disadvantageously antigenic. Processed nonviable alloimplants are acellular but contain bone morphogens, tissue antigens, enzymes, and structural proteins, chiefly collagen (43). Freezing and freeze-drying diminish but do not eliminate antigenicity of the implant (4, 7, 11, 43). Both humoral responses with cytotoxic antibodies and more importantly a cellular response with small round cells, plasma cells, and reticulocytes block the osteoinductive and osteoconductive phases of allogeneic bone incorporation. This delayed hypersensitivity reaction occurs 14 days after a fresh allograft and 21 to 28 days after a nonviable alloimplant is placed (43). Techniques designed by Urist (44) to reduce the antigenicity of allogeneic bone and preserve its morphogenetic protein by chemical processing have resulted in a fusion rate in lumbar fusions equivalent to that with fresh autogeneic bone.

As neurosurgeons an area of primary interest is anterior cervical fusions. Although the debate continues over whether there is a relationship between radiographic fusion and clinical result (10, 15, 19, 34), after discectomy alone the rate of fusion in two very small series is 63 and 72% (23, 25). The rate of fusion with both autogeneic and allogeneic bone in larger and more significant series is about 90% (3, 20, 33, 38). After fusion the cervical alignment is superior (23). There is immense benefit to the patient, however, with the use of processed alloimplants, wherein pain and other morbidity from the iliac crest donor site is eliminated and hospitalization is shortened.

DURA MATER

Freeze-dried allogeneic dura mater has successfully been used in human transplantation since June 1954 (31). After sterilization with gaseous ethylene oxide and then freeze-drying for removal of toxic residues and storage, this membrane along with allogeneic fascia lata prepared in a similar fashion is ideal for repair of pachymeningeal defects over the brain and spinal cord. It is inert, does not adhere to the brain, and gradually becomes penetrated by fibroblasts until it eventually becomes indistinguishable from adjacent dura of the host (35) (Fig. 22.1).

Neuroskeletal Transplantation Laboratory

Over the past 3 years 2428 implants of allogeneic bone, dura mater, and fascia lata have been harvested from suitable donors, cleansed of debris, sterilized with ethylene oxide, and freeze-dried. During this period

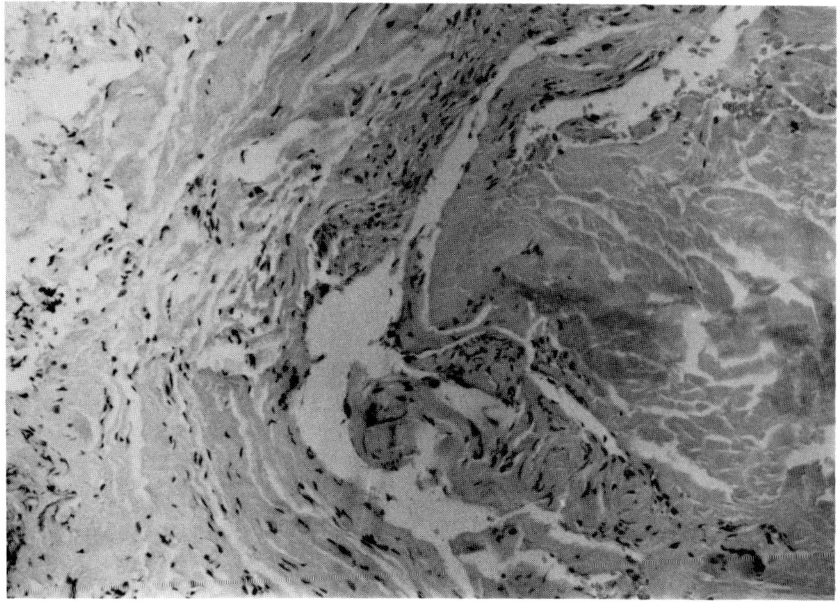

FIG. 22.1. Photomicrograph demonstrates junction of recipient's dura (*left*) and freeze-dried allogeneic dura (*right*) 10 months after implantation. The inert acellular matrix of the cadaver dura is eventually invaded by vessels and fibroblasts such that eventually the alloimplant becomes indistinguishable from adjacent dura without evidence of inflammation or a foreign body reaction, H & E, ×40. (Courtesy of M. Herrick, M.D.)

1673 segments of bone fashioned in various forms, 664 deposits of dura, and 91 sections of fascia lata have been implanted by surgeons throughout the United States. There have been no documented cases of infection among these implants. A preliminary review of the data returned by 14 surgeons to our laboratory reveals that for anterior cervical arthrodeses allogeneic bone dowels have resulted in the fusion of 160 interspaces out of a total of 166 (96%) among 115 patients. We conclude, therefore, from information retrieved so far that allogeneic bone has a fusion rate equivalent to that of fresh autogeneic bone.

A unique application of cadaver skull has been the use of small discs to fill bur holes in areas of cosmetic importance after craniotomy. Over the past 2½ years 48 such discs have successfully been implanted in 22 patients. In one individual who expired 3 months subsequent to the craniotomy, the predominately cortical skull disc was being incorporated with newly formed bone entering the disc from adjacent skull (Fig. 22.2).

In summary, it may be concluded that for some neurosurgical applications properly selected and processed cadaver bone is equivalent to fresh autogeneic bone and advantageously avoids a second painful wound for donor bone. Freeze-dried allogeneic dura mater and fascia lata are the

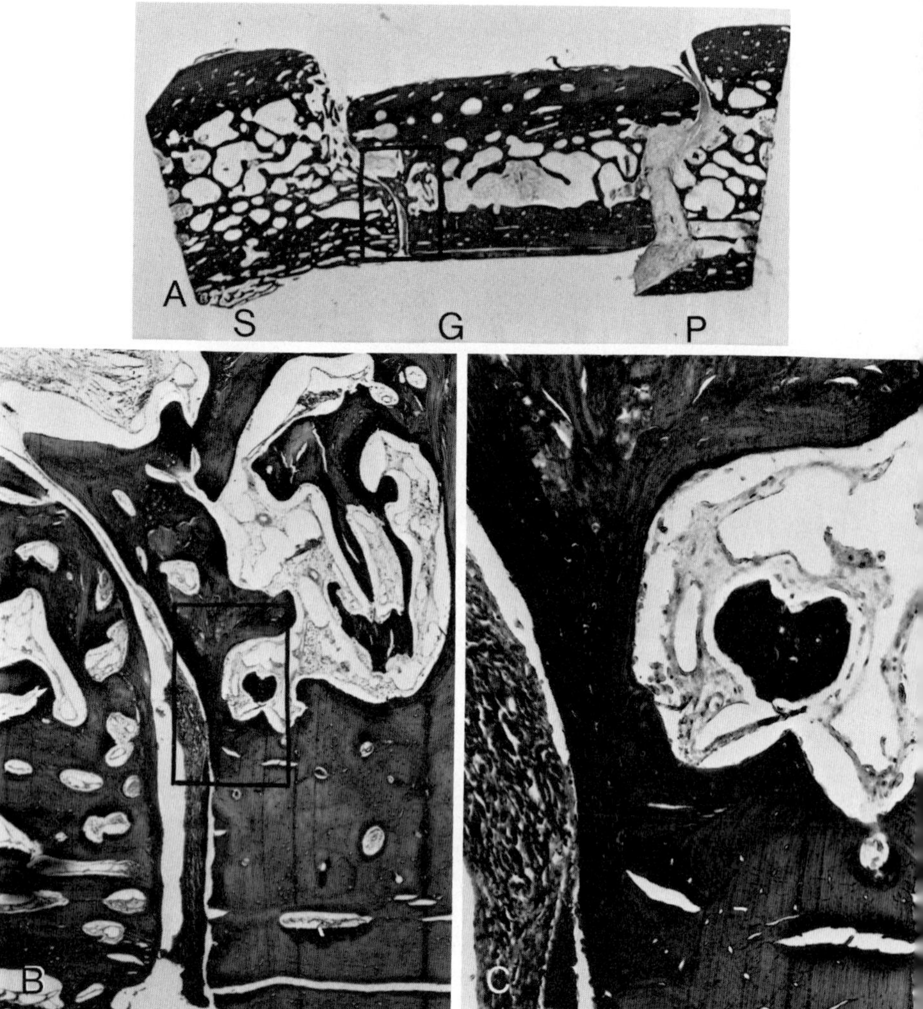

FIG. 22.2. (*A*) In this cross-sectional view of human skull the bur hole defect was replaced with a disc of processed allogeneic (human) skull at the time of craniotomy 3 months before death. *S* designates host skull bordering the craniotomy defect. *P* represents the free skull segment removed during the craniotomy. *G* is the alloimplant of human cadaver skull filling the defect. *Enclosed area* is magnified in *B*. (*B*) Photomicrograph shows living bone of adjacent skull on *left*, vertical fibrous tissue within kerf or junction slightly to *left of center*, and cadaver disc on *right* containing acellular matrix of dead bone at the *lower right* and viable bone and bone marrow at the *upper and right* portions of the illustration. Enclosed area is magnified in *C*. H & E, ×10. (Courtesy of A. Christensen, M.D.) (*C*) Magnification (×40) of area enclosed in *B* demonstrates living fibous tissue within kerf on *left*, viable osteocytes within lacunae (*above*), living bone marrow (*center right*), and acellular dead matrix of alloimplant being resorbed (*below right*).

most physiological and in practice the most effective membranes for repair of dural defects.

Bellwethers among neurosurgeons will recognize that once the life of their patient is beyond recall that their own self-interest demands heraldic resourcefulness in the acquisition of permission to harvest transplantable tissues.

REFERENCES

1. Bassett, C. A. L. Clinical implications of cell function in bone grafting. Clin. Orthop., *87:* 49–59, 1972.
2. Berger, A., and Millesi, H. Nerve grafting. Clin. Orthop., *133:* 49–55, 1978.
3. Brown, M. D., Malinin, T. I., and Davis, P. B. A roentgenographic evaluation of frozen allografts versus autographs in anterior cervical spine fusions. Clin. Orthop., *119:* 213–236, 1976.
4. Burchardt, H., Jones, H., Glowczewskie, F., Rudner, C., and Enneking, W. F. Freeze-dried allogeneic segmental cortical bone grafts in dogs. J. Bone Joint Surg. (Am.), *60A:* 1082–1090, 1978.
5. Buring, K. Ionizing radiation for sterilization of bone. *In* Sterilization and Preservation of Biological Tissues by Ionizing Radiation, pp. 71–78. Panel on Radiation Sterilization of Biological Tissues for Transplantation, International Atomic Energy Agency, Vienna, 1970.
6. Burwell, R. G. The fate of bone grafts. *In* Recent Advances in Orthopedics, edited by A. G. Apley, pp. 115–207. Churchill, London, 1969.
7. Burwell, R. G. The fate of freeze-dried bone allografts. Transplant. Proc. (Suppl.), *8:* 95–111, 1976.
8. Campbell, J. B. Peripheral nerve repair. Clin. Neurosurg., *17:* 77–98, 1970.
9. Cloward, R. B. Gas-sterilized cadaver bone grafts for spinal fusion operations. Spine, *5:* 4–10, 1980.
10. Dunsker, S. B. Anterior cervical discectomy with and without fusion. Clin. Neurosurg., *24:* 516–521, 1977.
11. Friedlaender, G. E. The antigenicity of preserved allografts. Transplant. Proc. (Suppl.), *8:* 195–200, 1976.
12. Gye, R. S., Hargrave, J. C., Loewenthal, J., McLeod, J. G., Pollard, J. D., and Booth, G. C. Use of immunosuppressive agents in human nerve grafting. Lancet, *1:* 647–650, 1972.
13. Haase, J., Bjerre, P., and Simesen, K. Median and ulnar nerve transections treated with microsurgical interfascicular cable grafting with autogenous sural nerve. J. Neurosurg., *53:* 73–84, 1980.
14. Heiple, K. G., Chase, S. W., and Herndon, C. H. A comparative study of the healing process following different types of bone transplantation. J. Bone Joint Surg. (Am.), *45A:* 1593–1616, 1963.
15. Hirsch, C., Wickbom, I., Lidström, A., and Rosengren, K. Cervical-disc. resection. A follow-up of myelographic and surgical procedure. J. Bone Joint Surg. (Am.), *46A:* 1811–1821, 1964.
16. Kao, C. C., Chang, L. W., and Bloodworth, J. M. B., Jr. Axonal regeneration across transected mammalian spinal cords: an electron microscopic study of delayed microsurgical nerve grafting. Exp. Neurol., *54:* 591–615, 1977.
17. Komender, J., Komender, A., Dziedzic-Goclawska, A., and Ostrowski, K. Radiation-sterilized bone grafts evaluated by electron spin resonance technique and mechanical tests. Transplant. Proc. (Suppl.), *8:* 25–37, 1976.

18. Lance, E. M. Bone and cartilage. *In* Transplantation, edited by J. S. Najarian, and R. L. Simmons, pp. 655–697. Lea & Febiger, Philadelphia, 1972.
19. Lunsford, L. D., Bissonette, D. J., Jannetta, P. J., Sheptak, P. E., and Zorub, D. S. Anterior surgery for cervical disc disease. J. Neurosurg., *53:* 1–11, 1980.
20. Malinin, T. I., Rosomoff, H. L., and Sutton, C. H. Human cadaver femoral head homographs for anterior cervical spine fusions. Surg. Neurol., *7:* 249–251, 1977.
21. Marmor, L. Regeneration of peripheral nerves by irradiated homografts. J. Bone Joint Surg. (Am.), *46A:* 383–394, 1964.
22. Marmor, L. Nerve grafting in peripheral nerve repair. Surg. Clin. North. Am., *52:* 1177–1187, 1972.
23. Martins, A. N. Anterior cervical discectomy with and without interbody bone graft. J. Neurosurg., *44:* 290–295, 1976.
24. Millesi, H. Treatment of nerve lesions by fascicular free nerve grafts. *In* Traumatic Nerve Lesions of the Upper Limb, edited by J. Michon and E. Moberg, Ch. 16 (or pp. 91–100). Churchill Livingstone, Edinburgh, 1975.
25. Murphy, M. G., and Gado, M. Anterior cervical discectomy without interbody bone graft. J. Neurosurg., *37:* 71–74, 1972.
26. Pappas, A. M., and Beisaw, N. E. Bone transplantation: correlation of physical and histological aspects of graft incorporation. Clin. Orthop., *61:* 79–91, 1968.
27. Perry, V. P. Freeze-drying for the preservation of human tissues. Transplant. Proc. (Suppl.), *8:* 189–193, 1976.
28. Pollard, J. D., and Fitzpatrick, L. An ultrastructural comparison of peripheral nerve allografts and autografts. Acta Neuropathol., *23:* 152–165, 1973.
29. Pollard, J. D., and Fitzpatrick, L. A comparison of the effects of irradiation and immunosuppressive agents on regeneration through peripheral nerve allografts: an ultrastructural study. Acta Neuropathol., *23:* 166–180, 1973.
30. Prolo, D. J., Burres, K. P., McLaughlin, W. T., and Christensen, A. H. Autogenous skull cranioplasty: fresh and preserved (frozen), with consideration of the cellular response. Neurosurgery, *4:* 18–29, 1979.
31. Prolo, D. J., Pedrotti, P. W., and White, D. H. Ethylene oxide sterilization of bone, dura mater, and fascia lata for human transplantation. Neurosurgery, *6:* 529–539, 1980.
32. Richardson, P. M., McGuinness, U. M., and Aguayo, A. J. Axons from CNS neurones regenerate into PNS grafts. Nature, *284:* 264–265, 1980.
33. Rish, B. L., McFadden, J. T., and Penix, J. O. Anterior cervical fusion using homologous grafts: a comparative study. Surg. Neurol., *5:* 119–121, 1976.
34. Robertson, J. T. Anterior removal of cervical disc without fusion. Clin. Neurosurg., *20:* 259–261, 1973.
35. Rosomoff, H. L., and Malinin, T. I. Freeze-dried allografts of dura mater-20 years experience. Transplant. Proc. (Suppl.), *8:* 133–138, 1976.
36. Russell, P. S., and Monaco, A. P. The Biology of Tissue Transplantation. Little, Brown, Boston, 1965.
37. Samii, M. Modern aspects of peripheral and cranial nerve surgery. *In* Advances and Technical Standards in Neurosurgery, edited by H. Krayenbühl, Vol. 2, pp. 33–85. Springer-Verlag, New York/Wein, 1975.
38. Schneider, J. R., and Bright, R. W. Anterior cervical fusion using preserved bone allografts. Transplant. Proc. (Suppl.), *8:* 73–76, 1976.
39. Singh, R. Reappraisal of homologous nerve grafts. Clin. Neurol. Neurosurg., *2:* 136–141, 1974.
40. Singh, R., Vriesendorp, H. M., Mechelse, K., and Stefanko, S. Nerve allografts and histocompatibility in dogs. J. Neurosurg., *47:* 737–743, 1977.
41. Terzis, J. K., and Strauch, B. Microsurgery of the peripheral nerve: a physiological approach. Clin. Orthop., *133:* 39–48, 1978.

42. Triantafyllou, N., Sotiropoulos, E., and Triantafyllou, J. N. The mechanical properties of the lyophilized and irradiated bone grafts. Acta Orthop. Belg. (Suppl.), *41:* 35–44, 1975.
43. Urist, M. R. Practical applications of basic research on bone graft physiology. *In* Instructional Course Lectures, American Academy of Orthopedic Surgeons, edited by B. Evans, Vol. 25, pp. 1–26. C. V. Mosby, St. Louis, 1976.
44. Urist, M. R., and Dawson, E. Intertransverse process fusion with the aid of chemosterilized autolysed allogeneic (AAA) bone. Clin. Orthop., *154:* 97–113, 1981.
45. Urist, M. R., Mikulski, A., and Boyd, S. D. A chemosterilized antigen-extracted autodigested alloimplant for bone banks. Arch. Surg., *110:* 416–428, 1975.
46. Zalewski, A. A., and Silvers, W. K. An evaluation of nerve repair with nerve allografts in normal and immunologically tolerant rats. J. Neurosurg., *52:* 557–563, 1980.

CHAPTER

23

Guidelines for Noninvasive Evaluation of Asymptomatic Carotid Bruits

MARK M. KARTCHNER, M.D., and LORIN P. McRAE, Ph.D.

The carotid bruit is a significant clinical finding which poses a quandary regarding appropriate further diagnostic and therapeutic measures. Advocates of the aggressive surgical approach cite the high incidence of strokes without transient ischemic attacks in asymptomatic bruit patients (6, 9). The conservative approach entails following the carotid bruit until frank clinical symptoms indicate cerebrovascular insufficiency before proceeding with arteriography (4, 5). Advocates of the conservative approach argue that surgery may precipitate a stroke but cannot alleviate symptoms which do not exist. Concern for the asymptomatic carotid bruit is further heightened in those patients who are anticipating other major surgery (2, 3).

SIGNIFICANT BRUITS

It is a serious mistake to discuss asymptomatic bruits as though there is a common agreement as to the definition of significant carotid bruit since some seem to feel that a bruit is a bruit.

Starting with the most significant bruits, of greatest consequence is the bruit which is shown by carotid phonoangiography, or CPA, to extend beyond systole into diastole (Fig. 23.1). Diastolic carotid bruits are from the internal carotid artery and indicate poor collateral circulation with low distal hemispheric blood pressure or a more severe carotid stenosis on the contralateral side.

Next is the pansystolic bruit of a crescendo nature where the maximal amplitude recorded by CPA is at midsystole. This contrasts to the bruit which is pansystolic but maximal by CPA at the beginning of systole (Fig. 23.1). The crescendo pansystolic bruit generally indicates carotid stenosis greater than 70%, whereas a decrescendo pansystolic bruit may be present with as little as 40% stenosis. The carotid bifurcation level bruit which terminates before the end of systole (not pansystolic) is not considered significant when determining the degree of carotid stenosis.

Bruits of greatest significance are those localized to or of maximal duration at the level of the carotid bifurcation (Fig. 23.2). Bruits that are

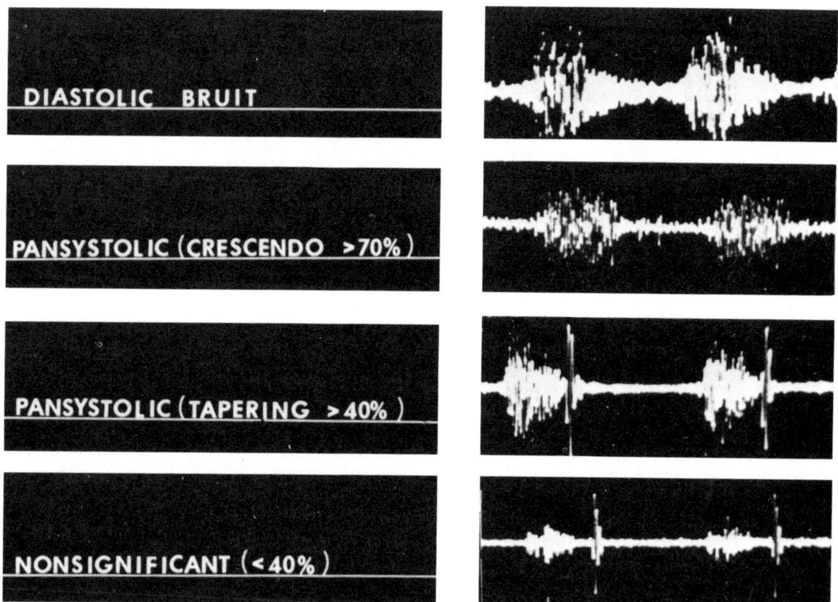

FIG. 23.1. Four types of carotid bruits of varying significance.

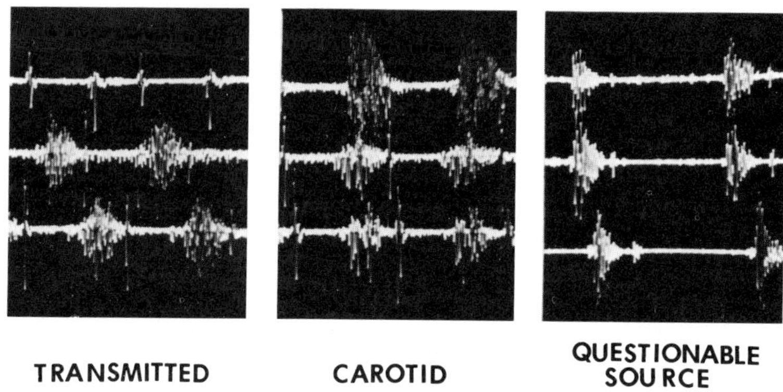

FIG. 23.2. Differentiating transmitted bruits from carotid bifurcation bruits. (The *top*, *middle*, and *bottom* recordings are from the angle of the jaw, area of the bifurcation, and base of the neck, respectively.)

maximal at the base of the neck or equal throughout the carotid distribution are of probable noncarotid origin. Pitch is also helpful in determining the origin of the bruit since the higher frequencies fade more rapidly with distance from the underlying stenosis. Using split-trace carotid phonoangiography (Fig. 23.3), higher frequencies are selectively shown above the baseline and indicate close proximity to the underlying stenosis.

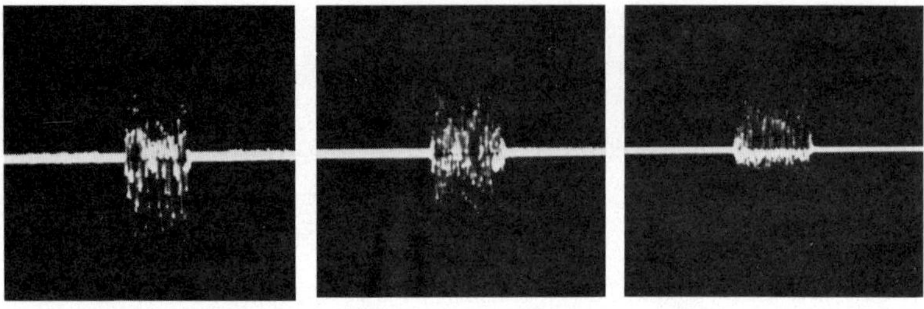

FIG. 23.3. Split-trace carotid phonoangiography (CPA) representation of bruits with emphasis on higher frequencies above and lower frequencies below the baseline.

High-pitched bruits which are not pansystolic usually originate from the external carotid artery. However, in general, except for diastolic bruits, there are no general rules for distinguishing external carotid from internal carotid or common carotid bruits.

Incorrectly interpreted by some as significant carotid bruits are venous murmurs, late systole bruits in young patients, and cardiac murmurs heard over the course of the cervical carotid arteries. For the remainder of this discussion, **cervical bruit** relates to any of the many murmurs or bruits that one might hear in auscultation over the neck, whereas **significant carotid bruit** is reserved for pansystolic bruits with maximal duration at or above the carotid bifurcation.

"ASYMPTOMATIC" BRUIT

In evaluating 4,000 patients for asymptomatic cervical bruits we found cervical bruits with total absence of neurologic symptoms in 590 (7). An additional 697 had generalized nonhemispheric or vertebral basilar neurologic symptoms, such as dizziness, lightheadedness, blackout, drop attack, or bilateral transient visual disturbance. Clinical follow-up of these patients ranged from 6 to 70 months with an average of 24 months. No significant difference was noted in the development of transient ischemic attacks (TIAs) or stroke when comparing patients with total absence of neurologic symptoms and those with nonhemispheric neurologic symptoms. In referring to "asymptomatic" bruit patients, therefore, we include all patients without present or past transient lateralized or fixed neurologic deficits.

HEMODYNAMICALLY SIGNIFICANT STENOSIS

A stenosis narrowing the internal carotid artery lumen by at least 40% is generally required to reduce blood flow and produce a pansystolic bruit.

However, even 40% stenosis will not result in blood flow reduction or pressure gradient if the residual lumen has a diameter greater than 2.5 mm (1).

From Fig. 23.4 note that a 40% diameter stenosis corresponds to a 64% reduction in cross-sectional area. Further note that a 70% diameter stenosis corresponds to a 91% area reduction. It is often unclear in the literature and in medical reports whether 70% stenosis refers to diameter or cross-sectional area. For noninvasively evaluating the hemodynamic significance of carotid bruits, we use our version of oculoplethysmography, or OPG, consisting of the differential time delay analysis of ocular pulses recorded from a fluid-filled system (8). This OPG method is sensitive to 40% stenosis if the lumen is less than 2.5 mm in contrast to most other noninvasive hemodynamic tests which are sensitive at the 70% diameter stenosis level.

A stenosis of from 40 to 70% should alert patients and physicians alike to the possibility of focal TIAs, and more frequent noninvasive testing should be used to determine the stability or progressive nature of such stenoses. Arteriography is not generally indicated at this level of stenosis except for specific symptoms.

Plaques causing greater than 70% diameter stenosis (greater than 90%

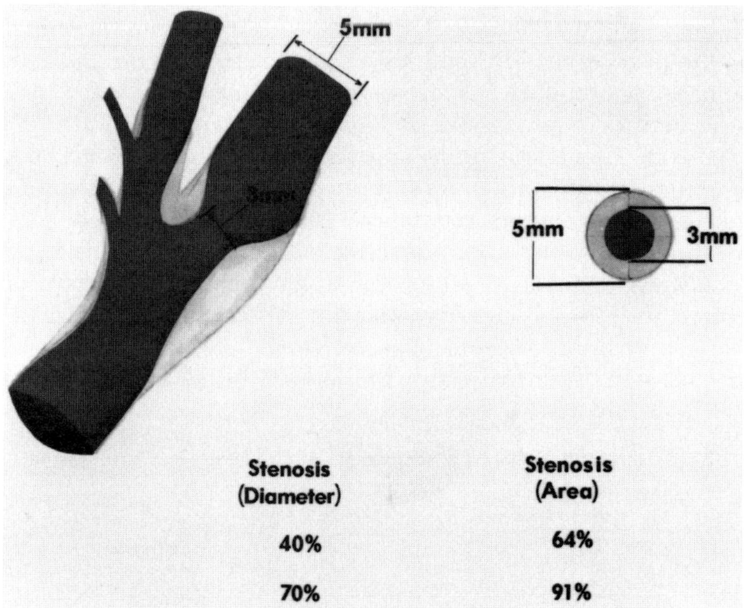

FIG. 23.4. Measurement of carotid stenosis by diameter compared to cross-sectional area.

reduction in cross-sectional area) have a profound influence on blood flow through the affected internal carotid artery. The potential for embolic or ischemic neurologic symptoms is greatly increased by this degree of stenosis. Carotid surgery is generally indicated since it is not possible to follow the progression of such stenoses with sufficient confidence of preventing the stroke which occurs without recognized antecedent symptoms.

It is important to detect asymptomatic bruits early and follow them objectively to determine the rate of progression, because rapidly developing plaques have a greater potential for releasing emboli, and collateral circulation may not keep pace with the rate of plaque development.

We have devised a grading chart for roughly quantifying carotid stenoses and following their progression (Table 23.1). Patients in grades 1 and 2 are generally treated similarly except for the frequency of follow-up. Grade 5 represents those patients severely positive by oculoplethysmography but without significant bruit. Grade 4 constitutes the bulk of patients who have both significant bruit and hemodynamically and clinically significant stenosis.

PROTOCOL FOR "ASYMPTOMATIC" BRUITS

Asymptomatic bruit patients may be divided into two major categories by noninvasive oculoplethysmographic evaluation—those that are negative or only mildly positive by OPG (grades 1 and 2) and those in grade 4 who are positive by OPG and have significant bruit (Fig. 23.5). Those in the negative group we elect to follow, watching carefully for transient ischemic attacks or progression noted by subsequent OPG/CPA. We feel that those asymptomatic bruits which are positive in a grade 4 category merit strong consideration for arteriography in anticipation of endarterectomy if the appropriate stenotic lesion is demonstrated.

Since many consider a carotid bruit a prestroke lesion, is it safe to follow asymptomatic bruits which do not have associated flow reduction and therefore are not hemodynamically significant? In our review of asymptomatic bruit patients followed from 3 to 70 months without endarterectomy, those patients with cervical bruits and with negative

TABLE 23.1

Kartchner/McRae Scoring Chart for Internal Carotid Occlusive Disease

Grade	CPA (Stenosis)	OPG (Flow reduction)	Interval follow-up
1	<40%	<20%	12 mo
2	40–60%	20–30%	6–12 mo
3	60–70%	30–40%	3–6 mo
4	70–85%	>40%	Arteriography or 2–4 mo
5	85–100% (no bruit)	>40%	Clinical judgement

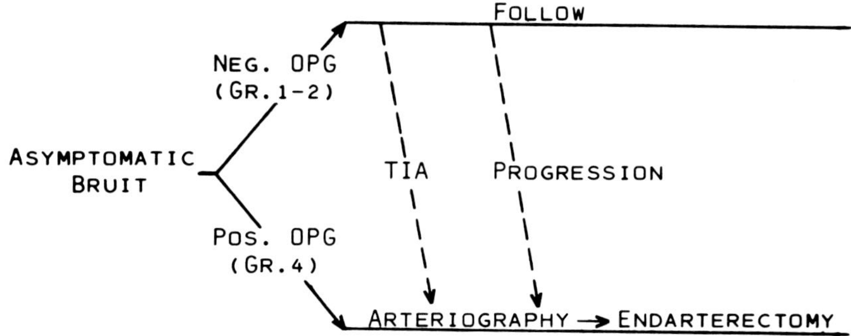

FIG. 23.5. Approach to the "asymptomatic" bruit.

OPG demonstrated a 0.7% incidence of stroke of apparent carotid origin (Table 23.2). Further narrowing this group and reviewing only those with pansystolic bifurcation bruit and negative OPG, there is still a stroke incidence of only 1.1%. This clearly demonstrates that patients being evaluated for asymptomatic carotid bruits, even those with a pansystolic carotid bruit, who do not have associated flow reduction, can be safely followed with minimal stroke risk over a significant period of time.

The 0.7% stroke incidence for cervical bruits negative by OPG/CPA contrasts vividly with the 20.4% incidence of strokes in patients with greater than 70% stenosis (grade 4) by OPG. This clearly indicates a very significant risk of stroke in those asymptomatic bruit patients with a grade 4 or greater than 70% stenosis by OPG. Hence, in those centers with a low risk in arteriography and surgery, prophylactic carotid endarterectomy would appear to be warranted for this group.

Grade 5 patients are those with markedly positive OPG and absence of significant bruit. Significant carotid bruit greatly increases the probability that the internal carotid is not totally occluded and that the stenotic lesion is localized to the carotid bifurcation. In our experience, there is 80% probability of surgical benefit for grade 4 patients which drops to 30% for grade 5 because of the higher incidence of total occlusion (Table 23.3). Obviously, all asymptomatic carotid bruit patients who have positive OPG are not candidates for surgery. Hence it is appropriate to review clinical background and the probability of surgical relief when considering prophylactic carotid endarterectomy.

PROGRESSION

The rate and degree of progression of stenosis underlying asymptomatic bruits can be validly documented by serial OPG/CPA evaluations. Arteriography is impractical for evaluating rapidly developing stenosis in "asymptomatic" patients, but we have a few patients with repeat arteri-

TABLE 23.2

"Asymptomatic" Bruit Patients Followed 3 to 70 Months without Endarterectomy (Average, 24 mo)

	Strokes of carotid origin*
Cervical bruits with negative OPG	0.7% (6/832)
Pansystolic carotid bruit with negative OPG	1.1% (1/91)
Pansystolic carotid bruit with >70% stenosis by OPG	20.4% (10/49)

* Strokes of obvious intracranial or cardiac derivation excluded.

TABLE 23.3

Anticipated Yield from Arteriography

OPG/CPA results	Stenotic surgical lesion (%)	Internal occlusion, external bruit (%)	Ophthalmic artery stenosis or false positive (%)
Grade 4 (significant bruit)	80	15	5
Grade 5 (no significant bruit)	30	55	15

ography which documents the accuracy of OPG/CPA for following progression. In 32 patients with progressively positive OPG/CPA and with repeat arteriography, we have observed an average increase of 53% degree of stenosis over an average 28-month interval. The minimal intervals for progression from grade 2 to grade 4 by OPG/CPA were 4 to 6 months. The value of serial baseline OPG/CPA studies to establish a trend upon which future follow-up studies can be recommended is clearly apparent.

Fig. 23.6 illustrates a patient first observed in an asymptomatic state with 30% stenosis. Fifteen months later OPG/CPA indicated greater than 70% stenosis and a diastolic bruit. Repeat arteriography demonstrated a 76% stenosis of the internal carotid artery.

ASYMPTOMATIC BRUITS AND MAJOR SURGERY

Another group of asymptomatic bruit patients at risk of stroke are those facing other major surgery. An evaluation of 234 patients prior to cardiovascular surgery indicated there is no increased risk of stroke in those patients with transient ischemic attacks or residual stroke deficit compared with those who were asymptomatic or had nonhemispheric symptoms (Table 23.4).

Fig. 23.7 clearly shows that the risk of perioperative stroke with major cardiovascular surgery is primarily related to the presence of a hemodynamically significant carotid stenosis. There were only two nonischemic strokes in 192 patients who had no OPG evidence of hemodynamic carotid stenosis as contrasted to seven ischemic strokes and two operative deaths in the 41 patients with significant flow reduction by OPG (grade 3 or greater).

It should be noted that only one ipsilateral and two contralateral pansystolic bruits were present relative to the positive OPG in seven perioperative ischemic strokes demonstrating the ineffectiveness of auscultation alone for detecting stroke risk in these patients. In our opinion, any patient undergoing major blood loss, hypotension, or hypoxia will be at risk of stroke in the presence of positive OPG demonstrating a hemodynamically significant carotid stenosis. We believe these noninvasive studies to be a good prognosticator of the relative risk of stroke in patients undergoing major surgery.

RISK OF ULCERATIVE LESIONS IN "ASYMPTOMATIC" BRUIT PATIENTS

The question has been raised as to whether the inability of the current noninvasive techniques to detect nonstenotic ulcerative lesions constitutes a major deficiency of these noninvasive testing modalities. It is our opinion that ulcerative lesions are important in terms of their clinical

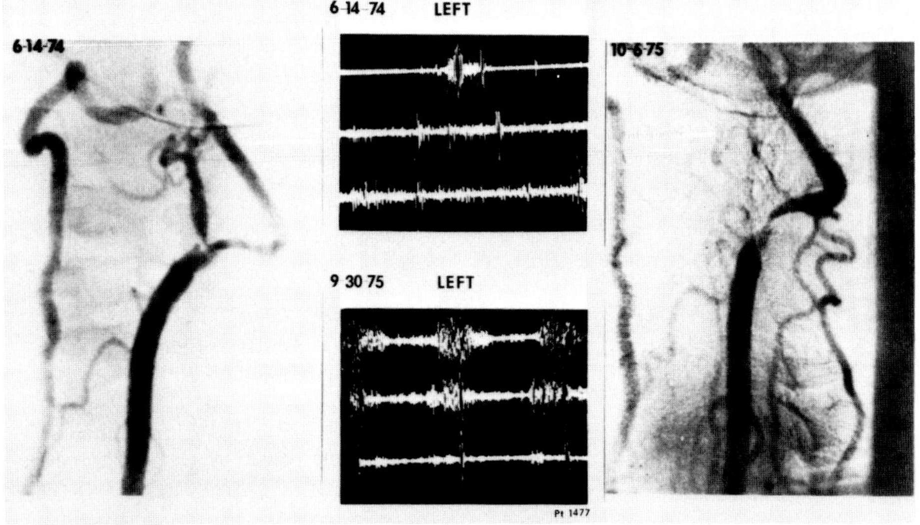

FIG. 23.6. Rapid progression of asymptomatic bruit and underlying stenosis.

TABLE 23.4
Evaluation of 234 Patients prior to Cardiovascular Surgery

Neurologic symptoms	Patients	Perioperative strokes
Asymptomatic	110	4
Nonhemispheric symptoms	64	4
Transient ischemic attacks	42	1
Residual stroke deficit	18	0

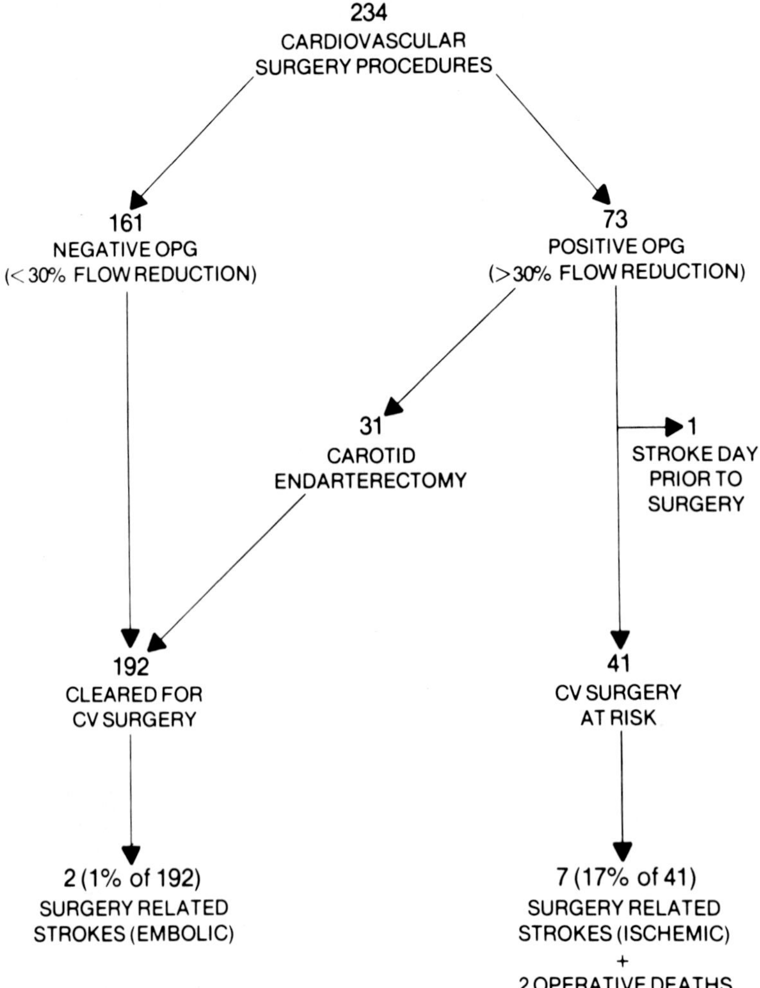

FIG. 23.7. Flow chart of OPG evaluations prior to cardiovascular surgery and perioperative strokes.

manifestations and are rarely of significance in the asymptomatic patient unless associated with an underlying hemodynamic stenosis. This has been well demonstrated by the relative safety in following a large number of patients who do not have associated flow-reducting lesions as contrasted to the high risk in those patients followed with a marked stenosis (Table 23.2). Hence, in ulcerative lesions it seems safe to await the onset of symptoms or progression to significant stenosis before pursuing invasive diagnostic measures. The newer noninvasive ultrasound imaging techniques show promise for demonstrating nonhemodynamic and ulcerative lesions but the results of Table 23.2 suggest that the decision for carotid endarterectomy in asymptomatic patients should still rely heavily on OPG/CPA.

SUMMARY

Basic recommendations for follow-up utilizing OPG/CPA results are as follows:

Grade 1: Repeat studies in 12 months in the absence of specific focal TIAs or increase of bifurcation level bruit.

Grade 2: Serial studies in 6 to 12 months in the absence of focal TIAs which provide their own indications for evaluation. If stability is established, 12-month interval testing is adequate.

Grade 3: Serial studies in 3 to 6 months until a progression trend is established. Anticipation of major surgery with possible hypotension or severe blood loss is an indication for arteriography and possible endarterectomy.

Grade 4: If repeat studies confirm grade 4 status, prophylactic carotid arteriography and endarterectomy should be seriously considered. If surgery is not employed, repeat OPG/CPA evaluations at 2 to 4 month intervals detects further progression toward total occlusion.

Grade 5: Indications for arteriography in anticipation of surgery are tempered by the lower probability (30%) of a surgically correctable stenosis and the clinical status of the patient

In conclusion, we feel that OPG/CPA represents one valid means of noninvasively evaluating the presence and underlying hemodynamic significance of an asymptomatic bruit with sufficient reliability to justify angiography and prophylactic carotid endarterectomy on the basis of appropriate findings.

REFERENCES

1. Brice, J. G., Dowsett, D. J., and Lowe, R. D. Haemodynamic effects of carotid artery stenosis. Br. Med. J., *2:* 1363, 1964.
2. Carney, W. I., Stewart, W. B., DePinto, D. J., *et al.* Carotid bruit as a risk factor in aortoiliac reconstruction. Surgery, *81* (5): 567–570, 1977.
3. Evans, W. E., and Cooperman, M. The significance of asymptomatic unilateral carotid bruits in preoperative patients. Surgery, *80:* 521–522, 1978.
4. Fields, W. S. Current concepts of cerebrovascular disease—stroke: the asymptomatic carotid bruit-operate or not? Stroke, *XIII:* January–February, 1978.
5. Grindal, A. B., and Toole, J. F. Surgical treatment of carotid and vertebral artery disease: an updating to 1974. Ann. Intern. Med., *81:* 647, 1974.

6. Javid, H., Ostermiller, W. E., Hengesh, J. W., *et al.* Carotid endarterectomy for asymptomatic patients. Arch. Surg., *102:* 389, 1971.
7. Kartchner, M. M., and McRae, L. P. Noninvasive evaluation and management of the "asymptomatic" carotid bruit. Surgery, *82* (6): 840–847, 1977.
8. Kartchner, M. M., McRae, L. P., Crain, V., and Whitaker, B. Oculoplethysmography: an adjunct to arteriography in the diagnosis of extracranial carotid occlusive disease. Am. J. Surg. *132*, December 1976.
9. Thompson, J. E., Patman, R. D., and Persson, A. V. Management of asymptomatic carotid bruits. Am. Surg., *42* (2), February 1976.

CHAPTER

24

Neurosurgical Applications of the Cyanoacrylate Adhesives

BRUCE E. MICKEY, M.D., and DUKE SAMSON, M.D.

The rapid development of the technology of synthetic organic polymers in the period since World War II has produced a wealth of plastics and adhesives which have revolutionized modern industry and manufacturing. Relatively few of these compounds have been accepted for permanent implantation in humans due to the inherent cytotoxicity of many synthetic organic compounds and solvents, their potential carcinogenicity, and the requirement that they perform reliably over time periods as long as the human life span. In neurosurgery, the use of compounds which could be applied in liquid form to harden *in situ* was stimulated by the search for materials for reinforcing aneurysms. The first materials used for this purpose were awkward to apply and have not received general acceptance. The cyanoacrylate adhesives which provide ease of application and what was initially felt to be lack of histotoxicity have been widely investigated in a number of neurosurgical settings. Initially used to reinforce aneurysms and to seal cerebrospinal fluid leaks, they have recently been evaluated as liquid emboli for intracranial and intraspinal vascular lesions.

The Cyanoacrylate Adhesives

The cyanoacrylate adhesives are a group of homologous organic monomers which undergo a rapid addition polymerization in the presence of weak bases, including water (8, 41). When interposed between two surfaces in the liquid monomeric state, these adhesives thoroughly "wet" them both, then solidify by polymerizing, bonding them together. Modern adhesive theory holds that the strength of an adhesive bond lies in *van der Waals* forces attracting closely opposed molecules of adhesive and adherend, not in a chemical reaction between the two (65). Chemical bonding, when present, may improve flexibility, water resistance, or other secondary characteristics of the adhesive bond. Rapid hardening by polymerization is the mechanism by which the cyanoacrylates function in neurosurgery, both as adhesives and as structural plastics for reinforcing or embolizing vascular lesions.

The tendency of the pure cyanoacrylate monomers to polymerize on contacting atmospheric moisture or a variety of surfaces renders their storage and application in this form impractical. The medical grade cyanoacrylates which have been studied in a neurosurgical setting (Fig. 24.1) are all pure monomers, to which an acidic inhibitor, usually sulphur dioxide, has been added. The commercial grade cyanoacrylates, marketed under several names as "super" glues, usually contain the methyl and ethyl monomers, plus a variety of plasticizers and stabilizers.

The individual cyanoacrylate monomers, distinguished by their alkyl side chains, differ significantly in their physical and chemical properties and in their biological activity. A series of investigations conducted on the sulphur dioxide-inhibited pure monomers at Walter Reed has revealed that the polymerization time of a single drop of monomer placed on an aqueous solution (Table 24.1) and the bond strength of the polymer to proteinaceous substrates increase as the length of the alkyl side chain increases (8, 45). Polymerization times on protein-containing solutions, the rate of hydrolytic degradation, and histotoxicity in animal models, tend to decrease as the side chain lengthens (41, 42). *In vitro* in aqueous solutions, and *in vivo*, the polymers are degraded by a hydrolytic mechanism to formaldehyde and the appropriate alkylcyanoacetate (42, 71). As noted above, the rate of this degradation decreases as the side chain lengthens, so that in extracranial implantation studies in animals the methyl polymer is completely degraded in 4 to 8 weeks (36, 76) while 50% of the initial mass of the butyl polymer remains at 2 years (39). Although the structural integrity of none of the currently available cyanoacrylate

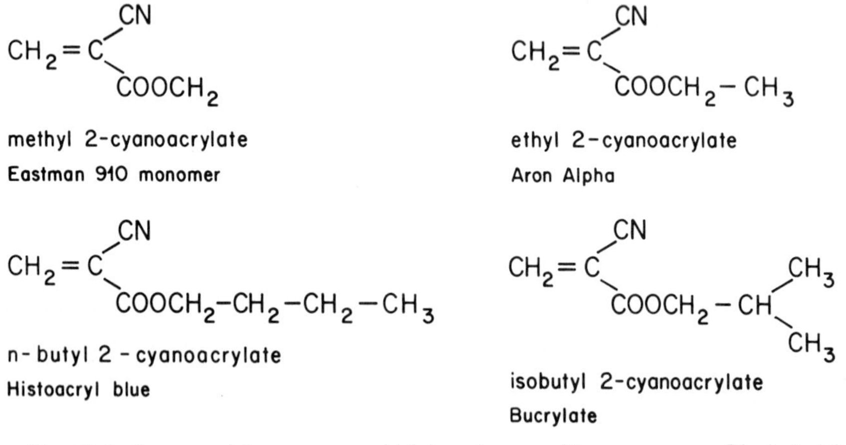

$CH_2{=}C(CN)\text{—}COOCH_2$

methyl 2-cyanoacrylate
Eastman 910 monomer

$CH_2{=}C(CN)\text{—}COOCH_2{-}CH_3$

ethyl 2-cyanoacrylate
Aron Alpha

$CH_2{=}C(CN)\text{—}COOCH_2{-}CH_2{-}CH_2{-}CH_3$

n-butyl 2-cyanoacrylate
Histoacryl blue

$CH_2{=}C(CN)\text{—}COOCH_2{-}CH(CH_3)(CH_3)$

isobutyl 2-cyanoacrylate
Bucrylate

FIG. 24.1. Cyanoacrylate monomers which have been used in neurosurgery. The isobutyl monomer (Bucrylate, Ethicon, Inc., Somerville, N.J.) is currently available in the United States for investigational use. The similar *n*-butyl monomer (Histoacryl blue, B. Braun Melsungen AG, Melsungen, West Germany) is marketed in Europe.

TABLE 24.1
*Average Spreadability and Polymerization Times for Water and Citrated Blood**

Monomer	H_2O (pH 7.1)		Citrated blood	
	Spreadability (cm)	Polymerization (sec)	Spreadability (cm)	Polymerization (sec)
Methyl	20	10	0.5	>300
Ethyl	14.5	10	0.5	>300
n-Propyl	10	10	2	20
n-Butyl	18	10	5	1
n-Amyl	16	15	14	2
n-Hexyl	16	64	14	2.5
n-Heptyl	20	>300	11	2
n-Octyl	18	>300	15	4

* After Leonard (41).

polymers can be relied upon permanently, they are replaced by connective tissue in the process of their degradation.

The more rapid *in vivo* hydrolysis of the lower cyanoacrylate homologues, by producing higher local concentrations of formaldehyde and the alkylcyanoacetates, probably underlies their greater histotoxicity. It was noted initially that methyl 2-cyanoacrylate elicits a marked acute inflammatory response, which subsides to be replaced by a dense fibrotic reaction as the polymer is degraded. The benign appearance of this fibroblastic response, and the capacity of injured tissues for self-repair, led some early investigators, looking only for evidence of long-term cytotoxicity, to overestimate the safety of the methyl and ethyl monomers (4, 7). Further studies in the rabbit, cat, dog, and chimpanzee revealed that surface application of the methyl monomer can produce cortical neuronal necrosis, demyelination of peripheral and optic nerves, and transmural necrosis of peripheral and intracranial arteries (17, 35, 38, 69, 74). In 1966 Sachs *et al.* (58) reported a fatal rebleed in the early postoperative period after coating an aneurysm with methyl 2-cyanoacrylate; a recent acute necrosis of the wall of the aneurysm was noted at autopsy. On the basis of chronic toxicity studies in the rabbit and cat, ethyl 2-cyanoacrylate was recommended for the reinforcement of intracranial aneurysms (7). The appearance of reports implicating this monomer in postoperative arterial thrombosis (6, 47) and two reports of visual impairment following its use to coat ophthalmic artery aneurysms (6) prompted reevaluation of its toxicity. In a later report, cats examined 2 weeks after cortical application of the ethyl monomer revealed neuronal and axonal degeneration and vascular wall necrosis (12).

The most thorough investigation of the intracranial toxicity of the cyanoacrylates is that conducted by Lehman and Hayes (38) at Walter Reed with the sulphur dioxide-inhibited pure methyl, ethyl, *n*-propyl, isobutyl, and *n*-octyl monomers. Using a fronto-temporal approach to the optic chiasm in rhesus monkeys (weighing from 2.1 to 5.7 kg), 0.2 to 0.3 ml of the liquid monomer was dropped on the superolateral aspect of the chiasm so as to coat the anterior communicating artery complex and the origin of the middle cerebral artery. Frequent deaths, usually preceded by a period of coma lasting from the time of operation, were noted in the methyl and ethyl groups. In the survivors, the incidence of demyelination in the optic chiasm and frontal cortex and of vascular wall necrosis in the circle of Willis was much greater with the ethyl monomer than with the higher homologues. Intimal proliferation and thrombosis in small perforating vessels were thought to underlie the postoperative deaths and the deep frontal lobe lesions noted in some survivors. While the higher homologues were shown to be safer than the methyl and ethyl monomers, all of the monomers tested produced significant CNS injury.

The results of acute toxicity studies performed on animals with cyanoacrylates cannot be directly extrapolated to man. While application of the methyl and ethyl monomers to the circle of Willis produced frequent fatalities in rhesus monkeys due to occlusion of perforating vessels (38), these same monomers have been reported for human use in this region to coat aneurysms with minimal morbidity and mortality (4, 7, 48, 75). The greater caliber and wall thickness of the human perforators and the more deliberate surgical application of the adhesive probably accounts for much of the difference in this case. The relative toxicities of these monomers can be accurately assessed from animal studies. Lehman and Hayes (38) found the isobutyl monomer to be significantly less toxic to neural and vascular tissue than the methyl and ethyl monomers. They found no significant difference between the toxicities of the *n*-propyl, isobutyl, and *n*-octyl monomers, but noted that the isobutyl monomer had the optimal polymerization speed for clinical use. Extracranial animal studies at the same institution have revealed that the *n*-butyl and isobutyl monomers are similar in histotoxicity and speed of polymerization (2, 36).

The chronic toxicity of the cyanoacrylates for man, specifically their carcinogenic potential, is difficult to evaluate due to the long latent period proposed for plastic carcinogens in man (28). Polymethylmethacrylate, structurally similar to the cyanoacrylate polymers (Fig. 24.2), produces

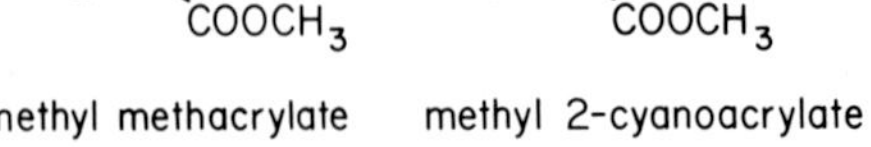

$$CH_2{=}C(CH_3)COOCH_3 \qquad CH_2{=}C(CN)COOCH_3$$

methyl methacrylate — methyl 2-cyanoacrylate

FIG. 24.2. The structural similarity between methyl methacrylate and methyl 2-cyanoacrylate.

local sarcomas in rats when implanted intramuscularly, subcutaneously, or intraperitonally as discs (28). A mechanism of physical carcinogenesis has been proposed as an etiology for these tumors, which may be related more to the size and shape of the implants than to their chemical makeup (28, 55). Despite widespread use in cranioplasties and total joint replacements, polymethylmethacrylate has not been causally related to any human malignancy (55). The butyl cyanoacrylate monomers and polymers have not proven carcinogenic in animals (38). Humans have been exposed to various cyanoacrylates intraperitoneally and intracranially since the 1960's, without developing evidence of an increased risk for neoplasms in these areas. The cyanoacrylate monomers and polymers are probably not carcinogenic in man, but greater experience with their use must be accumulated before definite conclusions can be reached.

Of the currently available cyanoacrylates, the butyl monomers are the safest for clinical use. The rapid polymerization times of these monomers in both aqueous (CSF) and protein-containing (blood) environments makes them valuable both as adhesives and as liquid emboli. Firm adhesion, when desired, requires a dry field, as a thin film of interposed blood or CSF will prevent adequate contact between the polymer and a surface. The butyl monomer available in the United States, isobutyl 2-cyanoacrylate (Bucrylate, Ethicon, Inc., Sommerville, N. J.) is approved by the Food and Drug Administration for investigational use only. The medical use of commercial cyanoacrylate adhesives, which usually contain the more toxic methyl and ethyl monomers, in addition to unknown additives, should be avoided.

The Reinforcement of Intracranial Aneurysms

The risk of repeat subarachnoid hemorrhage is maximum within the first 3 weeks of an initial aneurysmal bleed but persists throughout the remainder of the patient's life. A clip or ligature which excludes the aneurysm from the circulation offers both immediate and indefinite protection against rebleeding and is therefore considered optimal treatment. Occasionally, due to the broadness of its neck or the proximity of large atherosclerotic plaques or essential vessels, an aneurysm cannot be safely clipped or ligated. Because it is often not possible to identify these aneurysms preoperatively, an alternate form of therapy should be available at each operation.

Theoretically, an adherent patch applied so as to cover the point at which the aneurysm had ruptured would offer some protection against rebleeding. Such a technique would not prevent further growth of the aneurysm at its neck, nor would it prevent rupture at some other thin-walled portion of the dome. Complete encasement of an aneurysm and its parent vessel would reinforce the fundus at all points and prevent both rupture and further growth. Clinical experience with various techniques and materials used to reinforce aneurysms supports these concepts.

In 1933 Norman Dott (13) reported the first planned operation for an intracranial aneurysm, wrapping it with gauze into which bits of muscle had been hammered. Dott proposed that his muscle and gauze wrapping would provide a framework for fibrous encasement of the aneurysm, preventing enlargement and rupture. Attempts at reinforcing aneurysm with bits of muscle have been unsuccessful; Drake reported three fatal bleeds in six patients so treated (15). Theoretically, any wrapping which relied on a reactive fibrosis for its strength would provide some protection once this process was complete. Such a process would not be effective immediately and therefore would not be able to prevent rebleeding in the time period shortly after rupture. Gillingham (21), in 1958, proposed covering aneurysms with small squares of fine mesh cotton gauze or muslin. Although one would not predict early protection from this procedure, two investigators have recently reported good long-term results with its use. Taylor and Choudhury (67) in 1977 reported 35 patients whose ruptured middle cerebral artery aneurysms had been completely dissected then wrapped with small pieces of muslin gauze. They noted one fatal rebleed on postoperative day 5 but no further bleeding in 31 survivors followed 2 to 15 years. Mount and Antunes treated 21 aneurysms unsuitable for clipping using a similar technique with no documented postoperative bleeds during a varying follow-up period (50).

Dutton in 1956 reported the first clinical experience using a plastic substance, methyl methacrylate, to encase intracranial aneurysms (18). His technique, which required a dry field and experience in the preparation of the compound, was criticized because the resulting encasement was rigid and nonadherent. Selverstone and Ronis (62) in 1958 reported the development of a strong and flexible adherent coating for aneurysms. Their elaborate technique involved spraying the aneurysm with a latex emulsion using an artist's airbrush, then coating it with an epoxy-polyamide resin using a spatula. Both methods, while unwieldy, have proven effective. Dutton later reported the use of methyl methacrylate in 106 cases followed 1 to 10 years with no rebleeds (16). Hayes and Leaver (24) have reported its use in 40 patients followed from 3 to 7 years with no rebleeds. Selverstone (61) reports that he has used his technique to coat "approximately 200 aneurysms" and that "rebleeding after an aneurysm has been fully coated has not been documented." The phenomenon of adherence has played a large role in the development of plastic compounds for the reinforcement of aneurysms. The good results achieved with methyl methacrylate would suggest that adherence is not necessary when an aneurysm is completely encased. Incomplete encasement with nonadherent compounds, however, can be dangerous. Todd and Crue (68) using a nonadhering, rapid hardening silicone rubber in 18 cases noted two rebleeds. In one the intact rubber jacket was found to have "blown off" the aneurysm as it ruptured.

The search for an adherent coating which obviates the need for complete encasement has centered on the cyanoacrylate glues. As noted earlier these substances adhere well to dry surfaces, but all are histotoxic to some degree and all are biodegradable. Methyl 2-cyanoacrylate, the first monomer used clinically, was abandoned after numerous reports of histotoxicity in animals. Realizing its potential as an adhesive, Handa *et al.* (23) incorporated this monomer with a nitrile rubber and a polyisocyanate to form a compound "EDH adhesive" (Biobond). Although minimally histotoxic, this compound was noted in one study to become pliable and nonadherent 3 months after intracranial application in the rabbit (76). Handa reported the use of Biobond in 42 cases over a 6-year period with one recurrent hemorrhage, due, he felt, to incomplete coating of the fundus (23). There have been other clinical reports of its successful use (66).

In 1967 ethyl 2-cyanoacrylate (Aron Alpha) was reported to be superior to Biobond in long-term adherence and ease of application (75). Chou *et al.* (7) reported its use in 42 aneurysms with one rebleed, believed to be due to incomplete coating of the dome. Reports of human and animal toxicity, discussed earlier, have raised doubts about the safety the application of this monomer in the vicinity of the optic chiasm or the anterior communicating artery (6, 12, 38).

As noted earlier, extensive testing of the cyanoacrylates at Walter Reed has revealed the butyl monomer to be the least histotoxic. Studies performed in our laboratory on the internal carotid artery-posterior communicating artery junction in the dog have confirmed their claim that optimal adherence requires a dry surface (Mickey and Samson, unpublished data). When applied to the moist vessel wall, the glue in many cases polymerizes on a film of moisture, leaving a nonadherent cast which flakes off with ease. Drying the vessel wall with air blown from a commercial hairdryer seems to improve adhesion. Some authors have mentioned the use of this monomer for the reinforcement of unclippable aneurysms (64, 73), but no one has reported extensive experience with it for this application.

The value of the cyanoacrylate glues in the reinforcement of aneurysms is uncertain. One or two drops of glue applied to the moist dome of an aneurysm may deceptively appear to firmly surround it in plastic, but in many cases this coating will be nonadherent and will not completely encase the lesion. There have been numerous reports of rebleeding following incomplete reinforcement of aneurysms with both adherent and nonadherent plastics (7, 23, 50, 61, 68). Attention paid to drying the surfaces of the aneurysm and parent artery may permit firm adhesion, but one is then faced with the problem of completely coating it without applying a histotoxic material to the optic nerve, or to small but essential perforating vessels. The minimal toxicity of the butyl monomers is encouraging, but one should recall that both the methyl and ethyl monomers were felt to be safe until clinical experience suggested otherwise. Muslin gauze wrapping appears at this time to offer an effective method for reinforcing aneurysms pending further investigation of the cyanoacrylates.

Cerebrospinal Fluid Fistulae

For those cerebrospinal fluid leaks that require operative intervention, a variety of surgical approaches, both intracranial and extracranial, have been developed to seal the fistulous tract (25, 49, 52). Recurrences are high in those cases in which the site of fistula cannot be definitely identified. Most intracranial and some extracranial approaches to these fistulae are designed to identify and directly repair the underlying dural defect (3, 30). It is in these cases, which often require suturing synthetic or autogenous grafts to friable dura in an awkward exposure, that the use of tissue adhesives has proven to be of value. While several authors have reported successful repairs of CSF fistulae using tissue adhesives, investigators at Walter Reed have reported one of the largest series (40, 70). Using isobutyl 2-cyanoacrylate to seal grafts of lyophylized dura, pericranium, or fascia lata, in cases where sutures alone were felt to be inadequate, they reported one recurrence in 22 cases. There were two postoperative deaths attributed to preexisting meningitis. They emphasized the necessity of operating in a dry field, noting that bonding was poor or nonexistent in the presence of blood or CSF. Maxwell and Goldware (46) have since reported similar success using this adhesive in 12 cases.

While some extracranial approaches to CSF fistulae involve direct visualization and repair of the dural defect (29), others rely on obliterating the fistulous path through an involved sinus or bony defect using autogenous fat, cartilage, or muscle (5). The value of the cyanoacrylate adhesives in these latter cases is questionable. Due to the irregular surfaces involved and the difficulty of keeping them dry, the glue rarely forms an adherent bond despite its generous application. Young and Gates, using ethyl 2-cyanoacrylate to aid in reconstituting the sella floor following transsphenoidal hypophysectomy, noted postoperative CSF rhinorrhea in five of 28 cases, requiring reoperation in two (77). The incidence of this complication without the use of tissue adhesives is 3 to 6% in large series (22, 37). In our unpublished experience with the cyanoacrylate adhesives in transsphenoidal surgery, in those cases requiring reexploration the glue has been found in nonadherent flakes lying within the sphenoid sinus. We have seen one case of a fulminant (but asymptomatic) chemical osteitis of the body of the sphenoid 3 years after the application of a commercially obtained cyanoacrylate in the closure of a transsphenoidal hypophysectomy.

The use of the cyanoacrylates in the closure of CSF fistulae should be limited to the application of the medical grade butyl monomer in the direct repair of dural defects. These adhesives have not been proven effective in preventing CSF rhinorrhea following transsphenoidal hypophysectomy. The use of commercial grade adhesives containing histotoxic monomers or unknown additives may be unsafe.

Intravascular Applications of the Cyanoacrylates

ARTERIOVENOUS MALFORMATIONS

Of the arteriovenous malformations presently coming to clinical attention, 10 to 25% are not considered amenable to the optimal treatment, which is complete surgical excision (53, 54). Neurosurgeons and neuroradiologists have begun to study the effects of embolization of these malformations with a variety of substances. The arterial feeders of an AVM may be embolically occluded using various solid particles injected via a catheter placed in the internal carotid or vertebral artery. These occlusions are rarely permanent, as new feeders develop. Small catheters, capable of entering the feeding vessels directly, would theoretically allow the delivery of emboli into the fistula itself while preserving important parent vessels. Such catheters and techniques for their placement have now been developed, but due to the small diameters involved particulate embolization is not feasible, and has been replaced by liquid embolization with substances which can be made to polymerize and harden intravascularly. The first such substances used, the silicone rubbers, are viscous and require the addition of a catalyst to initiate polymerization (11, 26). Due to their low viscosity and rapid polymerization in blood, the cyanoacrylates appear to be better polymers for this purpose.

Isobutyl 2-cyanoacrylate (IBC), the least histotoxic of the cyanoacrylate monomers, polymerizes in 1 to 2 seconds on contacting blood. One study has reported vascular wall necrosis following the injection of IBC in the visceral circulation of the pig (72). It should be noted that commercial as well as medical formulations of this monomer were studied and that the authors did not comment on the differences in the histotoxicity of the two glues. Other studies in the cerebral and visceral vascular beds of humans and animals have revealed acutely only a mild inflammatory response, contained entirely within the vessel lumen (20, 64, 78).

On intravascular polymerization, IBC has been noted to entrap red blood cells within a sponge-like matrix (64). Chronically, a mild fibroblastic response ensues, so that these areas are noted to be filled with fibroblasts, collagen, and scattered foreign body giant cells at 2 months (20).

The addition of iophendylate (Pantopaque) to the IBC monomer in varying concentrations reproducibly prolongs its polymerization time (10). In addition to providing radiographic visualization of the polymer mass, this technique may enhance the obliteration of lower flow fistulae by enabling further penetration before polymerization takes place. Tantalum dust disbursed within the glue renders it radiopaque without altering its polymerization characteristics (10).

Kerber, a pioneer in the use of IBC for the transcatheter embolization of intracranial vascular lesions, recently reviewed his experience. Of 15 intracranial AVMs treated none were completely obliterated, but ischemic systems were improved, and in some cases, surgical removal was facilitated (32). He reported one parietal lobe infarction, and three cases in which catheters were glued into place without referable symptoms. Two of these catheters were subsequently removed. In his initial animal studies, occluding high-flow direct arteriovenous fistulae in dogs, enough of this polymer reached the dogs' lungs to cause three fatalities (31). By using a balloon-tipped catheter to occlude the arterial feeder being injected, he has been able to slow flow to prevent this complication (32). Kerber and others (34, 44) have reported similar results using these techniques to embolize spinal AVMs.

Due to the technical difficulty of catheterizing all of the arterial feeders of an AVM, especially those derived from the anterior and posterior cerebral arteries, transcatheter embolization has only rarely been reported to effect the complete obliteration of one of these lesions (19, 43, 56). Drake (14), using Pantopaque-soaked gelfoam pledgets (14), and Cromwell and Harris (9), using a 50% mixture of IBC and Pantopaque (9), have directly injected and embolized these feeders at craniotomy to facilitate surgical excision. The latter group reported the 30% obliteration of an AVM following direct injection without surgical excision. Samson *et al.* (59) have recently reported their experience with the direct injection of IBC in the management of AVMs in 10 patients. Four of these lesions were excised at the same operation. Of the six that were not amenable to resection, four were completely obliterated by injection alone, although one of these required reinjection at a second operation. No operative mortality and no permanent neurologic morbidity were noted.

Transcatheter embolization of intracranial and intraspinal AVMs with IBC appears to provide a safe method of improving ischemia-related symptomatology and facilitating surgical resection in selected cases. Direct injection of this polymer into the feeding vessels of an AVM at operation may prove to be an effective means of completely obliterating those lesions considered unresectable due to large size or critical location.

CAROTID-CAVERNOUS FISTULAE

Early operative approaches to carotid-cavernous fistulae attempted to decrease the arterial flow to the lesion by sacrificing the internal carotid artery (57). While often effective, these procedures were occasionally complicated by cerebral infarction and death (51). More recently, induced thrombosis of the venous portion of the fistula has been reported to be both highly effective and safe, while preserving normal internal carotid flow (27, 51). By introducing a variety of thrombogenic substances directly into the cavernous sinus, Mullan (51) has reported successful obliteration of 33 fistulae in 31 patients while sacrificing carotid patency in only one case. His elaborate technique, which involves a subtemporal approach to the lateral wall of the sinus, requires intraoperative angiography and a thorough familiarity with the anatomy of the region. Using a similar technique we have occluded four fistulae by directly injecting IBC into the cavernous sinus, maintaining carotid patency in all cases (60).

Recent advances in angiographic catheter technology have made it possible to approach the sinus indirectly, via the fistulous opening in the internal carotid artery in many cases, and via the jugular vein in some. Serbinenko (63) first reported the transarterial placement of a detachable balloon in the sinus to occlude a carotid-cavernous fistula. In the experience of Debrun *et al.* (11) this technique is not possible in most spontaneous fistulae and in some posttraumatic fistulae, due to the small size of the fistulous opening. He was able to enter 14 of 17 posttraumatic fistulae with a detachable balloon catheter and to maintain carotid patency in 12 cases. While Debrun has filled his balloons with a silicone polymer in most cases to maintain their volume, the detachable balloon technique does not involve the deposition of a free-flowing polymer into the sinus. Kerber *et al.* (33) have reported entering the sinus transarterially in three cases using a flow-guided microcatheter and injecting IBC to occlude the fistula. All three patients developed transient neurologic deficits consistent with cortical ischemia during or after the procedure.

All of the methods described above for occluding the venous component of a carotid-cavernous fistula while maintaining carotid patency are technically complex. Each owes its efficacy and safety to the extensive laboratory and clinical experience of the investigators employing it, not to the materials and techniques used. Isobutyl 2-cyanoacrylate has been injected both directly and transarterially into the cavernous sinus to effect fistula occlusion with good success, but in only a few cases with limited follow-up. Its usefulness and relative safety in this clinical setting has yet to be determined.

INTRACRANIAL ANEURYSMS

Despite the suitability of isobutyl 2-cyanoacrylate as an intravascular occlusive agent, its use in the obliteration or thrombosis of intracranial arterial aneurysms has proven to be technically difficult. Due to the fact that the glue "expands" as it polymerizes by the inclusion of red blood cells in its mass, it is difficult to estimate the volume of IBC required to completely fill an aneurysm. On the basis of their experience with intraluminal thrombosis with horse hair and wire, as well as with cyanoacrylate, Drake and Vanderlinden (15) concluded that incomplete occlusion of the aneurysm lumen does not protect against rebleeding. On the other hand, overfilling an aneurysm may occlude or embolize its parent vessel.

Sheptak *et al.* (64) reported their experience using IBC to occlude aneurysms thought to be unclippable by direct injection at craniotomy in 18 cases and by stereotactic injection in two cases. The volume of glue to be injected was estimated from the size of the aneurysm as it appeared on angiography. They noted one death in the immediate postoperative period due to a thrombosis extending from an overfilled internal carotid artery aneurysm. Of the 18 survivors, 11 had incompletely occluded aneurysms. Two nonfatal rebleeds and one fatal rebleed were noted in this group during a follow-up period of 1 to 6 years.

Alksne and Smith (1) have recently reported better results using iron powder dispersed in methyl methacrylate to stereotactically inject anterior communicating artery aneurysms in patients with medical problems thought to prohibit craniotomy. Using intraoperative angiography to monitor filling and a magnet to restrict the material to the lumen of the aneurysm, they reported complete occlusion in 17 of 22 cases with two cases of postoperative hemiparesis and no operative mortality. None of the 22 patients has rebled in a follow-up period ranging from 6 months to 4½ years.

Isobutyl 2-cyanoacrylate may be inferior to methylmethacrylate for the intraluminal occlusion of aneurysms because its rapid speed of polymerization requires that the total volume of glue used be injected as a single bolus. Using intraoperative angiography and a slowly polymerizing substance, it may some day be feasible to gradually occlude some aneurysms by direct injection at craniotomy or via transarterial catheterization. At the present time intraluminal occlusion with polymeric plastics is a highly experimental procedure.

SUMMARY

The cyanoacrylate adhesives are a biologically heterogenous group, some of which are potentially valuable additions to the neurosurgical armamentarium. The commercially available cyanoacrylates usually contain the more toxic methyl and ethyl monomers. The safer butyl monomer, isobutyl 2-cyanoacrylate, is approved in the United States by the Food and Drug Administration for investigational use only. Isobutyl 2-cyanoacrylate may prove to be useful for the extravascular reinforcement of intracranial aneurysms and for the intravascular occlusion of carotid-cavernous fistulae. Safe and effective alternatives exist for the management of these two problems. The sealing of certain cerebrospinal fluid fistulae and the intravascular occlusion of certain arteriovenous malformations may be more effectively accomplished with isobutyl 2-cyanoacrylate than with other currently available techniques. The ultimate role of this and of other as yet untested cyanoacrylates in neurosurgery remains to be determined.

REFERENCES

1. Alksne, J. F., and Smith, R. W. Stereotaxic occlusion of 22 consecutive anterior communicating artery aneurysms. J. Neurosurg., *52:* 790–793, 1980.
2. Bhaskar, S. N. Butyl cyanoacrylate as a surface adhesive in human oral wounds. *In* Adhesion in Biological Systems, edited by R. S. Manly, pp. 201–208. Academic Press, New York, 1970.
3. Calcaterra, T. C. Extracranial surgical repair of cerebrospinal rhinorrhea. Ann. Otol. Rhinol. Laryngol., *89:* 108–116, 1980.
4. Carton, C. A., Kennady, J. C., Heifetz, M. D., and Ross-Duggan, J. K. The use of a plastic adhesive (methyl 2-cyanoacrylate monomer) in the management of intracranial aneurysms and leaking cerebral vessels: a report of 15 cases. *In* Intracranial Aneurysms and Subarachnoid Hemorrhage: A Cooperative Study, edited by A. L. Sahs and W. S. Fields, pp. 372–443. Charles C Thomas, Springfield, Ill., 1965.
5. Charles, D. A., and Snell, D. Cerebrospinal fluid rhinorrhea. Laryngoscope, *89:* 822–826, 1980.
6. Chou, S. N. Use of cyanoacrylates (Letter). J. Neurosurg., *46:* 266, 1977.
7. Chou, S. N., Ortiz-Suarez, H. J., and Brown, W. E. Technique and material for coating aneurysms. Clin. Neurosurg., *21:* 182–193, 1974.
8. Collins, J. A., Pani, K. C., Lehman, R. A., and Leonard, F. Biological substrates and cure rates of cyanoacrylate tissue adhesives. Arch. Surg., *93:* 428–432, 1966.
9. Cromwell, L. D., and Harris, A. B. Treatment of cerebral arteriovenous malformations: a combined neurosurgical and neuroradiological approach. J. Neurosurg., *52:* 705–708, 1980.
10. Cromwell, L. D., and Kerber, C. W. Modification of cyanoacrylate for therapeutic embolization: preliminary experience. A.J.R., *132:* 799–801, 1979.
11. Debrun, G., Lacour, P., Caron, J. P., Hurth, M., Comoy, J., and Keravel, Y. Detachable balloon and calibrated-leak balloon techniques in the treatment of cerebral vascular lesions. J. Neurosurg., *49:* 635–649, 1978.
12. Diaz, F. G., Mastri, A. R., and Chou, S. N. Neural and vascular tissue reaction to aneurysm-coating adhesive (ethyl 2-cyanoacrylate). Neurosurgery, *3:* 45–49, 1978.
13. Dott, N. M. Intracranial aneurysms: cerebral arterio-radiography: surgical treatment. Edin. Med. J., *40:* 219–234, 1932–1933.
14. Drake, C. G. Cerebral arteriovenous malformations: considerations for and experience with surgical treatment in 166 cases. Clin. Neurosurg., *26:* 145–208, 1979.
15. Drake, C. G., and Vanderlinden, R. G. The later consequences of incomplete surgical treatment of cerebral aneurysms. J. Neurosurg., *27:* 226–238, 1967.

16. Dutton, J. Acrylic investment of intracranial aneurysms. A report of 12 years' experience. J. Neurosurg., *31:* 652–657, 1969.
17. Dutton, J., and Yates, P. O. An experimental study of the effects of a plastic adhesive, methyl 2-cyanoacrylate monomer (M2C-1) in various tissues. J. Neurosurg., *24:* 876–882, 1966.
18. Dutton, J. E. Intracranial aneurysm. A new method of surgical treatment. Br. Med. J., *2:* 585–586, 1956.
19. Fox, J. L., Al-Mefty, O. Embolization of an arteriovenous malformation of the brain stem. Surg. Neurol., *8*(1): 7–9, 1977.
20. Freeny, P. C., Mennemeyer, R., Kidd, C. R., and Bush, W. H. Long-term radiographic-pathologic follow-up of patients treated with visceral transcatheter occlusion using isobutyl 2-cyanoacrylate (bucrylate). Radiology, *132:* 51–60, 1979.
21. Gillingham, F. J. The management of ruptured intracranial aneurysm. Hunterian lecture. Ann. R. Coll. Surg. Engl., *23:* 89–117, 1958.
22. Hamlin, H. The case for transsphenoidal approach to hypophysial tumors. J. Neurosurg., *19:* 1000–1003, 1962.
23. Handa, H., Ohta, T., and Kamijyo, Y. Encasement of intracranial aneurysms with plastic compounds. Prog. Neurol. Surg., *3:* 149–192, 1969.
24. Hayes, G. J., and Leaver, R. C. Methyl methacrylate investment of intracranial aneurysms. A report of seven years experience. J. Neurosurg., *25:* 79–80, 1966.
25. Henry, R. C., and Taylor, P. H. Cerebrospinal fluid otorrhoea and otorhinorrhoea. Following closed head injury. J. Laryngol. Otol., *92:* 743–756, 1978.
26. Hilal, S. K., Sane, P., Michelson, W. J., and Kosseim, A. The embolization of vascular malformations of the spinal cord with low-viscosity silicone rubber. Neuroradiology, *16:* 430–433, 1978.
27. Hosobuchi, Y. Electrothrombosis of carotid-cavernous fistula. J. Neurosurg., *42:* 76–85, 1975.
28. IARC Working Group. Some monomers, plastics and synthetic elastomers, and arcrolein. IARC Monogr. Eval. Carcinog. Risk Chem. Hum., *19:* 513, 1979.
29. Ito, H., Ishikura, A., Marukawa, S., and Yamamoto, S. Repair of cerebro-spinal fluid rhinorrhoea with pedicled dural flap. Acta Neurochir. (Wien), *45:* 237–246, 1979.
30. Jamieson, K. G., and Yelland, J. D. Surgical repair of the anterior fossa because of rhinorrhea, aerocele, or meningitis. J. Neurosurg., *39:* 328–331, 1973.
31. Kerber, C. Experimental arteriovenous fistula. Creation and percutaneous catheter obstruction with cyanoacrylate. Invest. Radiol., *10:* 10–17, 1975.
32. Kerber, C. Use of balloon catheters in the treatment of cranial arterial abnormalities. Stroke, *11:* 210–216, 1980.
33. Kerber, C. W., Bank, W. O., and Cromwell, L. D. Cyanoacrylate occlusion of carotid-cavernous fistula with preservation of carotid artery flow. Neurosurgery, *4:* 210–215, 1979.
34. Kerber, C. W., Cromwell, L. D., and Sheptak, P. E. Intraarterial cyanoacrylate: an adjunct in the treatment of spinal/paraspinal arteriovenous malformations. A.J.R., *130:* 99–103, 1978.
35. Kline, D. G., and Hayes, G. J. An experimental evaluation of the effect of a plastic adhesive, methyl 2-cyanoacrylate, on neural tissue. J. Neurosurg., *20:* 647–654, 1963.
36. Lamborn, P. B., Jr., Soloway, H. B., Matsumoto, T., and Aaby, G. W. Comparison of tensile strength of wounds closed by sutures and cyanoacrylates. Am. J. Vet. Res., *31:* 125–130, 1970.
37. Laws, E. R., and Kern, E. B. Complications of transsphenoidal surgery. Clin. Neurosurg., *23:* 401–416, 1976.
38. Lehman, R. A., and Hayes, G. J. The toxicity of alkyl 2-cyanoacrylate tissue adhesives: brain and blood vessels. Surgery, *61:* 915–922, 1967.

39. Lehman, R. A., Hayes, G. J., and Leonard, F. Toxicity of alkyl 2-cyanoacrylates. I. Peripheral nerve. Arch. Surg., *93:* 441–446, 1966.
40. Lehman, R. A., Hayes, G. J., and Martins, A. N. The use of adhesive and lyophilized dura in the treatment of cerebrospinal rhinorrhea (Technical Note). J. Neurosurg., *26:* 92–95, 1967.
41. Leonard, F. Hemostatic applications of alpha cyanoacrylates: bonding mechanism and physiological degradation of bonds. *In* Adhesion in Biological Systems, edited by R. S. Manly, pp. 185–199. Academic Press, New York, 1970.
42. Leonard, F., Kulkarni, R. K., Brandes, G., Nelson, J., and Cameron, J. J. Synthesis and degradation of poly (alkyl-alpha cyanoacrylates). J. Appl. Polymer Sci., *10:* 259–272, 1966.
43. Leussenhop, A. J., and Presper, J. H. Surgical embolization of cerebral arteriovenous malformations through internal carotid and vertebral arteries. Long term results. J. Neurosurg., *42:* 443–451, 1975.
44. Margolis, M. T., Freeny, P. C., and Kendrick, M. M. Cyanoacrylate occlusion of a spinal cord ateriovenous malformation. Case report. J. Neurosurg., *51:* 107–110, 1979.
45. Matsumoto, T., Nemhauser, G. M., Soloway, H. B., Heisterkamp, C., and Aaby, G. Cyanoacrylate tissue adhesives: an experimental and clinical evaluation. Milit. Med., *134:* 247–252, 1969.
46. Maxwell, J. A., and Goldware, S. I. Use of tissue adhesive in the surgical treatment of cerebrospinal fluid leaks. Experience with isobutyl 2-cyanoacrylate in 12 cases. J. Neurosurg., *39:* 332–336, 1973.
47. Mazur, J. B., and Salazar, J. L. Late thrombosis of middle cerebral artery following clipping and coating of aneurysms. Surg. Neurol., *10:* 131–133, 1978.
48. Messer, H. D., Strenger, L., and McVeety, H. J. Use of plastic adhesive for reinforcement of a ruptured intracranial aneurysm. J. Neurosurg., *20:* 360–362, 1963.
49. Morley, T. P., and Hetherington, R. F. Traumatic cerebrospinal fluid rhinorrhea and otorrhea, pneumocephalus, and meningitis. Surg. Gynecol. Obstet., *104:* 88–98, 1957.
50. Mount, L. A., ano Antunes, J. L. Results of treatment of intracranial aneurysms by wrapping and coating. J. Neurosurg., *42:* 189–193, 1975.
51. Mullan, S. Treatment of carotid-cavernous fistulas by cavernous sinus occlusion. J. Neurosurg., *50:* 131–144, 1979.
52. Ommaya, A. K. Spinal fluid fistulae. Clin. Neurosurg., *23:* 363–392, 1976.
53. Parkinson, D., and Bachers, G. Arteriovenous malformations. Summary of 100 consecutive supratentorial cases. J. Neurosurg., *53:* 285–299, 1980.
54. Perret, G., Nishioka, H. Report on the cooperative study of intracranial aneurysms and subarachnoid hemorrhage, section VI. Arteriovenous malformations. An analysis of 545 cases of cranio-cerebral arteriovenous malformations and fistulae reported to the cooperative study. J. Neurosurg., *25:* 467–490, 1966.
55. Poss, R., Thilly, W. G., and Kaden, D. A. Methylmethacrylate is a mutagen for Salmonella typhimurium. J. Bone Joint Surg. (Am), *61:* 1203–1207, 1979.
56. Prager, R. J., Debrun, G., and Wolpert, S. M. Intracranial hemorrhage as a complication of therapeutic embolization. Presented at the 1980 Annual Meeting of American Society of Neuroradiology, Los Angeles, California, March 16–21, 1980.
57. Prolo, D. J., and Hanbery, J. W. Intraluminal occlusion of a carotid-cavernous sinus fistula with a balloon catheter (Technical Note). J. Neurosurg., *35:* 237–242, 1971.
58. Sachs, E., Jr., Erbengi, A., Margolis, G., and Wilson, D. H. Fatality from ruptured intracranial aneurysm after coating with methyl 2-cyanoacrylate (Eastman 910 Monomer, M2 C-1). Case report. J. Neurosurg., *24:* 889–891, 1966.
59. Samson, D., Ditmore, Q. M., and Beyer, C. W. The intravascular use of isobutyl 2-cyanoacrylate in the treatment of intracranial arteriovenous malformations. Neurosurgery, *8:* 43–51, 1981.

60. Samson, D., Ditmore, Q. M., and Beyer, C. W. The intravascular use of isobutyl 2-cyanoacrylate in the treatment of carotid-cavernous fistulas. Neurosurgery, *8:* 52–55, 1981.
61. Selverstone, B. Coating of intracranial aneurysms with nontoxic adherent plastics. *In* Current Techniques in Operative Neurosurgery, edited by H. H. Schmidek, and W. H. Sweet, pp. 31–40. Grune & Stratton, New York, 1977.
62. Selverstone, B., and Ronis, N. Coating and reinforcement of intracranial aneurysms with synthetic resins. Bull. Tufts-N.E. Med. Cent., *4:* 8–12, 1958.
63. Serbinenko, F. A. Ball-on catheterization and occlusion of major cerebral vessels. J. Neurosurg., *41:* 125–145, 1974.
64. Sheptak, P. E., Zanetti, P. H., and Susen, A. F. The treatment of intracranial aneurysms by injection with a tissue adhesive. Neurosurgery, *1:* 25–29, 1977.
65. Skeist, I. Handbook of Adhesives, Ed. 2. Van Nostrand Reinhold, New York, 1977.
66. Sugar, O., and Tsuchiya, G. Plastic coating of intracranial aneurysms with "EDH-Adhesive." J. Neurosurg., *21:* 114–117, 1964.
67. Taylor, J. C., and Choudhury, A. R. Reinforcement with gauze wrapping for ruptured aneurysms of the middle cerebral artery. J. Neurosurg., *47:* 828–832, 1977.
68. Todd, E. M., and Crue, B. L. The coating of aneurysms with plastic materials. *In* Intracranial Aneurysms and Subarachnoid Hemorrhage: A Cooperative Study, edited by A. L. Sahs and W. S. Fields, pp. 357–371. J. B. Lippincott, Philadelphia, 1969.
69. Tsuchiya, G., Sugar, O., Yashon, D., and Hubbard, J. Reactions of rabbit brain and peripheral vessels to plastics used in coating arterial aneurysms. J. Neurosurg., *28:* 409–416, 1968.
70. VanderArk, G. D., Pitkethly, D. T., Ducker, T. B., and Kempe, L. G. Repair of cerebrospinal fluid fistulas using a tissue adhesive. J. Neurosurg., *33:* 151–155, 1970.
71. Vezin, W. R., and Florence, A. T. In vitro heterogeneous degradation of poly (n-alkyl alpha-cyanoacrylates). J. Biomed. Mater. Res., *14:* 93–106, 1980.
72. White, R. I., Strandberg, J. V., Gross, G. S., and Barth, K. H. Therapeutic embolization with long-term occluding agents and their effects on embolized tissues. Radiology, *125:* 677–687, 1977.
73. Yasargil, M. G., and Fox, J. L. The microsurgical approach to intracranial aneurysms. Surg. Neurol., *3:* 7–14, 1975.
74. Yashon, D., Jane, J. A., Gordon, M. C., Hubbard, J. L., and Sugar, O. Effects of methyl 2-cyanoacrylate adhesives on the somatic vessels and the central nervous system of animals. J. Neurosurg., *24:* 883–888, 1966.
75. Yashon, D., White, R. J., Arias, B. A., and Hegarty, W. E. Cyanoacrylate encasement of intracranial aneurysms (Technical Note). J. Neurosurg., *34:* 709–713, 1971.
76. Yodh, S. B., and Wright, R. L. Experimental evaluation of four synthetic adhesives for possible treatment of aneurysms. J. Neurosurg., *26:* 504–510, 1967.
77. Young, W. C., and Gates, G. A. The use of cyanoacrylate in transsphenoidal hypophysectomy. Laryngoscope, *88:* 1784–1788, 1978.
78. Zanetti, P. H., and Sherman, F. E. Experimental evaluation of a tissue adhesive as an agent for the treatment of aneurysms and arteriovenous anomalies. J. Neurosurg., *36:* 72–79, 1972.

CHAPTER

25

Cranial Nerve Vascular Compression Syndromes (Other than Tic Douloureux and Hemifacial Spasm)

PETER J. JANNETTA, M.D.

The present concepts of vascular compression of neural structures are based on major contributions made in the past by Dandy, Sir Sidney Sunderland, and James Gardner. Dandy (4–7) noted vessels, tumors and other abnormalities in a high percentage of patients upon whom he sectioned the nerve for classical tic douloureux and what he termed "trigeminal neuralgia." Dandy lumped these two groups together in his operative series. Trigeminal neuralgia, to him, was a syndrome of constant unilateral focal facial pain, burning in character, occurring more commonly in women and more frequently in the right V_2 distribution. Mild facial numbness was frequently present. Neurologists and neurosurgeons have unfortunately lumped this group with our atypical facial pain patients, who have another syndrome. Dandy removed the tumors but did not, to my knowledge, ever move a blood vessel away from the nerve as treatment, nor could he clarify the relationships with the technology available to him. Sunderland (30), in an extensive and orderly series of studies of cadaver brains, noted the elongation of arteries at the base of the brain and collated these relationships to some of the cranial nerves. The brains were from an older population and were without clinical correlation. Sunderland, therefore, could not and did not correlate these common neurovascular relationships with any disease process. Gardner (11) and Gardner and Sava (12) in 1962 published two especially important papers concerning their experience with trigeminal neuralgia (TN) and hemifacial spasm (HFS), noting abnormal neurovascular relationships in some cases and treating a few patients by vascular decompression but also with nerve trauma (11, 12).

With the introduction of the binocular microscope to clinical neurosurgery in 1957 by Kurze, a new world opened up which is altering neurosurgical practice and, more importantly, is altering some of our concepts of disease. It is on these new concepts that this paper is focused. Trigeminal neuralgia and hemifacial spasm, the abnormal hyperactive symptom complexes which form the now generally accepted basis of our current concepts of cranial nerve vascular compression, will not be considered in the present paper. Many investigators have published series and case reports of patients who underwent microvascular decompression for these problems (1–3, 9, 10, 13, 22–28, 31, 32).

The purpose of the present paper is to describe our findings in various cranial nerve disorders which are primarily or frequently due to abnormal neurovascular contact. Table 25.1 is a summary of the current state of knowledge concerning vascular compression of cranial nerves. In this table, the cranial nerves save for the olfactory are listed on the left with the function of the nerve adjacent. In the next column are listed the hyperactive dysfunction syndromes due to vascular compression at the root entry zone (REZ) or further distally on the nerve. In the last column are listed the hypoactive dysfunction syndromes about which less is known. Areas about which we have no clinical evidence are listed with a question mark. These areas demand investigation. In the discussion of these problems, we will first consider the REZ syndromes other than trigeminal neuralgia and hemifacial spasm, then the more peripheral chronic vascular compression syndromes. Lastly, we will discuss the hypoactive dysfunction syndromes.

TABLE 25.1

Cranial Nerve Dysfunction Caused by Vascular Compression

Nerve	Function	Hyperactive dysfunction	Hypoactive dysfunction
II	Vision	?	Visual failure
III	Motor—EOMs	?	Palsy
	Autonomic—pupil	?	Pupillary dilatation
IV	Motor—EOMs	Trochlear myokymia?	Palsy
V	Somatic sensory	Trigeminal neuralgia	Neuropathy
		Atypical trigeminal neuralgia	
	Somatic motor	Trismus?	Denervation
VI	Motor—EOMs	?	Palsy
VII	Somatic motor	Hemifacial spasm	Palsy
VIII	Special sensory		
	Hearing	Tinnitus	Hearing Loss
	Balance	Vertigo	Vestibular neuropathy
IX–X	Somatic sensory	Glossopharyngeal neuralgia	Palate and gag reflexes
	Glutition	?	Palsy
	Autonomic	Essential hypertension (L)	?
		? (R)	?
XI	Motor	? Some torticollis	?
XII	Motor	?	Neuropathy

Root Entry Zone Syndromes

These consist of somatic sensory (V, IX–X) somatic motor (VII), special sensory (VIII), and autonomic nervous system dysfunction (X) due to vascular cross compression of the REZ of the nerve in question. Cranial nerves VIII, IX, and X will be discussed. It should be emphasized that the symptoms are caricatures of the normal function of the nerve and that loss of function gradually accompanies the hyperaction function in all these problems and may occasionally supervene. Lastly, the reader should notice that only one vagus nerve, the left, has been studied regarding autonomic dysfunction. The right vagus, which has a different distribution than the left, deserves attention.

ACOUSTIC NERVE

Thirty eight patients with acoustic nerve dysfunction have undergone retromastoid craniectomy (RMC) and microvascular decompression (MVD) for intractable vertigo and/or tinnitus (Table 25.2). These patients carried the diagnosis of vestibular Meniere's disease, cochlear Meniere's disease, unqualified Meniere's disease, benign paroxysmal vertigo, positional vertigo, or uncategorizable tinnitus and/or vertigo. There was a clear clinical-pathological correlation of the symptoms with the location of the vascular compression in all 38 patients: Cross compression of the vestibular nerve REZ caused vertigo; of the cochlear nerve REZ, tinnitus; of both, both tinnitus and vertigo (Table 25.3). In our early experience, the relief of tinnitus was not generally satisfactory but has improved with improved techniques and the use of softer implant materials. The results of operation are tabulated in Table 25.4. Not shown in the table are two points of interest: First, our results with the treatment of tinnitus are improving; second, it may take weeks or months for symptoms to improve and gradually disappear. Complications are noted in Table 25.5. Two patients, neither with useful hearing, had serious permanent decrease in hearing immediately postoperatively. One older woman developed an internuclear ophthalmoplegia with increased vertigo

TABLE 25.2
*Eighth Nerve Vascular Compression in 38 Patients**

Sex	
Females	24
Males	14
Side	
Right	17
Left	21

* Age at onset, 15 to 59 years. Three patients were teenagers; five were in their 20s; seven were in their 30s; 12 in their 40s; 10 in their 50s; one, unknown.

TABLE 25.3

Eighth Cranial Nerve Dysfunction

Operative findings					Total
Offending vessel					
Artery*					26
Cochlear	6	Cochlear + AICA	1		
AICA	5	Vertebral	2		
PICA	5	Superior cerebellar	2		
Unidentified artery	4	AICA + PICA	1		
Vein					8
Artery and vein					4
Total					38

* AICA, Anterior inferior cerebellar artery; PICA, posterior inferior cerebellar artery.

TABLE 25.4

Eighth Cranial Nerve Dysfunction: Results of Operation

Symptoms	Relieved	Mild improvement	Recurred or no relief	Worse
Vertigo and tinnitus	13	0	6	1
Vertigo	6	1	0	0
Tinnitus	5	0	6	0
Totals	24	1	12	1

TABLE 25.5

Eighth Cranial Nerve Dysfunction: Complication

Temporary	1 Epidural hematoma postoperative, with n. VI paresis*
	1 X cranial nerve paresis*
	2 Aseptic meningitis
	1 Urinary tract infection
Permanent	1 Internuclear ophthmoplegia and worsening of vertigo
	2 Deterioration of hearing

* Same patient.

on her 2nd postoperative day. Both of these symptoms have persisted and she is, if anything, worse than she was preoperatively.

GLOSSOPHARYNGEAL NEURALGIA

Seventeen patients have undergone RMC (Table 25.6), 11 by the author (21). Operative findings are noted in Table 25.7. Note that vessels were not identifed at operation in two of the 17 patients. One of them, operated upon by the author, had undergone prior section of nerve IX only, with brief pain relief. The area was densely scarred and the REZ could not be inspected. The author was not present at the second procedure when an only questionable vascular compression was seen and, therefore, called "negative." Operation, treatment, and results of operation in the patients treated by the author are tabulated in Table 25.8. Recurrences occurred in two patients treated using small fragments of muscle as the implants. It is presumed that this muscle tissue eroded away by continuing pulsation of the arterial loops which did not have their axes altered. Shredded Teflon felt is now used and should be more satisfactory in the tight spaces where major mobilization of an artery is not feasible. Fifteen patients in the total series are now free of pain, but two of them underwent subsequent nerve section. Two patients died. One of them underwent nerve section on the left and never awoke from anesthesia (patient not personally known to the author). Another (Table 25.8) died of a hypertensive stroke after right IX to X nerve medullary MVD. This tragic patient, operated upon in 1973, is the first of two patients who aroused the interest of the author in hyperactive autonomic dysfunction by vascular compression as a cause of hypertension (21).

TABLE 25.6

Glossopharyngeal Neuralgia: Patient Population

Sex	10 women, 7 men
Age	30–68 yr
Age at Onset	1, 30s; 3, 40s; 9, 50s; 4, 60s
Side	10 right, 7 left

TABLE 25.7

Glossopharyngeal Neuralgia: Offending Vessel

Vessel	Number
Posterior inferior cerebellar artery	9
Anterior inferior cerebellar artery	1
PICA + vertebral	1
Unidentified small arterial loop	1
No vessel identified	2
Vertebral artery and vein	1
Vertebral artery	1
Vein	1

TABLE 25.8

Glossopharyngeal Neuralgia: Personal Series (11 Patients)

Treatment	Microvascular decompression	9
	Nerve section	2
Results	Pain free, MVD	6
	No relief or recurrence, MVD	2
	Pain free, section	2
	Dead, hypertensive stroke	1

"ESSENTIAL" HYPERTENSION

The question of arterial compression of the left vagus nerve and adjacent medulla oblongata was pursued beginning in 1973 with the patient noted above. This 55-year-old woman had no significant history of hypertension save for blood pressure of 150/90 at one time preoperatively. She died postoperatively from a hypertensive crisis with a huge right intracerebral hemorrhage (21). At postmortem examination, she had left ventricular concentric hypertrophy consistent with hypertension. Her problem may have been spuriously or only indirectly related to the present consideration as she had a right sided lesion, and we now understand that left vagal-medullary arterial compression appears to be the common denominator of essential hypertension (15, 18, 19, 29). The patient population with essential hypertension who underwent RMC and MVD is tabulated in Table 25.9. Operative findings are tabulated in Table 25.10. Note that arteries were causal in all patients, that no compression was seen on the right (five patients), and that left vagus-external medulla oblongata arterial compression was clearly seen in 20 of 22 patients on the left side. In addition to vascular compression of the cranial nerve REZ for which the patient was operated upon, left lateral medullary-vagal decompression was attempted in 14 of 22 patients. It was not felt that vascular transsection and anastomosis of the offending arterial loop were indicated in these patients in our present state of knowledge, and only those vessels were mobilized in whom it was felt that a vascular decompression could be performed safely, rapidly, and easily. Eleven of the 14 patients are improved; six are normotensive,

TABLE 25.9
Essential Hypertension (28 patients)

Sex	20 Women, 8 men
Age	2, 30s; 7, 40s; 7, 50s; 11, 60s; 1, 70s
Side of operation	5 Right, 23 left

TABLE 25.10
Essential Hypertension: Operative Findings

	Number
Right side	5 (No vessel)
Offending vessel (all left side)	
A. Vertebral artery	13
"normal"	9
ectatic	4
B. PICA*	7
C. Vertebral and PICA	1
D. AICA and PICA†	1

* One questionable, no. 19, anterior.
† Questionable, no. 28, very caudal.

three are normotensive on medication, and two are significantly improved.

Syndromes due to Chronic Vascular Compression Distal to the Root Entry Zone

As we age and the arteries at the base of the brain elongate, they loop about; a fact known to all neurosurgeons. If we are unlucky, the REZ will be cross-compressed giving the symptom of hyperactive dysfunction discussed above. Many patients who develop peripheral cranial nerve vascular compression have no major symptoms. Many may be subject to mild progressive loss of function. Some patients may develop a pain syndrome in the trigeminal distribution which is not classical tic douloureux and which was called "trigeminal neuralgia" by Dandy, who grouped these patients together in his operative series. This terminology and his combined series have led to some confusion. These patients are more commonly women, at an age younger than those with classical tic douloureux. They develop constant pain, usually described as "burning" in character, most frequently located in the V_2 distribution and more commonly on the right. Some patients have mild and evanescent tic-like pain. The pain is mild and not memorable at onset but gradually worsens. Mild hypalgesia and/or hypesthesia may be noted in the region of the nasolabial fold on careful testing. Just as in classical tic douloureux, this finding is frequently missed. These patients are usually labelled as psychoneurotics as they are lumped with the "atypical face pain" group, another entity entirely. They ultimately become neurotic.

Another group of patients have pain in the trigeminal distribution which includes the upper molar region, temple, and ipsilateral V_1 distribution which may be associated with variable nasal stuffiness, lacrimation, tearing, and ultimately a pounding headache. All of these patients have carried multiple diagnoses depending upon the discipline of the physician or dentist who has seen them and depending upon when they are seen. These diagnoses consist of myofacial-pain syndrome, temporomandibular joint syndrome or disease, Horton's cephalalgia (cluster headaches), vidian, sphenopalatine, or Raeder's paratrigeminal neuralgia. We have classified these as "atypical trigeminal neuralgia" and "atypical trigeminal neuralgia with (variable) hyperautonomic dysfunction."

Over 75 patients have been operated upon in this series. All were desperately ill with intractable constant pain and had undergone vigorous therapy with high doses of all known medications. My former colleague, R. Laha, and I have collated the data concerning the first 30 patients and these data will be reviewed (21). These patients have been followed from 4 to 8 years.

The series consisted of 20 women and 10 men, ranging in age from 15 to 59 years, with a mean age of 44 years. Nine patients were under 40 years of age. The duration of symptoms varied from 1 to 19 years (mean 6.6 years). The pain was on the right in 18, the left in 12, and bilateral (more severe on the right) in two. Mild sensory abnormalities were noted in 21 patients (Table 25.11). The abnormalities found at operation are collated in Table 25.12 and the results of operation in Table 25.13. One patient died unexpectedly in this series. She had an unsuspected arterio-venous malformation in the cerebellum which ruptured in the postoperative period. Other complications were transient. Despite extensive review of these patients, we still cannot predict who will do well and who will not after MVD for atypical trigeminal neuralgia.

One subgroup of acoustic nerve disorder is that caused by peripheral vascular compression of the 8th cranial nerve by the meatal loop of the

TABLE 25.11

Atypical Trigeminal Neuralgia (1972 through June 1976)

Physical Examination					
A. Trigeminal motor weakness—2					
B. Sensory abnormality—18					
	V_1	V_2	V_{1-2}	V_{2-3}	$V_{1,2,3}$
Hypalgesia		2	1	4	3
Hypalgesia-hypesthesia		3		1	4
Corneal↓	3				

TABLE 25.12

Atypical Trigeminal Neuralgia (1972 through June 1976)

Operative findings		Total
A. Vascular compression		28
Artery alone	14	
Artery and vein	7	
Vein alone	6	
Artery and enostosis	1	
B. Other		2
Ridge-Meckel's cave and brain sag	1	
Tumor (neurilemmoma)	1	

TABLE 25.13

Operative Results: Atypical Trigeminal Neuralgia

Results	No. of patients
Relief of pain	15
Partial relief*	5
No benefit	9
Death†	1

* Persistence of varying degree of background pain.

† Postoperative rupture of undiagnosed intracerebellar arteriovenous malformation.

anterior inferior cerebellar artery when it lies on the underside of the VII to VIII nerve bundle at the meatus, gives a branch to the porus, and is accompanied by "brain sag" causing stretch of nerve VIII over the artery.

This syndrome consists of tinnitus with progressive hearing loss, and progressive decrease in vestibular function without vertigo. It is surprising that the five patients operated upon have had no vertigo. It is most difficult to treat this problem and very easy to harm the cochlear nerve. The data on these patients are included with the tinnitus group noted above.

Vascular Compression Syndromes and Sudden Loss of Function

Several "idiopathic" cranial nerve dysfunction syndromes consist of rapid or sudden loss of function with a high (80% or better) increase of complete or significant recovery. These entities include trigeminal neuropathy, idiopathic abducens nerve palsy, Bell's palsy, vestibular neuritis, idiopathic sensorineural hearing loss, and hypoglossal neuropathy. Observations have been made in most of these entities (14–17, 20, 21, 33). Many of these problems appear to be caused by shift of an elongated arterial loop in the cerebellopontine angle, which stretches a cranial nerve causing loss of function. A stretched peripheral nerve has generally an 80% or better chance of recovery, the same sequency noted in these "idiopathic" cranial nerve palsies. Only intractable cases with persistent problems have undergone RMC and MVD in this series. A total of 17 patients, five with trigeminal neuropathy, 11 with Bell's palsy, and one with hypoglossal neuropathy are discussed.

Five patients with intractable unilateral facial numbness, two with accompanying face pain, were examined. Four were operated upon. All were found to have significant stretch of the trigeminal nerve by an arterial loop which had apparently shifted. The nerve was decompressed. Numbness was relieved totally in three and significantly in the fourth with measurable improvement beginning in the immediate postoperative period. Face pain was relieved in both patients. The fifth patient (no. 2) recovered gradually and spontaneously over a 2-year period (Table 25.14).

Eleven patients with intractable Bell's palsy have been operated upon. Ten of the 11 had significant stretch of the facial nerve by a looping artery which had apparently shifted. Patient data operative findings and results are collated in Table 25.15.

One patient (case 4 of the trigeminal neuropathy series) also had left hypoglossal neuropathy. This was caused by stretch and compression of the left hypoglossal nerve against the occipital bone by a small medullary arterial loop. Gradual but complete recovery of left tongue function, strength, and bulk followed vascular decompression. These patients are described in more detail in several publications (14–17, 20, 21, 33).

TABLE 25.14

Trigeminal Neuropathy: Summary of Five Patients

Patient no.	1	2	3	4	5
Age	39	28	53	29	56
Sex	M	F	F	M	F
Side	L	L	R	L	R
Distrib. numbness	$V_{1\text{-}2\text{-}3}$	$V_{2\text{-}3}$	$V_{1\text{-}2\text{-}3}$	$V_{2\text{-}3}$	$V_{1\text{-}2\text{-}3}$
Pain	−	−	+	−	+
Operation	+	0	+	+	+
Artery*	SCA AICA	No oper.	SCA	SCA	SCA
Result in numbness	+		+	+	Significant improvement
Pain			None		None

* SCA, superior cerebellar artery.

TABLE 25.15

Bell's Palsy: Patient Data: Operative Findings and Results

11 patients	
Age	29–73
Sex	8 Male, 3 female
Side	3 Right, 8 left
Duration of symptom	11 Days to 8 yr
Operative findings	Nerve stretched by arterial loop, 8 patients
	Nerve also swollen, 2 patients (11 and 41 days)
Operative results	No improvement, 3
	No treatment, 1 (initial observation)
	Improved, 7
	Synkinesis, 5 of 7
	Weakness, 6 of 7
	Crocodile tears, better on awakening

Conclusion

It now appears that a number of cranial nerve problems, some of which may cause systemic illness, are the result of the aging process in a very specific sense. With arterial degeneration and elongation due to arteriosclerosis, the small arteries around the base of the brain may cause neural compression of cranial nerves peripherally in the cerebellopontine angle, at the root entry zone, or even of the brain stem itself. This pulsatile compression may cause hyperactive dysfunction, loss of function, or a combination of both. It is usually progressive but may be self-limited. Of some interest perhaps is the vascular compression syndrome of the left vagus nerve and anterolateral medulla oblongata causing "essential" hypertension. It appears that this common entity is not a "disease" as the symptoms mentioned above are not diseases. Fein and Frishman (10) have recently verified these findings in two patients in whom they did left sided posterior circulation bypass procedures and one who had a left posterior circulation aneurysm. The hypertension disappeared postoperatively in the first two patients and was unchanged in the aneurysm patient in whom the aneurysm was not clipped. The authors noted that arteries stretching the left vagus nerve were mobilized away from the nerve during the bypass preocedure. One wonders if the mechanism in these patients was the same as in the laterally medullary group or whether hind brain ischemia and subsequent relief of the ischemia by the bypass could have played a role.

The left vagus carries the servo-mechanism control of the left heart. Disruption of this control by pulsatile compression may cause the left heart, the pump, to overwork. Compensatory mechanisms come into play: renal, endocrine, peripheral vascular, perhaps even emotional. The pump ultimately fails. The compensatory mechanisms ultimately fail. My colleagues and I have developed a self-contained pump, the "balloon-balloon," a chronic model in baboons (16). We hope to study the above entities and others, which by logical extension of the above noted findings, should lead us to a further appreciation of a number of diseases of the aging process.

REFERENCES

1. Apfelbaum, R. I. A comparison of percutaneous radiofrequency trigeminal neurolysis and microvascular decompression of the trigeminal nerve for the treatment of tic douloureux. Neurosurgery, *1:* 16, 1977.
2. Bland, J. E., Lazar, M. L., and Naarden, A. L. Treatment of pain syndromes. *In* Current Treatment of Neurological Diseases, edited by R. Rosenberg, p. 589. Spectrum Publications, Holliswood, N.Y., 1978.
3. Briani, S., and Ammannati, F. Patologia dei nervi craniaci da compressione vasale diretta. Riv. Neurobiol., *24:* 285, 1978.
4. Dandy, W. E. Section of the sensory root of the trigeminal nerve at the pons. Bull. Johns Hopkins Hosp., *36:* 105–106, 1925.
5. Dandy, W. E. Operation for cure of tic douloureux; partial section of the sensory root at the pons. Arch. Surg., *18:* 687–734, 1929.
6. Dandy, W. E. Treatment of trigeminal neuralgia by the cerebellar route. Ann. Surg., *96:* 787–795, 1932.
7. Dandy, W. E. Surgery of the brain. A monograph. *In* Practice of Surgery, edited by Lewis, Vol. 12, pp. 167–187. Prior, Hagerstown, 1945.
8. Dujovny, M., Osgood, C. P., Faille, R., Bennett, M. H., and Kerber, C. Posterior fossa AVM producing hemifacial spasm: a case report. Angiology, *30*(6): 425, 1979.
9. Fabinyi, G. C. A., and Adams, C. B. T. Hemifacial spasm: treatment by posterior fossa surgery, J. Neurol. Neurosurg. Psychiatry, *41:* 829, 1978.
10. Fein, J. M., and Frishman, W. Neurogenic hypertension related to vascular compression of the lateral medulla. Neurosurgery, *6:* 615–622, 1980.
11. Gardner, W. J., and Sava, G. A.: Hemifacial spasm: a reversible pathophysiologic state. J. Neurosurg., *19:* 240–247, 1962.
13. Hankinson, H. L., and Wilson, C. B. Microsurgical treatment of hemifacial spasm. West. J. Med., *124:* 191, 1976.

14. Jannetta, P. J. Observations on the etiology of trigeminal neuralgia, hemifacial spasm, acoustic nerve dysfunction and glossopharyngeal neuralgia. Definitive microsurgical treatment and results in 117 patients. Neurochirurgia, *20:* 145–154, 1977.
15. Jannetta, P. J. Microsurgery of cranial nerve cross compression. Clin. Neurosurg., *26:* 206–207, 1979.
16. Jannetta, P. J. Neurovascular compression in cranial nerve and systemic disease. Ann. Surg., *192:* 518–525, 1980.
17. Jannetta, P. J., and Bissonette, D. J. Bell's palsy: a theory as to etiology: observations in six patients. Laryngoscope, *88:* 849–854, 1978.
18. Jannetta, P. J., and Gendell, H. M. Neurovascular compression associated with essential hypertension. Neurosurgery, *2:* 165, 1978.
19. Jannetta, P. J., and Gendell, H. M. Clinical observations on etiology of essential hypertension. Surg. Forum, *30:* 431–432, 1979.
20. Jannetta, P. J., and Robbins, L. Trigeminal neuropathy: new observations. Neurosurgery, *7*(7): 347–351, 1980.
21. Laha, R. K., and Jannetta, P. J. Glossopharyngeal neuralgia. J. Neurosurg., *47:* 316–320, 1977.
22. Lazar, M. L. Trigeminal neuralgia: recent advances in management. Tex. Med., *74:* 45, 1978.
23. Loeser, J. D. What to do about tic douloureux. J.A.M.A., *239*(12): 1153, 1978.
24. Maroon, J. C. Hemifacial spasm. a vascular cause. Arch. Neurol., *35:* 481, 1978.
25. Petty, P. G. Arterial compression of the trigeminal nerve at the pons as a cause of trigeminal neuralgia. Inst. Neurol. Madra. Proc., *6:* 93, 1976.
26. Petty, P. G., and Southby, R. Vascular compression of lower cranial nerves: observations using microsurgery, with particular reference to trigeminal neuralgia. Aust. N.Z. J. Surg., *47*(3): 314, 1977.
27. Rhoton, A. L. Microsurgical neurovascular decompression for trigeminal neuralgia and hemifacial spasm. J. Fla. Med. Assoc., *65:* 425, 1978.
28. Sato, O., Kanazawa, I., and Kokunai, T. Trigeminal neuralgia caused by compression of trigeminal nerve by pontine vein. Surg. Neurol., *11:* 285, 1979.
29. Segal, R., Gendell, H. M., Canfield, D., Dujovny, M., and Jannetta, P. J. Cardiovascular response to pulsatile pressure applied to ventrolateral medulla. Surg. Forum, *30:* 433–435, 1979.
30. Sunderland, S. Neurovascular relationships and anomalies at the base of the brain. J. Neurol. Neurosurg. Psychiatry, *11:* 243–247, 1948.
31. Waga, S., Morikawa, A., and Kojima, T. Trigeminal neuralgia: compression of the trigeminal nerve by an elongated and dilated basilar artery. Surg. Neurol., *11:* 13, 1979.
32. Weidman, M. J. Trigeminal neuralgia. Med. J. Aust., *2:* 628, 1979.
33. Yonas, H., and Jannetta, P. J. Neurinoma of the trigeminal root and atypical trigeminal neuralgia: their commonality. Neurosurgery, *6*(3): 273–277, 1980.

CHAPTER

26

Assessment of Sensory Function in the Operating Room Utilizing Cerebral Evoked Potentials: A Study of Fifty-Six Surgically Anesthetized Patients*

A. ALLEN, M.D., ARNOLD STARR, M.D., and K. NUDLEMAN, M.D.

The use of sensory evoked potentials in the evaluation of patients with neurological and sensory disorders provides the clinician with a set of objective measures of nervous system function (see refs. 5 and 13 for reviews of the field). The techniques of electrode application, computer averaging, and evoked response measures are relatively straightforward. The application of evoked potential techniques to patients in the operating room has had only limited application. Feinsod *et al.* (6) first reported the use of visual evoked potentials to monitor optic nerve function in a patient with a pituitary adenoma during surgical decompression. A shortening of the latency of the potentials occurred on removal of the tumor, and there was an improvement in the patient's visual function postoperatively. There have been several papers on the use of somatosensory evoked potentials to monitor spinal cord function during placement of Harrington rods and a variety of other surgical procedures (4, 9, 11). Changes in the evoked components were correlated with mechanical changes (distraction) in the spinal column and cord. Raudzens (12) has recently reported on the use of evoked potentials to monitor neurosurgical patients, and Hashimoto *et al.* (8) describe the use of auditory brainstem potentials to monitor brainstem function in patients during exploration of the posterior fossa.

We will summarize in this report the results of studies over 2 years (1977 and 1978) of intraoperative monitoring of evoked potentials using auditory, visual, and somatosensory stimuli.

METHOD

Fifty-six patients with neurological or orthopedic disorders were studied with evoked potentials during surgery. A request for monitoring

* Presented in preliminary form at the April 1977 meeting of the American Academy of Neurology. Supported by the National Institutes of Health (Grant NS11876).

evoked potentials in the operating room originated with the responsible surgeon. Their anticipation was that evoked potentials may help define changes in neurophysiological functions resulting from surgery. The patients' neurological status was defined both preceding and following the operative procedures. The stimulating and recording techniques used in the operating room were only slightly modified from those used in the clinical evoked response laboratories.

Monocular visual stimuli was produced by an array of 10 light-emitting diodes placed in a black eyepatch and positioned over the closed eye. A flash rate of 3/sec was used. The active electrode was placed at Oz and a reference at Cz. Activity was amplified 50,000 times and filtered at a band pass of 1 to 100 Hz (3 db down). One hundred twenty-eight trials were sufficient to provide clear potentials during the 250-msec sample time following the flash (Fig. 26.1). Both pre- and postoperative visual evoked potentials to a patterned signal were also tested using an alternating checkerboard stimulus in which the size of the visual field field tested was 10°, the checks were 32 minutes, and the pattern reversal rate was 1.8/sec (Fig. 26.1).

Acoustic signals were clicks produced by 0.1 msec square wave pulses applied monaurally to insert ear mold speakers (hearing aid type) at an intensity of 65 db or 75 db HL re normal and at a rate of 10/sec. Electrodes were attached to Cz and the earlobe ipsilateral to the stimulus using collodion-saturated gauze patchers with an interelectrode impedance of <4 kohms. The scalp recorded potentials were amplified 100,000 times and filtered at a band pass of 100 Hz to 3 kHz (3 db down). One thousand trials were usually sufficient to extract a well-formed series of brainstem components during the 10 msec following the click (Fig. 26.1).

Somatosensory signals were constant current stimuli applied to a mixed peripheral nerve through surface discs or subcutaneous needle electrodes. The nerves stimulated were either the median nerve at the wrist, the peroneal nerve at the fibular head, or the posterior tibial nerve at the medial malleolus. The intensity of current used was adjusted to be just sufficient to produce a twitch in the appropriately innervated muscle. Recordings were made between C_3 or C_4 referenced to the ipsilateral mastoid (when stimulating the median nerve) or Cz referenced to the ipsilateral mastoid (when stimulating the nerve in the leg). The scalp recorded signal was amplified 50,000 times and filtered at a band pass of 3 to 300 Hz (3 db down). Two hundred fifty-six trials were usually sufficient to produce reproducible cortical components (Fig. 26.1). During this study we did not attempt to define the far-field spinal cord and brainstem somatosensory evoked potentials (Fig. 26.1, *bottom two traces*).

When possible, pre- and postoperative recordings were made in the laboratory or at the bedside, except in those instances when advance

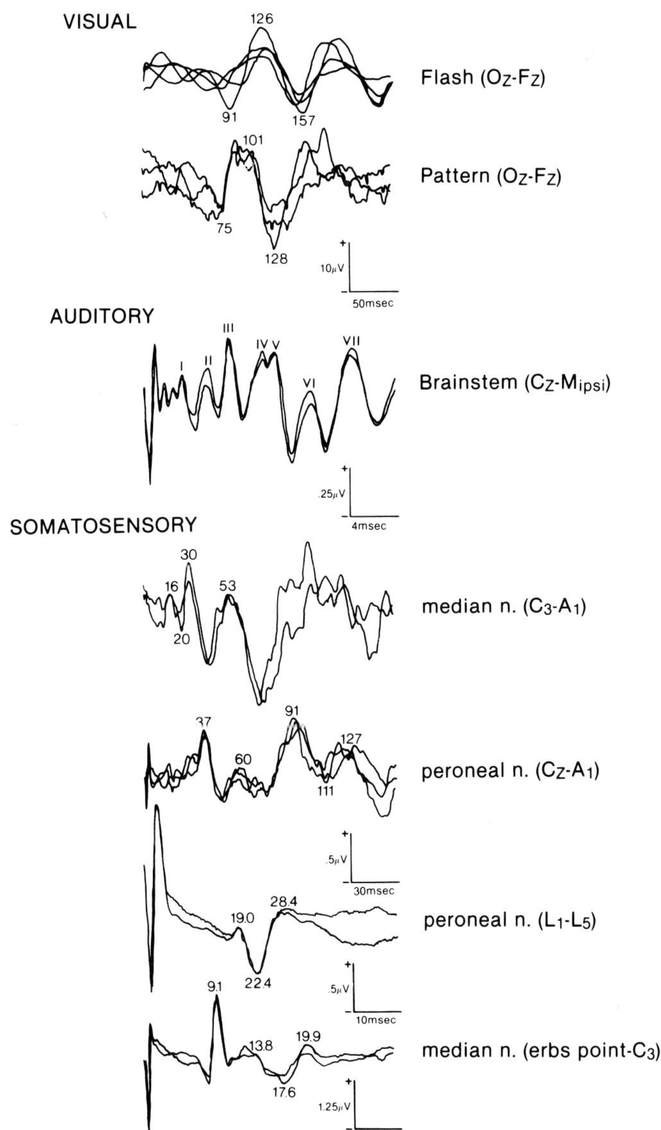

FIG. 26.1. Sensory evoked potentials available for monitoring brain function during surgery. The stimulus (visual, auditory, somatosensory) and recording montage are included with representative normal responses.

warning was not sufficient. In the operating room base line studies were made in all patients after the induction of anesthesia and prior to the initial incision.

During the surgical procedure, blood pressure, pulse rate, respiratory rate, temperature, and EKG were continuously monitored. Arterial blood gases, arterial pressure (via catheter), and CO_2 analysis were monitored in complex neurosurgical cases.

A variety of anesthetic agents were utilized. In general the patients received pentobarbital and atropine as a preoperative medication. A combination of barbiturate, N_2O, halogenated hydrocarbon (halothane, fluothane), and a neuromuscular blocking agent (Pavulon) was used.

Evoked potentials were continuously monitored during the surgical procedure, but only selected averages were plotted. During the approach to or the manipulation of neural structures adjacent to the sensory pathways, particular attention was paid to any change in the component's latency or amplitude. If potentials were significantly altered or lost, the operative procedure would be halted temporarily until additional averages were made. In general, this would require 2 to 3 minutes. Changes in the evoked potentials were considered transient if they reversed within 15 minutes.

RESULTS

In Table 26.1 an analysis of the patient population and evoked potential test modality is made. The most frequent request for evoked potential monitoring entailed the use of visual stimulation (25 cases) and, in particular, to monitor visual pathway function during removal of tumors near or in the sella turcica (19 cases).

The next most frequent request for evoked potential monitoring utilized somatosensory stimulation during placement of Harrington rods for severe scoliosis (38% of somatosensory evoked potential requests.). Maximal distraction of the Harrington rods can be complicated by spinal cord injury (5, 11), and somatosensory evoked potentials provide evidence of dorsal column function of the spinal cord during the procedure. Evoked potential monitoring was considered superior to the traditional methods of briefly "awakening" the patient to determine if movements of the lower extremities were still possible after distraction and prior to closing the incision.

Eighteen percent of the cases studied involved the use of auditory brainstem potentials. The two most frequent indications were in surgery for trigeminal neuralgia (section of $V_{2,3}$) and acoustic neuroma. In both instances injury to the brainstem can occur during the operative procedures.

Table 26.2 contains an analysis of both the feasibility and utility of evoked potentials monitoring during surgery. Satisfactory records were obtained in 77% of the patients tested. Of the patients with unsatisfactory records, almost three fourths had low amplitude potentials even prior to

TABLE 26.1

Evoked Potential Monitoring in the Operating Room: Stimulus Modality and Patient Diagnosis

Visual evoked potentials	No. of patients
Pituitary tumor	14
Craniopharyngioma	2
Optic glioma	2
Pituitary abscess	1
Orbital pseudotumor	1
Fracture of optic canal	1
Internal carotid aneurysm	1
Basilar artery aneurysm	1
Occipital arteriovenous malformation	1
Cerebrospinal fluid rhinorrhea	1
	25
Somatosensory evoked potentials	**No. of patients**
Scoliosis (Harrington rod)	8
Cervical cord compression (spondylosis)	3
Fractured spine	3
Spinal cord tumor	2
Herniated disc	1
Fractured odontoid	1
Tethered cord	1
Thalamic tumor	1
Sciatic nerve exploration	1
	21
Auditory brainstem potentials	**No. of patients**
Section of trigeminal nerve for neuralgia	3
Acoustic neuroma	3
Posterior fossa meningioma	2
Hemifacial spasm	1
IV ventricular tumor	1
	10

TABLE 26.2

Evaluation of Evoked Potential Monitoring in the Operating Room

	No. of patients*	Technically satisfactory recordings†	Transient evoked potential changes/postoperative neurological changes	Persistent evoked potential changes/postoperative neurological changes
Stimulus				
Visual	25	22 (88%)	15/0	7/2
Auditory	10	9 (90%)	5/0	3/2
Somatosensory	21	12 (59%)	11/0	1/1

* Total, 56.

† Total, 43 (77%).

surgery. In these patients it is likely that the sensory pathways were so compromised by disease that evoked potentials could only be resolved with difficulty. In the remaining one fourth of the patients, the unsatisfactory recordings obtained in the operating room were due to technical problems such as line voltage artifact, "electrode slippage" due to repositioning and moving the head, artifacts from the electrocautery, and potentials generated by movements of the electrodes from manipulation of supporting structures such as the spine during testing of somatosensory evoked potentials.

Among the various evoked potential procedures, the somatosensory potentials evoked by stimulation of the nerves in the leg were the most difficult to define. In contrast, somatosensory evoked potential to stimulation of the median nerve and visual and auditory evoked potentials were all obtained with little difficulty.

Visual Evoked Potentials

In normals, the potentials evoked by the light-emitting diode eyepatch consisted of a negative-positive-negative complex in which the main positive component peaked at approximately 120 msec. This same morphology was elicited by the alternating checkerboard stimulus with the latency of the positive component being normally 100 msec (Fig. 26.1). The potentials arise from activity in visual cortex, and changes in latency and amplitude can reflect disorders anywhere along the visual pathway.

Satisfactory evoked potentials to diffuse flash were obtained in 88% of the patients during the operative procedures. Alterations in the evoked potentials' morphology, amplitude, and/or latency occurred on a transient basis (persisting up to 15 minutes) in 68% of the patients and on a persisting basis for the duration of the operation in 32% of the patients. Visual function postoperatively was unaffected in those patients with transient evoked potential alterations. In contrast, 2 of the 7 patients with persisting modifications had an improvement in their vision postoperatively.

Many of the evoked potential changes accompanied pressure or traction on the optic nerve or chiasm or closely related supporting structures. These manipulations may have adversely affected the evoked potentials as a result of direct contact with the optic nerve or interference with its blood supply. Alternatively, sudden decompression of the optic nerve during removal of adhesions, a deforming tumor, or bone fragment could be associated with an immediate growth in amplitude and/or shortening of latencies of the evoked potentials. A dramatic appearance of potentials in the operating room was observed in 4 patients with blindness: in 2 of these patients there was a return of some vision in the affected eye postoperatively.

There were other events not directly related to the trauma and surgery that were associated with transient loss in evoked potentials such as irrigation of the region of the optic nerves, a drop in blood pressure, or changes in levels of anesthesia. The changes in the evoked potential accompanying these events were only distinguished from the changes accompanying tissue manipulation by knowledge of what had just occurred (Fig. 26.2). In 2 patients the loss of evoked potentials persisted

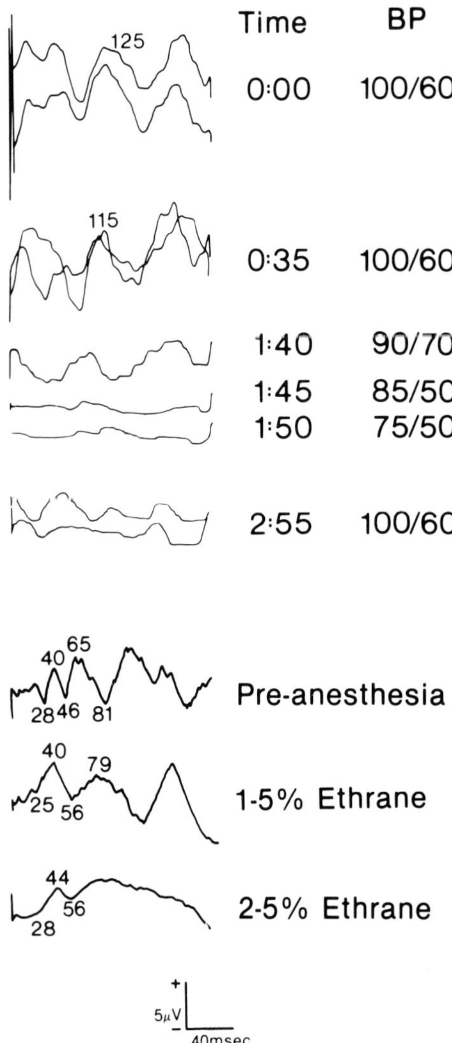

FIG. 26.2. The effect of some systemic factors that can influence evoked potentials in the operating room. Note the loss of the visual evoked components when blood pressure drops. At the bottom, there is a decrease in amplitude, a lengthening of latency, and a loss of later components of somatosensory potentials as anesthetic level is raised.

throughout the remainder of the operative period. However, during the postoperative period normal evoked potentials were again detected, and there were no persisting changes in function.

CASE HISTORIES

Patient 1. This 36-year-old right-handed male developed a loss of vision in the right eye for 4 months which culminated in total blindness 1 month prior to hospitalization. Radiological tests were compatible with a pituitary tumor. Visual acuity in the left eye was 20/20, with a small superior temporal quadrantic defect. He was blind in the right eye without pattern reversal or diffuse flash evoked potentials. The electroretinogram was normal. During surgical decompression of the right optic nerve, visual evoked potentials abruptly appeared at a latency of 170 msec and persisted through the procedure (Fig. 26.3). Postoperatively, the patient regained partial vision, and the evoked responses to the alternating checkerboard and diffuse flash stimulation of the previously blind eye were present but were of broadened morphology and low amplitude.

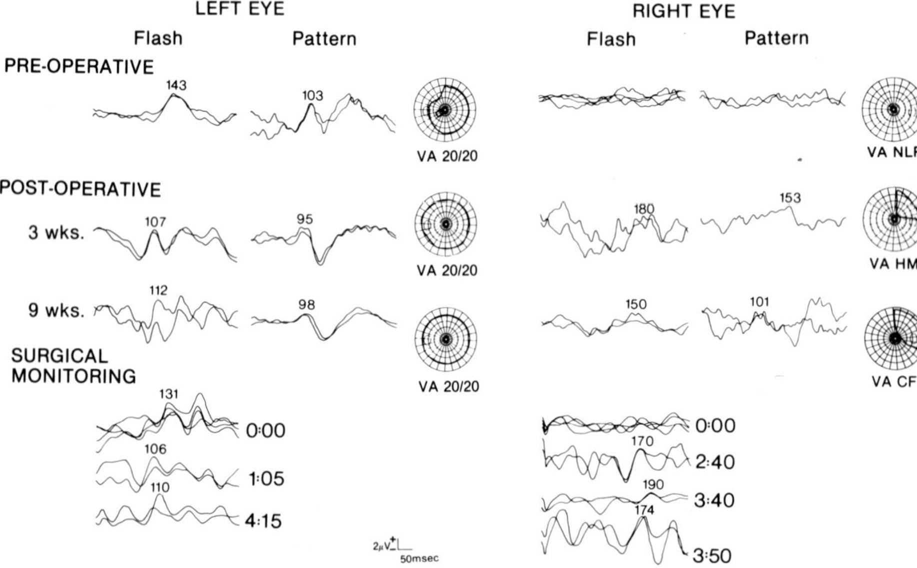

FIG. 26.3. Visual evoked potentials, pituitary tumor. Visual fields, flash and pattern-reversal evoked potentials from patient 1 (visual evoked potentials) recorded preoperatively, during surgery, and postoperatively. Preoperatively there was no light perception (*NLP*) in the right eye; postoperatively at 3 weeks hand movement (*HM*) could be distinguished and at 6 weeks counting of fingers (*CF*) was possible. The numbers above the positive component of the evoked potential wave forms is its latency in msec. Note the appearance of potentials at 170 msec from stimulating the previously unresponsive right eye at 2:40 into the surgery.

Patient 2. This 20-year-old woman complained of blurring of her vision 1 year prior to admission. A "black spot" in the middle of her vision developed when she used the left eye which then progressed 1 month prior to admission to total blindness. On admission the visual acuity was 20/20 in the right eye, with a right temporal field defect, and the left eye was blind to light. There were no clear potentials evoked from stimulating the left eye (Fig. 26.4). Following decompression of the optic nerve (at 2: 30 in Fig. 26.4) potentials abruptly appeared with a positive component at approximately 160 msec. Postoperatively, the patient was able to count fingers. Over the subsequent 3 weeks, visual acuity in the left eye

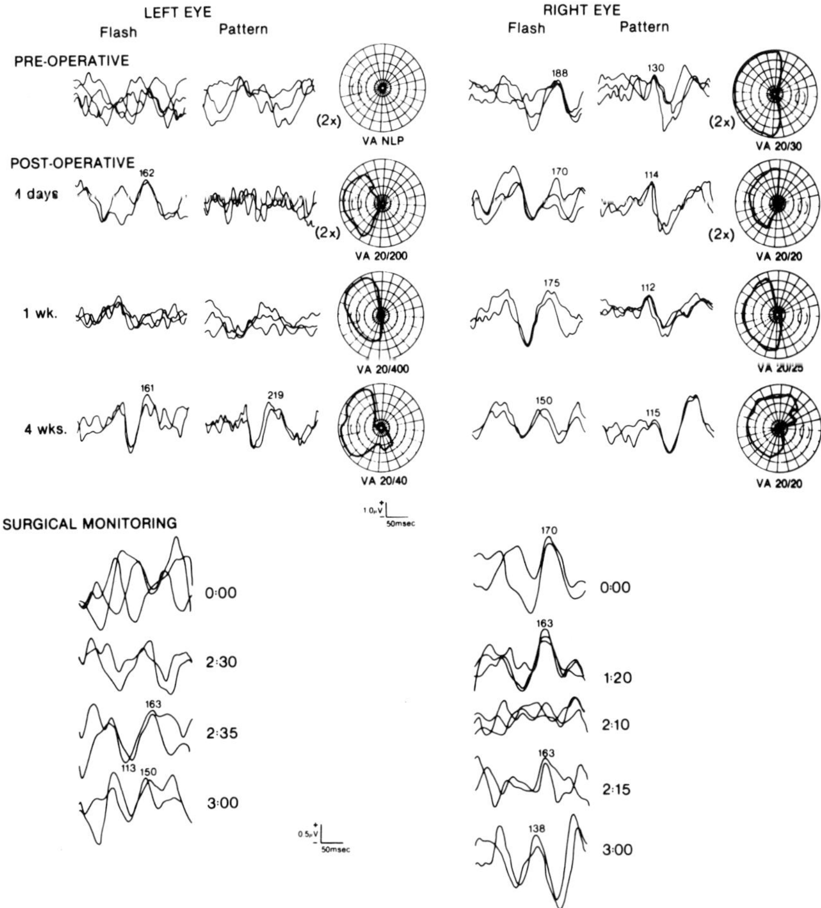

FIG. 26.4. Evoked potentials from case 2 (visual evoked potentials, pituitary tumor). The format is the same as in the preceding figure. Note the appearance of reproducible components on stimulating the left eye at 2:35 from a previously unresponsive state.

improved to 20/40, and the positive component's latency to the diffuse flash was 161 msec and to the checkerboard 219 msec. The visual field defect in the right eye was gone after surgery, and the latency of the positive component from stimulating that eye also decreased from 130 msec preoperatively to 115 msec.

Patient 3. This 50-year-old male had the abrupt onset of blindness in the left eye 6 weeks prior to admission. On admission the visual acuity in the right eye was 20/20, and there was no light perception with the left eye. No reliable potentials to light flash could be defined from stimulating the left eye (Fig. 26.5). At surgery the optic nerves were surrounded by extensive adhesions with a small amount of necrotic material within the sella. As the left optic nerve was freed from adhesions (at 3:15 in Fig. 26.5), visual evoked potentials appeared with a positive peak at 103 msec which persisted for the remainder of the surgery. However, postoperatively no visual evoked potentials could be obtained, and the patient remained totally blind.

Patient 4. This 25-year-old male sustained a basilar skull fracture and a loss of vision in the left eye presumably secondary to an orbital fracture. Visual acuity was 20/20 in the right eye. Six days following injury the patient was taken to surgery. There was a fracture of the optic canal with bony fragment impinging on the optic nerve. Following decompression of the left optic nerve, visual evoked potentials appeared for the first time with a positive peak at 110 msec. However, near the end of the surgery the potentials were again lost. Postoperatively, the patient remained blind, and visual evoked potentials were not evident.

Patient 5. This 25-year-old male had a 1-month history of headaches and loss of peripheral vision. Visual acuity on admission was 20/20 bilaterally and a superior quadrantic defect was detected. During surgery a pituitary abscess was evacuated. Near the end of surgery the base of the brain was irrigated with cool saline, resulting in a loss of the evoked potentials (Fig. 26.6). The potentials did not return during the remainder of the surgical procedure. The following day the patient's visual acuity was 20/20, and the latency of visual evoked potentials to both flash and alternating checkerboard were normal.

Patient 6. This 27-year-old male (Fig. 26.7) complained of headaches and decreased vision in the right eye. Angiography revealed a large basilar artery aneurysm. At surgery the aneurysm protruded forward and impinged on the right optic nerve. To facilitate clipping of the aneurysm the level of anesthesia was increased, producing an abrupt drop in blood pressure to 85/58. The visual evoked potentials were lost following the fall in blood pressure and did not reappear for almost 90 minutes. Postoperatively, the patient's visual acuity was 20/20, and the positive component evoked by alternating checkerboard stimulus at 150 msec was narrower than preoperatively.

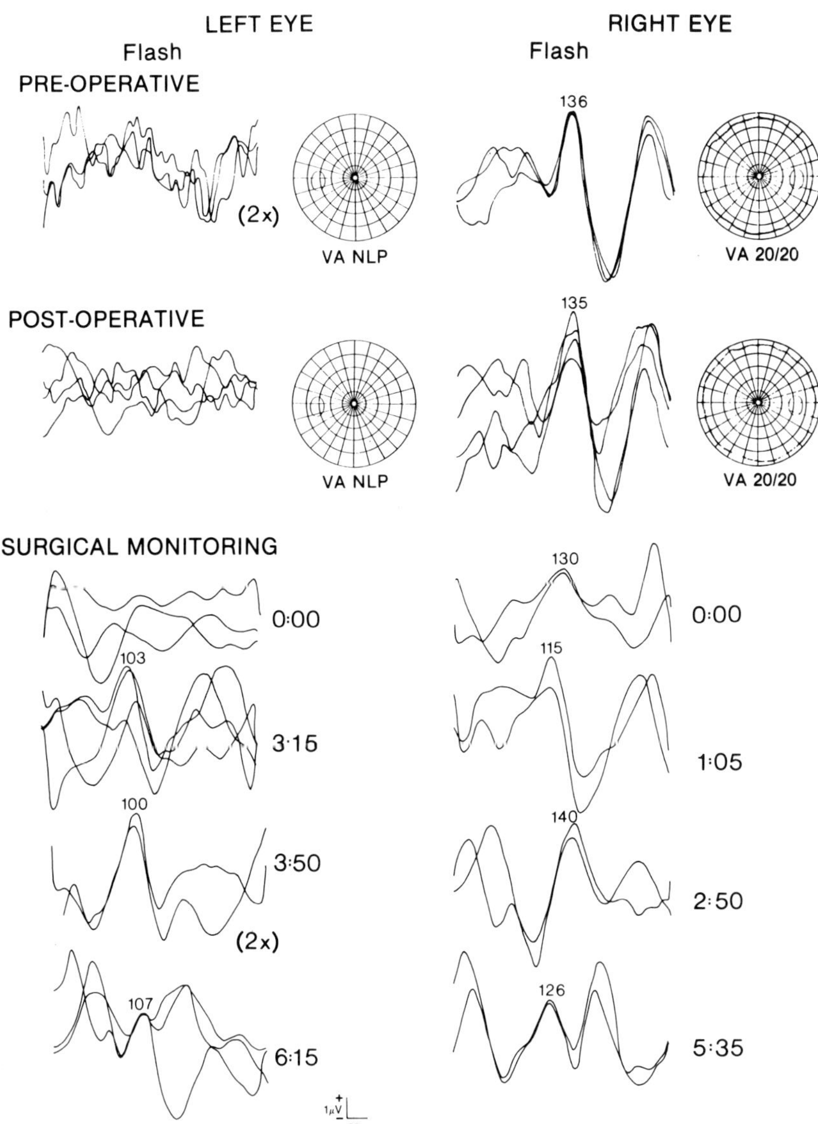

FIG. 26.5. Evoked potentials from case 3 (visual evoked potentials, arachnoiditis). Note appearance of reproducible components on stimulating the left eye at 3:15 and 3:50, and their attenuation at 6:15. No evoked potentials were detected on stimulating the left eye postoperatively. *NLP*, no light perception.

Patient 7. This 45-year-old man had a 10-year history of headaches which ceased 1 year prior to admission. Preoperative studies revealed a massive pituitary tumor with suprasellar extension and erosion into the sphenoid sinus. During surgical decompression the chiasm was manipu-

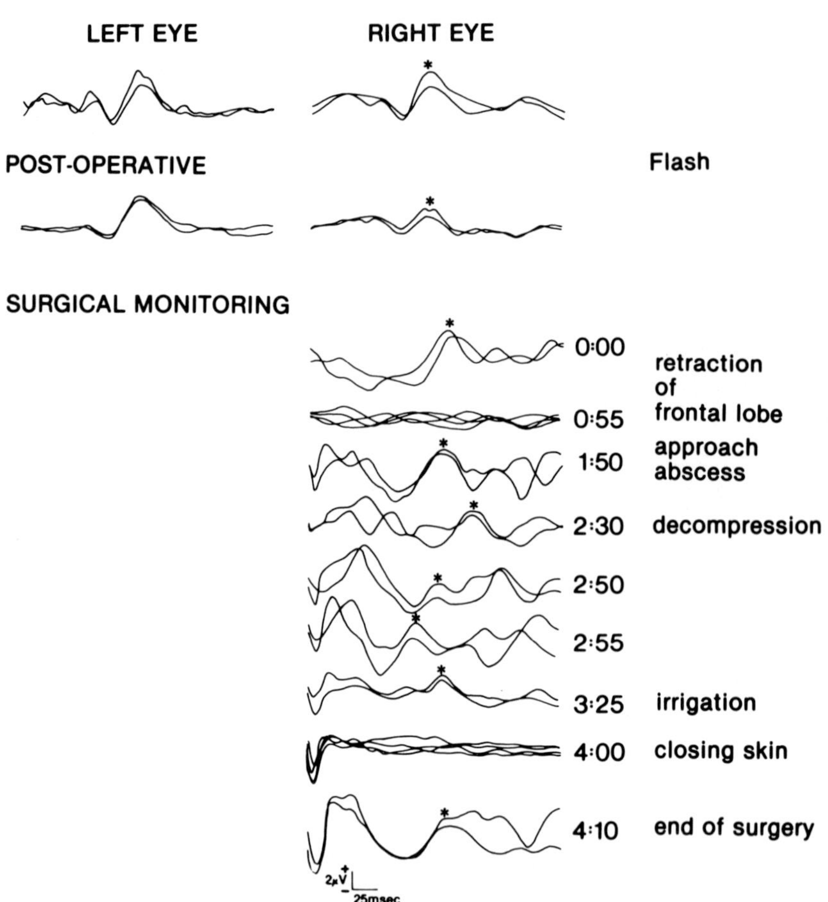

FIG. 26.6. Evoked potentials from case 5 (visual evoked potentials, pituitary abscess). * indicates the peak of the positive component to diffuse light flash. The tracings in the top line are the preoperative recordings. Note the fluctuation in its latency during surgery and the loss at 0:55, and again at 4:00.

lated, resulting in a transient loss of the evoked potentials (Fig. 26.8, *left eye*, 6:30). Throughout the surgery there were other transient changes in the latency and morphology of the evoked potentials accompanying various operative procedures. Postoperatively, vision and evoked potentials were normal.

Summary of Visual Evoked Potentials in the Operating Room

The first four patients illustrate a persistent return or improvement of visually evoked potentials occurring during surgery. In the first two cases, the appearance of potentials from a previously unresponsive state was correlated with a degree of return of vision postoperatively. In the latter two patients, the potentials appeared during surgery, on decompression of the optic nerve, but were absent once again postoperatively, and the patients remained blind. Cases 5 and 6 illustrate changes in evoked potentials accompanying changes in the level of anesthesia, blood pres-

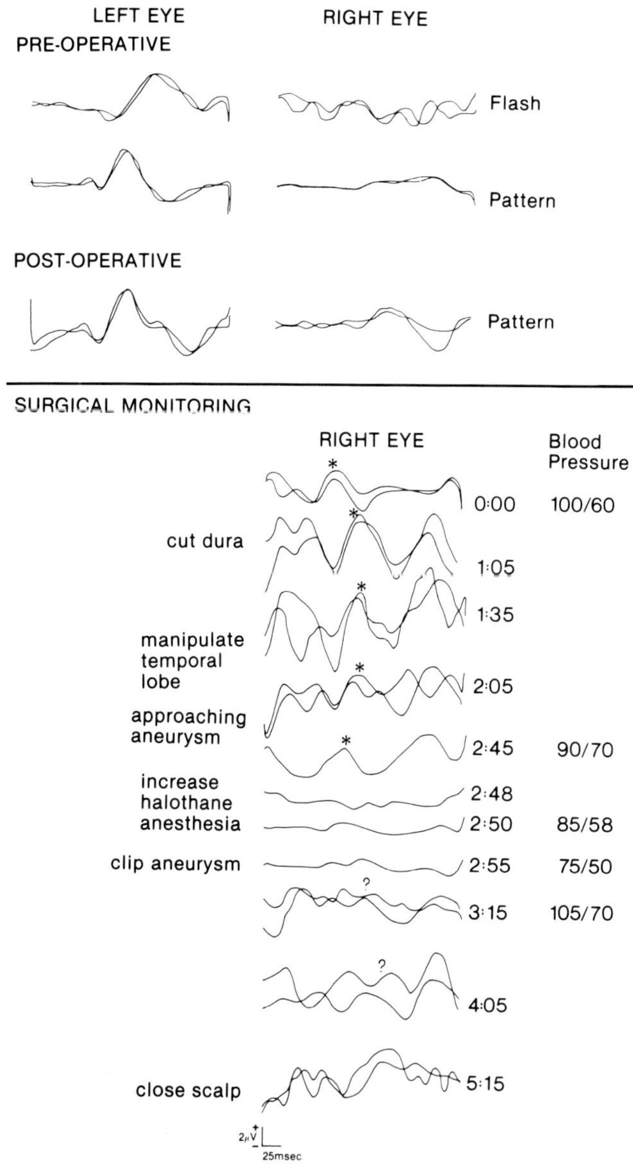

FIG. 26.7. Evoked potentials for case 6 (visual evoked potentials, basilar artery aneurysm). Note the loss of components at 2:48 when anesthesia was increased and blood pressure dropped.

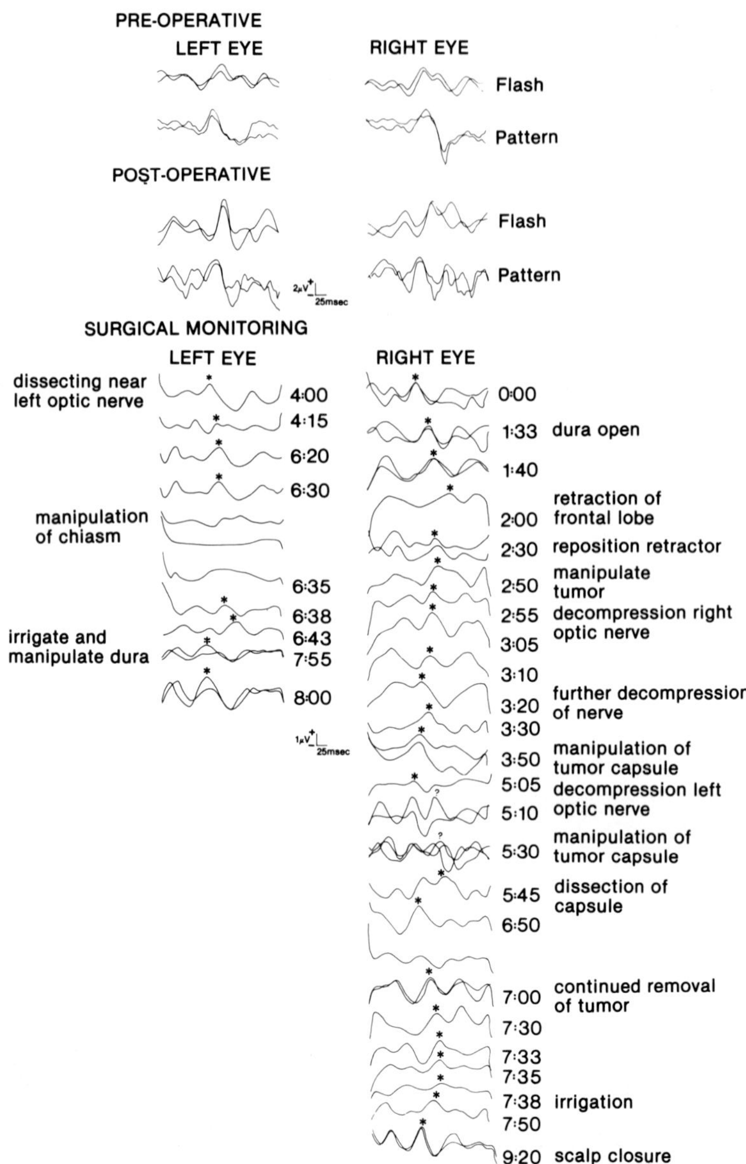

FIG. 26.8. Evoked potentials from case 7 (visual evoked potentials, pituitary adenoma). There are transient fluctuations of the potentials throughout the course of surgery related to various operative interventions. * designates the peak of the positive component to diffuse light stimulation monitored through the surgery.

sure, and irrigation around the optic nerves that persisted through the surgery but were not associated with any postoperative change of visual function. Case 7 illustrates a wide variety of transient changes in evoked potentials that can occur without any postoperative visual deficit.

Auditory Evoked Potentials

Auditory brainstem responses (ABR) consist of a series of up to seven components of submicrovolt amplitude which are thought to originate from sequential activation of the nuclei and tracts of the brainstem auditory pathway (10) (Fig. 26.1). The latency of these components changes in an orderly fashion with signal intensity whereas the interpeak latencies, reflecting transmission within the brainstem pathway, are unaffected by signal levels (14).

Technically satisfactory auditory brainstem potentials were obtained in 90% of the patients at surgery. There were persistent worsening of the potentials in 3 patients that correlated in two with changes in their postoperative neurologic findings. There were 5 patients who had transient changes in evoked potentials which were unassociated with postoperative changes or new neurologic deficit.

CASE HISTORIES

Patient 1. This 45-year-old woman with a 10-year history of trigeminal neuralgia was operated upon for an intracranial section of the trigeminal nerve. During surgery the cerebellum was retracted, and immediately thereafter the auditory brainstem potentials after Wave I were lost (Fig. 26.9). Subsequently, these components reappeared but their amplitudes were reduced, and the central conduction time (I–V) was prolonged from 4.1 msec to 6.0 msec. On recovery from surgery, the patient was deaf in the right ear and had a partial right facial paralysis. Three days postoperatively, the I–V interval of the auditory brainstem potentials were still abnormal.

Patient 2. This 14-year-old boy had a menigioma near the left cerebellopontine angle and presented with a history of progressive weakness of his left face, decreased sensation in the trigeminal distribution, and absent hearing in the left ear. Preoperatively, no auditory brainstem potentials were elicited to left-sided stimulation, whereas normal potentials were evoked from right-sided stimulation. During the surgical procedure, auditory brainstem potentials to right-sided stimulation were lost during aspiration of cerebrospinal fluid from the posterior fossa at the time blood pressure fluctuations and tachycardia occurred. The surgical procedure was temporarily halted until cardiac rhythm and blood pressure stabilized. However, during the remainder of the surgical procedure, no

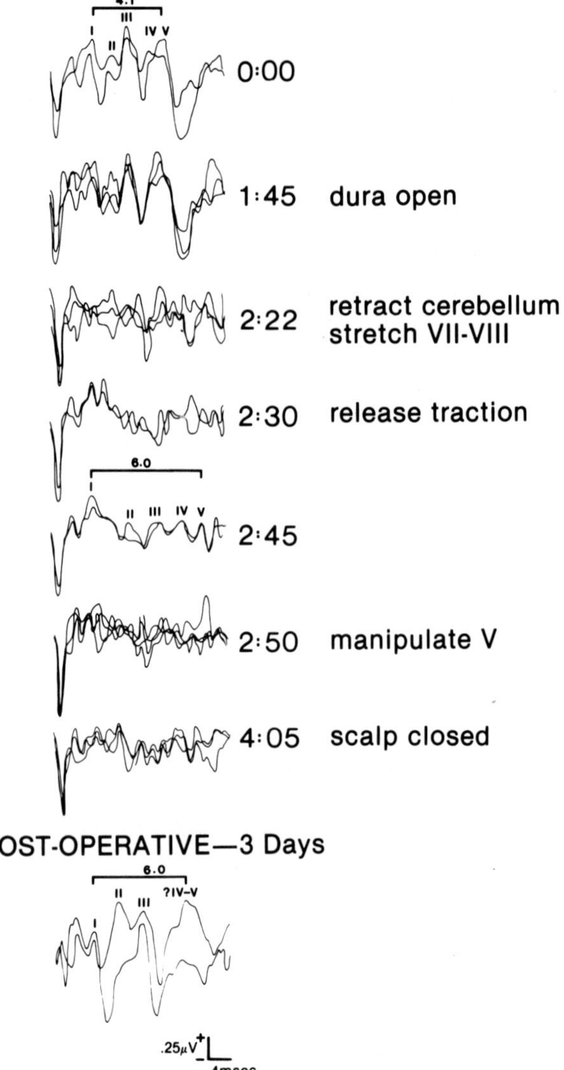

FIG. 26.9. Auditory brainstem responses section of trigeminal nerve. Evoked potentials from case 1 (auditory evoked potentials). Auditory brainstem components with peak designation and I–V interpeak latency were recorded during section of the trigeminal nerve. Note the loss of components at 2:22 and their reappearance at 2:45 but with prolonged I–V intervals.

auditory brainstem potentials could be recorded bilaterally. Postoperatively, the patient had improvement of the left Vth and VIIth cranial nerves and hearing was present in the left ear. Auditory brainstem potentials postoperatively were normal from stimulation of the right ear, and components were evident from stimulation of the left ear compatible with a 40-db hearing loss.

Patient 3. This 60-year-old male had a progressive loss of hearing in the right ear due to an acoustic neuroma. Preoperatively, auditory brainstem potentials were normal on stimulating the left ear, and showed a 20- to 30-db hearing loss on the right with normal interpeak conduction times. During removal of the tumor the potentials were obliterated transiently on both sides. As the tumor was removed, the potentials evoked by stimulating the affected ear became abnormal with only a small amplitude wave I still evident at a delayed latency. The responses from stimulating the contralateral ear were normal. The loss of ABR was thought to be associated with damage to the VIIIth nerve coincident with tumor removal. Audiometry, performed 1 week following surgery, revealed a totally deaf right ear, and auditory brainstem potentials were absent.

Patient 4. This 50-year-old female was originally admitted to the psychiatric unit because of confusion. Additional history was of a gait disturbance of approximately 1-year duration. Examination revealed multiple cranial nerve deficits on the right. Auditory brainstem potentials tested preoperatively revealed prolonged central conduction times of 4.7 msec on the right, and 5.1 msec on the left (normal values for our laboratory are 4.0 ± 0.2 msec). At surgery a large posterior fossa meningioma was found compressing and thinning the cerebellum with distortion of cranial nerves. Obliteration of brainstem potentials occurred transiently during removal of the central portion of the tumor. During removal of the tumor capsule there was a further transient prolongation of central conduction time of 0.2 msec. Postoperatively the patient had improvement of the Vth and VIIth cranial nerves, but there were no significant changes in auditory function or evoked potentials. The tumor had most likely produced a persisting alteration in auditory brainstem functions due to chronic pressure.

Summary to Auditory Brainstem Potentials in the Operating Room

Changes in auditory brainstem potentials correlated with postoperative symptoms with one exception (Patient 2). In this individual the ABRs were inexplicably lost following changes in blood pressure accompanying aspiration of CSF from the posterior fossa.

Somatosensory Evoked Potentials

Somatosensory evoked potentials consist of both submicrovolt components of short latency that reflect activity in spinal cord and brainstem pathways and of high amplitude long latency components that reflect activity in thalamic and cortical structures (Fig. 26.1). The scalp recording montage used in this study (Cz or C3, C4 referenced to the mastoid) enhances detection of the long latency events. Stimulation of the median nerve typically elicits a small positive component at 15 msec, a negative component at 19 msec, a positive component or components at 25 to 30 msec, and subsequent negative and positive waves at 35 and 45 msec, respectively. Stimulation of the nerves in the lower extremity leads to the same sequence of components but is delayed approximately 10 msec. In the operating room it was unpredictable which of the long latency cortical components would be sufficiently robust to serve as a marker of somatosensory function during the operative procedure. In general, P25 from median nerve and P40 from peroneal nerve were sufficiently stable and of high enough amplitude to serve as a monitor while in other instances the later positive waves at 70 to 80 msec were preferable. In only rare instances was the initial short latency positive and negative component (P15, N19 from median nerve stimulation) of sufficient amplitude to allow reliable monitoring during surgery.

Somatosensory stimulation evoked clear evoked potentials in 57% of the patients studied. The small number of useful responses during surgery was related to a large proportion of patients (24%) who had abnormal preoperative recordings. In addition 19% of the patients had intraoperative responses that were too contaminated by artifact or too variable, limiting their utility.

Transient changes in the evoked potentials were detected in all but 1 patient. These changes consisted of reduction in amplitude and or a prolongation in latency of the various components. These alternations were particularly evident with the later cortical components. Anesthetic level and blood pressure were significant variables affecting the cortical components of the somatosensory potentials (Fig. 26.2). Manipulation of the spinal cord was associated with transient loss of potentials. In one patient these changes persisted and were correlated with a postoperative deficit. The most dramatic changes in the evoked potentials occurred whenever the dura was open and direct contact was made with the spinal cord.

CASE HISTORIES

Patient 1. This 25-year-old male sustained head injuries resulting in an unstable odontoid process. The patient did not have neck pain and was without deficits. During surgery, median nerve stimulation produced well-formed N17, P29, and N56 components. There were transient minor alterations in morphology and a 50% reduction in amplitude of the N56 wave during the operation. Postoperatively the patient had an uneventful recovery with no neurological deficits.

Patient 2. This 4-year-old female with multiple congenital defects complained of back pain. A tethered cord was demonstrated on myelography. At surgery a fibrous strand was evident which upon stimulation evoked no potentials (Fig. 26.10). In contrast, peroneal nerve stimulation evoked a positive component at 85 msec both prior to and after section of the tethering band. Postoperatively the child had no neurologic deficits.

Patient 3. This 20-year-old female with idiopathic scoliosis of 80° was admitted for surgical correction. The neurologic examination revealed an inconsistent diminution of pin sensation in the lower extremities with a variable pattern of weakness. During anesthesia the initial positive component at 35 to 40 msec was unclear whereas P80 and P120 were prominent (Fig. 26.11). Postoperatively, no deficits were detected.

Patient 4. This 45-year-old male with a 2-year history of progressive weakness in his arms and legs was found to have cerfical spondylosis with a narrow spinal canal. There was wasting of the intrinsic muscles of the hands and a spastic paraparesis. At surgery the patient had an abrupt drop in blood pressure which obliterated the P80 wave of the somatosen-

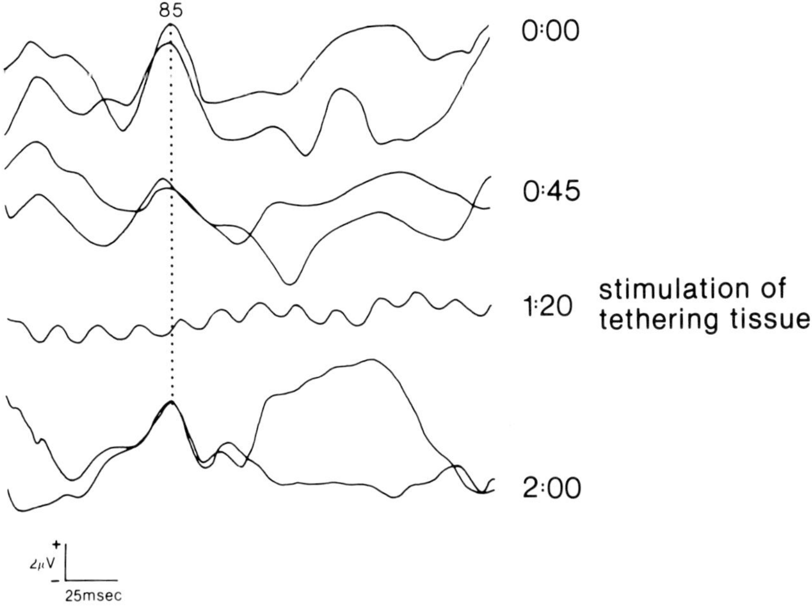

FIG. 26.10. Evoked potentials from case 1 (somatosensory evoked potentials, tethered spinal cord). Components P85 is present on stimulating the peroneal nerve but absent when the tethered strand is stimulated at 1:20.

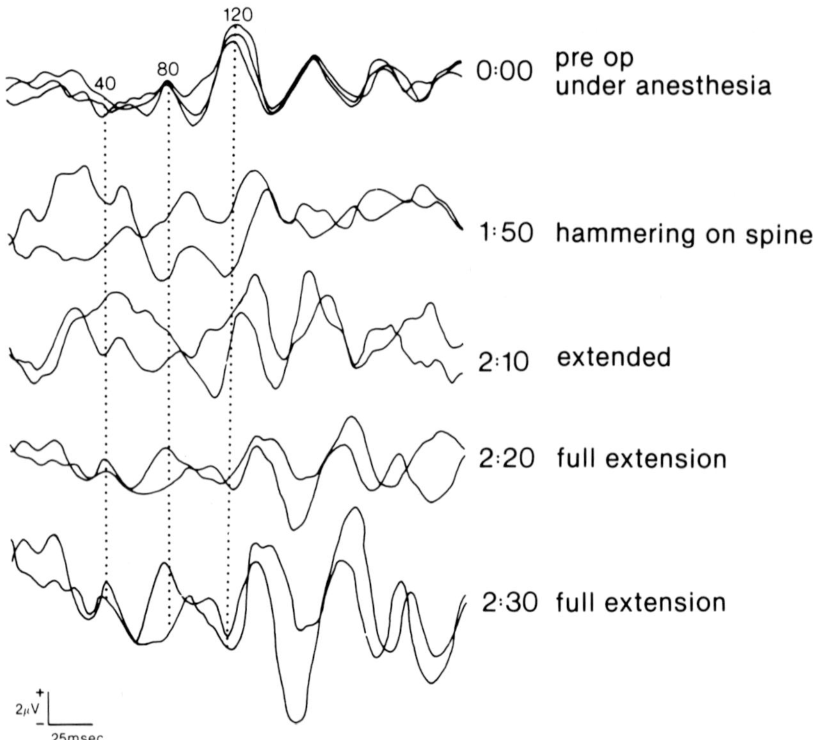

FIG. 26.11. Evoked potentials from case 3 (somatosensory evoked potentials, Harrington rod placement). Components P40, P80, and P120 are designated, but only the latter is clearly evident throughout the operation.

sory evoked potential but was without affect on the initial P15, N20, and P25 components (Fig. 26.12). Following reestablishment of adequate blood pressure the evoked potential returned to baseline. The balance of the procedure revealed fluctuations in potentials, especially when the dura was compressed with shifts of up to 10 msec in the P25 wave. Postoperatively no new deficits were noted.

Patient 5. This 27-year-old male presented with 5 years of progressive spastic paraparesis. Some 15 years previously he had been transiently quadriplegic. On examination he had marked spastic paraparesis, with intact position and vibratory senses bilaterally. At surgery there was an intrinsic spinal cord tumor at the cervical-thoracic junction. The P40 and P70 components of the potentials to stimulating the peroneal nerve were monitored. These components fluctuated in amplitude and latency throughout the procedure and became unobtainable at the time of tumor manipulation and removal. Postoperatively the patient was weak in his left lower extremity and paralyzed in the right lower extremity. Some 9 months later the evoked potential had returned to normal. His strength and proprioception were normal at the time on the right side (Fig. 26.13).

Summary of Somatosensory Evoked Potentials in the Operating Room

Somatosensory evoked potentials proved to be the most difficult of the sensory systems to study in the operating room. The components fluctuated in latency and amplitude with changes in level of anesthesia and blood pressure as well as when spinal cord transmission was affected by manipulation. Nevertheless, the method proved of value in assessing spinal cord function during the extension of Harrington rods and during operation on the spine and cord itself.

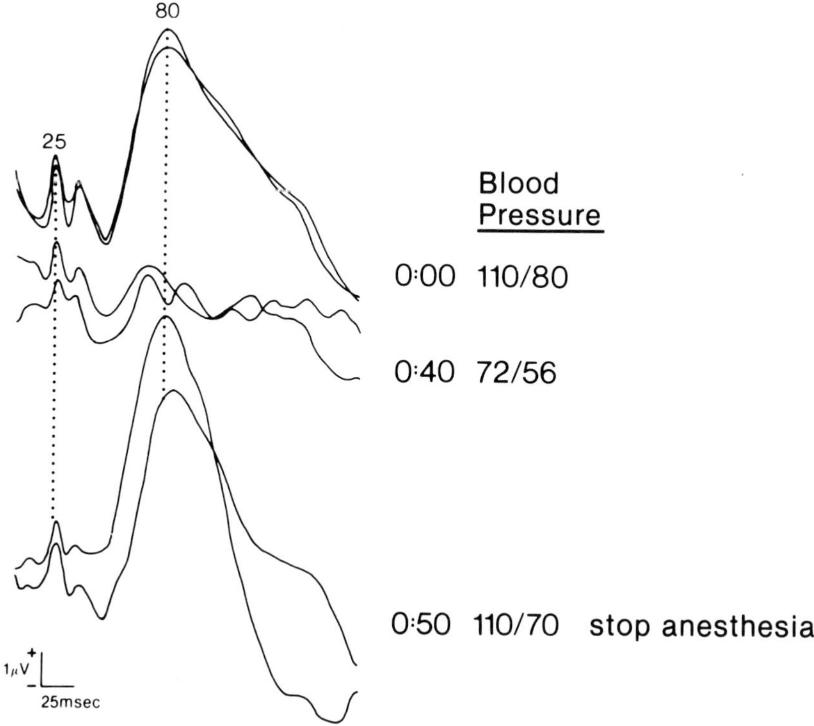

FIG. 26.12. Evoked potentials from case 4 (somatosensory evoked potentials, cervical spondylosis). Components P25 and P80 are designated. Note the loss of the latter when blood pressure dropped at 0:40 into the operation.

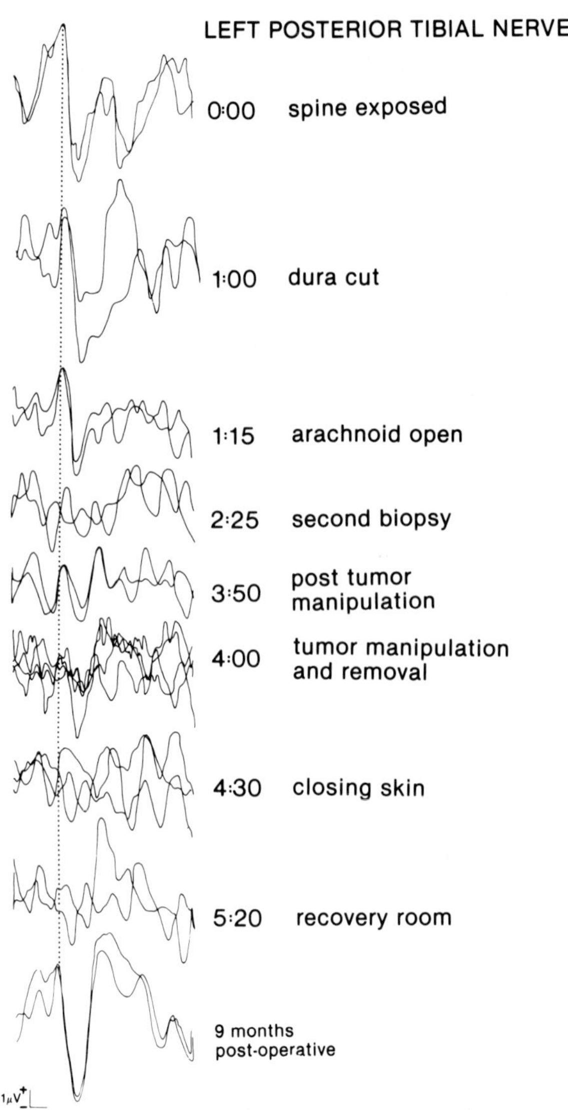

FIG. 26.13. Evoked potentials from case 5 (somatosensory evoked potentials, surgical monitoring of spinal cord tumor). Note the loss of reproducible responses at 4:00 when the spinal cord tumor was removed.

DISCUSSION

Monitoring of sensory pathways in the operating room using computer averaging techniques is a challenging area of clinical research. Previously, the integrity of the sensory pathway could only be examined clinically when the patient recovered from anesthesia. Evoked potentials provide an immediate assessment of the effects of surgery on the nervous system with implications for modifying surgical techniques. During this study we applied evoked potential techniques in a variety of circumstances to demonstrate their feasibility to assist the surgeon. Useful recordings were obtained in the majority of patients, and the resulting changes could be correlated to some extent with postoperative morbidity and improvement.

The most dramatic results occurred monitoring visual function during operations near the optic nerve and chiasm. The abrupt appearance of potentials from stimulating a previously blind eye occurred in 4 patients. In 2 of these patients vision was restored postoperatively. In the other 2 patients vision was not restored even though neural conduction, albeit temporary, did occur when the optic nerve was decompressed. The failure for useful conduction to persist postoperatively is unclear and indicates that additional information is needed as to the effects of chronic compression and its removal on nervous system function.

Evoked potentials recordings in the operating room should utilize those components that are primarily sensitive to focal changes in the functions of the sensory pathway and that are only slightly affected by systemic factors such as level of anesthesia, BP, and CO_2. It would seem that components arising from spinal cord, brainstem, and subcortex are best suited for these requirements whereas cerebral cortically generated components are unsuitable.

The visual and somatosensory components of the evoked potentials measured in the present study have as their generators cerebral structures. In contrast the ABR components originate from the brainstem. The well-known sensitivity of the cerebrum and the primary sensory cortex to anesthetic agents is most likely responsible for a large portion of the fluctuation in latency and amplitude of the visual and somatosensory potential during the operations (16). In contrast, the ABR is remarkably stable even under doses of anesthetic that can produce absence of cerebral electrical activity as manifested by an isoelectric EEG (15). Thus, it would be preferable to study the spinal cord, brainstem, and subcortical evoked potential components to somatosensory stimuli as a way of minimizing the influence of anesthetics. In the visual system, the identification of the response of subcortical visual structures from scalp recordings has only begun to be examined, and the results are preliminary (3, 7).

During manipulation of the neural structures at surgery there were considerable fluctuations in the evoked potentials. Changes in latency and even total obliteration of the response did not necessarily signify a poor outcome. In general, if the changes were transient (less than 15 minutes), no postoperative deficits were present. When evoked potential changes persisted, the probability of alterations in neurological status was increased. Notable exceptions occurred in 4 patients who had persistent changes in the evoked potentials during surgery but no postoperative deficits. The evoked potential changes occurred when there was change in brain temperature associated with irrigation with cold solution, drop in blood pressure, or increased levels of anesthesia. Thus, knowledge of the events associated with the evoked potential changes is paramount for correct interpretation of their significance.

In general the difficulties encountered in recording evoked potentials in the operating room are greater than those found in the laboratory. Constraints of space and difficulty in verifying electrodes and cables once the patient has been prepped can pose problems. Moreover, there are major problems related to artifacts from surgical manipulation and electrocautery. On the other hand, the recordings are easier in some respects since the patient is paralyzed, removing the confounding influence of muscle potential artifacts.

Of paramount importance in the operating room is the establishment of good rapport between the surgical team and the individual measuring evoked potentials since it is necessary at times to request that the operation briefly halt to obtain recordings not contaminated by artifact. This is particularly true when abrupt changes in the potentials are noted and their significance is not understood. The actual length of time that the surgical procedure may be prolonged by monitoring must be weighed against the savings in an unsuspected permanent neurologic deficit. In our experience the surgical procedure has never been extended more than 15 minutes beyond what was required by the actual procedure.

Certainly the technique of evoked potential monitoring in the operating room needs much additional development. The effects of variety of anesthetic agents and a host of other parameters (blood pressure, temperature, CO_2, pH, etc.) have on evoked potentials components remain to be systematically investigated. How do traction and manipulation affect nerve conduction in normal and chronically compressed neural tissue? When do transient changes in function become significant?

We believe it is evident that the application of these relatively new computer techniques offers the surgeon an important means of assessing ongoing physiological activity in specific sensory pathways during critical portions of the surgery. We expect that as the validity of this information is established, the surgeon will certainly be influenced in his operative approach.

SUMMARY

Sensory evoked potentials (visual, auditory, and somatosensory) were recorded from 56 patients at the time of surgery to monitor neural function during critical portions of the operation. Fluctuations in latency and amplitude of the components occurred with changes in depth of anesthesia, blood pressure, irrigation, and neural tissue manipulation. Most of these changes were only transient. Permanent changes in evoked potentials occurred with decompression of neural tissue and prolonged retraction. Transient changes were not associated with any change in postoperative neurological function whereas changes in evoked potentials that persisted through the operation were highly likely to be associated with a postoperative change.

ACKNOWLEDGMENTS

We wish to express our appreciation to the neurosurgeons Dr. John Kusske, Dr. Don DeFeo, and Dr. Eldon Foltz, and the orthopedic surgeons, Dr. Ted Waugh and Dr. William McMasters, for their interest and helpful comments throughout these studies.

REFERENCES

1. Achor, L. J., and Starr, A. Auditory brain stem responses in the cat. I. Intracranial and extracranial recordings. Electroencephalogr. Clin. Neurophysiol., *48:* 154–173, 1980.
2. Achor, L. J., and Starr, A. Auditory brain stem responses in the cat. II. Effects of lesions. Electroencephalogr. Clin. Neurophysiol., *48:* 174–190, 1980.
3. Cracco, R. Q., and Cracco, J. B. Visual evoked potential in man: early oscillatory potentials. Electroencephalogr. Clin. Neurophysiol., *45:* 731–739, 1978.
4. Engler, G. L., Spielholz, N. I., Bernhard, W. N., Danziger, F., Merkin, H., and Wolff, T. Somatosensory evoked potentials during Harrington instrumentation for scoliosis. J. Bone Joint Surg. (Am.), *60:* 528–532, 1978.
5. Evoked potentials. *In* Proceedings of ... edited by C. Barber, International Evoked Potentials Symposium, Nottingham, England, 1978. University Park Press, Baltimore, 1980.
6. Feinsod, M., Selhorst, J., Hoyt, W. F., and Wilson, C. Monitoring optic nerve function during craniotomy. J. Neurosurg., *44:* 29–31, 1976.
7. Harding, G. F. A., and Rubinstein, M. P. The scalp topography of the human visually evoked subcortical potential. Invest. Ophthalmol. Vis. Sci., *19:* 318–321, 1980.
8. Hashimoto, I., Ishiyama, Y., Totsuka, G., and Mizutani, H. Monitoring brainstem function during posterior fossa surgery with brainstem auditory evoked potentials. *In* Evoked Potentials, edited by C. Barber, Ed. 1, Chapter 43. MTP Press Limited, Lancaster, 1980.
9. Hattori, S., Saiki, K., and Kawai, S. Diagnosis of the level and severity of cord lesion in cervical spondylotic myelopathy. Spine, *4:* 478–485, 1979.
10. Jewett, D. L., and Williston, J. S. Auditory-evoked far fields averaged from the scalp of humans. Brain, *94:* 681–696, 1971.
11. Nash, C. L., Lorig, R. A., Schatziner, L. A., and Brown, R. H. Spinal cord monitoring during operative treatment of the spine. Clin. Orthop., *126:* 100–105, 1977.
12. Raudzens, P. Intracranial pressure effects on brainstem potentials (meeting abstract). *51*(3S)*:* S40, 1979.
13. Starr, A. Sensory evoked potentials in clinical disorders of the nervous system. Annu. Rev. Neurosci., *1:* 103–127, 1978.
14. Starr, A., and Achor, L. J. Auditory brainstem responses in neurological disease. Arch. Neurol., *32:* 761–768, 1975.
15. Stockard, J. J., Stockard, J. E., and Sharbrough, F. W. Nonpathologic factors influencing brainstem auditory evoked potentials. Am. J. EEG Technol., *18:* 177–209, 1978.
16. Uhl, R. R., Squires, K. C., Bruce, D. L., and Starr, A. Effect of halothane anesthesia on the human cortical visual evoked response. Anesthesiology, *53:* 273–276, 1980.

CHAPTER

27

Computed Tomography: Basic Principles of Operation

KENNETH R. MARAVILLA, M.D., and ROBERT C. MURRY, JR., PH.D.

INTRODUCTION

In the few short years since the introduction of computed tomography (CT), the rapid evolution of this technology has been truly remarkable. One has only to compare cross-sectional pictures of the brain obtained from the original CT scan unit with those obtainable with today's state-of-the art CT equipment in order to verify this (Fig. 27.1). As a result of the vastly improved image quality has come increased sensitivity of the CT method and improved diagnostic ability. Nevertheless, the full potential of CT has not yet been realized.

The main emphasis of CT research during the past 7 years has been directed toward two major objectives: first, faster scanning speed through more efficient methods of data (x-ray measurement) collection and, second, more sophisticated mathematical reconstruction algorithms which provide better picture quality and improved suppression of artifacts (1, 2). The results of these endeavors have been astounding, as can be seen from the technical comparisons listed in Table 27.1. However, we are now beginning to reach a plateau in our ability to further improve the quality of the CT image. Although some further improvements will no doubt be forthcoming, I believe the major emphasis of research and the greatest CT advances in the next few years will center mainly on computer manipulation and analysis of the massive amounts of data obtained from each scan. Techniques to provide dynamic information (6), more specific information regarding chemical composition of tissues (14), and three-dimensional interactive display of the CT image (7, 16, 17) are all active fields of research at the present time. In order to appreciate present as well as potential future applications of CT technology, one must understand the basic principles of the CT method as well as its inherent limitations. In the discussion which follows, we will look at these principles and also speculate briefly on where the technique may be headed in the not-too-distant future.

Principles of CT Operation

All of the various x-ray computed tomographic scanners work on the same basic principles as the original CT unit designed by Godfrey Hounsfield and built by EMI Limited (8). The basic operations of a CT scanner can be divided into three broad steps, namely: (a) data acquisition in which multiple measurements or "views" of x-ray absorption through the scanned object are obtained at different angles; (b) mathematical processing of the data in order to reconstruct a cross-sectional image of the scanned object; and (c) display of the mathematically reconstructed image on the video screen. The CT scanner measures x-ray absorption within a body by passing narrowly collimated pencil beams of x-ray from the source (x-ray tube) through the object being scanned to a precision x-ray detector. The amount of x-ray which is produced at the source minus the quantity transmitted through the body and registered by the detector provides a measurement of the amount absorbed within the body. Individual absorption measurements are taken at equally spaced intervals as the x-ray tube and detector traverse or "scan" across the patient. The x-ray tube and detector are then rotated and the scanning motion repeated at many different angles. Similar measurements are taken for each angle and the data is stored in the computer. These multiple pencil beam measurements form a lattice of intersecting points (Fig. 27.2) within the scan object. The data is then processed through a series of simultaneous equations (algorithm) in order to calculate relative absorption coefficients (Hounsfield numbers or CT numbers) for each intersecting point within the lattice. The result is a mathematical cross-sectional map of the object or body scanned. By assigning gray scale levels to the calculated numerical values, an image of the scanned object can be displayed on a video monitor.

The original EMI scanner utilized a single x-ray source and single detector to record each individual pencil beam measurement. A total of 28,800 measurements were taken, and a scan took approximately 300 seconds (8). At present all CT scanners use a fan-shaped beam of x-rays and multiple detectors to record a large number of pencil beam measurements simultaneously (Fig. 27.3). This greatly improves speed and efficiency of data collection so that a scan can be completed is as short as 2 to 5 seconds during which time several hundred thousand measurements may be taken! The types of CT equipment is use today can be divided into three broad categories (Fig. 27.4):

1. Rotate-Translate System (Fig. 27.4*A*). This is the earliest design of a fan beam scanner and is essentially a modification of the original first generation EMI Mark I scanner in which a fan-shaped beam has been

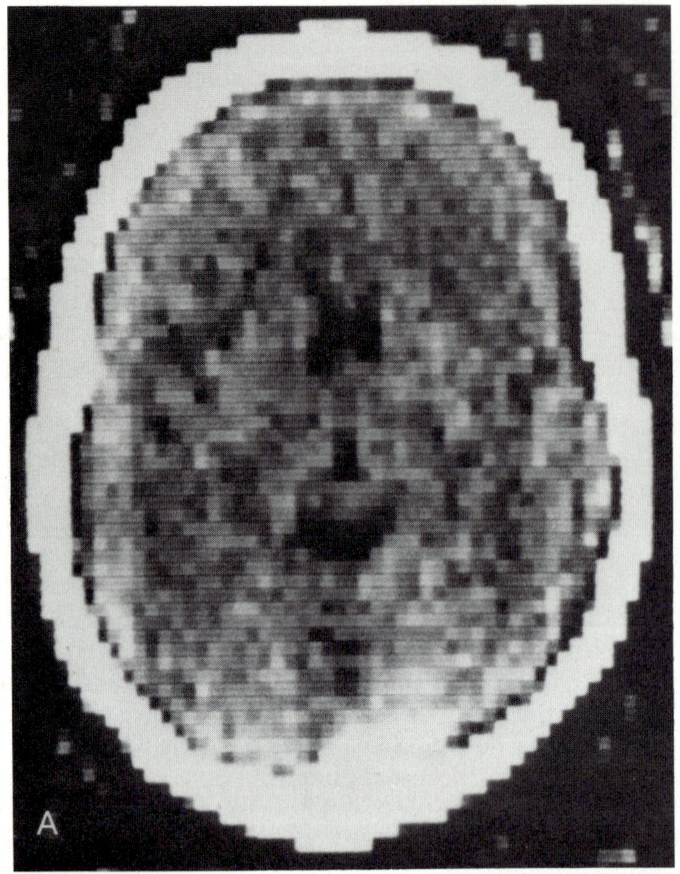

FIG. 27.1. Comparison of CT scans taken at similar anatomical levels using a first generation EMI scanner with an 80 × 80 matrix (*A*) versus the high quality picture obtainable with today's state-of-the-art equipment (*B*).

substituted for the single pencil beam. This design, although slower than the rotating fan beam scanners described below, is capable of performing a scan in approximately 18 seconds.

2. Rotating Tube-Rotating Detectors (Fig. 27.4*B*). In this design a pulsed fam beam of x-ray encompasses the entire patient, and multiple pencil-beam measurements (as many as 523) of the patient are obtained simultaneously with each pulse of the x-ray tube. The number of pencil beams encompassed in the fan beam is dictated solely by the number of detectors in the system. The x-ray tube and detectors are fixed to a wheel and rotate together 360° around the patient while measurements are obtained continuously. The system is fast (scans are obtained in 3 to 10 seconds), provides excellent resolution, and is highly reliable.

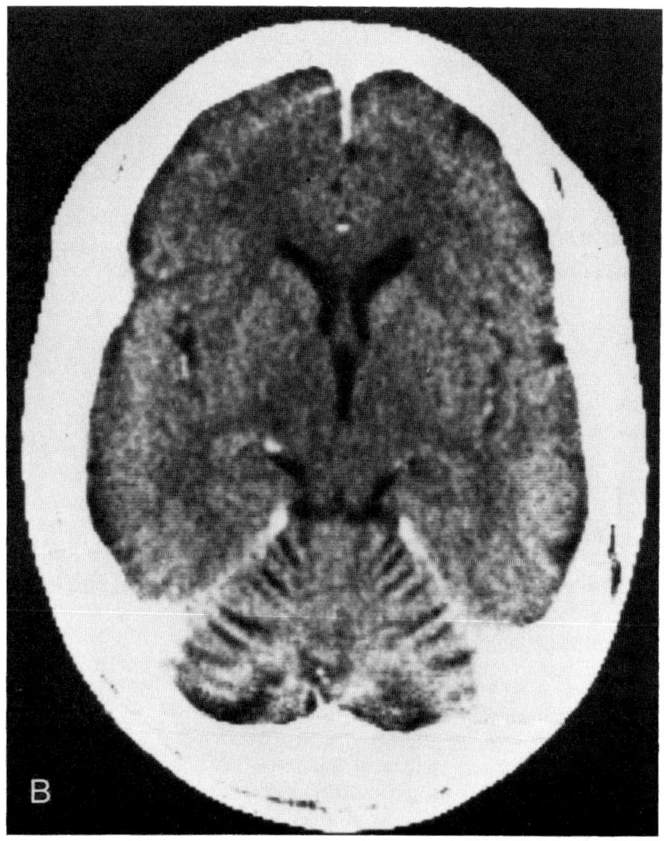

FIG. 27.1. (*B*)

TABLE 27.1
State of the Art of Computed Tomography

	1973	1980
Scanning time	300 sec	2–10 sec
Reconstruction time	300 sec	3–30 sec
No. of x-ray measurements	28,800	Several hundred thousand
Picture matrix	80 × 80	512 × 512
Pixel size	3 mm × 3 mm	0.5 mm × 0.5 mm
Slice thickness	13 mm	1–10 mm
Gray/white matter discrimination	Very poor	Excellent

3. Rotating X-Ray Tube-Fixed Ring of Detectors (Fig. 27.4*C*). Similar to the system described in 2, this type of machine also uses a fan beam of x-rays which encompasses the entire patient. However, unlike the previous system, the detectors do not move, but rather a ring of stationary detectors surrounds the patient. This type of system is also very fast and

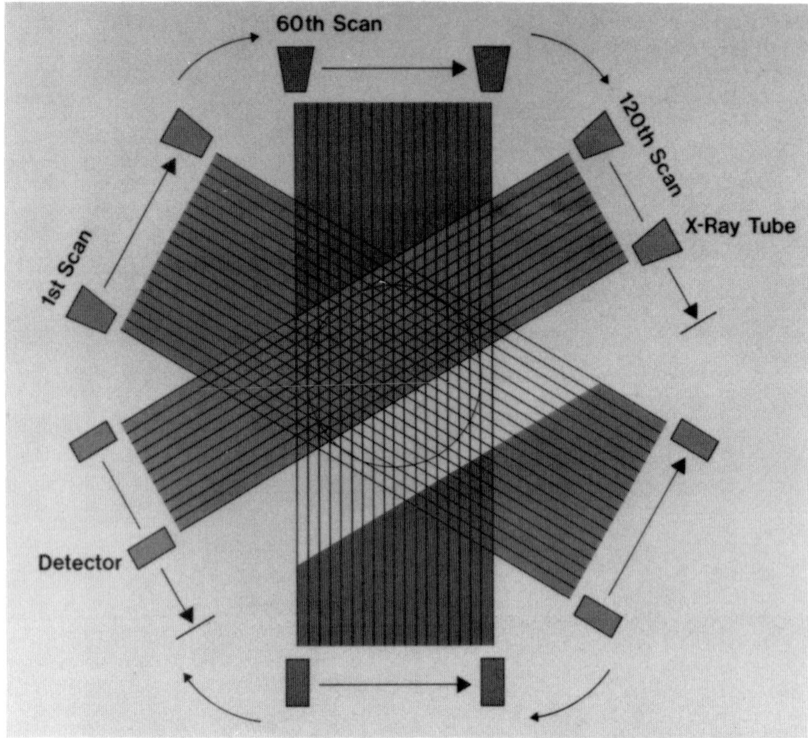

FIG. 27.2. Diagrammatic representation illustrating operation of original EMI CT scanner. A scan of equally spaced pencil beam measurements is obtained from multiple angles around the patient. These multiple measurements form a lattice of intersecting points within the head which can be used to calculate relative absorption coefficients. (From K. R. Maravilla and M. S. Pastel. Computed Tomography, *2:* 137–144, 1978. Published with permission.)

can scan in 2 to 10 seconds. Resolution is excellent, but the very large number of detectors needed to completely surround the patient can become very expensive. One of the advantages with the system is that the individual detectors can be collimated to varying degrees to provide either scans of high density resolution or scans of high spatial resolution at a fixed patient dose.

Resolution

Let us diverge at this point from geometric considerations of equipment design in order to consider the problem of resolution as it applies to the CT scan image. When one speaks of CT resolution, two different and inversely related types of resolution must be considered (9, 13). These are: spatial resolution, also called high contrast resolution, and density resolution, which is also called low contrast resolution.

Spatial resolution may be defined as the ability of a CT scanner to correctly reproduce small objects of relatively high density difference compared with the surrounding structures. Spatial resolution is related to the pixel (picture element) size to which the image has been reconstructed (9, 15). By convention spatial resolution is usually measured for objects having approximately a 10% difference in density compared with the surrounding tissue (13). High contrast spatial resolution in some of the more sophisticated CT machines available today is great enough to resolve parallel pinholes as small as 0.6 mm in diameter which are separated by a distance of 0.6 mm (Fig. 27.5). An example of high spatial resolution applied to clinical CT scanning includes visualization of major vessels at the base of the brain when enhanced with intravenous iodine

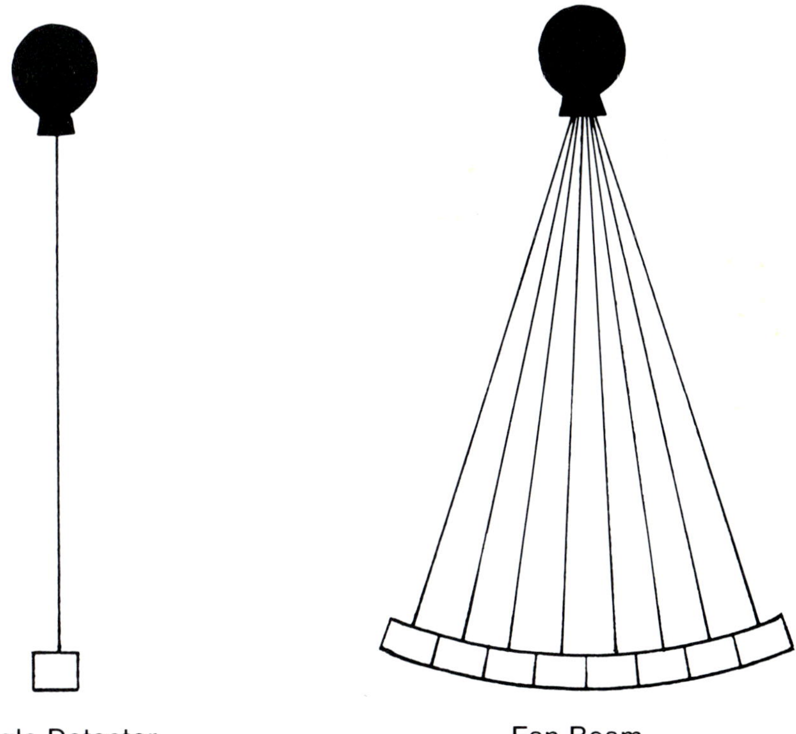

FIG. 27.3. The original CT scanner used a single detector to record data for each scan slice. All present day CT scanners use a fan-shaped beam with multiple detectors to record a large number of measurements simultaneously.

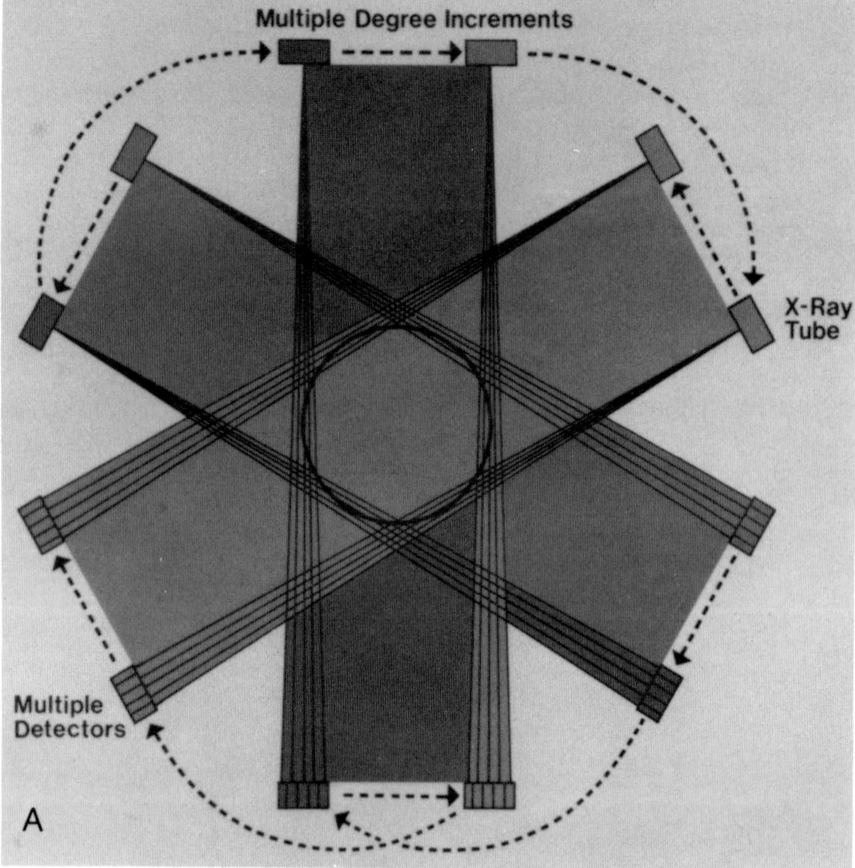

FIG. 27.4. Schematic representation of the various types of fan beam scanners available today: (*A*) Rotate-translate system; (*B*) Rotating tube-rotating detector system; and (*C*) Rotating X-ray tube-fixed detector system. (From K. R. Maravilla and M. S. Pastel. Computed Tomography, *2:* 137–144, 1978. Published with permission.)

contrast, or visualization of the optic nerves and individual intraorbital structures which are outlined by fat.

Density resolution, on the other hand, may be thought of as the ability of a CT scan unit to detect structures possessing a very small difference in density relative to the surrounding tissues. Thus, one looks at the ability of a scanner to distinguish structures possessing differences in density of about 1%. The ability of a given scan design to accomplish this is related to the inherent noise present within the CT image (9, 12, 21). Modern CT scan units can, under optimal conditions, separate differences in density as small as 0.5%. Clinical examples whereby this amount of

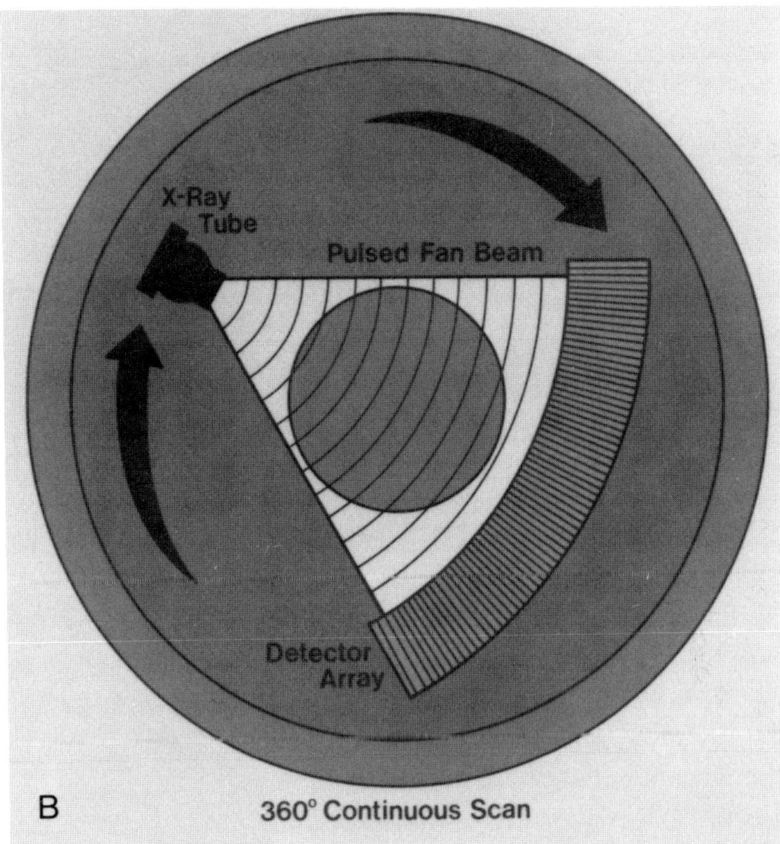

FIG. 27.4. (*B*)

precision is utilized can be found in the differentiation of gray and white matter within the brain or the differentiation of metastatic nodules in the liver.

Now that we have defined what we mean by density and spatial resolution, let us consider how they affect one another and how they interrelate with a third important consideration in clinical CT scanning, that is, radiation dose to the patient. These three factors are closely interrelated and we cannot alter one without having an effect upon the other two (3, 18) (Fig. 27.6).

As stated earlier, spatial resolution is directly related to pixel size. Each pixel or picture element in the CT image corresponds to a cross-sectional area of tissue in the patient. The pixel size (*i.e.*, the area of tissue represented by each picture element) can be calculated by taking the diameter of the scanning field and dividing by the size of the picture

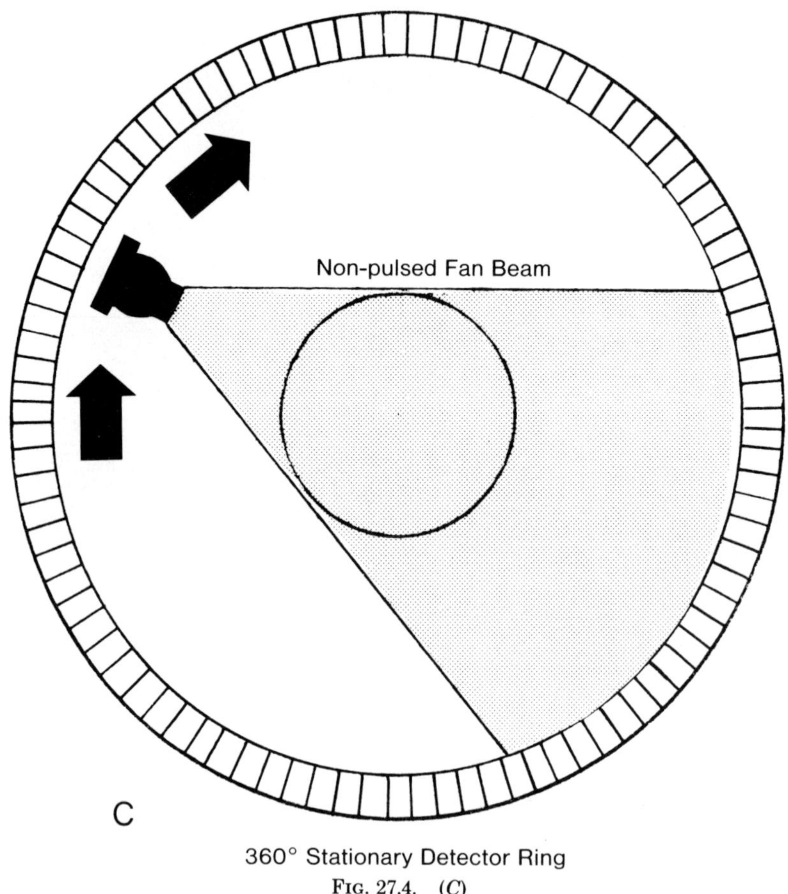

FIG. 27.4. (*C*)

matrix. Thus, a 25-cm scan field (average field size for head CT) which is reconstructed to a 512 × 512 matrix yields a pixel size of approximately 0.5 mm × 0.5 mm. It should also be kept in mind that to talk of resolution in only two dimensions is not sufficient. One must also consider resolution in the third plane or Z-axis which is determined by the scan slice thickness. Thus, each element composing a CT picture element actually represents a volume element determined by X- and Y-axes representing the surface area of a pixel, and a Z-axis which represents the depth of the slice. These volume elements which make up the picture are referred to as voxels, and the volume represented by an individual voxel is given by the product of the pixel area and the slice thickness (Fig. 27.7). Modern CT scanners have variable slice thicknesses of between 1 and 13 mm. If we consider the pixel size in the example cited above, using a 1-mm slice

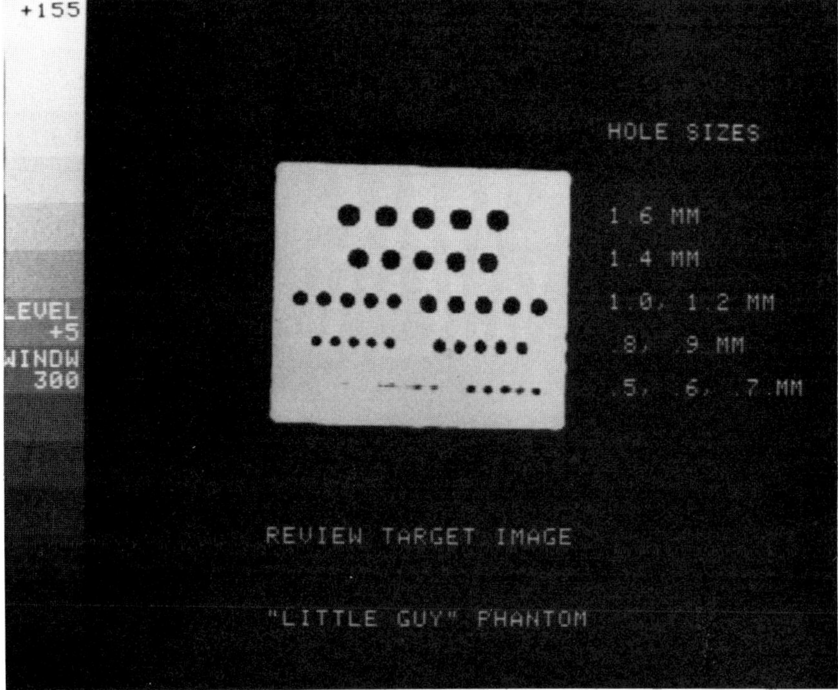

FIG. 27.5. CT scan of parallel pinhole phantom in which one can just barely see the holes which are 0.6 mm in size. This illustrates the high resolution capability of modern CT equipment. (Photo compliments of General Electric Co., Medical Systems Division)

thickness the volume of tissue (voxel size) represented on the video display is $0.5 \times 0.5 \times 1$ mm, or 0.25 mm^3. This compares with the voxel size of the original EMI CT unit whose parameters measured 3 mm $\times$ 3 mm $\times$ 13 mm, corresponding to a volume element size of 117 mm^3. Thus, we can see that, citing the best case, the size of the resolution element compared with the original CT scanner has been improved by a factor of 468! However, as we shall now see, this remarkable spatial resolution is obtained only at the expense of density resolution and increased patient radiation dose.

As described above, our ability to resolve structures possessing densities which differ only slightly from surrounding tissue is highly dependent upon the noise present in the CT picture. Noise can also be thought of as picture grain or irregularity and has been synonymously referred to as quantum mottle or statistical variation.

Consider a CT scan of a perfectly homogeneous material such as a water phantom. If there was no noise present within the CT scan, then

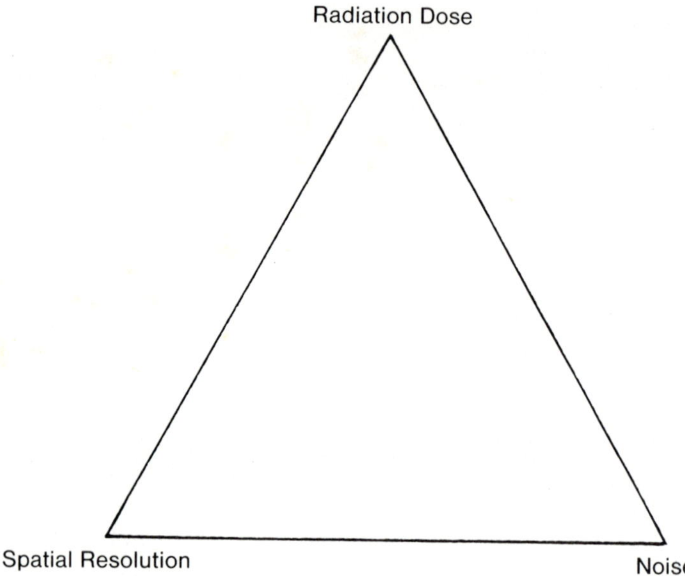

FIG. 27.6. Radiation dose, spatial resolution, and system noise are all closely interrelated, and a change in any one of these factors will have a direct impact on the other two.

the picture obtained would be perfectly uniform and every pixel which makes up the image of the water bath would have an identical CT number. In real life, we know that these numbers are not perfectly homogeneous, but there are some random statistical variations between adjacent pixel values in a homogeneous medium (Fig. 27.8). It is this statistical variation which we term "noise," and it is the magnitude of this variation which limits the ability of the CT method to discriminate between structures which have small differences in density.

If the noise level is higher than the density difference of two objects, then their definition will be obscured. The magnitude of this variation is directly dependent upon the number of x-ray photons which contribute to the calculation of an individual pixel. The noise can be stated as being proportional to plus or minus the square root of the average number of x-ray photons which contribute to the calculation of an individual picture element. The higher the number of measured photons, the lower the percentage of a statistical fluctuation and, thus, the lower the noise.

For example, if the average number of photons contributing to each pixel calculation is 10,000, then the statistical fluctuation is roughly equivalent to:

$$\sqrt{10{,}000} = 100$$

which represents a variation of ±1%. If 100,000 photons are measured to

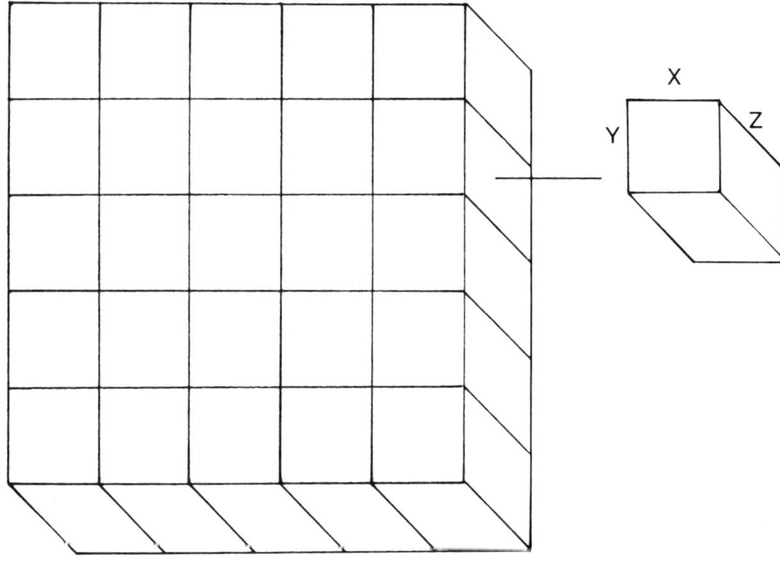

FIG. 27.7. Each picture element in the CT scan matrix represents a volume of tissue defined by the cross-sectional area of each pixel and the CT scan slice thickness. This resolution element is called a voxel.

calculate each pixel, then we obtain:

$$\sqrt{100{,}000} = 316$$

which represents a variation of only ±0.3%. Thus, we can significantly decrease noise and increase low contrast resolution in CT scan pictures by increasing the number of photons per unit volume which is passed through the patient. This, of course, raises the amount of radiation to the patient and has practical clinical considerations. Assuming all other factors constant, noise and x-ray dose form an inverse square relationship (9).

$$\text{Noise } \alpha \frac{1}{\sqrt{\text{dose}}}$$

What happens as spatial resolution is increased by decreasing pixel size? Consider the X,Y planes of a picture element and assume that it has dimensions 1 mm × 1 mm on each side. Assume that 100,000 photons pass through this picture element and contribute to the calculation of relative attenuation coefficient for this pixel. If the spatial resolution is doubled by halving the pixel size to 0.5 mm × 0.5 mm, then the original pixel is composed of four of the smaller pixels (Fig. 27.9). If the x-ray

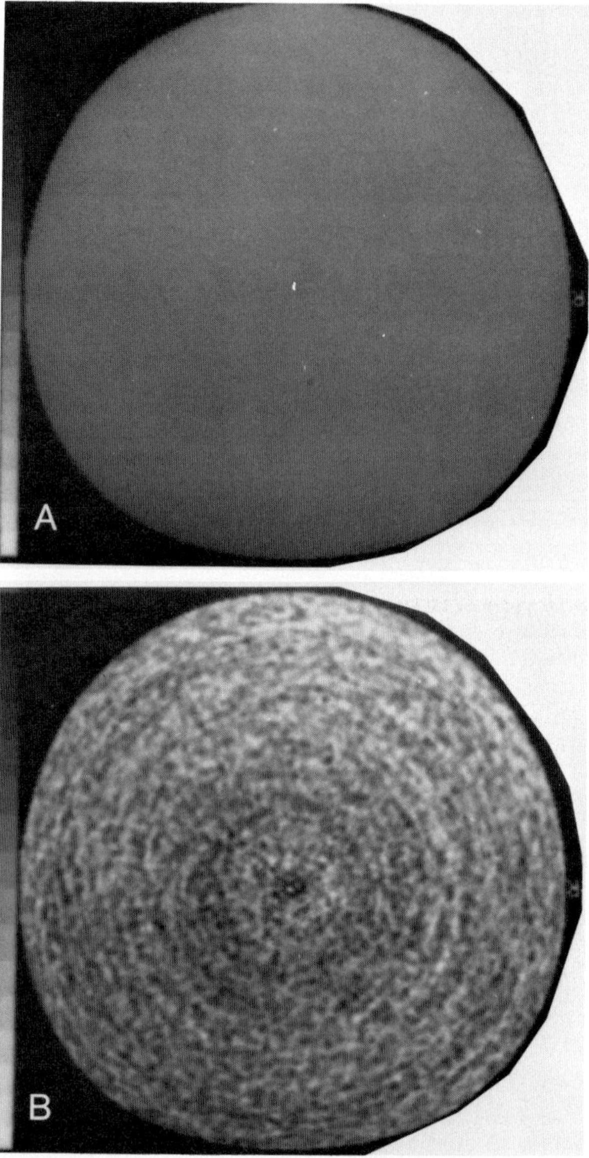

FIG. 27.8. CT scan of water bath appears perfectly homogeneous (*A*). However, when viewed at a very narrow window width this same water bath shows course irregularity or grain within the picture due to statistical variation of CT numbers between adjacent pixels (*B*). This variation is referred to as CT noise.

level remains constant, then only 25,000 photons will pass through each of the new, smaller pixels. Thus, for this increased spatial resolution, if we maintain all other factors constant, the noise is increased and the density resolution is decreased (2).

Noise levels are also increased if the Z-axis or slice thickness for a scanner is decreased while holding the pixel area and the amount of radiation constant. This, however, bears a directly inverse relationship. Thus, comparing a 10-mm slice thickness for a given pixel size with a slice thickness which is decreased to 5 mm, then the number of photons contributing to the calculation of the smaller voxel is likewise halved. Decrease in slice thickness causes less degradation of the final image than doubling the matrix size.

The limiting factor in selecting optimum scanning parameters is patient dosage. Since radiologists must deal in tradeoffs between spatial resolution and density resolution, it is important to individualize CT parameters for each individual clinical problem. Certain situations demand high spatial resolution while at the same time density resolution can be compromised. Such a situation occurs in CT scanning of the orbit where we are dealing with very small structures surrounded by fat, which possesses a large density difference relative to the soft tissues and bone

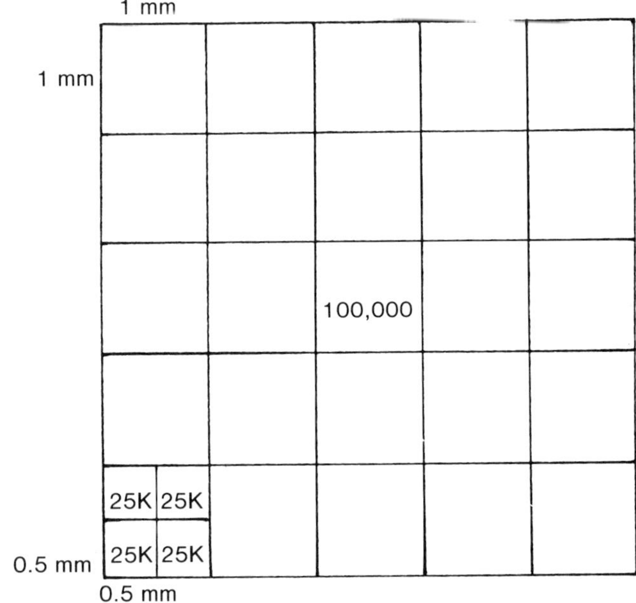

FIG. 27.9. Graphic illustration representing changes which occur in photon statistics when spatial resolution is doubled by decreasing the pixel size by a factor of 2.

of the orbit. Conversely, definition of white and gray matter of the brain requires exquisite density resolution since these structures vary in density by only about 0.8% (20). Small sellar lesions often require both high spatial *and* high density resolution, necessitating an increased radiation dose in some cases.

The foregoing discussion assumes that all CT noise is a function of random variation of x-ray photons. This is not the case. Electronic noise originating from signal detection, amplification, and transmission within the CT machine also contributes to the final noise level of the image. However, refinements in equipment design and quality control have minimized these contributions. In the past several years both density resolution and spatial resolution have been significantly improved while maintaining tolerable patient dosages mainly through better engineering design, more efficient x-ray detectors, and more accurate reconstruction algorithms. We are now beginning to approach the theoretical limit of photon utilization and measurement for a given radiation dose, and it is for this reason that the magnitude of improvements in picture quality will begin to plateau.

Future Innovations

This is not meant to imply that CT technology has reached its ultimate level of sophistication. Remarkable advances may be made in manipulation of the massive amounts of data which are collected during a CT scan. Among potential applications of data manipulation currently being explored are more accurate analysis of tissue composition within a lesion and dynamic CT scanning to reveal rapidly occurring changes, such as regional cerebral blood flow. Early attempts at these two techniques have been done in the laboratory, and in the case of dynamic scanning, in early clinical trials as well.

DUAL ENERGY CT SCANS

Several groups have attempted to define tissue composition by comparing CT absorption numbers calculated from scans obtained at two different x-ray energy levels (14, 22). The principles upon which this analysis is possible are based upon the fact that tissues with different chemical composition may show similar absorption patterns when exposed to a beam of x-ray at one energy level, but display differing absorption patterns when exposed to a beam of x-ray at a different energy. This is due to a differential change in the ratio between the amount of radiation deflected (Compton scattering) versus the amount absorbed (photoelectric interaction) for each substance at the two energy levels. Clinical use of this phenomenon can be made by performing CT scans at two separate energy levels (kilovoltage or kVp) and reconstructing the data from each scan. By subtracting the CT numbers calculated from data obtained at one kVp from the reconstructed data obtained at a second kVp, a shift of the CT numbers will be observed. It is then possible to make predictive judgements as to the probable composition of some lesions.

Marshall *et al.* (11) demonstrated the ability to separate high density lesions experimentally by scanning brains at 100 and 140 kVp. His contention was that lesions possessing an effective atomic number near water should show no significant change in absorption in this kVp range, while lesions of high atomic number (calcium or iodine) would show decreased absorption at the higher kVp. By comparing data measurements from the dual kVp scans, Marshall showed that it was possible to reliably separate acute hematoma from calcified lesions or contrast-enhanced lesions by observing the magnitude and direction of shift of the CT numbers (Table 27.2). They also proposed an equipment design modification for performing dual kVp scans in a clinical setting (22). Such a unit would utilize an x-ray source which is pulsed at alternating energy levels. During one scan enough data would be collected to reconstruct two images from the partial data sets obtained from alternate pulses. Since the images are obtained simultaneously, they can be subtracted electronically and computer-analyzed.

DYNAMIC CT

Dynamic CT scanning has also been described (4, 6, 19) and is currently being introduced into clinical practice through software and hardware modifications of existing CT units. To perform meaningful dynamic scanning requires a machine which will perform multiple fast scans in rapid sequence, together with reconstruction programs which have been modified to do reconstructions from partial sets of data. One such system which currently has units in field operation has been modified to perform

TABLE 27.2

*Partial Summary of Lesions Studied at 140 and 100 kVp**

Lesion	Diagnosis	Avg CT no. at 140 kVp	CT no. difference (100 kVp–140 kVp)
1	Calcified meningioma	47.2	5.36
2	Calcified meningioma	43.4	4.46
3	Contrast-enhanced sarcoma	56.8	6.14
4	Calcified oligodendroglioma	51.6	8.18
5	Intracerebral hemorrhage	44.0	0.35
6	Intracerebral hemorrhage	57.8	−0.76
7	Cerebellar hematoma	54.2	0.74

* Adapted from Marshall (11).

rapid sequential 5-second scans with 1-second interval between each successive scan. Data from each 360° scan can be subdivided and reconstructed into as many as three individual pictures. This is accomplished by taking data measurements from three portions of the scanning circle and reconstructing each of these subsets of data into an individual picture (Fig. 27.10). Since 180° is the minimum scan angle from which one can reconstruct a picture, these three partial reconstructions share overlapping data points. This method for the example illustrated results in three individual pictures with the midpoint of data collection for each picture spaced by 1.2 seconds. Since dynamic changes in regional cerebral blood flow are a continuum throughout the entire 5 seconds of scanning, the individual pictures reconstructed from data obtained at different times during one scan sequence truly do show temporal changes which are occurring during that time.

At this time we have only begun to explore the clinical application for the types of data manipulation possible. No doubt with future advances

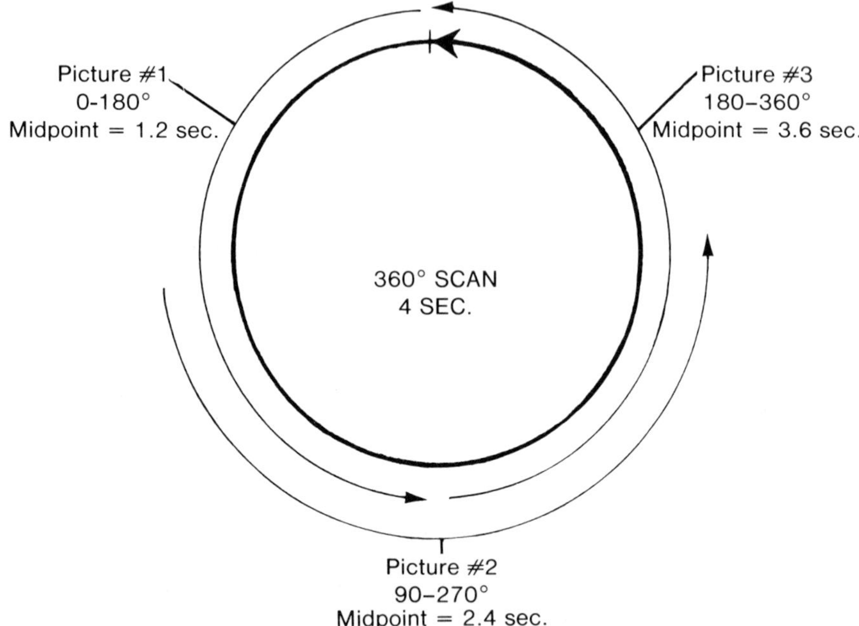

FIG. 27.10. Diagrammatic representation of how data obtained during a single, continuous 4.8-second scan can be subdivided and individual pictures obtained using overlapping subsets of data. While a *single picture* reconstructed from the full 360° of data will average any changes which may have occurred during the scan, the individual pictures reconstructed from the subsets of data will separate out dynamic changes which have occurred between each portion of the scanning cycle.

in software programming, even more astounding things may become possible.

The next major advance in CT machine design may come in several years with the introduction of a subsecond scanner capable of performing a scan in the range of 25 to 50 msec. This will allow stop action pictures of rapidly moving structures such as the heart and will enable far more accurate dynamic scanning through repetitive stop action pictures. One such machine design has been proposed (10), and a modification of this

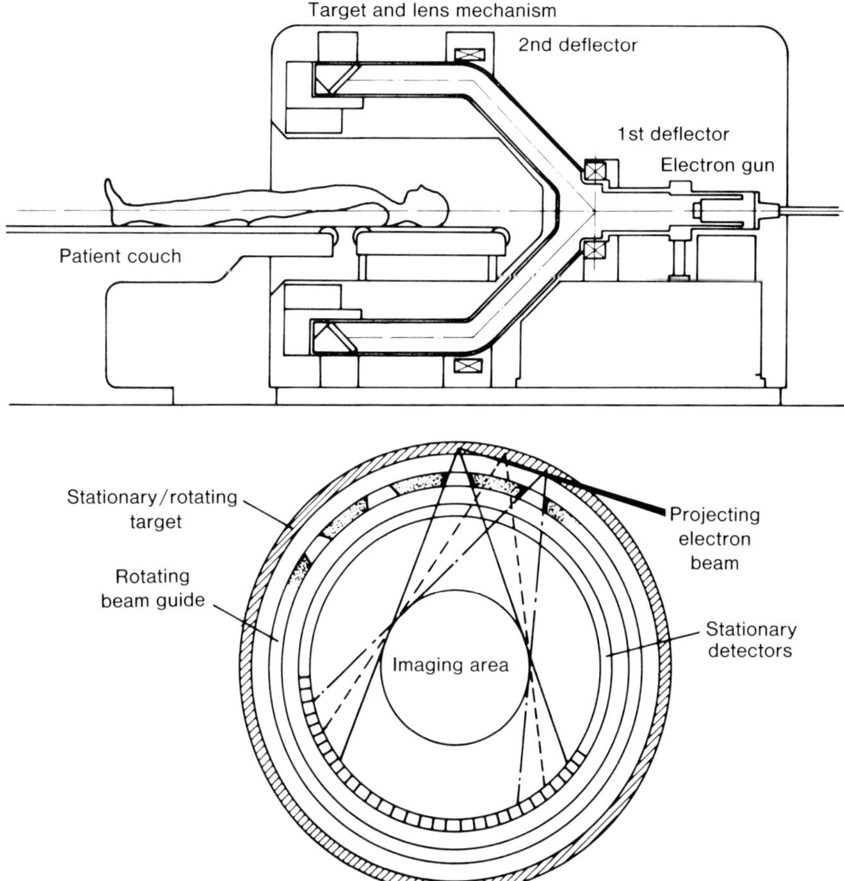

FIG. 27.11. Cross-sectional diagrams of side (*top*) and en face (*bottom*) views of a proposed ultrafast CT scanner design. This system would utilize a focused electron beam which is deflected to a circular target anode surrounding the patient and then electronically "scanned" around the perimeter of this target in 25 to 50 msec. A circular ring of detectors surrounding the patient records the data in much the same fashion as today's rotating x-ray tube-fixed detector ring systems. This design appears feasible but will require several years of development. (From T. A. Iinuma *et al.* (10). Published with permission.)

design is currently under construction in at least one center. The main principle behind the design of a subsecond CT unit involves the elimination of moving parts. The x-ray source is scanned around the patient electronically by using a focused beam of electrons which is swept across a giant circular tungsten target. The detectors are placed opposite this circular target, and once again the basic principles of operation remain the same as with today's conventional machines (Fig. 27.11). Essentially, instead of rotating the x-ray tube around the patient, the patient lies within a giant x-ray tube and the x-ray beam moves electronically. The cost of research and development of such a system is high, and the problems to be overcome are formidable. However, the possibilities of noninvasive dynamic imaging, very rapid data accumulation, and elimination of all artifact caused by motion make such an endeavor worth undertaking.

REFERENCES

1. Boyd, D. P., Korobkin, M. T., and Moss, A. Engineering status of computerized tomographic scanning. Optical Eng., *16:* 37–44, 1977.
2. Brooks, R. A., and Di Chiro, G. Principles of computer assisted tomography (CAT) in radiographic and radioisotopic imaging. Phys. Med. Biol., *21:* 689–732, 1976.
3. Chesler, D. A., Riederer, S. J., and Pelc, N. J. Noise due to photon counting statistics in computed x-ray tomography. J. Comput. Assist. Tomogr., *1:* 64–74, 1977.
4. Dobben, G. D., Valvassori, G. E., Mafee, M. F., and Berninger, W. H. Evaluation of brain circulation by rapid rotational computed tomography. Radiology, *133:* 105–111, 1979.
5. Drayer, B. P., Heinz, E. R., Dujovny, M., Wolfson, S. K., Jr., and Gur, D. Patterns of brain perfusion: dynamic computed tomography using intravenous contrast enhancement. J. Comput. Assist. Tomogr., *3:* 633–640, 1979.
6. Heinz, E. R., Dubois, P., Osborne, D., Drayer, B., and Barrett, W. Dynamic computed tomography study of the brain. J. Comput. Assist. Tomogr., *3:* 648–649, 1979.
7. Herman, G. T., and Liu, H. K. Display of three-dimensional information in computed tomography. J. Comput. Assist. Tomogr., *1:* 155–160, 1977.
8. Hounsfield, G. N. Computerized transverse axial scanning (tomography). Part I. Description of system. Br. J. Radiol., *46:* 1016–1022, 1973.
9. Hounsfield, G. N. Picture quality of computed tomography. A.J.R., *127:* 3–9, 1976.
10. Iinuma, T. A., Tateno, Y., Umegaki, Y., and Watanabe, E. Proposed system for ultrafast computed tomography. J. Comput. Assist. Tomogr., *1:* 494–499, 1977.
11. Marshall, W. H., Jr., Easter, W., and Zatz, L. M. Analysis of the dense lesion at computed tomography with dual kVp scans. Radiology, *124:* 87–89, 1977.
12. McCullough, E. C. Factors affecting the use of quantitative information from a CT scanner. Radiology, *124:* 99–107, 1977.
13. McCullough, E. C., Payne, J. T., Baker, H. L., Jr., Hattery, R. R., Sheedy, P. F., Stephens, D. H., and Gedgaudus, E. Performance evaluation and quality assurance of computed tomography scanners, with illustrations from the EMI, ACTA, and Delta scanners. Radiology, *120:* 173–188, 1976.
14. McDavid, W. D., Waggener, R. G., Dennis, M. J., Sank, V. J., and Payne, W. H. Estimation of chemical composition and density from computed tomography carried out at a number of energies. Invest. Radiol., *12:* 189–194, 1977.

15. Ommaya, A. K., Murray, G., Ambrose, J., Richardson, A., and Hounsfield, G. Computerized axial tomography: estimation of spatial and density resolution capability. Br. J. Radiol., *49:* 604–611, 1976.

16. Pelc, N. J., and Chesler, D. A. Utilization of cross-plane rays for three-dimensional reconstruction by filtered backprojection. J. Comput. Assist. Tomogr., *3:* 385–395, 1979.

17. Rhodes, M. L., Glenn, W. V., and Azaawi, Y. M. Extracting oblique planes from serial CT sections. J. Comput. Assist. Tomogr., *4:* 649–657, 1980.

18. Rice, J. F., and Banks, T. E. Normal and high accuracy computed tomography of the brain: dose and imaging considerations. J. Comput. Assist. Tomogr., *3:* 497–502, 1979.

19. Traupe, H., Heiss, W. D., Hoeffken, W., and Zulch, K. J. Hyperperfusion and enhancement in dynamic computed tomography of ischemic stroke patients. J. Comput. Assist. Tomogr., *3:* 627–632, 1979.

20. Weinstein, M. A., Duchesneau, P. M., and MacIntyer, W. J. White and gray matter of the brain differentiated by computed tomography. Radiology, *122*(2 Suppl)*:* 699–702, 1977

21. Zatz, L. M. Image quality in cranial computed tomography. J. Comput. Assist. Tomogr., *2:* 336–346, 1978.

22. Zatz, L. M., and Alvarez, R. E. An inaccuracy in computed tomography: the energy dependence of CT values. Radiology, *124:* 91–97, 1977.

CHAPTER

28

Computed Tomography vs. Angiography in the Diagnosis of Intracranial Neoplasms

STANLEY FREDRIC HANDEL, M.D.

Since the development of computed tomography (CT) the indications for and use of angiography in the diagnosis of intracranial neoplasms have undergone marked change. In this presentation I shall compare the advantages of CT to those of angiography. I shall emphasize the complimentary roles of these modalities in specific clinical situations and also present instances when angiography may be reasonably omitted.

Aspects Influencing Diagnostic Success

The net result from both CT and angiography is largely dependent on the quality of performance and interpretation. If these are practiced at the "state-of-the-art" level, then results are superior to those obtained from a lesser level of practice. In the case of CT, this clearly will result in lesser dependence on angiography.

Factors which may influence the CT diagnosis include the CT machine and its characteristics: scan speed, resolution, collimator size and software capabilities; artifacts due to motion and those inherent to the machine; use and amount of contrast; timing of scan in relation to contrast administration; window and center settings; camera adjustment; clinical data; and interpretative skill. The factors influencing angiographic diagnosis include: the equipment characteristics; film quality; selectivity of vascular contrast injection; amount and rate of contrast injection; use of magnification and subtraction technique; clinical data; and interpretative skill.

Diagnostic Content: CT vs. Angiography

A review of the diagnostic content of computed tomograms and angiograms is important to clarify the perspective of CT as a more direct method and angiography as a more indirect method for demonstrating brain neoplasm. CT findings which imply presence of an intracranial neoplasm are: abnormal attenuation coefficients in brain: either low, implying tumor and/or concomitant pathology, such as infarction, inflammation, encephalomalacia, cyst and edema; or high, implying calcification, hemorrhage, or other abnormally dense tissue; displacement and distortion of anatomical structures, such as the cisterns, ventricles, choroid; abnormal contrast enhancement; and bone changes. CT appearance alone cannot be translated into a histological diagnosis with anything approaching 100% accuracy. In diagnosing and evaluating intracranial neoplasms by angiography, the following angiographic findings are important: displacement of vessels; decreased or increased vascularity compared to normal brain; the presence of intrinsically abnormal and unusual vessels, *e.g.*, large meningeal vessels without normal tapering, irregular vessels typical of neovascularity and vascular tortuosity; and abnormalities of circulation time, such as arteriovenous shunting.

Advantages and Uses of CT vs. Angiography

The advantages of CT vs. those of angiography are intrinsic to the sensitivity, diagnostic content and methodology of data acquisition, and display of these techniques. CT allows direct visualization of brain including: differentiation of white and gray matter, the deep brain substance, periventricular region, CSF spaces, bone and the extracalvarial soft tissues. This is due to exquisite sensitivity to differences in tissue attenuation coefficients (high contrast difference resolution) which also allows direct visualization of many pathological processes, such as tumor, calcifications, blood clots, and edema in a fashion currently unparalled by any other technique (12). Intravenous iodine contrast enhancement further defines abnormalities, causing blood brain barrier defects and abnormal blood pools. For these purposes angiography does not rival CT and therefore has been relegated to the status of a secondary procedure for detection of intracranial neoplasm. Despite this, the essence of angiography, demonstration of blood vessels, remains unmatched by CT, although improvement in demonstration of blood vessels by CT has continued. Hence, we have the potential for a true complimentary situation when the angiographic and CT options are properly exercised. If we are considering the possibility of a structural change in the brain, then CT becomes the examination of choice for the reasons mentioned. It follows that brain tumors should rarely be first diagnosed by angiography. I stress that angiography, radionuclide scanning, EEG, and skull films separately or combined do not substitute for CT. On the other hand, vascular abnormalities will be diagnosed less effectively by CT.

The most thorough CT study is one performed without contrast followed by intravenous contrast. Ideally, a fast, high resolution scanner should be used and 80 gm of iodide (600 ml of 30% contrast) infused rapidly. The contrast scan can be obtained immediately after injection of contrast, a delayed scan performed 1 to 1½ hours after injection, or both. In most patients it is not practical or necessary to perform all three scans.

In the screening examination with low suspicion for an intracranial mass I perform only the immediate contrast scan. Recent experience strongly indicates that tumors are best defined on CT 1 to 1½ hours after high dose infusion of contrast (15, 28). Thus, when suspicion is high, a delayed scan may replace or follow the immediate postcontrast scan. A drawback to the use of delayed scans only is that some pathology, for example, some arteriovenous malformations (AVMs) may be less obvious on the delayed scan. For routine follow-up scans in patients with brain tumors little information is lost by obtaining only the immediate or delayed postcontrast scan.

If we summarize the possible functions of cerebral angiography for brain tumor work-up they are to: find the tumor, exclude coincidental or masquerading lesions, diagnose the type of tumor, and define important anatomy for planning the surgery. As discussed previously, angiography is a distant second to CT in finding tumor. Nevertheless, angiography may define a tumor not appreciated or only suspected on CT. In particular, angiography offers definite advantages for examining vessels at the skull base which may be involved by neoplasm not appreciated on CT scanning (Fig. 28.1). Patients with small tumors anywhere within the

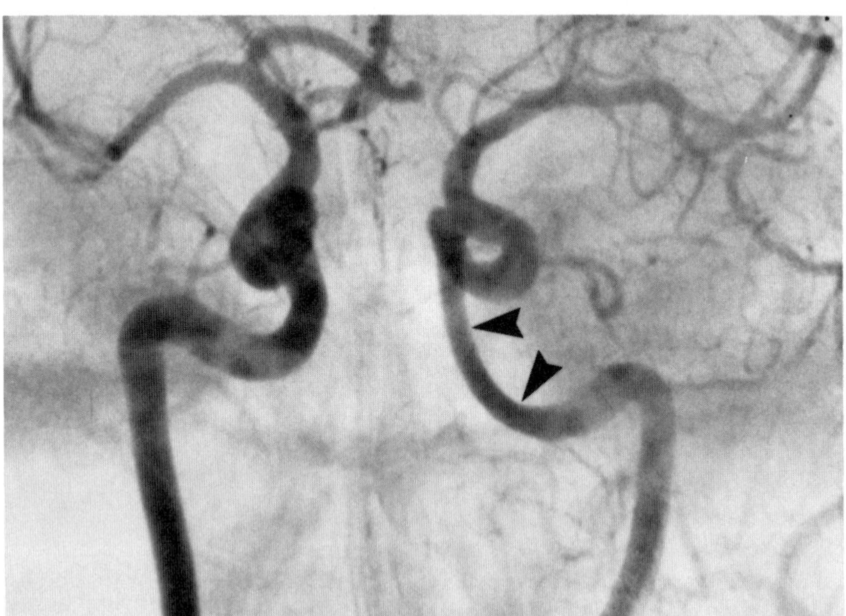

FIG. 28.1. Superimposed AP subtraction views of right and left internal carotid angiograms. The ganglionic portion of the left internal carotid is compressed and arced (*arrowheads*) by a chordoma. The CT scan was normal.

brain may have false negative scans due to any of the following reasons: adjacent to bone, below spatial resolution of the scanner, partial volume averaging, nonhomogeneity of slice thickness, and failure to use high dose iodide delayed scans. If the clinical suspicion is strong and focally directed, angiography may be helpful. A specific example would be in patients with suspected hemangioblastoma. These patients may have small secondary tumors or vascular anomalies not apparent on CT (6). Another use would be in those patients with hypernephroma and onset of seizures and normal or equivocal CT. Angiography could show a very small hypervascular metastasis.

As regards the exclusion of coincidental or masquerading lesion, I refer to atheromatous disease, aneurysms, and arteriovenous malformations (Fig. 28.2). If the clinical assessment and/or the CT suggest a vascular component to or etiology for the patient's problem then angiography is indicated.

The last two indications deal with the necessity for angiography when the CT scan is positive. When the clinical data and CT leave a reasonable doubt as to the diagnosis, angiography may improve the confidence level of our diagnosis. The fourth indication is the need for vascular information vital to planning and successfully performing the surgical procedure. If the tumor is vascular, then demonstration of origin, size, and course of

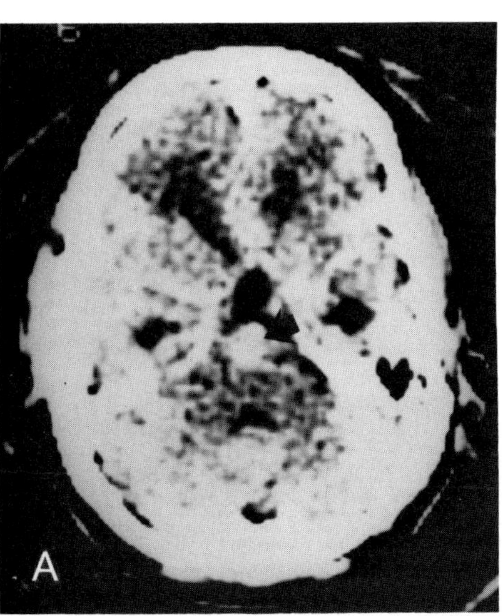

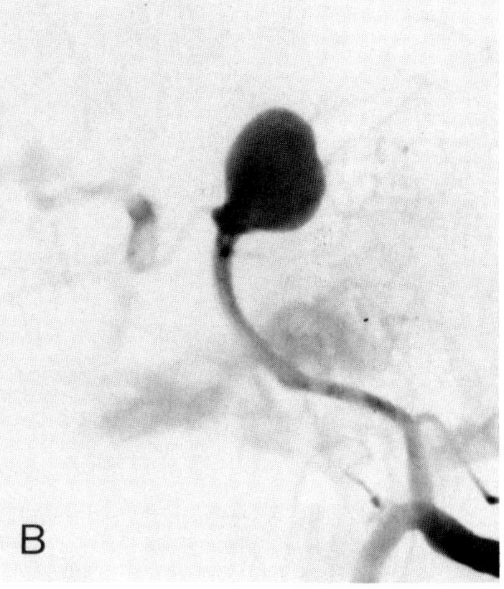

FIG. 28.2. (*A*) Patient with lung carcinoma and brain stem signs. An enhancing mass in the anterior pons region (*arrow*) was initially diagnosed as metastasis. (*B*) Lateral view vertebral angiogram. A basilar artery aneurysm is responsible for the enhancing CT lesion.

feeding arteries is frequently vital. Moreover, angiography will allow opportunity for embolization procedures as an alternative or as a prelude to surgery in selected patients (Fig. 28.3) (5). Angiographic demonstration of arterial encasement or occlusion may govern whether and how surgery is performed and if other treatment, such as radiotherapy, is to be used. Angiography will establish patency of collateral pathways of supply through the circle of Willis, through the external carotid system and the leptomeningeal route. Superficial temporal bypass feasibility may be assessed.

The venous system deserves emphasis equal to the arteries. Venous drainage pathways, dural sinus occlusion, collateral channels, and outflow of contrast from the brain are often key to successful surgical results when the neoplasm has involved the venous system. CT may provide good information, such as demonstration of superior sagittal sinus occlusion, but the precise preoperative anatomic detail remains in the province of angiography. Venous anatomy may also be important for the preop-

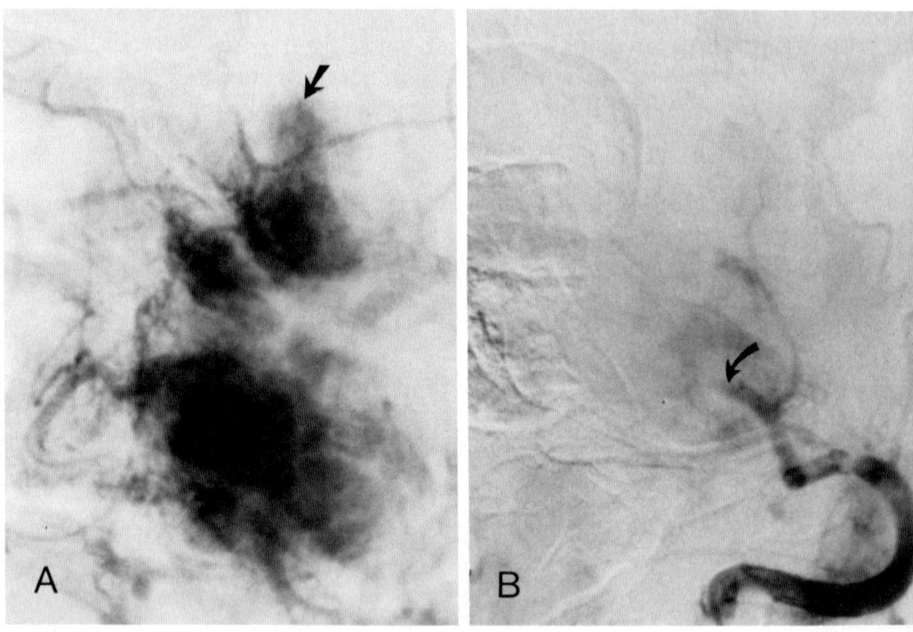

FIG. 28.3. (*A*) Lateral view, intermediate phase of an external carotid angiogram. A large vascular metastasis involves the skull base and extends intracranially (*arrow*). The tumor was inoperable. (*B*) Following embolization with gelfoam the external carotid artery is occluded (*arrow*). The patient had immediate relief of the facial pain he had been experiencing. (From V. P. Chuang *et al.* (5). Published with permission.)

erative planning of the flap. Finally, angiography will define the anomalously located vessel which is best identified before rather than during surgery.

The Unnecessary Angiogram

If an enhanced scan of satisfactory quality is normal, angiography is usually not indicated to search for tumor. I do not recommend angiography for patients with suspected metastases if the primary tumor is not a highly vascular type. I prefer that they be followed with CT, as the diagnostic yield with angiography tends to be quite low. Metastases that are of low vascularity and not obvious on CT are unlikely to be diagnosable with consistent confidence at angiography. Similarly, the primary brain tumor not seen on a high quality CT scan is unlikely to be diagnosed angiographically. In these instances serial CT scans seem more appropriate. Overriding all of this may be the idea of doing everything possible to make a diagnosis when the clinical judgment calls for additional evaluation. I do not oppose angiography in this context, but would emphasize that without strong clinical or CT indications the diagnostic yield from angiographic fishing expeditions is very low.

We should refrain from angiography in those instances when treatment will not be influenced by the angiographic findings, e.g. the patient is not an operative risk or he will receive whole head irradiation regardless of the angiographic findings. Angiography is of little value for tumors demonstrated by CT to be within brain substance, not abutting on a dural surface and not suggested as being markedly hypervascular on CT. Angiography is generally not indicated to localize tumors for surgery after the tumors have been diagnosed on CT, as localization techniques are available using the CT scanner or plain films (4, 10).

Specific Applications: CT and Angiography

GLIOMAS

Based on the clinical information and CT scan, supratentorial gliomas can be diagnosed with 85 to 90% accuracy (13, 16). Mass effect, location and precontrast appearance, enhancement pattern, and edema contribute to the diagnosis. Grade of glioma is also indicated with some accuracy. Low grade gliomas tend to have little edema and scant enhancement while higher grade gliomas are associated with more edema and dense contrast enhancement. This latter finding is based on the pathological features of the tumor which correlate with malignancy, most importantly vascularity and necrosis (2). This is not always the case, and high grade gliomas may have little edema or enhancement. We can speculate that histological variation in a given tumor may be in part responsible for this discrepancy. If the diagnosis seems secure from the clinical data and CT, and the tumor's location and appearance meet the qualifications mentioned in the previous section, then angiography can be omitted. If surgery or biopsy are not performed, then angiography may be useful to make the radiotherapist more comfortable if typical angiographic findings of neovasculature, staining, and arteriovenous shunting are demonstrated. If the diagnosis of glioma is in question because of atypical clinical or CT features, angiography becomes almost mandatory. Angiography will often distinguish glioma from infarction, giant aneurysm, angiomas, meningiomas, and other lesions which may simulate or be simulated by gliomas (3, 14, 16, 21, 31).

If CT demonstrates complex ring or garland enhancement (Fig. 28.4), then diagnosis of glioblastoma is highly accurate (29). Similarly, irregular ring enhancement with nodular areas strongly indicates tumor. Otherwise, ring enhancement is quite nonspecific, being seen with varying frequency in most of the entities previously mentioned (7). Hematomas and infarctions with ring enhancement may be diagnosed by serial scanning. Separation of glioma from metastasis or from abscess may only

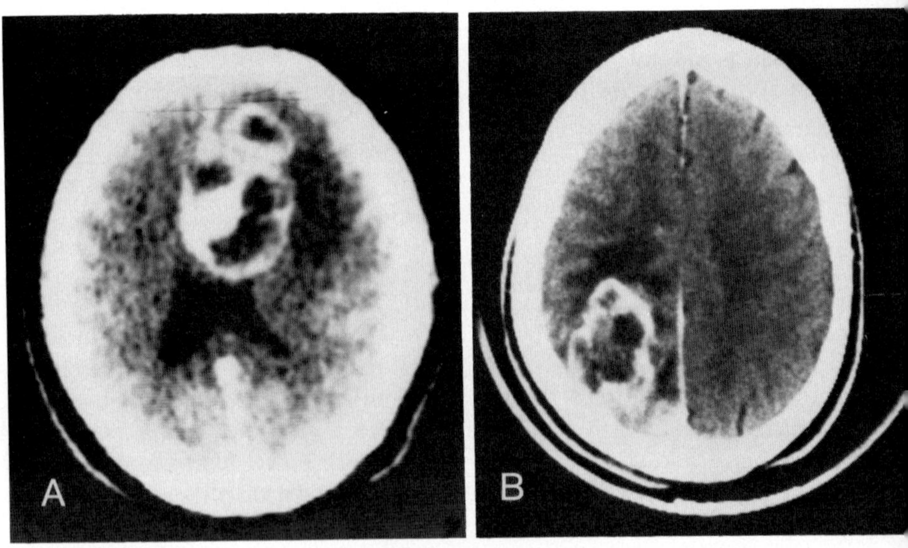

FIG. 28.4. Two patients with enhanced scans strongly indicative of glioblastoma. (*A*) Butterfly glioblastoma. Note the confluent, irregular rings. (*B*) Right parietal glioblastoma with a garland-shaped ring of irregular thickness.

be finalized by tissue sample. The operating surgeon is always well advised to be prepared for the unexpected brain abscess when operating on a lesion which ring enhances on CT, but has no other distinctive features whether on CT or angiography.

MENINGIOMA

Accuracy of CT diagnosis of meningioma is in the range of 90 to 95% (19). We tend to think of meningiomas as having very typical diagnostic CT and angiographic features. Calcifications, hyperostosis, dural abuttment, and increased tumor density are seen on the plain CT scan and homogenous enhancement expected on the contrast CT. Homogenous and prolonged tumor blush with meningeal arterial supply are typical on the angiogram, although the films must be carefully examined to avoid overlooking unusual meningeal supply such as middle meningeal artery origin from the ophthalmic artery. These features raise the confidence of diagnosis to virtually 100% when present; however, atypical, neuroradiologic features are not unusual and can lead to misdiagnosis (Fig. 28.5)

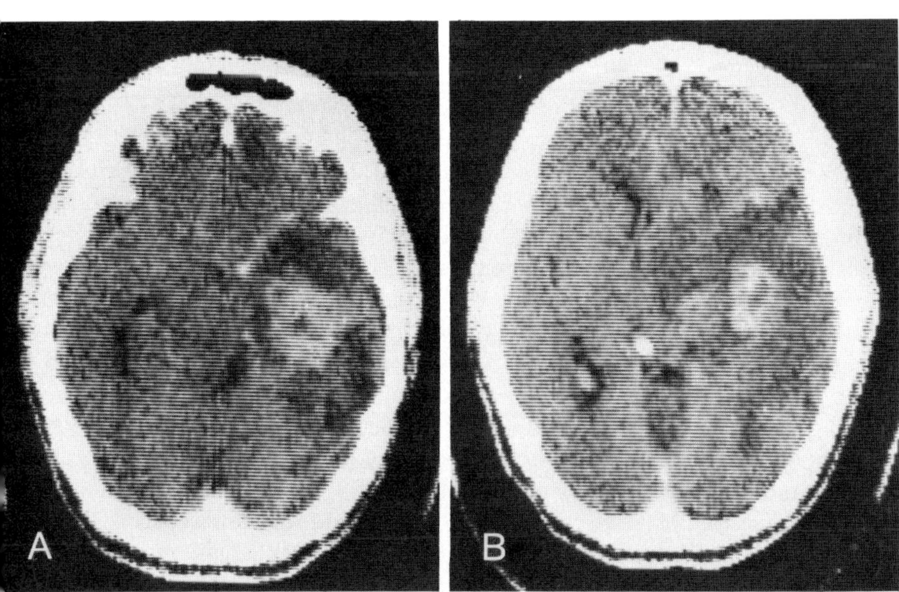

FIG. 28.5. Middle aged male with progressive neurological deterioration. An irregularly enhancing left temporal lobe mass with marked surrounding edema is present. Angiography failed to reveal meningeal supply or meningioma-type tumor stain. A preoperative diagnosis of glioblastoma was made, but meningioma was found at surgery.

(26). Atypical CT appearances can include focal areas in the tumor of low, iso-, or high density; marked surrounding low density, irregular, or ring enhancement, and absence of enhancement. These CT findings are due to such tumor changes as necrosis, cyst formation, hemorrhage of varying age, calcification, lipomatous degeneration, tumor scarring, and surrounding edema and brain atrophy. Thus, meningioma must be a constant question when intracranial masses are identified and angiography used liberally to help obtain the proper answer. We must acknowledge also that angiography may be misleading, and final diagnosis of malignant tumor based on the CT scan and angiography and a decision to omit surgery must be made cautiously. Ideally, tissue for pathological diagnosis should be obtained in every patient with presumed intracranial tumor. In particular, small middle cranial fossa meningiomas may cause a great deal of edema. The enhancement may be minimal and not apparent when volume is averaged with the edema or the skull base. The rare intraventricular meningioma and meningioma without obvious dural attachment are other possible diagnostic problems on CT scanning. In most cases, however, angiography will provide the needed information for clinching the diagnosis while demonstrating other important points, such as arterial encasement or occlusion at the brain base, and feeding arteries. Last, just as meningiomas may have varied appearances and simulate other types of pathology, other lesions may simulate meningioma on CT scan and perhaps less frequently on the angiogram (18).

METASTASES

When cerebral metastases are suspected, high volume contrast with a 1 to 1½ hour delay of the CT scan has the highest yield. Shalen *et al.* (28) found more information available on delayed scans than on immediate scans in a large series of tumor patients. Eleven percent of their patients would have had a false negative CT if a delayed scan had not been performed. Cerebral angiography adds little if a high quality CT scan is normal. While leptomeningeal tumor is not routinely demonstrable by CT scanning, it is even less reliably shown by angiography (9). In our experience, the presence of an equivocal metastatic lesion on the CT scan is usually not corroborated by angiography, nor is cerebral angiography indicated for searching for additional cerebral metastases after a single metastasis has been demonstrated by CT. More importantly, if the patient did not have a high dose iodine delayed scan, then one should be obtained prior to surgery on the presumed single metastasis.

SELLA AND PARASELLAR REGION

Detection of masses within and about the sella has greatly improved due to high resolution scanning. As a result, angiography no longer has a significant role in finding neoplasms in this area, being much less sensitive than CT. In particular, with infiltrative midline gliomas, the efficacy of angiographic demonstration is dismally low compared with CT. Plain films and CT characteristics usually lead to correct differentiation between tumor types, although craniopharyngioma, pituitary adenomas, and meningiomas may be virtually indistinguishable from each other (14). Moreover, parasellar aneurysms may also be mistaken for tumor. In these cases angiography may be essential to aid in the precise diagnosis, rule out coincidental aneurysm, and demonstrate the effect of the mass on the vessels at the brain base (Fig. 28.6). In a small number of cases neither routine CT or angiography may demonstrate small suprasellar tumors, *e.g.*, the nonenhancing craniopharyngioma isodense with brain or the suprasellar cyst isodense with CSF (30). In these cases, high resolution CT scanning with intrathecal metrizamide should provide the diagnosis (8). Alternatively, this remains a possible use for complex motion tomography with pneumoencephalography. We no longer perform angiography prior to transphenoidal approach for pituitary microadenoma (24). High resolution scans can exclude the presence of a large tumor, show that the cavernous sinus-carotid artery complex is not encroaching on the sella, and demonstrate the location of the internal carotid arteries above the cavernous sinus (Fig. 28.7). With densely enhancing larger tumors occupying the sella angiography is useful to exclude the coincidental aneurysm or the occasional medially located carotid siphon and to identify the internal carotid artery within the cavernous sinus (Fig. 28.8). Rapid sequence dynamic CT scanning may make additional inroads on angiography for these purposes in the next several years.

THIRD VENTRICLE REGION

In patients with enhancing third ventricular tumors typical of colloid cysts we have been performing angiography to exclude a solid tumor or aneurysm. If the scan is strongly indicative of colloid cyst and the clinical data support that diagnosis, angiography can be safely omitted if the CT satisfactorily separates the enhancing lesion from the suprasellar arteries. If doubt exists angiography should be performed. On occasion, colloid cysts may not be appreciated on CT scan, especially if a high resolution scanner isn't used (Fig. 28.9). In these cases, clinical suspicion or lateral ventricular dilatation would hopefully lead to pneumoencephalography or positive contrast ventriculography. If angiography is performed elevation of the anterior portion of the internal cerebral vein and/or posterior portion septal vein would strongly indicate the presence of a foramen of Monro region mass (Fig. 28.10). Hopefully, with high resolution scan-

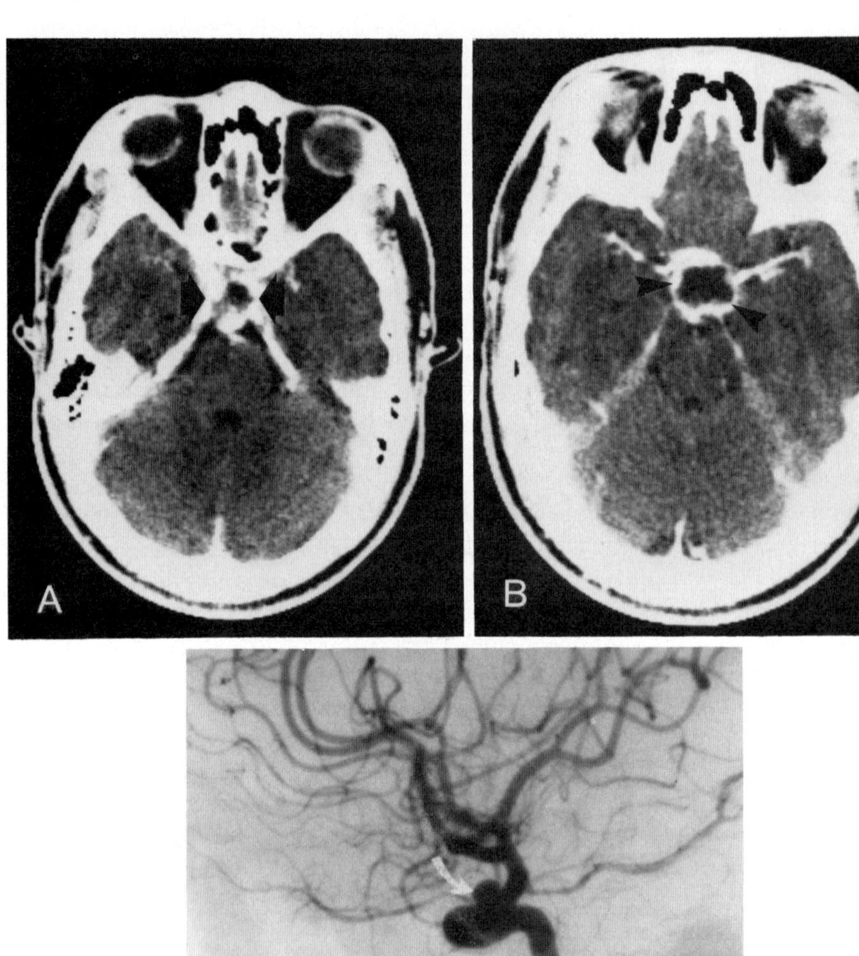

FIG. 28.6. Twenty-nine-year-old male with pilocytic glioma of hypothalamus. (*A* and *B*) Enhanced scans show partial sella (*arrows*) destruction and suprasellar ring enhancement (*arrowheads*) intimately associated with the vessels at the brain base. (*C*) Lateral angiogram, arterial phase reveals a coincidental aneurysm (*white arrow*) of the internal carotid artery contiguous with the tumor.

ning and multiplanar reconstruction, the misdiagnosis of colloid cysts will be rare.

Angiography is useful for posterior third ventricle region-tentorial incisural tumors. Obviously, vascular tumors and aneurysms will be

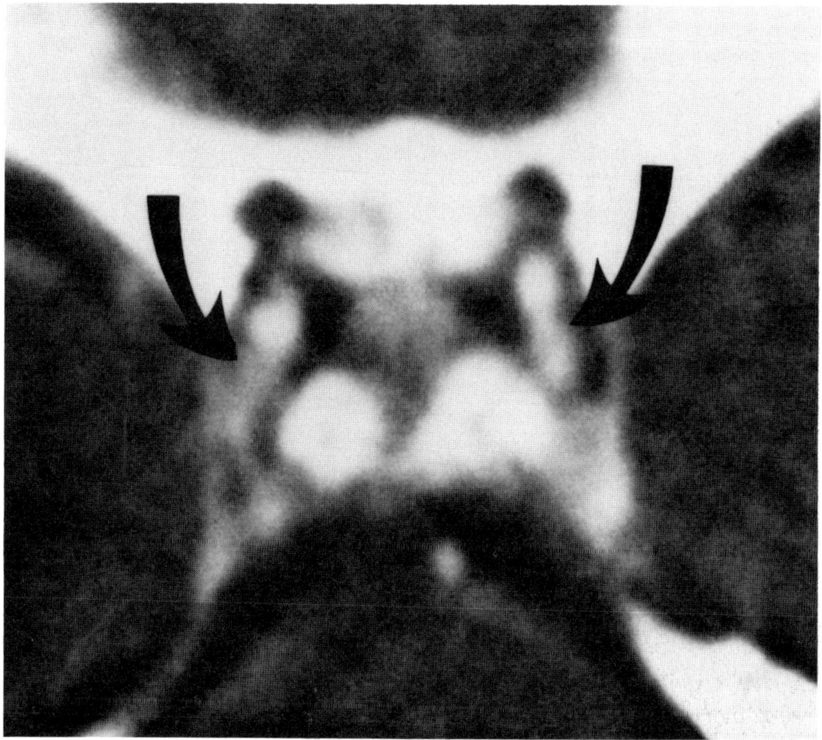

FIG. 28.7. Enhanced scan sharply defines the internal carotid arteries (*arrows*) from the pituitary just above the cavernous sinus.

identified and operative meningiomas distinguished from pinealomas prior to tissue sample.

CEREBELLOPONTINE ANGLE

Demonstration of cerebellopontine angle masses has moved almost entirely into the province of CT scans (25, 27). High resolution scans may be able to demonstrate enhancing masses as little as 6 mm in diameter in this area. Metrizamide cisternal and air contrast CT studies extend the capacity of CT within the internal auditory canals (1, 17). Angiography is useful for cases in which the presentation and appearance of the mass are not clearly typical of acoustic neuroma. Depending on size of the mass and the surgical approach chosen, angiography may be needed to define the vascularity and the blood supply to the tumor (20). Supply to cerebellopontine angle meningiomas and acoustic neuromas may be from vertebral, internal carotid, and external carotid branches. In cases in which the routine CT does not clearly distinguish between axial and extraaxial masses in this region, angiography may give the definite

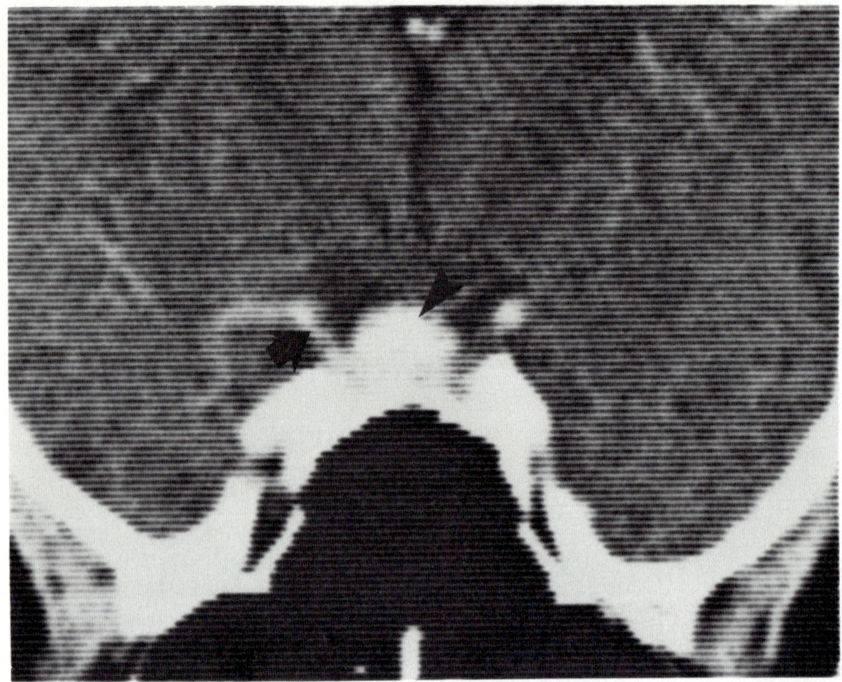

FIG. 28.8. Elderly female with Cushing's syndrome. CT shows an enhanced pituitary tumor with suprasellar extension (*arrowhead*). The internal carotid artery (*arrow*) is well shown on the right side but is not completely separable from the tumor. Angiography is mandatory for safe surgery.

information, especially if metrizamide cisternal CT is contraindicated. Appearance and position of the mass on CT and presence of internal auditory canal erosion are the most important findings in separating meningioma from acoustic neuroma. Venous abnormalities may also be important for angiographic differentiation (20).

CEREBELLUM AND BRAIN STEM

In posterior fossa masses in children, angiography has been found to add relatively little to differential diagnosis or to the successful surgery of the usual tumors, which include cerebellar astrocytoma, brain stem glioma, medulloblastoma, and ependymoma (22, 23). In those cases with an unusual CT appearance, *e.g.*, possible dural attachment or hypervascularity, angiography should be performed. Metrizamide-enhanced CT scans are helpful in questionable cases to separate intra- from extraaxial masses and in the diagnosis of brain stem tumor. Resolution is improved and artifacts are minimized in the posterior fossa with resultant sharper

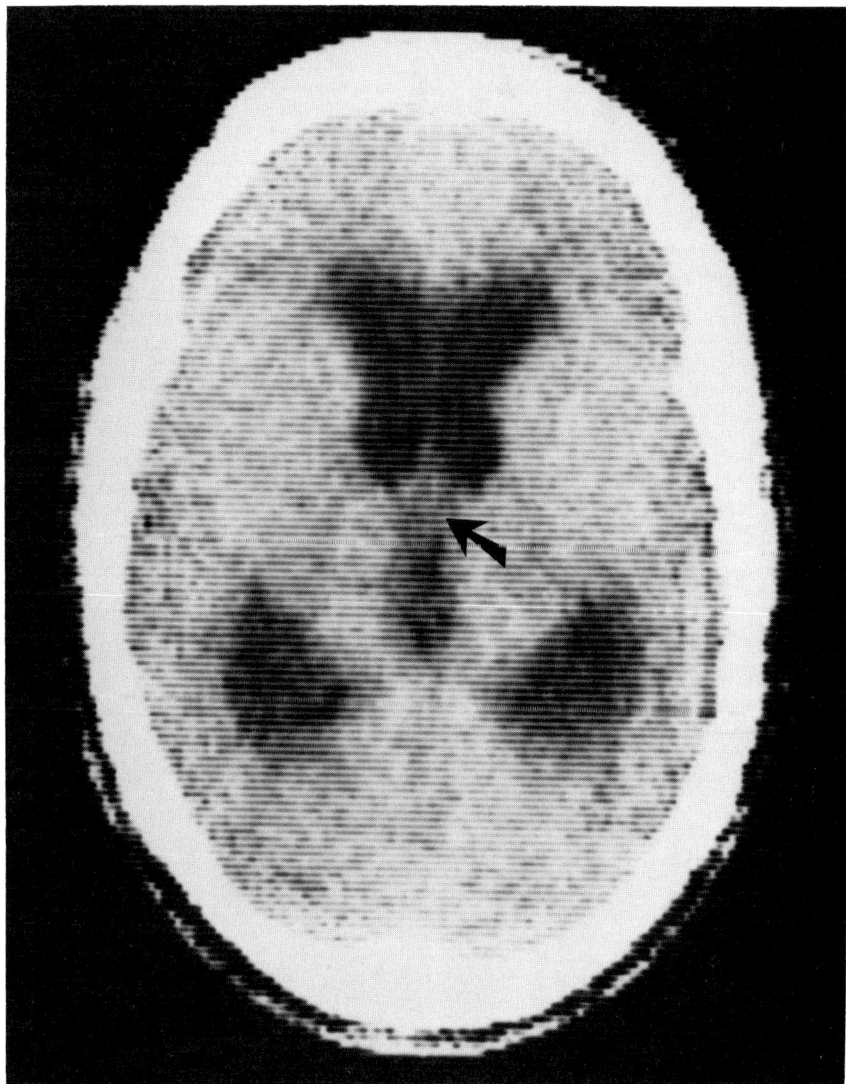

FIG. 28.9. CT scan in young, adult female. The third and lateral ventricles are enlarged. A colloid cyst (*arrow*) is present but poorly shown by CT. The cyst was found at autopsy.

delineation of the cisterns and brain substance (11) (Fig. 28.11). Delayed scans can also be helpful in defining the extent of tumor (Fig. 28.12).

SUMMARY

Computed tomography represents the examination of choice for detecting intracranial neoplasms. It is a screening procedure of great sen-

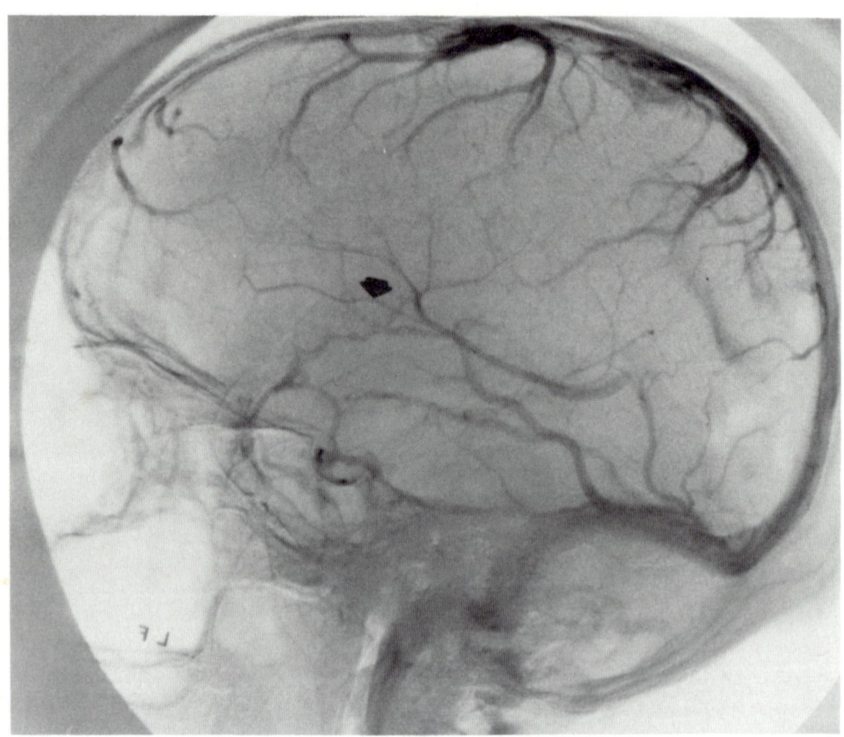

FIG. 28.10. Lateral view of angiogram, venous phase. The posterior portion of the septal vein (*arrow*) is elevated by a colloid cyst.

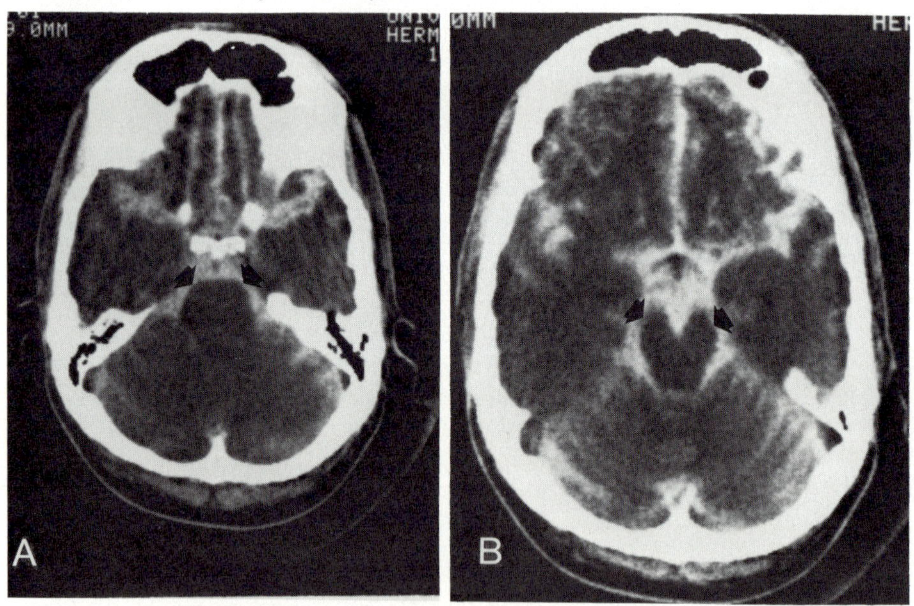

FIG. 28.11. CT metrizamide cisternography. The normal brain stem and peduncles (*arrows*) are well defined.

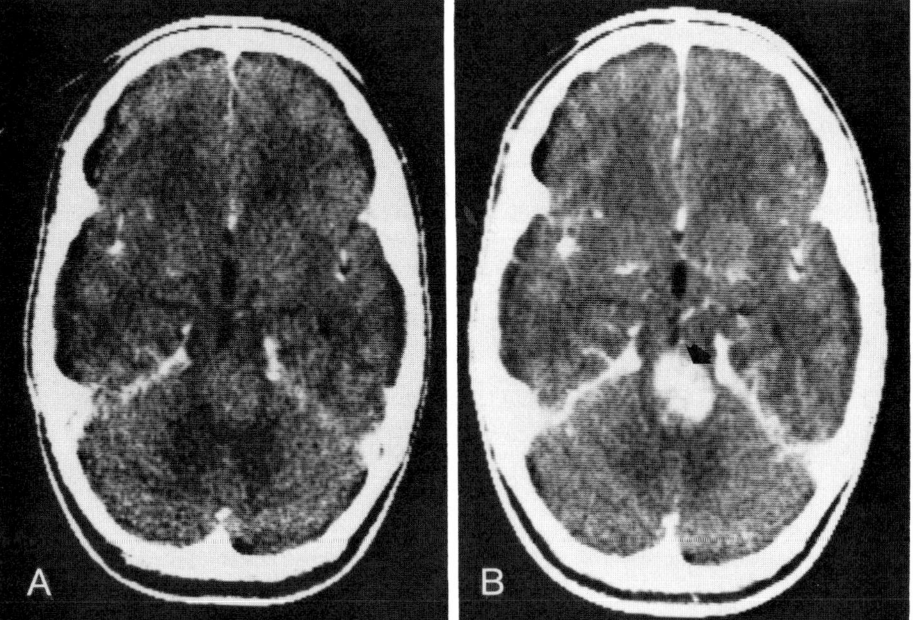

FIG. 28.12. Twelve-year-old girl with brain stem signs. (*A*) Scan immediately after 300 ml of 30% contrast. (*B*) One hour after 600 ml of 30% contrast. Marked upper brain stem enhancement definitively shows a glioma (*arrow*)

sitivity, and through proper analysis and use of clinical data, a correct diagnosis can be made in the great majority of cases.

Angiography as a complimentary modality for selected patients can carry us to a more confident pretreatment diagnosis. It can enable us to better characterize the vascular aspects of the tumor and demonstrate those important vascular anatomic relationships which may be the key to successful management.

REFERENCES

1. Bentson, J. R., Mancuso, A. A., Winter, J., and Hanafee, W. N. Combined gas cisternography and edge-enhanced computed tomography of the internal auditory canal. Radiology, *136:* 777–779, 1980.
2. Butler, A. R., Horii, S. C., Kricheff, I. I., Shannon, M. B., and Budzilovich, G. N. A statistical analysis of the parameters of malignancy and the positive contrast-enhanced CT scan. Computed tomography in astrocytomas. Radiology, *129:* 433–439, 1978.
3. Byrd, S. E., Bentson, J. R., Winter, J., Wilson, G. H., Joyce, P. W., and O'Connor, L. Giant intracranial aneurysms simulating brain neoplasms on computed tomography. J. Comput. Assist. Tomogr., *2*(3)*:* 303–307, 1978.
4. Cail, W. S., and Morris, J. L. Localization of intracranial lesions from CT scans. Surg. Neurol., *11*(1)1:35–37, 1979.
5. Chuang, V. P., Wallace, S., Swanson, D., Zornoza, J., Handel, S. F., Schwarten, D. A.,

and Murray, J. Arterial occlusion in the management of pain from metastatic renal carcinoma. Radiology, *133:* 611–614, 1979.

6. Cornell, S. H., and Hibri, N. S. The complementary nature of computerized tomography and angiography in the diagnosis of cerebellar hemangioblastoma (meeting abstract). Invest. Radiol., *13*(5)*:* 424, 1978.
7. Coulam, C. M., Seshul, M., and Donaldson, J. Intracranial ring lesions: can we differentiate by computed tomography? Invest. Radiol., *15:* 103–112, 1980.
8. Drayer, B. P., Rosenbaum, A. E., Kennerdell, J. S., *et al.* Computer tomographic diagnosis of suprasellar masses by intrathecal enhancement. Radiology, *123:* 339–344, 1977.
9. Enzmann, D. R., Krikorian, J., Yorke, C., and Hayward, R. Computed tomography in leptomeningeal spread of tumor. J. Comput. Assist. Tomogr., *2*(4)*:* 448–455, 1978.
10. Foley, W. D., Lawson, T. L., Scanlon, G. T., Heeschen, R. C., and DiBianca, F. Digital radiography of the chest using a computed tomography instrument. Radiology, *133:* 231–234, 1979.
11. Glanz, S., Geehr, R. B., Duncan, C. C., and Piepmeier, J. M. Metrizamide-enhanced CT for evaluation of brainstem tumors. Am. J. Neuroradiol., *1:* 31–34, 1980.
12. Grumme, T., Ebhardt, G., Lanksch, W., and Kretschmar, K. Intracranial space-occupying lesions with the density of brain tissue (meeting abstract). Acta Neurochir. (Wien), *44*(3/4)*:* 247–248, 1978.
13. Hacker, H., and Grau, H. The prediction of tumor pathology in computed tomography. Neurological surgery with emphasis on non-invasive methods of diagnosis and treatment. Proceedings of the Sixth International Congress of Neurological Surgery, Sao Paulo (Brazil), June 19–25, 1977, Carrea, R., Le Vay, D., (eds.). Amsterdam, Excerpta Medica, Excerpta Medica International Congress Series, 433, 1978.
14. Hatam, A., Bergstrom, M., and Greitz, T. Diagnosis of sellar and parasellar lesions by computed tomography. Neuroradiology, *18:* 249–258, 1979.
15. Hayman, L. A., Evans, R. A., Hinck, V. C. Delayed high iodine dose contrast computed tomography: cranial Neoplasms. Radiology, *136:* 677–684, 1980.
16. Kendall, B. E., Jakubowski, J. Pullicino, P., and Symon, L. Difficulties in diagnosis of supratentorial gliomas by CAT scan. J. Neurol. Neurosurg. Psychiatry, *42*(6)*:* 485–492, 1979.
17. Kricheff, I. I., Pinto, R. S., Bergeron, R. T., and Cohen, N. Air-CT cisternography and canalography for small acoustic neuromas. A.J.N.R., *1:* 57–63, 1980.
18. Naidich, T. P., Rifkin, M. D., Leeds, N. E., Lin, J. P., and Woodrow, P. Evaluation of meningiomas by computerized axial tomography (meeting abstract). Neuroradiology, *15*(2)*:* 128, 1978.
19. New, P. F. J., Aronow, S., and Hesselink, J. R. National Cancer Institute Study: evaluation of computed tomography in the diagnosis of intracranial neoplasms. IV. Meningiomas. Radiology, *136:* 665–675, 1980.
20. Numaguchi, Y., Kishikawa, T., Ikeda, J., Tsukamoto, Y., Fukui, M., Kitamura, K., and Matsuura, K. Angiographic diagnosis of acoustic neurinomas and meningiomas in the cerebellopontine angle—a reappraisal. Neuroradiology, *19:* 73–80, 1980.
21. Ostertag, C., and Mundinger, F. Diagnostic errors in the interpretation of cerebral infarction (meeting abstract). Acta Neurochir. (Wien), *44*(3/4)*:* 248–249, 1978.
22. Probst, F. P., and Liliequist, B. Assessment of posterior fossa tumors in infants and children by means of computed tomography. Neuroradiology, *18:* 9–18, 1979.
23. Rappaport, Z. H., and Epstein, F. Computerized axial tomography in the preoperative evaluation of posterior fossa tumors in children. Child's Brain, *4*(3)*:* 170–179, 1978.
24. Richmond, I. L., Newton, T. H., and Wilson, C. B. Indications for angiography in the pre-operative evaluation of patients with prolactin-secreting pituitary adenomas. J. Neurosurg., *52:* 378–380, 1980.

25. Rosenbaum, A. E., Drayer, B. P., Dubois, P. J., and Black, F. O. Visualization of small extracanalicular neurilemomas by metrizamide cisternographic enhancement. Arch. Otolaryngol., *104*(5): 239–243, 1978.

26. Russell, E. J., George, A. E., Kricheff, I. I., and Budzilovich, G. Atypical computed tomography features of intracranial meningioma. Radiologic-pathologic correlation in a series of 131 consecutive cases. Radiology, *135:* 673–682, 1980.

27. Schubiger, O., Valavanis, A., and Menges, H. Computed tomography for small acoustic neuromas. Neuroradiology, *15*(5): 287–290, 1978.

28. Shalen, P. R., Hayman, L. A., Wallace, S., and Handel, S. F. Protocol for delayed contrast enhancement in cranial computed tomographic evaluation of cerebral neoplasia. Unpublished data.

29. Steinhoff, H., Lanksch, W., Kazner, E., Grumme, T., Meese, W., Lange, S., Aulich, A., Schindler, E., and Wende, S. Computed tomography in the diagnosis and differential diagnosis of glioblastomas. A qualitative study of 295 cases. Neuroradiology, *14:* 193–200, 1977.

30. Volpe, B. T., Foley, K. M., and Howieson, J. Normal CAT scans in craniopharyngioma. Ann. Neurol., *3*(1): 87–89, 1978.

31. Weisberg, L. A. Cerebral computed tomography in the diagnosis of supratentorial astrocytoma. Comput. Tomogr., *4*(2): 87–105, 1980.

CHAPTER

29

CT Monitoring of Chemotherapeutic Agent Delivery after Osmotic Blood Brain Barrier Disruption*

EDWARD A. NEUWELT, M.D.†

INTRODUCTION

Recent successes in the management of a variety of cancers by multi-agent chemotherapy have provided the basis for an important refocus on the biology and therapy of malignant lesions identified in the central nervous system (CNS). Several types of disseminated systemic malignancies (*i.e.*, choriocarcinoma, oat cell carcinoma of lung, and breast cancer in women) managed with chemotherapy have demonstrated significant and durable complete response rates, even when the tumor is found in multiple metastatic sites. Therefore, it is indeed remarkable that when these same (responsive) neoplasms are identified as metastatic foci in the CNS, the effect of the chemotherapy at the CNS sites has been minimal (22). Similarly, systemic or intrathecal chemotherapy has not had a significant impact on primary (glial) CNS tumors.

The unique biologic circumstance of a blood brain barrier (BBB) provokes an important focus in the consideration of therapy of tumors in the CNS. A serious proposal relative to the documented therapeutic ineffectiveness in such lesions is that the presence of the BBB at the proliferating edge of primary and metastatic CNS tumors is at least one major factor that is responsible for this failure. It is the purpose of this study to consider some of the characteristics of this barrier and to evaluate the efficacy and toxicity of disruption of the barrier prior to the administration of systemic chemotherapy.

BBB LIMITS DELIVERY OF DRUGS

The BBB is created by tight junctions (zonulae occludentes) between endothelial cells in brain capillaries. These junctions restrict diffusion

---

* This work was supported by The Southwestern Medical Foundation, The Blanche Mary Taxis Foundation, The Veterans Administration, and Grants CA 23115, CA181132, and CA27191 from the National Cancer Institute, U. S. Public Health Service.

† The Departments of Surgery (Division of Neurosurgery) and Biochemistry.

between endothelial cells; they are found wherever there is physiological evidence of a barrier and are absent in the few areas that lack a BBB, such as the pineal gland, area postrema, and adenohypophysis (23).

Some oncologists view the "barrier hypothesis" as irrelevant because earlier studies of the BBB suggested that "the blood brain barrier was not a factor in the chemotherapy of brain tumors (30)". In general this thesis was based on the observation that the vessels inside metastatic cerebral tumors often have a fenestrated and discontinuous endothelium that is characteristic of the vessels of the primary tumor (9); similar fenestrated and gap junctions have also been seen in gliomas (30).

Nevertheless, current studies have confirmed that the "barrier" is far more complex than this all-or-none phenomenon. There may be loss of the BBB in the center of some tumors, but recent studies have provided important evidence that the tumor periphery has very different characteristics. For instance, Levin *et al.* (8) studied uptake of methotrexate (MTX) by intracerebral ependymoblastomas; the MTX level of normal brain was 3 to 4% of the plasma level, but in the center of the tumor it was 32%, and at the brain-tumor interface, 13% of the plasma level. Similarly, Tator (29) gave radiolabeled MTX intravenously to mice with intracerebral implants of ependymoblastoma; cells in the central mass were heavily labeled, while cells at the periphery and those infiltrating adjacent brain showed only scanty labeling. Shapiro *et al.* (28), using ^{14}C-labeled α-aminoisobutyric acid, also reported variability in the degree of BBB disruption in experimental brain tumors; they found a nearly normal BBB in small tumors and adjacent brain. Groothius and Vick (4) showed that intravascular peroxidase variably penetrated experimental gliomas in the brain but freely entered subcutaneous tumors. Walker and Weiss (31) posed a "sink effect" to explain the low concentration of drugs at the tumor periphery, that is, the "extra" drug that enters the periphery of the tumor rapidly diffuses into drug-free surrounding brain because of "mild disruption" of the BBB.

That the drug delivery problem is clinically significant was emphasized by Benjamin *et al.* (1), who described progressive increase in the size of brain metastases while other systemic metastases regressed with adriamycin chemotherapy. Posner (22) stated, "Drugs that appear to be successful in treating systemic metastases are ineffective against the same tumor when it is in the brain." It is not known whether these failures are the result of only a partially impaired barrier at the periphery of the tumor, the "sink effect," or both.

Two approaches have been utilized to overcome these problems in the chemotherapy of neoplasms in the CNS. First, since MTX normally penetrates the brain, albeit poorly, attempts to overcome the resistance of the BBB have involved the use of very high systemic doses of MTX

(27). Unfortunately, these resulted in only marginal therapeutic levels of MTX in brain. A second approach has involved direct instillation of drugs into neural spaces (*e.g.*, ventricular, subarachnoid). Kimelberg *et al.* (7) gave MTX by direct intraventricular infusion but failed to obtain therapeutic drug levels in the white matter deep to the cortex or the ependyma. With intrathecal or intraventricular chemotherapy, another problem is the certainty of drug dispersal, especially when there is blockage of spinal fluid circulation (in spinal cord or tentorial lesions).

REGULATION OF DRUG ENTRY INTO THE BRAIN

The two important factors determining drug-entry from blood into the brain are molecular weight and lipid solubility. The BBB normally prevents passage of ionized water-soluble drugs with a molecular weight of more than 180 daltons (3). Most currently effective chemotherapeutic agents have molecular weights between 200 and 1200 daltons (*i.e.*, MTX, 455; daunorubicin, 544; and cyclophosphamide, 261). Thus, on a molecular weight basis, the passage of many chemotherapeutic agents would be impeded by the BBB.

An even more important factor is lipid solubility. There is a linear correlation between the octanol/water coefficient of chemotherapeutic agents and cerebrovascular permeability. MTX, which has a pH of 4.7 and is 99.8% ionized at a blood pH of 7.4, is lipid insoluble; the normal CSF/plasma ratio is only 0.02 (23).

Entry of macromolecular water-soluble nutrients and drugs when the BBB is intact is also regulated by a number of transport mechanisms. The cerebrovascular endothelium can transport (by facilitated, stereospecific, saturable mechanisms) substances that are involved in brain metabolism.

REVERSIBLE DISRUPTION OF THE BBB

For effective therapy the BBB disruption must be reversible. Only a few techniques are known. Hypercarbia disrupts the BBB reversibly but inconsistently (23). MacDonell *et al.* (10) demonstrated reversible BBB disruption after intravenous administration of 5-fluorouracil, but barrier opening did not follow parenteral administration of MTX, cyclophosphamide, or vincristine. BBB disruption by intracarotid infusion of hypertonic solutions is the most thoroughly evaluated and most effective method for reversible BBB disruption (24).

Reversible osmotic BBB disruption is a threshold event with regard to either osmolality or duration of infusion (24). Osmotic barrier opening is essentially an all-or-nothing phenomenon. For instance, in the rat, using arabinose, the threshold was 1.6 osmolal, and the minimum infusion time 20 to 30 seconds (24). Similar thresholds have been observed in rabbit, cat, and primates. After "opening," the barrier remains open for less than 1 hour (17, 24).

The importance of the rate of carotid infusion was demonstrated by direct observation of the cerebral cortical surface when infusates were just above the threshold of osmolality (17, 24). Although this rate measurement is technically complex, it can be done by determining the rate of infusion which, by visual inspection, completely displaced blood from the cortical surface of the ipsilateral hemisphere. This rate is critical, since dilution of the infusate by blood from either the ipsilateral carotid artery or from collateral flow via the circle of Willis results in a subthreshold osmolality. Unfortunately, infusion rates higher than necessary result in intravascular hypertension, which can disrupt the barrier irreversibly.

Osmotic disruption of the BBB can be observed ultrastructurally. Brightman *et al.* (2) demonstrated opening of tight junctions to peroxidase tracer after intracarotid infusion of 3 M urea. When endothelial cells shrank because of the hypertonic environment, the membranes stressed the tight junctions and made them permeable to intravascular tracer. Separation of cerebral endothelial tight junctions of 0.1 μm was observed in rats after intracarotid infusion of arabinose (23).

Reversibility of barrier opening has been documented by administration of Evans' blue-albumin at different times after intracarotid hypertonic solution infusion. Following disruption the (Evan's) blue staining was not evident when dye was given 30 minutes after mannitol infusion (17, 24). Thus, for this 68,000 molecular weight marker, the barrier remains open for less than 30 minutes. However, slight permeability changes have been shown for smaller molecular weight markers for up to 2 hours after barrier disruption (17, 24).

The metabolic effects of hypertonic disruption of the BBB include transient increase of glucose metabolism and transient increase of brain water content by 1.5% (21). The slight increase in brain water (cerebral edema) requires up to 24 hours to resolve (24).

Several hypertonic solutions have been used to disrupt the BBB, including arabinose, mannitol, and radiographic contrast agents. They are all effective but with minor disadvantages. Mannitol (25%) is a nearly saturated solution at ambient temperature and must be filtered before use. Direct instillation of certain iodinated radiographic contrast agents into the internal carotid artery causes EEG changes that may persist for more than 2 hours (23).

Pappius *et al.* (21) observed conscious rats during and after osmotic disruption of the BBB. Transient behavioral changes, such as turning to one side and depressed activity, were seen. Rapoport *et al.* (26) did not observe neurological or behavioral sequelae in 7 of 8 rhesus monkeys given intracarotid infusions of 2.5 M D,L-lactamide, the eighth animal developed a right hemiparesis. After 48 hours, the animals were sacrificed. No cerebral edema was evident nor were there significant changes in brain water, Na+, or K+ content. However, intraocular pressure was reduced, and there was histologic evidence of severe damage to the ciliary epithelium of the eye (20). Eighteen months later, at least some visual acuity was retained (23a). In the rat, no such pathological eye changes have been observed (23a).

With reversible osmotic barrier disruption, permeability increases about 20-fold for substances which the brain normally excludes, such as sucrose, microperoxidase, penicillin, gamma globulin, and neurotransmitters (23, 25).

BBB DISRUPTION IN DOGS

Recently reported studies of reversible osmotic BBB disruption in the dog (17, 18) provides a working model with significant advantages over the previous small animal murine model (23, 25). First, the dog model permits an opportunity to obtain serial samples of CSF in sufficient quantity; second, the dog brain, in contrast to that of the rat, is large enough to be evaluated by computerized tomography (CT), which can monitor BBB disruption after intravenous administration of iodinated contrast material, thereby providing a noninvasive criterion of the success of the disruption; third, the dog is readily available and less costly than primates.

The dog, unlike the rat, has a small internal carotid (2 mm) artery located quite distally (just under the mandible), and a large distal external-to-internal carotid collateral circulation. In the early canine studies, hypertonic (25%) mannitol was infused through the common carotid artery, but resulted in variable BBB disruption as determined by transudation of Evans' blue given intravenously (15) and by variable levels of MTX in the brain. It is now clear that, in this model, mannitol infused into the common carotid artery produces inconsistent blanching of the ipsilateral cerebral cortex (15).

A major technical advance was made by simply altering the site of infusion. When the distally located internal carotid artery was cannulated, 42 ml of fluid infused over 30 seconds completely and consistently blanched the cerebral cortex of 25-kg mongrel dgs. By infusing into the internal carotid artery rather than the common carotid artery, brain levels of methotrexate rose from 1000 to 2000 ng of methotrexate per g of tissue to as high as 90,000 ng of methotrexate per g of tissue. Methotrexate levels in brain tissue of saline control animals, using internal carotid artery infusion, were about 1000 ng/g. The staining of brain parenchyma following intravenous Evans' blue infusion was also much more pronounced and consistent than it had been with common carotid artery infusion.

STUDIES OF THE USE OF THE CT SCAN AS A MEANS OF MONITORING BBB DISRUPTION

Enhanced CT is a noninvasive means of monitoring BBB disruption. It was used in a series of experiments to monitor the degree, distribution, extent, and reversibility of osmotic blood-brain barrier disruption in our canine model (17). The timing of administration of iodinated contrast agent was shown to be crucial to optimize "enhancement" by CT of the disrupted blood-brain barriers. Meglumine iothalamate given intravenously resulted in excellent enhancement on the CT scan (Fig. 29.1). Intracarotid infusion of the contrast agent was less satisfactory. Under similar conditions, enhancement due to metrizamide was less marked and more transient than that observed with meglumine iothalamate. Systemically administered methotrexate after osmotic blood-brain barrier disruption resulted in increased brain levels in areas that closely correlated with CT scan enhancement. Therefore, these results suggest that the CT scan provides an excellent noninvasive monitor of both blood-brain barrier disruption and the delivery of chemotherapeutic agents to the brain.

PHARMACOKINETICS OF METHOTREXATE ADMINISTRATION AFTER OSMOTIC BLOOD-BRAIN BARRIER DISRUPTION

The pharmacokinetics of methotrexate delivery to the brain and cerebrospinal fluid after osmotic blood-brain barrier disruption was evaluated next (16). One hour after mannitol and methotrexate infusion in experimental animals, there was a dramatic rise (about 10-fold) in the methotrexate level in the ipsilateral cerebral parenchyma, as compared with the levels in the ipsilateral hemisphere of control animals receiving saline instead of mannitol. The enhancement of drug delivery due to a combination of blood-brain barrier disruption (10-fold) and intracarotid methotrexate administration (5- to 10-fold) was, therefore, 50- to 100-fold. In short, combining osmotic blood-brain barrier disruption and intraarterial chemotherapy administration achieved maximum brain levels while the amount of drug in the systemic circulation was quite low, thereby limiting systemic toxicity. The pharmacokinetic studies evaluating serum, brain, and spinal fluid clearly indicated that assays of methotrexate levels in CSF are, unfortunately, an unreliable and inconsistent monitor of brain methotrexate levels after osmotic blood-brain barrier disruption. Indeed, on the basis of these studies, it was found that osmotic blood-brain barrier disruption appears to be an unsatisfactory method to enhance drug

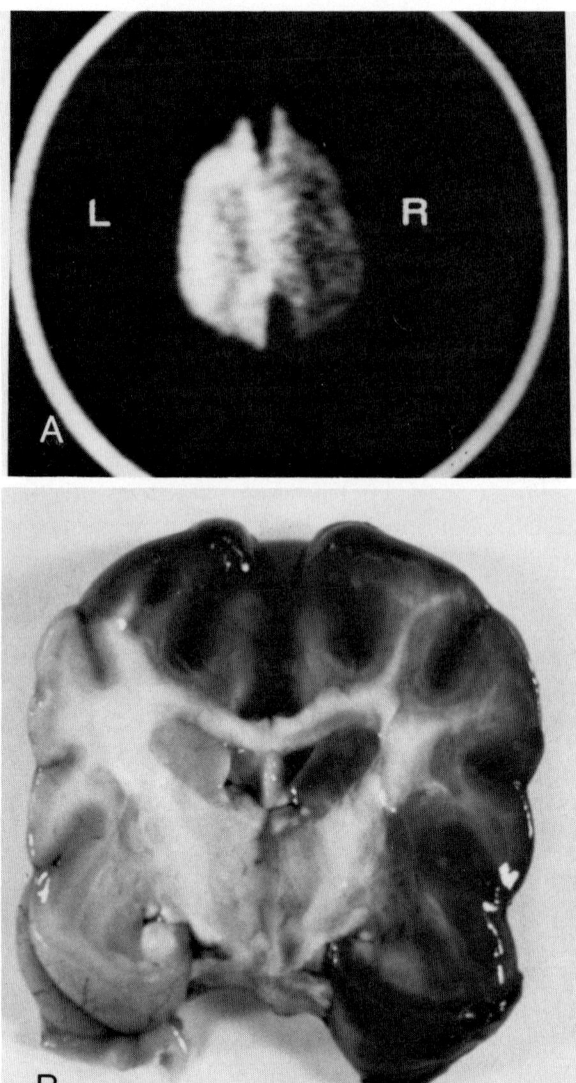

FIG. 29.1. (*A*) A computerized tomogram of canine brain 1 hour following osmotic BBB disruption of left cerebral hemisphere with 25% mannitol. Iodinated contrast material and Evans' blue were given I.V. prior to the intraarterial mannitol infusion. The image is a transverse section of the cerebrum. The *white (enhanced) area* is the result of iodinated contrast medium penetrating the BBB. The area which enhances includes the entire left hemisphere and the medial right hemisphere in the distribution of the right anterior cerebral artery. The *black areas* in both cerebral hemispheres are part of the ventricular system. (*B*) Unfixed canine brain 1 hour following osmotic BBB disruption of left cerebral hemisphere. The *dark areas* represent penetration across the BBB of Evans' blue-albumin (mol. wt. 68,500). The BBB was disrupted in the entire left cerebral hemisphere and in the distribution of the anterior cerebral artery of the right hemisphere. (From E. A. Neuwelt *et al.* (18). Published with permission.)

delivery to the CSF for potential lesions like carcinomatous meningitis. Conversely, it was found that CSF could not be used to monitor drug delivery to the cerebral parenchyma after osmotic blood-brain barrier disruption.

It should be noted that Ohno *et al.* (19) have observed a 10- to 50-fold increase in brain methotrexate levels in the rat model after osmotic BBB disruption. Similar results have been reported by Hasegawa *et al.* (5).

CLINICAL STUDIES

As summarized above, there is considerable evidence to support the view that the existence of the blood brain barrier may be a very significant factor for the poor chemotherapeutic responses seen in central nervous system malignant neoplasms. Recent observations in animals, including the rat, dog, and primates (16–18, 21, 23), have indicated that hypertonic solutions transiently and reversibly disrupt the blood-brain barrier with minimal evidence of permanent neurologic damage or dysfunction. These observations provided the basis for the therapeutic approach in our initial clinical studies in which methotrexate (100 mg) was given intraarterially after osmotic blood-brain barrier disruption. Of the 5 patients with primary and metastatic malignant brain tumors entered into this Phase I (toxicity) study, good to excellent blood brain barrier disruption was achieved in 4 patients (12–15). There was a single nontransient complication, that of a superficial wound infection at the burhole site in the first patient. There were 2 transient complications. One patient who has undergone blood brain barrier disruption 5 times and has a history of grand mal seizures had 2 episodes of seizures. These seizures followed osmotic blood brain barrier disruption, during which the documentation of disruption was evaluated by enhancement which used the parenteral administration of a double dose of contrast. It is of relevant interest that osmotic blood brain barrier disruption on 2 subsequent occasions in this patient was done with no contrast administration. The brain scan was used to document the blood brain barrier disruption, and no complications (seizures) were seen. A second patient with a large left temporal lobe glioblastoma had an increase in his nominal aphasia following osmotic blood brain barrier disruption; this reversed within a day after barrier disruption with steroid therapy. Therefore, on the basis of osmotic blood barrier disruption 28 times in 6 patients, it appears that reversible transient blood brain barrier disruption can be performed in man without significant toxicity. In addition, the technologic criteria which document blood brain barrier disruption can now be displayed by 2 noninvasive methods, computerized tomography and radionuclide brain imaging. The current studies further provide evidence that a metastasis or glioblastoma may have an intact or relatively intact blood brain barrier to an intravenous contrast agent (meglumine iothalamate) which only becomes permeable to this contrast agent (by CT scan) after osmotic blood barrier disruption. More specifically, evaluation of enhanced CT scan images (Fig. 29.2) and use of CT numbers (Table 29.1) in these patients with and without barrier disruption indicated that BBB disruption increased drug delivery to tumor as well as to surrounding brain. Neuroradiologic evaluation also demonstrated that drug persists in tumor longer after BBB disruption. As a result of an anatomic variation in the circle of Willis, barrier disruption extended into the posterior fossa in one patient without ill effect. Therefore, osmotic BBB disruption appears to be a relatively safe procedure in man capable of increasing drug delivery to both malignant brain neoplasms and to surrounding parenchyma (12–15).

The therapeutic implications of these clinical studies of methotrexate administration after osmotic blood brain barrier disruption need to be considered. Methotrexate, a phase-specific drug which acts during DNA synthesis (S) phase, is one of the agents used by the intrathecal route for the therapy of neoplastic lesions in the CNS. Because cell division is asynchronous, for a phase-specific drug such as methotrexate to be therapeutically effective, it should be present in therapeutic concentra-

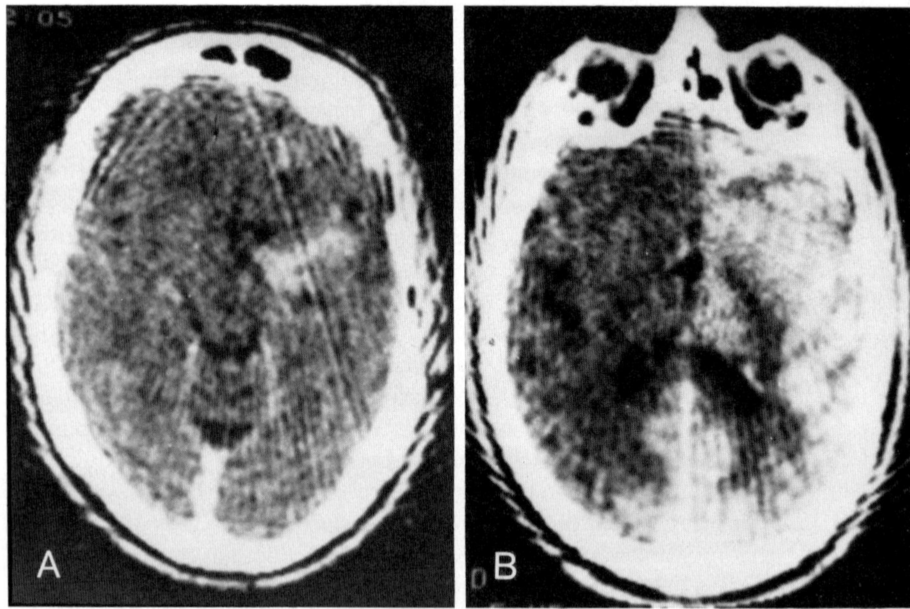

FIG. 29.2. Enhanced CT scans at the level of the lateral ventricles in patient D.R. with and without osmotic BBB disruption using a double dose of contrast agent. (*A*) Control enhanced CT scan at the level of residual glioblastoma in the left temporal lobe (*arrow*). (*B*) Enhanced CT scan after osmotic BBB disruption of the left hemisphere. There is a marked increase in enhancement in the region of the tumor (compare with *A*).

TABLE 29.1
Analysis of CT Number in Presence and Absence of BBB Disruption

	Control enhanced CT scan		Enhanced CT scan after osmotic BBB disruption	
	Normal hemisphere	Tumor hemisphere	Normal hemisphere	Tumor hemisphere
Gray matter	36	38	41	67
White matter	28	27	34	36
Tumor center		57		68

* The CT numbers listed on this table were derived from the CT scans of the patient illustrated in Fig. 29.2.

tions for at least 1 cell generation time (the time for 1 full cell cycle). Using glioblastoma as a typical example, *in vivo* studies have reported generation time values ranging from 57 hours to 6 to 8 weeks (16). Therefore, since osmotic blood brain barrier disruption is reversible and only opens the blood brain barrier for 30 to 60 minutes, a phase-specific drug such as methotrexate has definite theoretical disadvantages. On the other hand, the reversibility of osmotic blood brain barrier disruption also has a major advantage with respect to the use of methotrexate. The systemic effects of methotrexate can be minimized with folinic acid (citrovorum factor) rescue given after the blood brain barrier is reestablished since folinic acid does not appear to cross the blood brain barrier in significant concentrations. In addition, methotrexate is a drug that is easily assayed and that is still being evaluated in primary and metastatic brain tumors. Methotrexate and cytosine arabinoside are the two major chemotherapeutic agents which are placed intrathecally in man with clearly demonstrated efficacy and reasonably safety (11). Thus, despite a theoretical disadvantage of being a phase-specific drug, methotrexate appears to be a suitable candidate for at least initial Phase I trials.

FUTURE DIRECTIONS

Although the present studies provide an opportunity for reversible blood brain barrier disruption in man, it is clear at the present time that that we cannot be certain of the level of tolerance of the brain to increased concentrations of chemotherapeutic agents, the potential sensitivity of primary brain tumors to the available agents, or the effect of radiotherapy or other agents on drug accessibility after osmotic blood brain barrier disruption. These questions, as well as the applicability of such an approach in nonneoplastic neurological disorders (*e.g.*, infections, inborn errors of metabolism, etc.), are now under study in a series of animal models. Nonetheless, clinical studies of patients herein presented are continuing. The toxicity, pharmacokinetics, and efficacy of these chemotherapeutic studies with methotrexate and other drugs are continuing to be evaluated.

ACKNOWLEDGMENTS

Part of this manuscript was derived from a paper presented at the EORTC symposium on Treatment of Neoplastic Lesions of the Nervous System held in Brussels in April 1980, and which will be published in the European Journal of Cancer. The typographical expertise of Mary Ann Means in helping to prepare this manuscript was much appreciated.

REFERENCES

1. Benjamin, R. S., Wiernik, P. H., and Bachar, N. R. Adriamycin chemotherapy—efficacy, safety, and pharmacologic basis of intermittent single high dose schedule. Cancer, *33:* 19–27, 1974.
2. Brightman, M. W., Hori, M., Rapoport, S. I., Reese, T. S., and Westergard, R. Osmotic opening of tight junctions in cerebral endothelium. Comp. Neurol., *152:* 317–326, 1973.
3. Fenstermacher, J. D., and Johnson, J. A. Filtration and reflection coefficients of the rabbit blood-brain barrier. J. Physiol. (Lond.), *211:* 341–346, 1966.
4. Groothuis, D., and Vick, N. Differential permeability to horseradish peroxidase in intracerebral and subcutaneous tumors. Cancer Treat. Rep., in press, 1981.
5. Hasegawa, H., Allen, J. C., Mehta, B. M., Shapiro, W. R., and Posner, J. B. Enhancement of CNS penetration of methotrexate by hyperosmolar intracarotid mannitol or carcinomatous meningitis. Neurology, *29:* 1280–1286, 1979.
6. Hoshino, T. The cell kinetics of gliomas: its prognostic value and therapeutic implications. *In* Multidisciplinary Aspects of Brain Tumor Therapy, edited by P. Paoletti, M. D. Walker, G. Butti, and R. Knerich, Elsevier/North-Holland Biomedical Press, Amsterdam, 1979.
7. Kimelberg, H. K., King, D., Watson, R. E., Reiss, F. L., Biddlecome, S. M., and Bourke, R. S. Direct administration of methotrexate into the central nervous system of primates. Part I. Distribution and degradation of methotrexate in nervous and systemic tissue after intraventricular injection. J. Neurosurg., *48:* 883–894, 1978.
8. Levin, V. A., Clancy, T. P., Ausman, J. I., and Rall D. P. Uptake and distribution of ^{3}H-methotrexate by the murine ependymoblastoma. Natl. Cancer Inst. Monogr., *48:* 875–883, 1972.
9. Long, D. M. Capillary ultrastructure in human metastatic brain tumors. J. Neurosurg., *51:* 53–58, 1979.
10. MacDonell, L. A., Potter, P. E., and Leslie, R. A. Localized changes in blood-brain barrier permeability following the administration of anti-neoplastic drugs. Cancer Res., *38:* 2930–2934, 1978.
11. Neuwelt, E. A. Treatment of central nervous system neoplasms. *In* Treatment of Neurological Diseases, edited by R. Rosenberg, p. 205. 1979.
12. Neuwelt, E. A., Diehl, J. T., Vu, L. H., Frenkel, E. P., Hill, S. A., and Michael, A. J. Monitoring of methotrexate delivery in patients with malignant brain tumors after osmotic blood brain barrier disruption. Ann. Intern. Med. *94* (1): 449–454, 1981.
13. Neuwelt, E. A., Frenkel, E. P., Diehl, J. T., Maravilla, K. R., Vu, L. H., Clark, W. K., Rapoport, S. I., Barnett, P. A., Hill, S. A., Lewis, S. E., Ehle, A. L., Beyer, C. W., Jr., and Moore, R. J. Osmotic blood brain barrier disruption: pharmacodynamic studies in the canine and a clinical phase I trial in patients with malignant brain tumors. Third Conference on Brain Tumor Therapy at Asilomar, Monterey, Calif. Cancer Treat. Rep., in press, 1981.

14. Neuwelt, E. A., Frenkel, E. P., Diehl, J. T., Vu, L. H., and Hill, S. A. Reversible osmotic blood brain barrier disruption in man: implications for the chemotherapy of malignant brain tumors. Neurosurgery, *7:* 44–52, 1980.
15. Neuwelt, E. A., Frenkel, E. P., Hill, S., Barnett, P., Clark, K., Maravilla, K. R., Rapoport, S., and Diehl, J. Clinical and animal studies of reversible osmotic blood brain barrier disruption as a new means of increasing chemotherapy delivery to the central nervous system. Trans. Am. Neurol. Assoc., *104:* 1-5, 1979.
16. Neuwelt, E. A., Frenkel, E. P., Rapoport, S. I., and Barnett, P. A. The effect of osmotic blood brain barrier disruption on methotrexate pharmacokinetics in the canine. Neurosurgery, *7:* 36–43, 1980.
17. Neuwelt, E. A., Maravilla, K. R., Frenkel, E., Barnett, P., Hill, S., and Moore, R. The use of enhanced computerized tomography to evaluate osmotic blood brain barrier disruption. Neurosurgery, *5:* 576–582, 1979.
18. Neuwelt, E. A., Maravilla, K. R., Frenkel, E. P., Hill, S., Rapoport, S. I., and Barnett P. Osmotic blood-brain barrier disruption: computerized tomographic monitoring of chemotherapeutic agent deliver. J. Clin. Invest., *64:* 684–688, 1979.
19. Ohno, K., Fredericks, W. R., and Rapoport, S. I. Osmotic opening of the blood-brain barrier to methotrexate in the rat. Surg. Neurol., *12:* 323–328, 1979.
20. Okisaka, S., Kuwabara, T., and Rapoport, S. I. Selective destruction of the pigmented epithelium in the ciliary body of the eye. Science, *184:* 1298–1299, 1974.
21. Pappius, H. H., Savake, H. E., Feischi, C., Rapoport, S. I., and Sokoloff, L. Osmotic opening of blood-brain barrier and local cerebral glucose utilization. Ann. Neurol., *5:* 211–212, 1979.
22. Posner, J. B. Management of central nervous system metastases. Semin. Oncol., *4:* 81–91, 1977.
23. Rapoport, S. I. Blood-brain barrier in physiology and medicine. Raven Press, New York, 1976.
23a. Rapoport, S. I. Personal communication, 1976.
24. Rapoport, S. I., Fredericks, W. R., Ohno, K., and Pettigrew, K. D. Quantitative aspects of reversible osmotic opening of the blood-brain barrier. Am. J. Physiol., *235:* 421–431, 1980.
25. Rapoport, S. I., Ohno, K., Fredericks, W. R., and Pettigrew, K. D. Regional cerebrovascular permeability to ^{14}sucrose after osmotic opening of the blood-brain barrier. Brain Res., *150:* 653–657, 1978.
26. Rapoport, S. I., Matthews, K., Thompson, H. K., and Pettigrew, K. D. Osmotic opening of the blood-brain barrier in the rhesus monkey without measurable brain edema. Brain Res., *136:* 23–29, 1977.
27. Rosen, G., Ghavimi, F., Nirenberg, A., Mosende, C., and Mehta, B. M. High-dose methotrexate with citrovorum factor rescue for the treatment of central nervous system tumors in children. Cancer Treat. Rep., *61* (4): 681–690, 1977.
28. Shapiro, W. R., Mehta, B., Blasberg, R. G., Patlak, C. S., Kobayashi, T., and Allen, J. C. Pharmacodynamics of entry of methotrexate into brain of humans, monkeys, and a rat brain tumor model. Proceedings of the International Symposium on Multidisciplinary Aspects of Brain Tumor Therapy. Elsevier-North Holland Biomedical Press, Amsterdam, in press, 1981.
29. Tator, C. H. Chemotherapy of brain tumors: uptake of tritiated methotrexate by a transplantable intracerebral ependymoblastoma in mice. J. Neurosurg., *37:* 1–8, 1972.
30. Vick, N. A., and Bigner, D. D. Chemotherapy of brain tumors: The blood-brain barrier is not a factor. Arch. Neurol., *34:* 523–526, 1977.
31. Walker, M. D., and Weiss, H. Chemotherapy in the treatment of malignant brain tumors. Adv. Neurol., *31:* 149–191, 1975.

CHAPTER

30

Effects of Early Peripheral Lesions on the Somatotopic Organization of the Cerebral Cortex

LARRY V. CARSON, M.D.,
ANDREW M. KELAHAN, B.S., RICHARD H. RAY, PH.D.,
CLINTON E. MASSEY, M.D., GERNOT S. DOETSCH, PH.D.

Recent studies have shown that selective lesions of peripheral nerves or dorsal roots can produce dramatic changes in the normal functional organization of somatosensory areas of the brain (2, 4, 9, 12, 15). Common to most of these studies is the finding that such lesions cause the deafferented neural tissue to be "invaded" by inputs from other body regions; that is, neurons deprived of their usual somatic afferent drive often develop responsiveness to stimulation of neighboring skin regions. In some instances, these functional changes develop slowly over time while others may occur immediately following deafferentation; the effects appear to be more pronounced in young animals than in adults.

Chronic denervation of the forepaw in cats causes an age-dependent reorganization within somatosensory (SmI) cortex, such that deafferented neurons acquire new receptive fields in skin regions adjacent to the denervated areas (4). Selective dorsal root sections in cats result in a similar cortical rearrangement that progresses with time (2). Functional reorganization involving somatotopic disruption was observed in SmI cortex of monkeys following transection and subsequent regeneration of peripheral nerves innervating the hand (12, 15); when a transected median nerve was prevented from regenerating, reorganization occurred in an orderly somatotopic fashion (9). Disruptive changes occur in the topographic representation of mystacial vibrissae within SmI cortex in adult rats (6) and mice (13) after early destruction of individual vibrissal follicles. Perhaps most dramatic are several reports of immediate changes in the receptive field locations of single neurons following selective deafferentation; such rapid changes have been found in SmI cortex of cats during reversible epidural blocks of several dorsal roots (10) and also at lower CNS levels, such as in the dorsal column nuclei of cats after dorsal root sections (1, 11). The phenomenon of immediate switching of receptive field locations has been interpreted as "unmasking" or disinhibition of preexisting but normally latent neural connections; functional reorganization occurring more slowly may involve strengthening of such latent connections and possibly sprouting of intact afferents (8).

Compared with recent findings on somatosensory reorganization following nerve or dorsal root lesions, very little is known about the central physiological effects of amputation or other extensive damage to peripheral somatic structures. Functional changes within the CNS have been proposed to account for some of the perceptual phenomena reported after limb amputation in humans (14); however, direct physiological data from humans concerning possible reorganization within the cerebral cortex are very scarce (3, 7). The present study was undertaken to examine the central effects of peripheral somatic injury; the specific aim was to determine the consequences of early selective digit amputation on the functional organization of the hand representation within the adult somatosensory cerebral cortex.

Raccoons were used as experimental subjects because they have a highly developed somatosensory system, characterized by rather large and discrete functional representations of the forepaw digits within the dorsal column nuclei, thalamus, and cerebral cortex (17, 18). Fig. 30.1*A* shows the glabrous surface of the raccoon forepaw with the digits numbered 1 to 5 and the palmar pads lettered *A* to *E*. The basic plan of representation of the digits and pads within the cortex is illustrated in Fig. 30.1*B* (adapted from Welker and Seidenstein, ref. 18). The digits are sequentially represented lateral, anterior, and medial to the triradiate sulcus, and the pads are represented adjacent to their corresponding digit

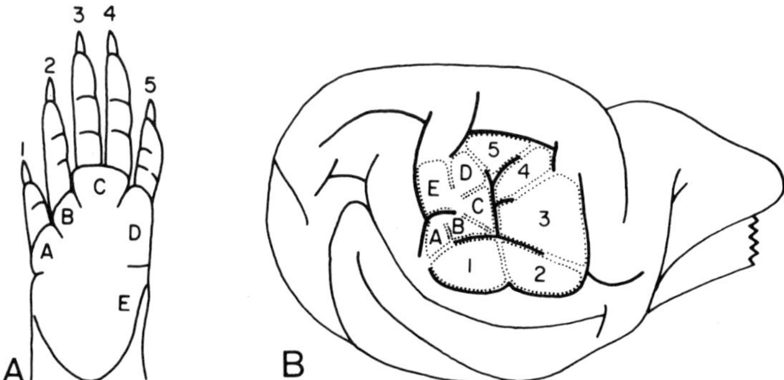

FIG. 30.1. Basic scheme of representation of the contralateral volar aspect of the forepaw in SmI cortex of the raccoon. (*A*) Ventral surface of the left forepaw, showing digits *1* to *5* and palmar pads *A* to *E*. (*B*) Digit and pad representations in the right SmI cortex. (Adapted from Welker and Seidenstein (18)).

areas, posterior to the triradiate sulcus. The cortical forepaw area makes up about 60% of the total SmI cortex and, as shown in Fig. 30.1*B*, the digit representations are often separated by sulci or dimples.

Methods

Electrophysiological data obtained from 10 adult raccoons subjected to digit amputation shortly following birth were compared with data obtained from eight normal adult raccoons. Using antiseptic procedures, the third digit of the left forepaw was locally anesthetized and then amputated at the metacarpophalangeal joint in four groups of neonatal raccoons at 2, 4, 6, and 8 weeks of age, respectively (the first two groups consisted of two animals each; the last two, of three animals each). After this procedure, the animals were housed together in a large enclosure which provided ample space for social interaction and various objects for manipulation. Nine to 12 months later, electrophysiological experiments were done on each animal to examine the functional organization of the SmI forepaw representation, with special emphasis on the somatotopic arrangement within digit 3 cortex and adjacent digit and pad areas. Each animal was anesthetized with sodium pentobarbital (35 mg/kg, i.p.), tracheotomized, and artificially ventilated with a respirator pump. The right femoral vein was cannulated for administering supplementary doses of anesthetic and infusing dextrose-saline to replace lost body fluids; arterial cannulation was performed to monitor blood pressure. Core temperature was maintained at 37.5 C° by a servoregulated heating pad placed underneath the animal. The animal's head was secured in a stereotaxic frame, and the right somatosensory cortex was surgically exposed. A dam was constructed around the cranial opening with gauze soaked in 3% agar solution; the dam was filled with warm mineral oil to prevent drying of the cortex.

Standard electrophysiological techniques were used to map the digit and pad areas of each animal. Recordings were made of primary cortical evoked potentials elicited by mechanical and electrical stimulation of the skin. Mechanical stimuli were applied manually with nylon filament probes. Electrical pulses of sufficient intensity to produce a maximum response were delivered through needle electrodes inserted into the distal glabrous portion of each digit and the stump of digit 3. Stimuli were presented at a frequency of 1/second, and the cortical responses were averaged over 60 trials using a signal averaging computer. Evoked potentials were recorded from cortical sites representing each digit and pad, but were concentrated over the digit 3 representation. The amplitude distributions of the primary responses to stimulation of each digit tip were later reconstructed on drawings of the cortical surface made from enlarged photographs of the exposed cortex. After the evoked potential recordings were completed, microelectrodes were used to record from single neurons and small clusters of neurons within the cortical digit and pad areas. The receptive fields of these neurons were carefully mapped at both threshold and suprathreshold (15 gm) intensities by punctate mechanical stimulation of the paw using nylon filaments calibrated for force. At the end of the experiment, the animal was sacrificed and perfused intracardially with 0.9% saline followed by 10% formalin-saline. The brain with the upper cervical spinal cord intact was removed and stored in 10% formalin-saline for subsequent histological study.

Results

Inspection of the exposed cortex at the beginning of each experiment revealed no obvious differences in gyral or sulcal patterns between the brains of amputated and normal animals. As shown in Fig. 30.2, the usual configuration of the triradiate sulcus was intact, and no abnormal vasculature was observed. These initial observations were confirmed by later, more careful examination of the brains after perfusion and fixation. In normal animals, considerable individual variation exists in the pattern of short sulci or dimples extending from the triradiate sulcus; allowing for such normal variation, no changes in the surface features of the cortex were detected as a result of neonatal digit amputation. Detailed histological study of the brains of all animals is currently in progress.

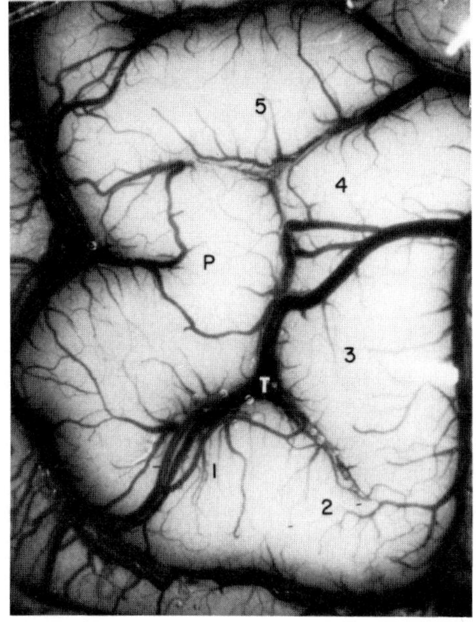

FIG. 30.2. Photograph of a por tion of the exposed right SmI corte: of an adult raccoon amputated at ‹ weeks of age. Major representation: of the digits (*1* to *5*) and pads (*P*) i relation to the triradiate sulcus (*T* are indicated.

Despite the absence of gross morphological changes, dramatic alterations were found in the functional organization of SmI forepaw cortex of amputated animals compared with normal animals, as described below. To determine whether such changes occur immediately after the injury, additional experiments were done on four animals (two adults and two neonates) which were studied just before and immediately after functional amputation by ligation of digit 3 at its base. Evoked potential data which are representative of the different groups of animals are shown in Fig. 30.3.

In normal animals, stimulation of each digit tip elicited a maximal primary evoked response over a small focal area within a different region (gyrus) adjacent to the triradiate sulcus (Fig. 30.3*A*). The response consisted of an initial surface-positive wave followed by a negative wave of longer duration; the mean latency of the positive peak of the responses to stimulation of the digit tips was 14.3 msec, averaged across all animals. This maximal response defines the cortical focus for any one digit tip; the amplitude of the responses obtained from that digit tip decreased gradually with distance from the focus. Although the focus for any one digit (or pad) was confined to a specific region, smaller responses to stimulation of that digit (or pad) could often be recorded near the focus for an adjacent digit (or pad). For example, stimulation of the digit 2 and 4 tips evoked large potentials near their respective foci, but also gave small off-focus responses near the digit 3 tip focus (Fig. 30.3*A*). The positive peak of the off-focus responses for all digits was more variable in latency than that of the on-focus responses, and occurred, on the average, 19.3 msec after the stimulus, about 5 msec later than that of the on-focus responses. Such off-focus responses revealed that some overlap exists among the digit and pad representations within normal cortex, certainly more than is implied by the schematic SmI cortical map of Fig. 30.1*B*.

The immediate effects of functional amputation by ligation of digit 3 are shown in Fig. 30.3*B*. No responses could be evoked by stimulation of digit 3 over its tip focus or at any other recording site. However, stimulation of adjacent digits 2 and 4 produced typical evoked potentials within their respective focal regions, and also gave small responses near the deafferented digit 3 tip focus. Again, these off-focus responses presumably reflected the overlap normally present within SmI tissue. Thus, functional amputation of digit 3 abolished cortical input from that digit, with no evidence of increased input or new inputs from adjacent digits or pads. No immediate functional reorganization seemed to occur, at least under the experimental conditions employed.

These findings contrast dramatically with the results obtained from animals studied 9 to 12 months after amputation as shown in Fig. 30.3*C*. The responses recorded from nondigit 3 areas (*e.g.*, near the foci for the digit 2 and 4 tips) were similar to those of normal animals. However, the

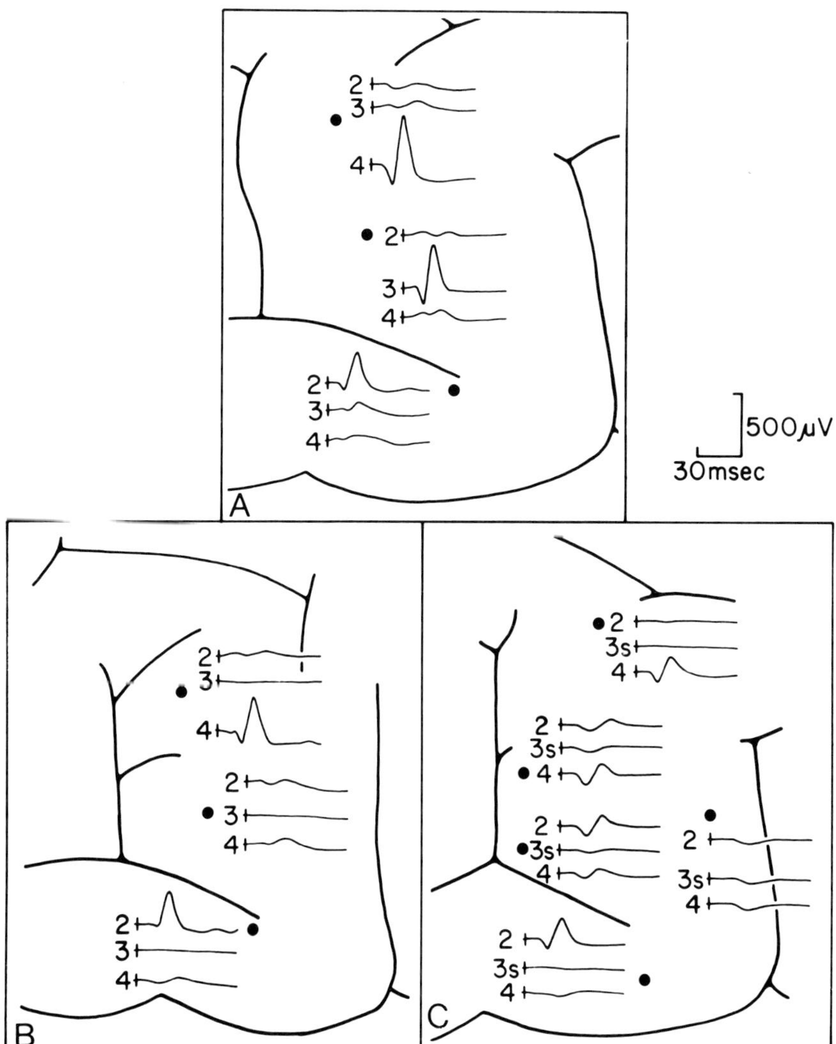

FIG. 30.3. Tracings of averaged primary cortical evoked responses recorded from a normal animal (*A*), an animal functionally amputated just prior to recording (*B*), and an animal amputated at 4 weeks of age (*C*). Cortical areas adjacent to the triradiate sulcus (see Fig. 30.2) are shown; recording sites are indicated by *solid circles*. Numbers beside each trace refer to digit tips (*2, 3, 4*) or digit 3 stump (*3s*) electrically stimulated. Positivity is down in all traces; time and voltage scales apply to *A*, *B*, and *C*.

deafferented digit 3 cortex showed a remarkable amount of functional reorganization; this tissue now gave responses in varying degrees to stimulation of all digits, pads, and the stump of digit 3. For example, stimulation of the digit 2 and 4 tips and the digit 3 stump all evoked some

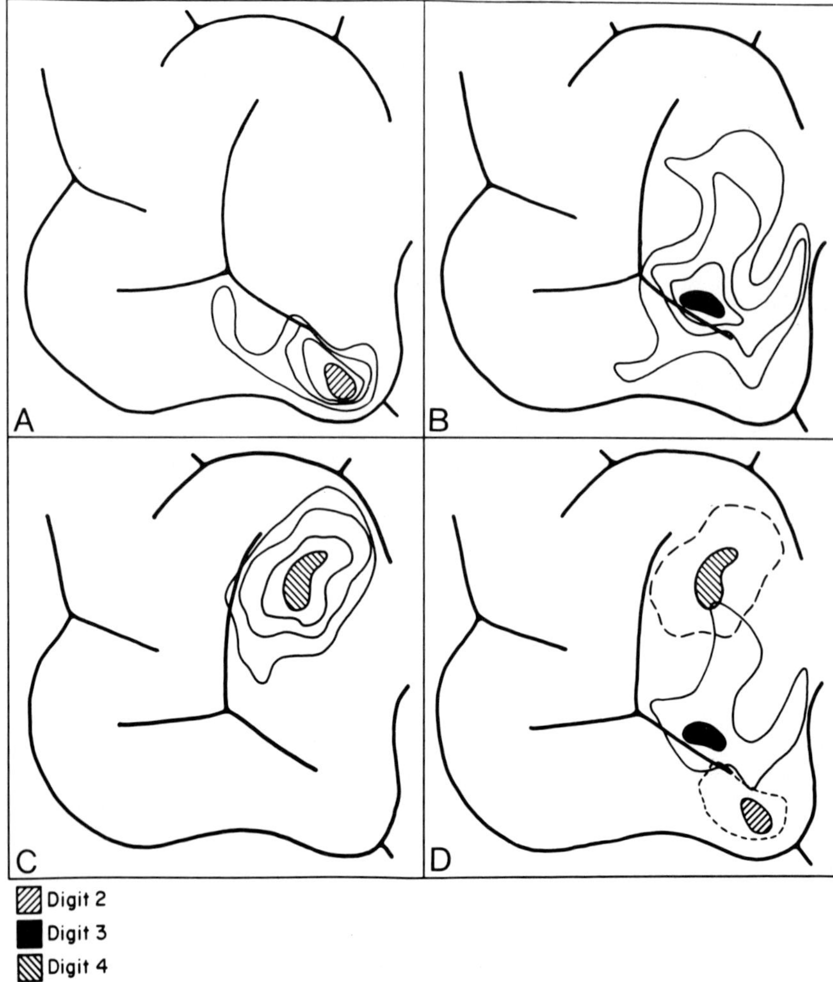

FIG. 30.4. Voltage contour maps based on primary evoked responses recorded from a normal animal. (*A* to *C*) Individual contour maps for digit tips 2 (*A*), 3 (*B*), and 4 (*C*). *Hatched* and *solid areas* represent focal sites giving response amplitudes ≥90% of maximum for a particular digit; surrounding contours enclose regions giving response amplitudes ≥ 70%, 50%, and 30% of maximum, respectively. (*D*) Composite voltage contour maps for digit tips 2, 3, and 4. *Hatched* and *solid* areas as above; surrounding contours enclose regions giving response amplitudes ≥50% of maximum. Code for different digits is given as *hatched* and *solid squares* at *lower left.*

response at each of the three recording sites within deafferented digit 3 cortex shown in Fig. 30.3*C*. In general, the off-focus digit responses within the deafferented region were considerably larger than off-focus responses obtained from normal tissue; yet, the mean latency of the positive peak of the off-focus digit responses was identical in deafferented cortex and in normal cortex (19.3 msec). The potentials evoked by stimulation of the digit 3 stump were relatively large, but smaller than the focal responses to stimulation of the intact digit 3 tip in normal animals. The positive peak of the stump response was quite variable in latency and occurred, on the average, 20.8 msec after the stimulus, a full 6.5 msec later than

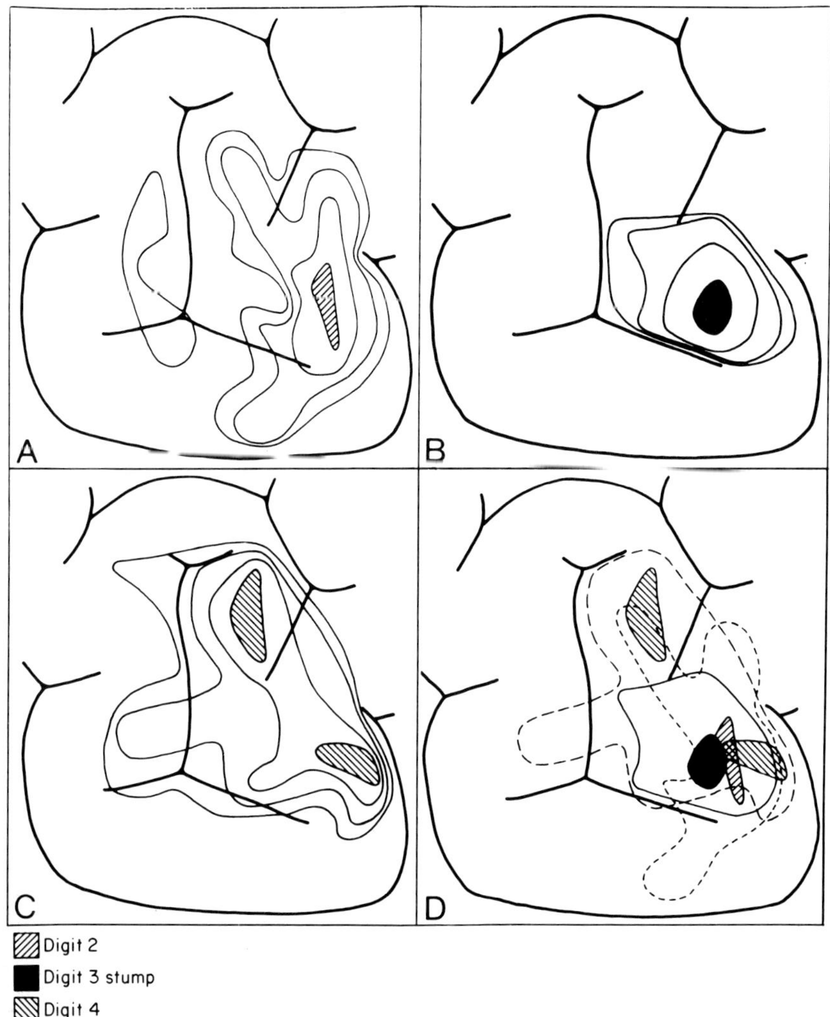

FIG. 30.5. Voltage contour maps based on primary evoked responses recorded from an animal amputated at 4 weeks of age. Contours in *A* to *D* as in Fig. 30.4*A* to *D*, except that contours with *solid areas* (*B*, *D*) are for the digit 3 stump. Code for digits and stump is given at *lower left*.

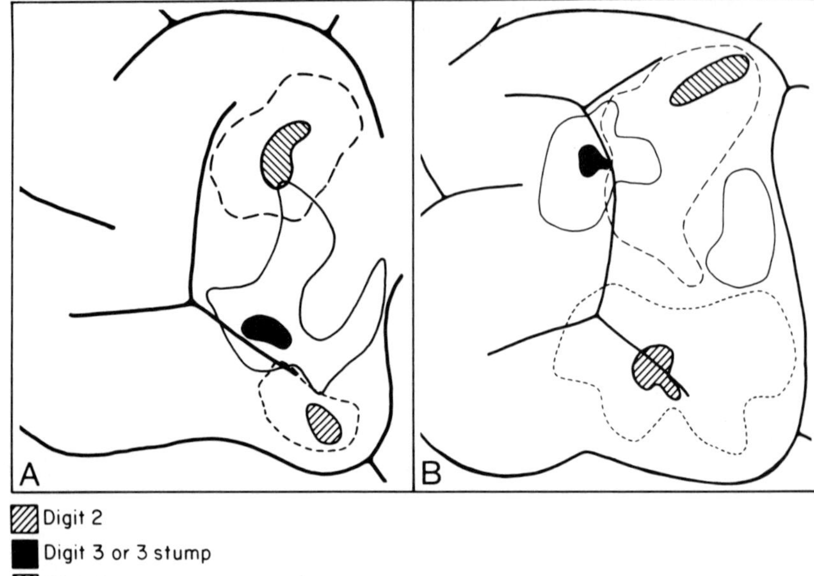

FIG. 30.6. Composite voltage contour maps based on primary evoked responses recorded from a normal animal (*A*) and animals amputated at 4 weeks (*B*), 6 weeks (*C, D*), and 8 weeks (*E, F*). Contours as in Figs. 30.4*D* and 30.5*D*. Code for digits and stump is given at *lower left* of *A*.

that of normal on-focus digit 3 potentials, but within the same range as that of normal off-focus responses ($\bar{X}$=19.3 msec). Thus, the responses within deafferented cortex to stimulation of the digit 3 stump behaved much like off-focus potentials, comparable in latency to the off-focus responses elicited by stimulation of the adjacent digits.

These evoked potential data show that, with time, the digit 3 cortex was "invaded" by widely overlapping inputs from most of the contralateral forepaw. To compare the amount of response overlap between normal and amputated animals, the amplitude distributions of the primary evoked potentials were plotted as voltage contour maps. The maps were constructed in the following manner: The maximum peak-to-peak focal potential for each digit tip or the digit 3 stump was arbitrarily given the value of 100; the amplitudes of all other responses for that same digit (or stump) were measured and scaled relative to this maximum. Voltage contour maps for each peripheral stimulus site were then constructed on drawings of the cortical surface by connecting isopotential points with lines representing voltage increments of 20%. The contour maps for digits 2, 3, and 4 of a normal animal are shown individually and as a composite in Fig. 30.4. As stated above, each digit representation had its own tip

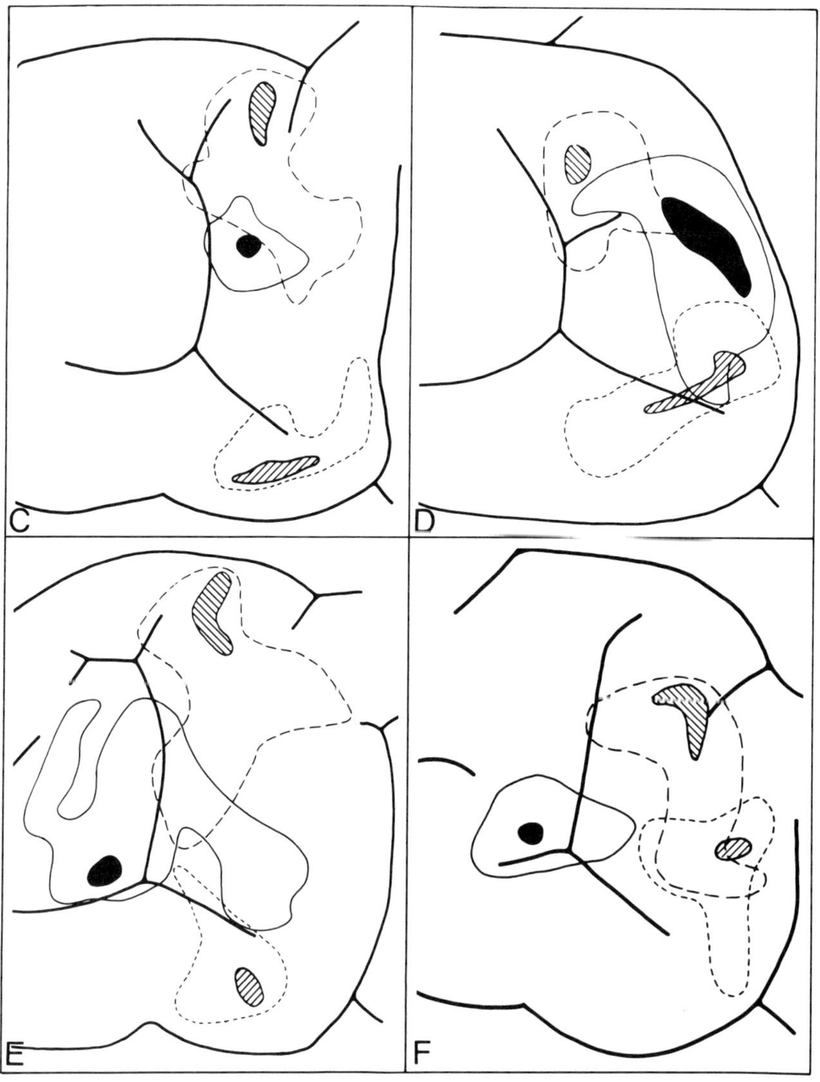

FIG. 30.6. (*C* to *F*)

focus (*hatched* and *solid areas*) which occupied a separate region or gyrus, but the entire representation was not confined to one region, nor segregated completely from adjacent digit tip areas. For example, responses as large as 50% of the maximum evoked by stimulation of the digit 3 tip were found across the anterolateral branch of the triradiate sulcus near the focus for the digit 2 tip. In general, the overlap of the digit tip areas was fairly extensive when measured at low voltages of the primary response; at higher voltages, *e.g.*, 50% of maximum, overlap was much less, in the range of 2 to 5%. It is clear that normal somatotopic organization within this tissue, as defined by the evoked potential technique, involves a focal representation for each digit (and pad) in a separate region with surrounding overlap.

For comparison, Fig. 30.5 shows individual and composite voltage contour maps for digits 2 and 4, and the digit 3 stump of an animal amputated at 4 weeks of age. As in normal animals, cortical foci were present for all intact digits; however, the digit 3 focus was replaced by a focal region responsive to stimulation of the digit 3 stump. The reorganization of digit 3 cortex found in this animal was typical with regard to considerable overlap of the stump and adjacent digit tip areas. A shift in the foci for the digit 2 and 4 tips toward, or at least partially into, the deafferented digit domain was also a common occurrence. However, the presence of two discrete regions of strong responsiveness to stimulation of the digit 4 tip was unusual; furthermore, the overlap of the stump focus with foci for *both* the digit 2 and 4 tips was not found in other animals. Thus, the contour maps of Fig. 30.5 illustrate an extreme case of overlapping reorganization. In general, the deafferented digit 3 cortex showed somewhat less overlap than illustrated here, but considerably more than in the normal cortex.

Examples of other contour maps showing overlapping digit and stump representations in the cortex of amputated animals are given in Fig. 30.6. These maps indicate that the overlap in the deafferented cortex was greater than normal at all voltages of the primary evoked responses. On the average, the overlap of the stump and digit tip areas at 50% of maximum was about 20% compared with 2 to 5% for digit tip areas in the normal cortex. The representation of the stump was found to be extremely variable in location and size; in some animals it involved most of the deafferented digit 3 region, and in others it shifted posteriorly into the palmar pad cortex. In any case, the maps make it clear that a focus was present for the digit 3 stump, and that there was greater than normal overlap of input to the deafferented digit 3 cortex.

The results of the evoked potential experiments thus indicate that the immediate effect of digit 3 amputation was to abolish digit 3 input to the cortex, with no obvious functional reorganization. The long-term effect of this amputation was the development of responsiveness to stimulation of extensive skin regions adjacent to the missing digit, with disruption of local somatotopic organization.

To examine the effects of amputation at the neuronal level, a comparison was made of the receptive fields of single neurons and clusters of neurons in normal and amputated animals. Representative receptive fields from these two groups of animals are shown in Fig. 30.7. At

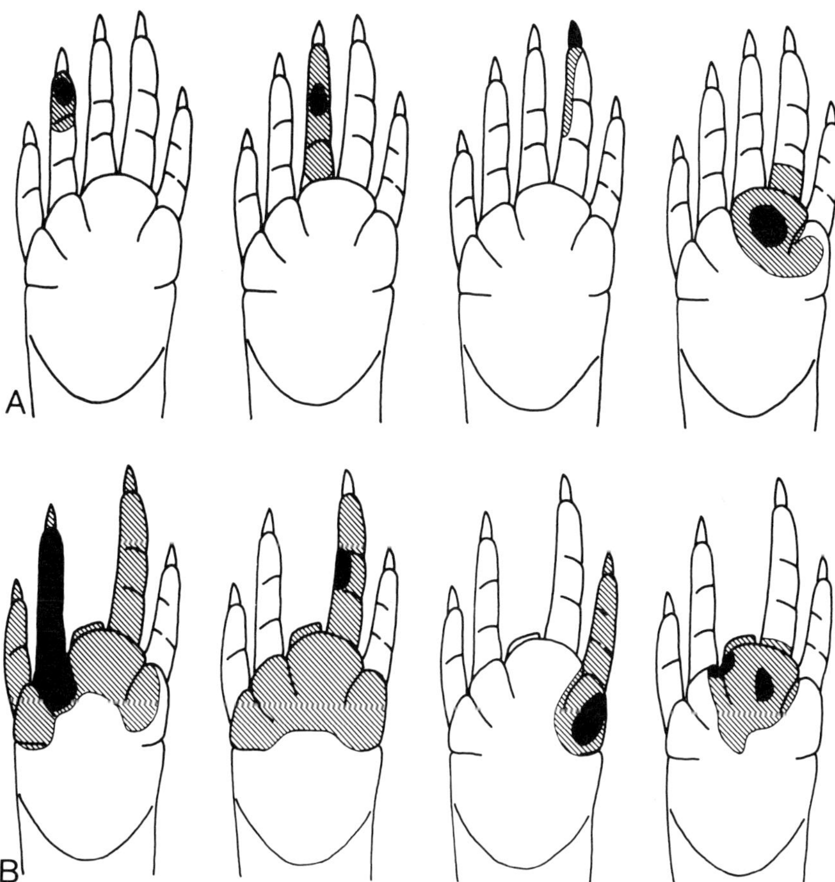

FIG. 30.7. Typical receptive fields of neurons within digit and pad cortex of normal (*A*) and digit 3 cortex only of amputated (*B*) animals. Fields mapped at threshold stimulus intensities are indicated by *solid areas*; fields mapped at the standard suprathreshold intensity (15 gm) are indicated by *hatched areas*.

threshold intensities of stimulation, the receptive fields of cells in normal cortex were typically small and confined to one contralateral claw, one palmar segment of a digit or to one pad (*solid areas*). Receptive fields mapped by suprathreshold stimulation (15 gm) are shown as *hatched areas* and were larger than the threshold fields, typically including the palmar surface of an entire digit and sometimes also involving an adjacent digit or pad. At all intensities of stimulation, the receptive fields of neurons in amputated animals tended to be larger than normal. Threshold fields often included continuous or discontinuous parts of digits 2 and 4 or an adjacent pad. With suprathreshold stimuli, field sizes were found to be even larger compared to normal. Suprathreshold fields often included two digits and adjacent pads, and sometimes included all four digits and the digit 3 stump or even the entire ventral paw. Suprathreshold fields also included the hairy dorsal surface of the paw considerably more often than in normal animals. Finally, there was greater variability in receptive field location both as a function of distance across the cortex and of depth within the cortex. A more detailed description of the receptive field data is presented elsewhere (5).

Summary and Conclusions

The results of these experiments demonstrate that early digit amputation had a profound effect on the subsequent functional organization of somatosensory cortex in adult raccoons, with no concomitant morphological changes in the surface features of the cerebral cortex. Cortical tissue normally representing the removed digit was "invaded" by widely overlapping inputs from adjacent intact skin regions, resulting in local disruption of normal somatotopy. In general, these findings are consistent with those of other studies of functional reorganization within SmI cortex following peripheral nerve or dorsal root lesions (2, 4, 9, 12, 15). The nontopographic reorganization which occurred in the raccoon was similar to that observed by Kalaska and Pomeranz (4) in cats after chronic paw denervation *without* peripheral nerve regeneration and in monkeys following peripheral nerve section but *with* subsequent regeneration (12, 15).

These findings differ from those of Merzenich *et al.* (9), who reported that, in monkeys, transection of the median nerve with prevention of regeneration was followed by a topographic functional reorganization; input from skin regions innervated by the ulnar and radial nerves progressively "invaded" the deafferented cortex in a somatotopic fashion. The reason for these differences is not entirely clear, given the variations among the animal species and experimental procedures involved. Dissection of the amputated raccoon paws after the present experiments revealed neuromas in the stump region with no evidence of extensive nerve regeneration; however, some reinnervation of tissue adjacent to the stump cannot be ruled out.

In any case, the new and strengthened inputs to the deafferented digit 3 cortex of the raccoon resulted in widely overlapping representations of both ventral and dorsal aspects of all remaining digits, palmar pads, and the stump. This increased overlap, as revealed by the evoked potential method, may be due to the observed increase in the sizes and/or topographic scatter of neuronal receptive fields. The finding in this study of unusual receptive field characteristics, such as discontinuous or multiple fields, exceptionally large fields, and topographically scattered fields has also been reported by others (2, 4, 12, 15).

The cortical reorganization observed in the raccoon did not occur immediately following amputation but required some, as yet undetermined, period of time to develop. Immediate switching of receptive field locations has been demonstrated in SmI cortex of cats during reversible epidural dorsal root blocks (10) and in monkeys following median nerve transection (9). The absence of such immediate changes in the present study may have been due to the type of anesthesia used or differences in the method of cortical deafferentation, or may reflect true species differences.

The functional reorganization found in the raccoon cortex has significant implications with regard to sensory phenomena associated with limb amputation and also congenital aplasia in man (14, 16). The entire cortical region normally containing the digit 3 focus became increasingly responsive to inputs from the digit 3 stump and adjacent forepaw tissue. The enhanced responsiveness reflects a magnification of the cortical representation of tissue in the stump region, which may be equivalent to a functional increase in "cortical innervation density;" this may account, at least in part, for stump hypersensitivity and better tactile discrimination on the stump than on corresponding regions of the opposite limb. This idea is consistent with the proposal made by Weinstein *et al.* (16) that enhanced sensitivity of the stump "derives from greater 'availability' of cortex." The representation within deafferented cortex of large regions of the forepaw in an overlapping nontopographic fashion may partially explain the phenomenon of false localization, such as referral of somatic stimuli to a phantom limb. However, the observed disorganization suggests that preservation of local somatotopy within SmI cortex may not be required for the subjective experience of a phantom limb.

The mechanisms underlying the functional reorganization of cortical tissue after amputation are presently unknown; both anatomical and functional changes may be involved. Possible mechanisms include some peripheral nerve sprouting and reinnervation, "unmasking" or disinhibition of normally latent neural connections, progressive strengthening of inputs via such latent pathways, and the development of new central connections (8). The fact that the responses within deafferented cortex to all inputs had mean latencies similar to those of off-focus responses within normal cortex suggests that strengthening of normal off-focus connections are involved in the functional reorganization revealed by this study.

ACKNOWLEDGMENTS

We wish to express our deep appreciation to George Holloman for his strong support of this project by providing a source for neonatal raccoons, caring for the animals during portions of this study, and for his illuminating raccoon stories. We also thank Brian Wilson for his technical assistance and photography, and Stephanie Doetsch for preparing the illustrations.

REFERENCES

1. Dostrovsky, J. O., Millar, J., and Wall, P. D. The immediate shift of afferent drive of dorsal column nucleus cells following deafferentation: a comparison of acute and chronic deafferentation in gracile nucleus and spinal cord. Exp. Neurol., *52:* 480–495, 1976.
2. Franck, J. I. Functional reorganization of cat somatic sensory-motor cortex (SmI) after selective dorsal root rhizotomies. Brain Res., *186:* 458–462, 1980.
3. Guillaume, MM. J., Bertrand, I., and Mazars, G. Un cas de moignon douloureux traite par myelotomie. Etude electroencephalographique et considerations physiopathologiques sur la douleur. Rev. Neurol., *77:* 145, 1945.
4. Kalaska, J., and Pomeranz, B. Chronic paw denervation causes an age-dependent appearance of novel responses from forearm in "paw cortex" of kittens and adult cats. J. Neurophysiol., *42:* 618–633, 1979.
5. Kelahan, A. M., Ray, R. H., Carson, L. V., Massey, C. E., and Doetsch, G. S. Functional reorganization of adult raccoon somatosensory cerebral cortex following neonatal digit amputation, submitted for publication.
6. Killackey, H. P., Ivy, G. O., and Cunningham, T. J. Anomalous organization of SMI somatotopic map consequent to vibrissae removal in the newborn rat. Brain Res., *155:* 136–140, 1978.
7. McComas, A. J., Sica, R. E. P., and Banerjee, S. Long-term effects of partial limb amputation in man. J. Neurol. Neurosurg. Psychiatry, *41:* 425–432, 1978.
8. Merrill, E. G., and Wall, P. D. Plasticity of connection in the adult nervous system. In Neuronal Plasticity, edited by C. W. Cotman, pp. 97–111. Raven Press, New York, 1978.
9. Merzenich, M. M., Kaas, J. H., Nelson, R. J., Wall, J., Sur, M., and Felleman, D. J. Progressive topographic reorganization of representations of the hand within areas 3b and 1 of monkeys following median nerve section. Soc. Neurosci. Abstr., *6:* 651, 1980.
10. Metzler, J., and Marks, P. S. Functional changes in cat somatic sensory-motor cortex during short-term reversible epidural blocks. Brain Res., *177:* 379–383, 1979.
11. Millar, J., Basbaum, A. I., and Wall, P. D. Restructuring of the somatotopic map and appearance of abnormal neuronal activity in the gracile nucleus after partial deafferentation. Exp. Neurol., *50:* 658–672, 1976.
12. Paul, R. L., Goodman, H., and Merzenich, M. M. Alterations in mechanoreceptor input to Brodmann's areas 1 and 3 of the postcentral hand area of *Macaca mulatta* after nerve section and regeneration. Brain Res., *39:* 1–19, 1972.
13. Pidoux, B., Diebler, M. F., Savy, Cl., Farkas, E., and Verley, R. Cortical organization of the postero-medial barrel-subfield in mice and its reorganization after destruction of vibrissal follicles after birth. Neuropathol. Appl. Neurobiol., *6:* 93–107, 1980.
14. Sunderland, S. Nerves and Nerve Injuries. Churchill Livingstone, Edinburgh, 1972.
15. Wall, J. T., Merzenich, M. M., Sur, M., Nelson, R. J., Felleman, D. J., and Kaas, J. H. Organization of the representations of the hand in areas 3b and 1 of postcentral somatosensory cortex of monkeys after section and regeneration of the median nerve. Soc. Neurosci. Abstr. *6:* 651, 1980.
16. Weinstein, S., Sersen, E. A., and Vetter, R. J. Phantoms and somatic sensation in cases of congenital aplasia. Cortex, *1:* 276–290, 1964–1965.
17. Welker, W. I., Johnson, J. I., Jr., and Pubols, B. H., Jr. Some morphological and physiological characteristics of the somatic sensory system in raccoons. Am. Zool., *4:* 75–94, 1964.
18. Welker, W. I., and Seidenstein, S. Somatic sensory representation in the cerebral cortex of the raccoon (Procyon lotor). J. Comp. Neurol., *111:* 469–501, 1959.

CHAPTER

31

Techniques of Intracranial Pressure Monitoring

MARC A. FLITTER, M.D.

INTRODUCTION

As our understanding of the relationship of intracranial pressure or ICP to specific disease states has grown, the efforts to develop techniques of intracranial pressure monitoring have continued. The individual practitioner who has made a decision to add ICP monitoring to his clinical management armamentarium may be uncertain as to the type of ICP device and monitoring techniques to utilize. In order for this uncertainty to be diffused, it is necessary to understand the basic functioning characteristics of ICP monitoring devices and their capacity to provide the type of ICP information desired. Data display alternatives, such as trend graph recordings, digital printouts, histogram constructions, or calculation of the standard deviation of the ICP pulse wave place requirements and restrictions in selecting the technique most appropriate to ICP monitoring in a particular patient.

The most fundamental clinical aspect differentiating techniques of ICP monitoring is whether or not the intracranial portion of the device system is fully implantable or requires a percutaneous lead. The implications to nursing care of the patient, risk of infection, and length of monitoring are obvious. As will be seen however, device accuracy, data display, and location of the intracranial portion of the device remain separate factors unrelated to whether the device is fully implantable or provided with a percutaneous lead.

Percutaneous Devices

Table 31.1 lists the major classification categories of percutaneous devices and examples of each.

A. PERCUTANEOUS HYDROSTATIC DEVICES

These devices have an intracranial component that transmits pressure to a remote physiologic transducer via a fluid-filled column. The pioneering effort of Lundberg (25) on continuous intraventricular pressure recording and control of ventricular fluid pressure in neurosurgical practice

TABLE 31.1
Percutaneous Devices

- A. Percutaneous hydrostatic
    1. Ventricular catheter
    2. Subdural cup catheter
    3. Subarachnoid bolt
    4. Epidural stopcock
    5. Implanted reservoir with ventricular catheter
- B. Percutaneous pneumatic
    1. Numoto switch
    2. Ladd fiberoptic monitoring device
- C. Implanted transducers with electrical leads
    1. Philips transducer

not only introduced the possibility of long-term ICP monitoring by this technique, but continues to serve as a standard against which other devices can be compared. Other percutaneous hydrostatic devices employ a cup catheter in the subdural space (41), a hollow bolt threaded into the skull with its tip opening into the subdural space (37), or a stopcock opening into the epidural space (21). All these devices require pressure-tight connections and high pressure tubing between the intracranial portion of the device and the remote transducer and display or recording module. Those systems employing an intraventricular catheter do provide the additional therapeutic option of cerebral spinal fluid drainage from the ventricle for the control of elevated intracranial pressure. Wright and Young (42) have described an ICP pressure regulator (Baxter Travenol Laboratory, Inc., Deerfield, Ill.) accomplishing this automatically as intraventricular pressure (IVP) reaches a predetermined level. A ventricular catheter specifically designed for use in ICP monitoring systems (Cordis Corporation, Miami, Fla.) has also been reported (13). It is possible to monitor ICP by tapping an implanted reservoir and ventricular cannula with a 23-gauge needle attached to high pressure tubing and a remote transducer (40). The risk of ventriculitis and the difficulty of placing a catheter in what may be called a collapsed ventricle are obvious factors which may mitigate against using the specific intraventricular catheter technique in certain clinical conditions. The Wilkinson cup catheter (Cordis Corporation, Miami, Fla.) is placed in the subdural space and is ribbon-shaped (3 × 8 mm) with a central lumen and a distal indented cup facing the brain (Fig. 31.1). It is made of barium-impregnated silatic rubber and is designed to permit use in postcraniotomy patients. When placed over an area of undisturbed pia arachnoid a short distance under the bony edge, the cup serves to seal the fluid column against the biological membrane directly beneath and helps to prevent catheter blockage. Additionally, if the catheter has been placed through a separate stab wound remote to the craniotomy incision, it can be withdrawn through this subcutaneous tunnel at the bedside without any additional surgery. The subcutaneous tunnel also serves as a barrier against intracranial sepsis and CSF leak. The need for q 2 hr fluid installation of sterile Ringer's solution with bacitracin (0.1 to .25 ml) to compensate for fluid leakage is of concern for reasons of infection, although preliminary reports suggest no increased risk of infection utilizing the device (41).

The cranial bolt described by Vries (Richmond Screw, Codman Corporation, Randolph, Mass.) permits rigid fixation to the skull by means of the threaded distal end of the device which engages in a ¼ inch twist drill hole (Fig. 31.2) (36). The proximal end consists of a standard Luer lock and hexagonal collar that allows the device to be threaded into the skull using a hexagonal screwdriver (37). The bolt is inserted after the dura has been opened. The lumen of the bolt is in communication with the subdural space. A saline-filled high pressure tubing then connects the bolt to a remote physiologic transducer. A bolt of similar design has been described with the lumen opening into the epidural space (6).

The remote transducers utilized in percutaneous hydrostatic devices are easily handled by nursing personnel familiar with monitoring peripheral arterial and pulmonary artery pressure. The devices are dependent upon water-tight connections for their accurate function. The presence

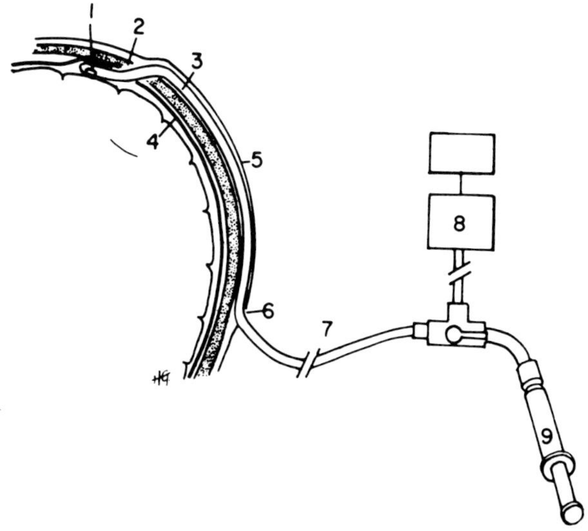

FIG. 31.1. Diagrammatic representation of the ICP-monitoring cup catherter in use: (*1*) sensing cup; (*2*) burr hole with beveled edges; (*3*) catheter in subcutaneous tunnel; (*4*) dura; (*5*) skin; (*6*) exit stab wound; (*7*) catheter tubing; (*8*) transducer and recorder; (*9*) syringe. (From H. A. Wilkinson (41). Published with pemission.)

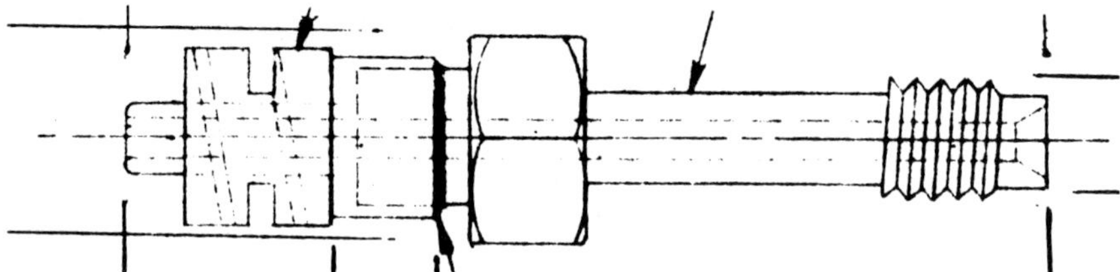

FIG. 31.2. Richmond subarachnoid screw. Note the threaded end of the device which screws into the previously placed ¼-inch twist drill hole. The accurate functioning of the device is dependent upon pressure-tight connections. (Courtesy of Codman and Shurtleff, Inc., Randolph, Mass.)

of microleaks may invalidate the pressure readings, and each portion of the system must be tested periodically during patient use in order to rule out a gradual and progressive loss or diminution of pressure recording. Dampening of the ICP pulse waves as visualized on a strip recorder is a manifestation of the partial occlusion of the bolt lumen by tissue or of air within the system and requires either removal of the air or a small fluid flush of sterile saline through the bolt to reestablish unattenuated pressure transmission. While the safety and clinical significance of changes in intracranial pressure following the addition of small measured amounts of sterile saline injected intracranially or via LP remain controversial, percutaneous hydrostatic devices easily permit such manipulations for determinations of cerebral elastance and compliance.

B. PERCUTANEOUS PNEUMATIC DEVICES

A second type of percutaneous device also utilizes a remote pressure transducer; however, it transduces a pneumatic rather than hydrostatic pressure in the cable linking the intracranial sensor to the external portion of the device (29). The Ladd intracranial pressure monitor (Roche Medical Electronics, Inc., Cranbury, N.J. 08512) generates a pneumatic pressure by an air bellows controlled by an electrooptical servo mechanism (Fig. 31.3) (23, 24). This servo mechanism is activated when a mirror contained within the intracranial sensor is deflected as a result of ICP and reflects light along fiberoptic bundles to a photoelectric cell controlling the air bellows. The pneumatic pressure generated by the air bellows then serves to reset the mirror to a point where the photoelectric cell is no longer activated by the change in reflected light. At this point the transduced pneumatic pressure is equal to the intracranial pressure. The mirror sensing element, 1 cm in diameter, is placed in the epidural space, although it has been used subdurally as well (Fig. 31.4). When utilized epidurally, a surrounding portion of dura must be freed from the inner table of the skull to prevent a so-called "wedge" effect producing artifactually high values of ICP. This device has also been utilized to detect

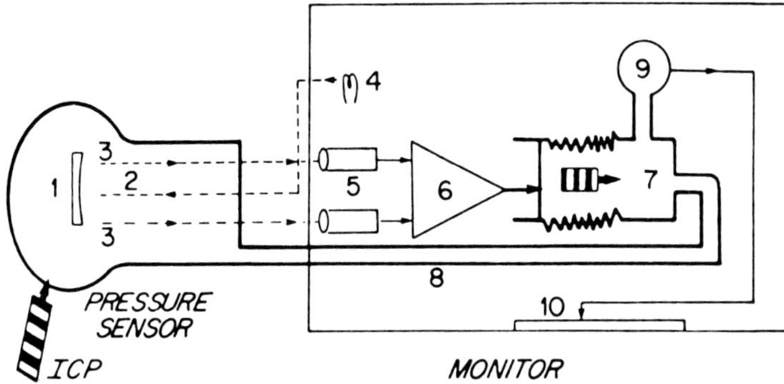

FIG. 31.3. Schematic diagram showing principle of operation of fiberoptic intracranial pressure sensor with monitor-control unit. (From A. Wald *et al.* (38). Published with permission.)

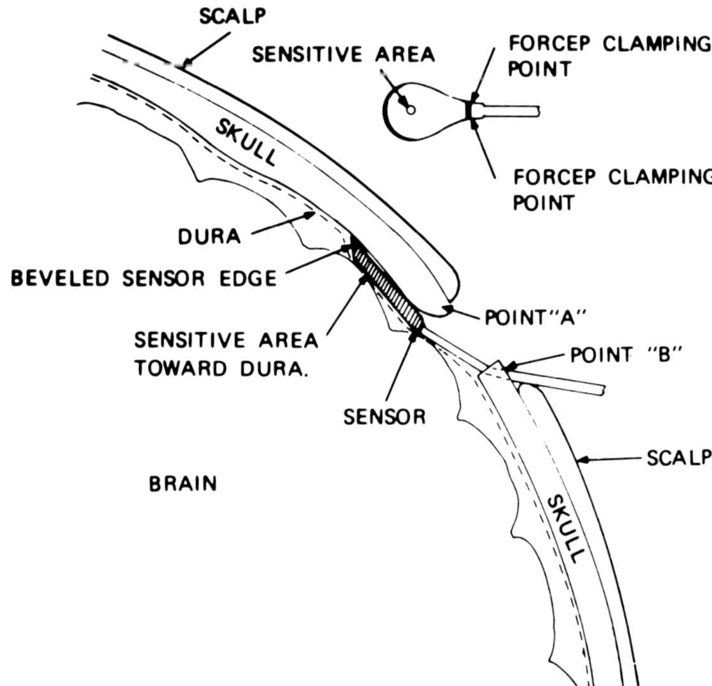

FIG. 31.4. Diagram demonstrating the epidural positioning of fiberoptic sensor of the percutaneous pneumatic device. (From A. B. Levin (24). Published with permission.)

intracranial pressure in the newborn with application of a sensor to the anterior fontanel (35). Clinical studies have demonstrated a correlation of 0.95 between ICP measured in this fashion and intraventricular or cisternal simultaneous pressure measurements. Rate of response of this system is 2.5 mm Hg/second.

C. IMPLANTED TRANSDUCERS WITH PERCUTANEOUS ELECTRICAL LEADS

The last group of percutaneous devices to be considered include those ICP device systems that place physiologic transducers directly into the intracranial compartment and utilize a percutaneous electrical lead to convey the output of the transducer to external amplifiers and display modules (3, 7, 8, 11, 12, 14, 18, 20, 22, 33, 34, 43, 44).

The placement of the transducers intracranially changes the technical requirements of the ICP monitoring device. *In vivo* zero calibration either cannot be accomplished or constitutes a major design characteristic of the transducer. Concern for zero or baseline drift (a change of output with no change in input) in sensitivity drift (a change in incremental output for a standard change in input) also become significant factors. One solution to *in vivo* calibration has been to surround the transducer with an inflatable balloon that could be inflated to atmospheric pressure at times of recalibration (14). Other devices have provided venting tubes as components of the percutaneous leads which permit equilibration between the outside atmosphere and the sensing chamber of the transducer (33). Alternatives to such *in vivo* calibrations have required efforts to design transducers to minimize factors contributing to zero and sensitivity drift, specifically thermal characteristics (drift associated with temperature change), hysteresis (discrepancy of output associated with approaching a particular value from different directions secondary to mechanical deformations of the transducing membrane), and those aspects of transducer construction associated with time-dependent stability. Although many prototype models of devices in this category have been reported, the Philips transducer (Philips Medical Systems, Inc., Shelton, Conn.) has had the most widespread clinical exposure (3, 22). This transducer has a ring-shaped sensing membrane fabricated with integrated circuit techniques in a slice of monocrystalline silicone. Strain gauge resistors and a wheatstone bridge configuration are integrated within the membrane structure. The sensing membrane is mounted on a stainless steel housing which fits into a stainless steel adapter 11 mm in width which initially and independently is placed in the burr hole with a special mounting tool (Fig. 31.5). Silicone rubber rings attached to the adapters assure a water-tight fit into the burr hole and are adjustable so that the adapter fits flush with the inner surface of the skull. After

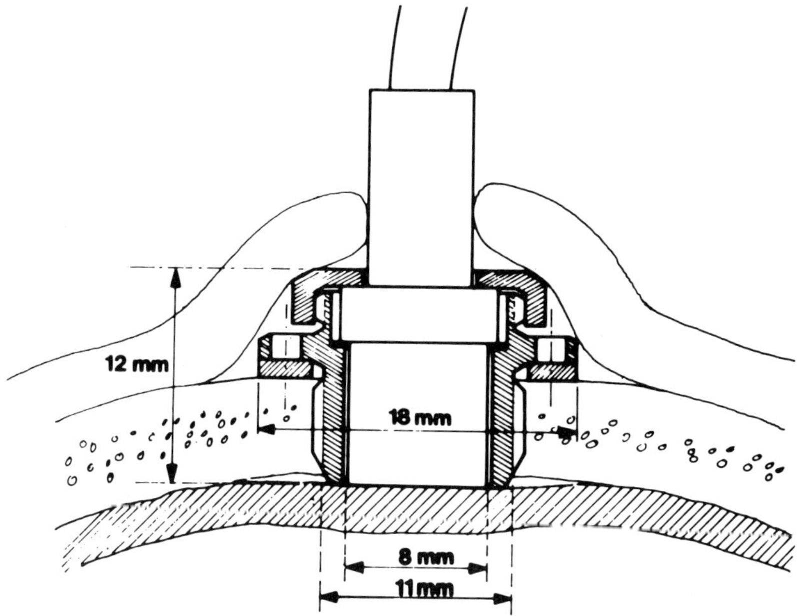

FIG. 31.5. A schematic design depicts the way the epidural transducer is placed. The adapter screw is introduced into the skull so that its ring stretches the dura mater. The transducer and a Teflon sealing ring are then introduced and fixed to the adapter screw. The transducer is dimensioned so that its sensitive part is flush with the ring of the adapter screw. (From W. G. Koster and M. H. Kuypers (22). Published with permission.)

insertion, the transducer is sealed in the adapter by means of a Teflon ring and an adjustable locking nut. The percutaneous polyurethane tube contains four Teflon-insulated leads and two thin teflon tubes which plug into the transducer to connect it with the remote pressure amplifiers. The transducer is able to refer intracranial pressure to atmospheric pressure by connecting the internal surface of the sensing membrane to atmospheric pressure by one of the two Teflon tubes contained within the cable. Accordingly, the transducer is not affected by alterations in atmospheric pressure. The sensitivity of the device is reported as −300 to +300 mm Hg, a sensitivity drift of less than 2.5% at 300 mm Hg per degree centigrade and a zero drift of less than 0.25% at 300 mm Hg per degree centigrade. Design of this transducer reflects the advances made by other workers, particularly in the field of detecting ICP from the epidural space. The device design reflects the principle that intracavitary pressure can be accurately measured through a surrounding biological membrane only if the stretching forces of that membrane itself have been absorbed (26). Accordingly, epidural transducer design construction has evolved to include an outer insensitive ring that surrounds the pressure-sensing membrane in current devices. This ring assures coplanarity of the sensing membrane of the transducer to the slack dura within the ring. Rigid fixation of the device is also required in order to maintain the coplanar approximation of the sensing membrane to the underlying dura.

Fully Implantable ICP Monitoring Devices

Table 31.2 lists the classification categories of fully implantable devices and examples of each.

ISOTOPE EMITTER

The Hittman-Meyer Intracranial Pressure Sensor (Hittman Corporation, Columbia, Md.) determines intracranial pressure with the aid of a radiation detector consisting of a sodium iodide-sensing crystal contained within a photomultiplier tube and connected to a scintillation counter. The intracranial portion of the device consists of both a subdural and a subgaleal sensing tambour in which the differential pressures (subdural ICP vs. subgaleal atmospheric) are transmitted to a fluid bathing a piston to which an isotope source, ^{145}Pm (38 kev, half-life 19 years), is attached (Fig. 31.6) (5, 27). Alteration of intracranial pressure results in a change of radiation emanating through a fixed collimator. This device is calibrated by manual compression of the subgaleal tambour which results in the least amount of radiation exposure and count. Since the subgaleal tambour is subject to increased pressure in the presence of tissue edema which could contribute to an error in the calculation of ICP and because such edema in the postoperative period makes the tambour difficult to palpate manually, the device is not suitable for acute ICP monitoring. A response time of 7 seconds limits the ability of this device to provide information about CSF dynamic pulse waves of shorter duration (28). Continuous ICP monitoring for the detection of Lundberg waves or other trends in ICP would also appear to be not readily accomplished. The

TABLE 31.2
Fully Implantable Devices

A. Isotope source
   1. Hittman-Meyer
B. Variable oscillator
   1. Battery powered
   2. Induction powered
C. Passive resonant devices
   1. Variable inductance
   2. Variable capacitance
   3. Differential pressure with balance meter

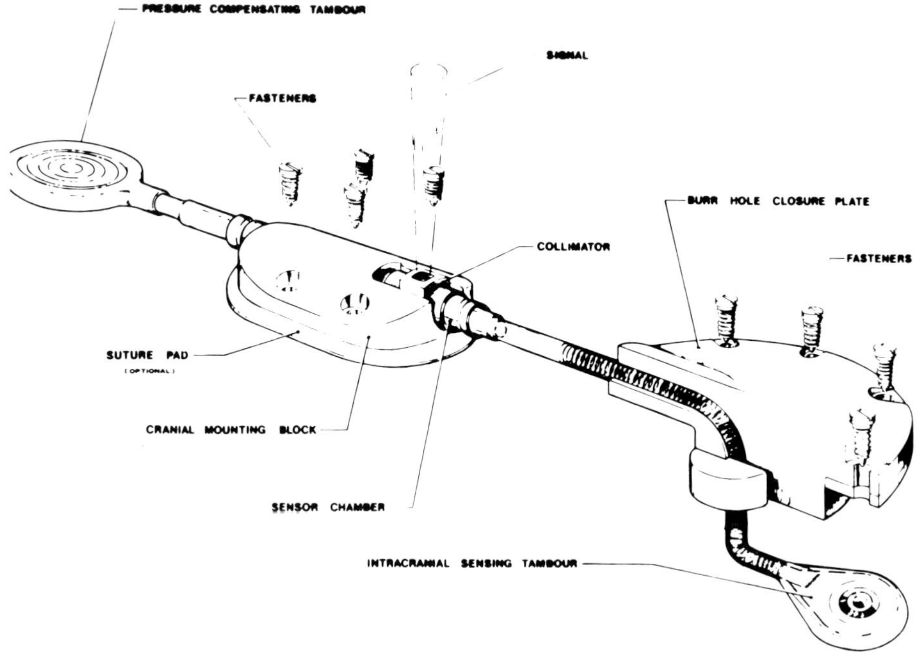

FIG. 31.6. The Hittman-Meyer intracranial pressure sensor (Hittman Corp., Columbia, Md.). The pressure-compensating tambour is subject to atmospheric pressure in the subgaleal space which provides a differential pressure to the intracranial sensing tambour located in the subdural space. (From P. R. Cooper *et al.* (9). Published with permission.)

device has been utilized in a group of patients with pseudotumor cerebri over a period of 14 months and has yielded information about the ICP in each patient that aided in their management (9).

VARIABLE OSCILLATOR DEVICES

Several devices have been devised that transmit radio waves from the fully implantable transducer that are detectable in the FM band and that can be demodulated to determine ICP (2, 4, 19, 31, 32, 39). Brock and Diefenthäler (4) have reported on such a device that utilizes a 4 volt disc mercury battery to energize the implanted transducer and transmitter, with signal detection possible up to 2 to 3 m. The implantable transmitter fits into a 16-mm burr hole and is fixed to the skull with two bolt screws. A high frequency oscillator emits signals at about 240 MHz in response to changes exerted on a capacitance sensor (copper beryllium membrane coated with silastic) in the epidural space. Although the device is fully implantable, a polyethylene tube connecting the sensor chamber with external atmospheric pressure is passed through the scalp to allow for quantitative measurements of ICP in reference to atmospheric pressure. This tube can also be used to perform a zero-point calibration by connecting it by means of a Y tube to a syringe and a mercury manometer. Negative pressure on the syringe causes the pressure sensor of the implanted portion of the device to short circuit. Since it is known that this "collapsing pressure" is 150 mm Hg, if the addition of the measured epidural pressure and the negative pressure measured in the syringe necessary to achieve a short-circuit exceeds 150 mm Hg, zero calibration is corrected by the mm Hg greater than 150. The device is suitable for detecting dynamic changes in ICP pulse waves as well as continuous monitoring to detect ICP trends and plateau waves. Overall precision of the device is reported to be ± 3 mm Hg over a scale of −10 to 100 mm Hg.

Watson has reported a similar battery-powered device that alters FM frequency and differs from the first transducer described in this category in that it responds to increased ICP by variable inductance as a result of pressures sensed by the transducing membrane rather than varied capacitance to produce changes in the oscillator frequency (39). The Watson device requires 24 hours in the active state to achieve stability characteristics for calibration prior to implantation. Zero drift can be corrected only in retrospect after removal of the device and reexposure to atmospheric pressure. The zero drift of the device has been reported to vary between ± 3 to 0.4 mm Hg per day.

The second category of fully implantable variable oscillator devices utilizes external radio frequency waves transmitted through the scalp to energize their implanted transmitters, thus obviating the need for an implanted battery source (2, 31, 32). Ream *et al.* (31) have reported on a capacitive pressure transducer energized at 420 kHz and radiating an FM signal at 10 MHz. They have constructed within their readout module that demodulates the FM signal to indicate ICP, compensations for both barometric pressure (by virtue of a matched transducer detecting atmospheric pressure at the bedside) and patient temperature (a thermistor included with the unit). Their transducer reflects the design modification that evolved with development of the implanted transducers with percutaneous leads, such as utilization of a guard ring to ensure dural coplanarity and to prevent edge loading, rigid fixation of the device to the skull, and utilization of a relatively large sensing surface to average out the effects of less than ideal smoothness and uniform thickness of the dura (Fig. 31.7). They report an average error of ± 3 mm Hg. A zero drift of ±0.1 mm Hg per day ± 2 mm Hg has proved suitable for studies up to 2 weeks, although linear compensation for extrapolated drift is required for chronic *in vivo* studies. The device does require a radio frequency

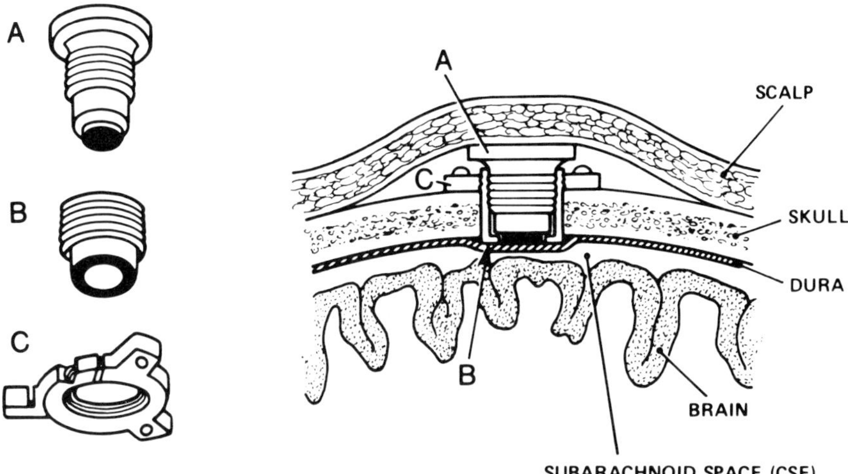

FIG. 31.7. The fully implantable capacitive pressure transducer of Ream and Silverberg. (*A*) pressure transducer and telemetry packages; (*B*) guard ring; (*C*) flanged bracket. The surfaces contacting the dura are blackened in diagram. (From G. Silverberg. Intracranial Pressure IV. Springer-Verlag, New York, 1980. Published with permission.)

antenna positioned on the scalp overlying the transducer for purposes of energizing the implanted portion of the system. The readout module may be several meters distant from the patient. This device is suitable for detecting dynamic CSF pulse waves and for continuous monitoring.

Rylander *et al.* (32) also defined a fully implantable system radiating FM waves and energized by an external RF source. His device differs from the Ream and Silverberg device in that a hermetically sealed air bellows serves as a transducer with compression of the bellows, producing a change of inductance of a resonant LC circuit to alter the frequency of the oscillator (Fig. 31.8). This allows for a greater baseline drift based on the stress factors associated with the bellows construction as opposed to the capacitive transducer of Ream and Silverberg which involves minimal physical movement of the sensing membrane. The Rylander device utilizes the same coil antenna to both energize the implant as well as detect the transmitted radio waves.

PASSIVE RESONANT DEVICES

An alternative technique for fully implantable devices that also precludes the need for an implanted battery with a limited life span is one in which the frequency of absorbed externally applied radio frequency electromagnetic energy can be detected and converted to a value representing intracranial pressure based on previous calibration data (1, 10,

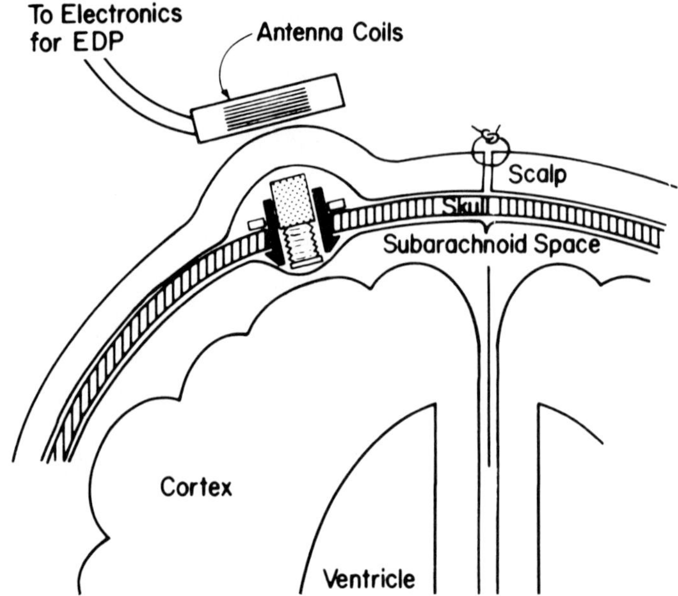

FIG. 31.8. Induction-powdered oscillator transducer. The antenna coils utilized in the Rylander device serve to energize the transducer via radio frequency waves and detect the radiated FM waves from the implanted device. (From H. G. Rylander *et al.* (32). Published with permission.)

17, 30). These devices utilize resonant LC inductance capacitor circuit transducers with pressure applied to the sensing membrane producing an alteration of the resonant frequency of the transducer. When the transducer is interrogated by an external source of radio frequency electromagnetic energy the frequency at which waves are absorbed by the transducer is directly proportional to the intracranial pressure. Gücer reported the use of such a device in 38 patients (Fig. 31.9) (17). Calibration errors in some of his devices detected after implantation, and a zero drift of 1 mm of water per day necessitated occasional lumbar punctures for required corrections. Continuous recordings were obtained displaying cerebral spinal fluid pulse wave changes, although specific values for intracranial pressure required the use of conversion charts by the intensive care unit nurses.

Atkinson described a similar technique using an implanted transducer of this design attached to a ventricular catheter (Fig. 31.10) (1). The variation of this passive resonant detection technique uses a feature of the Hittman-Meyer differential pressure apparatus. The device described by Zervas is a pressure balanced radiotelemetry system (Radionics, Inc., Burlington, Mass.) with two flexible diaphragms, one facing the subgaleal

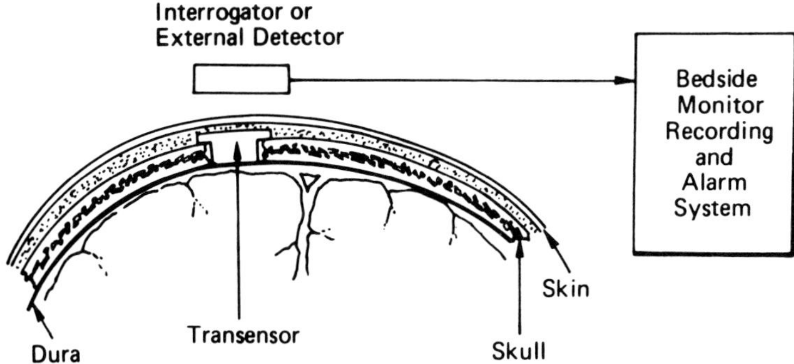

FIG. 31.9. The passive transensor absorbs electromagnetic energy at a resonant frequency determined by the ICP acting on the sensing membrane. (From G. Gücer and L. Viernstein (16). Published with permission.)

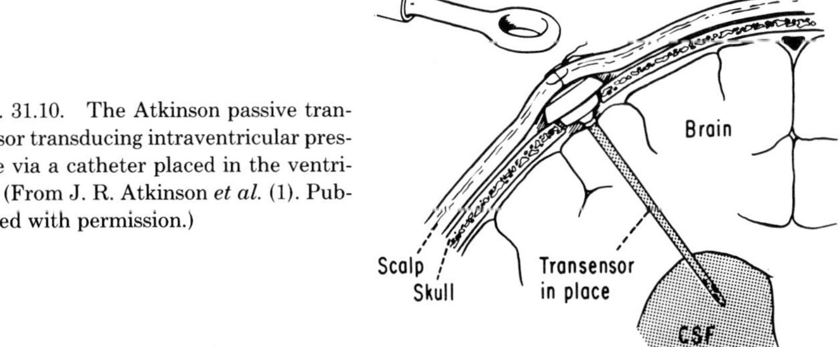

FIG. 31.10. The Atkinson passive transensor transducing intraventricular pressure via a catheter placed in the ventricle. (From J. R. Atkinson *et al.* (1). Published with permission.)

space and subject to atmospheric and externally applied cuff pressure, and one internal diaphragm positioned in the epidural space (Fig. 31.11) (45). The diaphragms are mechanically motion coupled by an induction tuning piston with a resonant LC tuned circuit. The balanced position of these diaphragms is achieved when intracranial pressure is equal to externally applied cuff pressure and can be detected by the energy absorption technique described above. An externally applied cuff is inflated until the balance meter indicates that the ICP has been equalized by the pressure of the cuff. The system can be repeatedly zero calibrated by inflating the cuff to a pressure of 600 mm of water which is sufficient to cause full downward displacement of the piston. In addition to the inflatable cuff, the antenna for the resonance frequency detection system must also be positioned on the scalp above the transducer. The zero displacement differential coplanar measurement has been analyzed on a mathematical basis and suggests an elimination of distortion factors seen

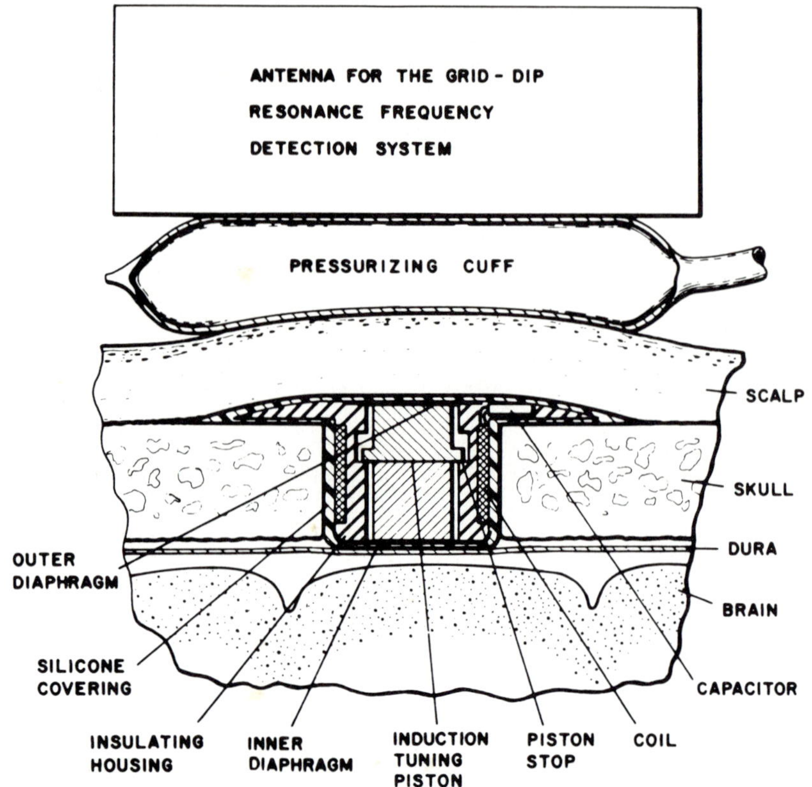

FIG. 31.11. Zervas pressure-balanced radiotelemetry system. The resonant frequency of the passive transensor achieves a predetermined rate when the pressurizing cuff is inflated to a pressure equal to ICP. (From N. L. Zervas, *et al.* (45). Published with permission.)

with surface deformation of other intracranial transducers. Continuous monitoring by this technique utilizing an automatically controlled continuously applied external pressure cuff would seem not to be practical in clinical conditions concerned with acute ICP measurements. A method of continuous recording based on deflection of the balance meter of the device applied without an externally applied pressure cuff can supply information concerning trends in ICP with specific values obtained with intermittent cuff inflation. The requirements of having sensors of variable lengths available at the time of surgical implant so that the deepest portion of the transducer is positioned exactly level with the inner table or no greater than 1 mm deeper have also been reported.

SUMMARY

A review of current techniques of ICP monitoring has stressed two major classifications, fully implantable and percutaneous devices. The most universally applied techniques continue to be those utilizing percutaneous hydrostatic devices. More sophisticated fully implantable and percutaneous devices are available and have received selective application. Future developments may be anticipated not only in instrumentation for ICP data acquisition, but in data analysis and display, as these factors assume increasing importance in specific clinical settings.

REFERENCES

1. Atkinson, J. R., Shurtleff, D. B., and Foltz, E. L. Radio telemetry for measurement of intracranial pressure. J. Neurosurg., *27:* 428–432, 1967.
2. Barbaro, V., and Macellari, V. Intracranial pressure monitoring by means of a passive radiosonde. Med. Biol. Eng. Comput., *17:* 81–86, 1979.
3. Beks, J. W. F., Albarda, S., Gieles, A. C. M., Kuypers, M. H., and Flanderijn, H. Extradural transducer for monitoring intracranial pressure. Acta Neurochir. (Wien), *38:* 245–250, 1970.
4. Brock, M., and Diefenthäler, K. A modified equipment for the continuous telemetric monitoring of epidural or subdural pressure. *In* Intracranial Pressure I, edited by M. Brock and H. Dietz, pp. 2–126. Springer-Verlag, New York, 1972.
5. Bustard, T. S., Lyon, W. C., and Moyer, G. A. A nuclear intracranial pressure sensor. IEEE Trans. Nucl. Sci., *21:* 697–701, 1974.
6. Cheek, W. R., Evans, A. F., Dennis, G. C., and Stein, F. Device for extradural monitoring of intracranial pressure. Technical note. Neurosurgery, *5:* 692–694, 1979.
7. Coe, J. E., Nelson, W. J., Rudenberg, F. H., and Garza, R. T. Technique for continuous intracranial pressure recording. Technical note. J. Neurosurg., *27:* 370–375, 1967.
8. Cohadon, F., LaBalme, M., Castel, J. P., and Vandendriessche, M. ICP microprobes series microfet. *In* Intracranial Pressure IV, edited by N. Lundberg, U. Ponten, and M. Brock, pp. 375–376. Springer-Verlag, New York, 1975.
9. Cooper, P. R., Moody, S., and Sklar, F. Chronic monitoring of intracranial pressure using an in vivo calibrating sensor: experience in patients with pseudotumor cerebri. Neurosurgery, *5:* 666–670, 1979.
10. de Jong, D. A., Berfelo, M. W., de Lange, S. A., and Maas, A. I. R. Epidural pressure monitoring with the so-called Rotterdam transducer. Further in vivo results. Acta Neurochir. (Wien), *45:* 301–309, 1979.
11. Dorsch, N. W. C., Stephens, R. J., and Symon, L. An intracranial pressure transducer. Biomed. Eng., *6:* 452–457, 472, 1971.
12. Dorsch, N. W. C., and Symon, L. A practical technique for monitoring extradural pressure. J. Neurosurg., *42:* 249–257, 1975.
13. Gilner, L. I. New catheter for intraventricular pressure monitoring. Surg. Neurol., *8:* 291–292, 1977.
14. Gobiet, W., Bock, W. I., Liesegang, J., and Grote, W. Experience with an intracranial pressure transducer readjustble in vivo. Technical note. J. Neurosurg., *39:* 272–276, 1974.
15. Gosch, H. H., and Kindt, G. W. Subdural monitoring of acute increased intracranial pressure. Surg. Forum, *23:* 405–406, 1972.
16. Gücer, G., and Viernstein, L., Long-term intracranial pressure recording in the management of pseudotumor cerebri. J. Neurosurg., *49:* 256–263, 1978.
17. Gücer, G., Viernstein, L. J., Chubbuck, J. G., and Walker, A. E. Clinical evaluation of long-term epidural monitoring of intracranial pressure. Surg. Neurol., *12:* 373–377, 1979.
18. Handa, H., Yoneda, S., Matsuda, M., and Handa, J. A miniature SFT transducer for continuous monitoring of intracranial pressure. *In* Intracranial Pressure II, edited by

N. Lundberg, U. Ponten, and M. Brock, pp. 378–379. Springer-Verlag, New York, 1975.

19. Heppner, F., Lanner, G., and Rodler, H. Telemetry of intracranial pressure. Acta Neurochir. (Wien), *33:* 37–43, 1976.
20. Ikeyama, A., Maeda, S., Nagai, H., Furuse, M., Igasaski, I., Inagaki, D., and Kitano, T. Epidural measurement of intracranial pressure by a newly-developed pressure transducer. Neurol. Med. Chir. (Tokyo), *17:* 1–7, 1977.
21. Kindt, G. W. Simplification of intracranial pressure monitoring. *In* Intracranial Pressure II, edited by N. Lundberg, U. Ponten, and M. Brock, pp. 381–383. Springer-Verlag, New York, 1975.
22. Koster, W. G., and Kuypers, M. H. Intracranial pressure and its epidural measurement. Med. Prog. Technol., *7:* 21–27, 1980.
23. Levin, A. B. The use of a fiberoptic intracranial pressure transducer in the treatment of head injuries. J. Trauma, *17:* 767–774, 1977.
24. Levin, A. B. The use of a fiberoptic intracranial pressure monitor in clinical practice. Neurosurgery, *1:* 266–271, 1977.
25. Lundberg, N. Continuous recording and control of ventricular fluid pressure in neurosurgical practice. Acta Psychiatr. Neurol. Scand. Suppl., *149:* 1–193, 1960.
26. MacKay, R. S., Marg, E., and Oechsli, R. Automatic tonometer with exact theory. Various biological applications. Science, *131:* 1 668–1,669, 1960.
27. Meyer, G. A., Lyon, W. C., and Bustard, T. S. Chronic in vivo testing of a fully implantable intracranial pressure sensor. IEEE Trans. Nucl. Sci., *21:* 702–706, 1974.
28. Meyer, G. A., Millis, R. M., and Budzinski, J. Validation of a new technique for measurement of intracranial pressure with a scintillation counter. Neurosurgery, *2:* 35–38, 1978.
29. Numoto, M., Slater, J. P., and Donaghy, R. M. P. An implantable switch for monitoring intracranial pressure. Lancet, *1:* 528, 1966.
30. Olsen, E. R., and Collins, C. C. Passive radio telemetry for the measurements of intracranial pressure. *In* Intracranial Pressure I, edited by M. Brock and H. Dietz, pp. 18–20. Springer-Verlag, New York, 1972.
31. Ream, A. K., Silverberg, G. D., Corbin, S. D., Schmidt, E. V., and Fryer, T. B. Epidural measurement of intracranial pressure. Neurosurgery, *5* (1 pt. 1): 36–43, 1979.
32. Rylander, G. H., Taylor, H. L., Wissinger, J. P., and Story, J. L. Chronic measurement of epidural pressure with an induction-powered oscillator transducer. J. Neurosurg., *44:* 465–478, 1976.
33. Schettini, A., McKay, L., Majord, R., Mahig, J., and Nevis, A. H. Experimental approach for monitoring surface brain pressure. J. Neurosurg., *34:* 36–47, 1971.
34. Tindall, G. T., McGraw, C. P., Wendenburg, H. O., and Peel, H. H. Evaluation of a subdural pressure transducer. Technical note. J. Neurosurg., *37:* 117–121, 1972.
35. Vidyasagar, D., and Raju, T. N. K. A simple noninvasive technique of measuring intracranial pressure in the newborn. Pediatrics, *59:* 957–961, 1977.
36. Vries, J. K., Becker, D. P., and Young, H. F. A subarachnoid screw for monitoring intracranial pressure. Technical note. J. Neurosurg., *39:* 416–419, 1973.
37. Vries, J. K., Becker, D. P., Young, H. F., Sakalas, R., Greenberg, R. F., and Rosner, J. J. The hollow screw technique for monitoring intracranial pressure. *In* Intracranial Pressure II, edited by N. Lundberg, U. Ponten, and M. Brock, p. 386. Springer-Verlag, New York, 1975.
38. Wald, A., Post, K., Ransohoff, J., Hass, W., and Epstein, F. A new technique for monitoring intracranial pressure. Med. Instrum., *11:* 352–354, 1977.
39. Watson, B. W., Currie, J. C. M., Riddle, H. C., and Meldrum, S. J. The long term recording of intracranial pressure. Phys. Med. Biol. *19:* 86–95, 1974.

40. White, R. J., and Takaska, Y. Chronic monitoring of head injury with an implantable ventricular module. J. Trauma, *17:* 521–525, 1977.
41. Wilkinson, H. A. The intracranial pressure monitoring cup catheter. Technical note. Neurosurgery, *1:* 139–141, 1977.
42. Wright, B. D., and Young, B. Automatic intracranial pressure regulation. Crit. Care Med., *6:* 373–375, 1978.
43. Yoneda, S., Matsuda, M., Handa, J., and Handa, H. Continuous measurement of intracranial pressure with SFT: clinical experiences. Surg. Neurol., *4:* 289–295, 1975.
44. Yoneda, S., Matsuda, M., Shimizu, Y., Handa, J., Handa, H., Oda, F., Matsuo, K., and Taguchi, N. SFT—a new device for continuous measurements of intracranial pressure. Technical note. Surg. Neurol., *1:* 13–15, 1973.
45. Zervas, N. T., Cosman, E. R., and Cosman, B. J. A pressure-balanced radio-telemetry system for the measurement of intracranial pressure. A preliminary design report. J. Neurosurg., *47:* 899–911, 1977.

CHAPTER

32

Electrical and Chemical Stimulation of the CNS by Direct Means for Pain Control: Present and Future

CHARLES D. RAY, M.D.

"It is not so amazing that the dancing bear can dance well or not but that he can dance at all." P. T. Barnum

Electrical Stimulation of the CNS for Pain Control

In Minneapolis in 1973 we held the first international symposium on the clinical applications of electrical stimulation methods for the control of pain (28). At that time there was a shroud of uncertainty about this technique. Much was said about "placebo effect." Much was unclear, confusing. The most important abiding element, however, was the fact that in clinical applications, stimulation worked. Indeed, several forms of electrical stimulation were helpful in controlling pain originating from several parts of the body. It had become apparent to a few of us that approximately one-half of the patients so treated would have a lasting relief of approximately 50% of their prestimulation pain. By and large, these numbers have remained or have improved. In the few dramatic years that followed, what with the discovery of the basic neurochemistry of pain, the once nearly black magic became respectable. Nevertheless, many clinicians today either do not know of or remain doubtful about practical uses of stimulation for pain control. Major reasons for this lie in the indecisions or uncertainties surrounding patient selection, appropriate techniques to be used, and determination of results.

Pain—We Are Ever Mindful of It

Pain is a necessary ingredient for survival. Like other complex functions important for survival, pain exhibits many states of order and disorder. The anatomy and physiology of pain has been so clouded with folklore that only within the last few decades has its true nature begun to be unraveled. Somewhat akin to the physiology of coagulation of the blood or respiration of cells, complex systems associated with survival represent major clusters of disease entities when their "normal" patterns are disrupted. Underlying all of these, there must be a disturbance in pain-associated neurophysiology or metabolism, local or distributed, which contributes to the pathological state.

The story of pain and its electrical treatment extends in Western literature to the 1st century A.D., when the curative powers of shocks obtained from electric fishes were first described (29). In the East, on the other hand, acupuncture has been known as a source of "energies" caused to flow in the body, somewhat akin to the earlier Franklin view of electricity as a fluid. With the recent political reopening of trade with China, there outflowed a revival of conflicting interests in acupuncture. Western neuroscience was instantly compelled, skeptical, repelled, and embarrassed at the inability to reasonably explain acupuncture analgesia. Further, with the rise of drug problems in our culture, there arose an intensification of pain-related research. A contemporary turning point for pain was the publishing of the gate-control theory by Melzack and Wall in 1965 (23). There shortly followed the identification of specific antipain substances in the CNS of animals and man. From there on the proverbial lid has blown off.

Before discussing the management of pain by CNS stimulation, we should review the anatomy and physiology of the pain systems, especially as to what structures need to be stimulated and what structures can be successfully stimulated.

Anatomy and Physiology of Pain

The search for abnormalities of nervous function through more accessible tissues, such as blood, is often fruitless. There are very few convincing animal models, either spontaneously occurring or laboratory induced, of diseases of the human nervous system. Further, some of the sensory system found in man is either different or poorly developed in lower animals. In the case of pain, it has been necessary to extrapolate from autopsy material but this has been quite misleading. Destructive lesions of the central nervous system that exert a marked influence on pain will commonly fail to maintain effectiveness for long periods of time. The use of nondestructive electrical stimulation in humans has provided an important source of new information about the organization of pain pathways. Of course, most important of all have been the development of techniques from molecular biology and immunochemistry, coupled with the discovery of neuroactive compounds such as the endorphins, substance P, and many others, that better understanding is finally coming (4, 14, 15, 36). I will make certain assumptions, principally that the schema given below has indeed been clarified and established. Further, I will present only a basic organizational sketch since anything else is beyond the scope of this paper or my own personal work. We must simultaneously bind together into one functional hypothesis the predominant subjective phenomena, the neuroanatomy/neurophysiology, and the neurochemistry of pain. In several places they will not combine easily, and indeed much of the present information may ultimately prove to be incorrect. The picture is unfolding at an incredibly fast rate in the scientific literature. Beyond pain, the ultimate goal lies in the chemistry of madness and all that this implies. Needless to say, these are giant clinical rewards and economic worlds to conquer for the pharmaceutical business, strong incentives to press ahead.

By experience, we learn that impulses arriving along Aδ and C fibers carry information associated with actual or threatened tissue damage. Yet, the perception of tissue threat or damage (nociception) is certainly not all there is to pain. There is in addition a remarkable affective state of agony, aversion, and unpleasantness. Unimodal nociceptors are those neurons which respond only to noxious stimuli. Polymodial nociceptors respond also to intense chemical, mechanical, or thermal effects. Some receptors never mediate pain even at maximal stimulation. It appears that the Aδ-fibers evoke sharp, pricking pain and that activity in the C-fibers results in a more burning sensation. Aδ pain is more severe, responding to a single stimulus, but C-fiber pain is more severe with repetitive stimulation.

A number of pain receptor substances have been identified and include histamine, bradykinin, kinin, somatostatin, substance P, prostaglandins, and K-ions. The receptor substance and the neurotransmitter best implicated for pain is substance P. It is elaborated in the dorsal root ganglion cell and flows to central synapses. These small axons enter via the lateral division of the dorsal root and pass through the tract of Lissauer and terminate in the marginal cells (lamina I) of the dorsal gray. The larger diameter fibers carrying other sensory input, such as pressure or vibration, enter through the lateral and medial divisions of the dorsal root and pass upward in the system of the dorsal column or terminate in the substantia gelatinosa (laminas II and III) (19). Some small inhibitory neurons are found between these and represent the "gate" as described by Melzack and Wall.

There is no doubt that the dorsal horn of the spinal cord is an important integrative area for sensory signal processing and not simply a relay station. We would expect, therefore, that most of the output from this system is modified or filtered, even suppressed.

Most of the neurons project to the contralateral side of the cord and rise as the lateral spinothalamic tract, and closely associate with the medial lemniscus, terminating in the posterior group of thalamic nuclei. This system is a fast conducting one important for temporal and spacial discriminative aspects of pain and pressure. This system, common only to man and higher primates, is known as the neospinothalamic system (Fig. 32.1). In the posterior thalamic nuclei the other sensory input arising through the dorsal columns is also integrated. The mechanoreceptive fibers in the dorsal columns are uncrossed until they reach the nuclei of the dorsal columns in the medulla. There they cross and join the lemniscal system to terminate in the posterior thalamus.

The system which is of much greater significance to pain is that which passes principally but not exclusively through the ventral (medial) spinothalamic tract. This is an indirect system which terminates first in the bulboreticular nuclei (principally the nucleus reticularis gigantocellularis), an important relay system for pain. Connections from here terminate in the hypothalamus and the limbic system, and they are involved in aversive, nondiscrimitative, motivational, and affective states of pain. Further, connections from the reticular neurons in the bulb pass to those of the mesencepalon and from there to the medial and intralaminar nuclei of the thalamus as well as to the periaqueductal central grey matter (PAG). This latter structure further communicates with a number of ascending and descending structures. This complex is known as the ancient or paleospinothalamic system which is found all the way down the genetic tree to the tiger salamander. We may say that the strain of pain lies mainly in the brain, the old brain, that is. It appears to be the only pain system for lower animals; the exquisitely localizing lateral spinothalamic pain system is not needed in hairy, leather, feather, or scale-covered species, even though localizing mechanoreception is otherwise intact. As mentioned earlier, the medial (including the paraventricular) and intralaminar (including the parafascicularis-center median) thalamic nuclei are involved in diffuse, nonsomatotopic, nondiscriminative aspects of pain and agony, especially in man (Fig. 32.2).

The entire human spinothalamic system is composed of perhaps 1,500 fibers, of which a great number are mechanoreceptors. Apparently, large numbers of fibers are not required for mediating nociception (4, 19).

Whereas the ventral nuclear complex of the thalamus is a terminus for representation of the neospinalthalamic tract and the dorsal column-medial lemniscal system, lesions here produce profound sensory discrimination defects with little influence on pain (19). The posterior thalamic nuclear complex receives fibers from similar input; this region, and in particular a small area posterior to the ventrobasal complex, is involved in the discriminative aspects of pain. As mentioned earlier, the medial (including the paraventricular) and intralaminar (including the parafascicular is and center median) thalamic nuclei are involved in a diffuse, nonsomatotopic, nondiscriminative aspects of pain.

As one might very well expect, stimulations in the posterior and lateral

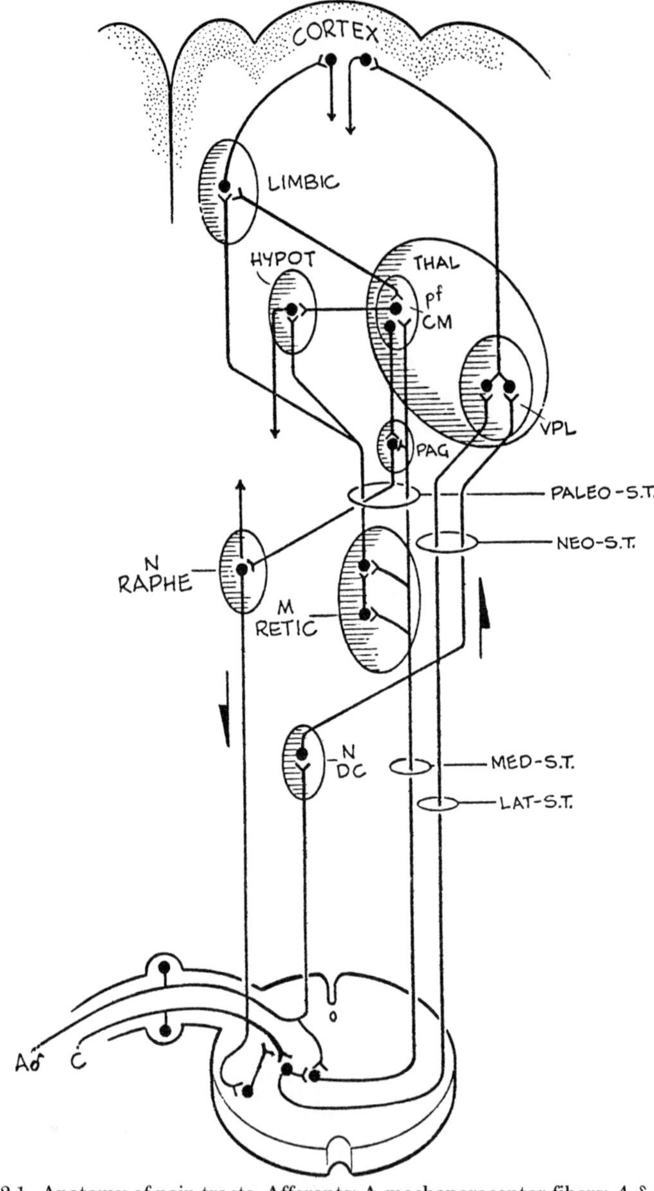

FIG. 32.1. Anatomy of pain tracts. Afferents: A-mechanoreceptor fibers; *A-δ* and *C* fiber nociceptor input. Ascending systems: *N DC*, nuclei of dosal columns; MED-S.T., medial spinothalamic tract; *LAT-S.T.*, lateral spinothalamic tract; *M RETIC*, mesencephalic reticular nuclei; *PALEO-S.T.*, paleospinothalamic; *NEO-S.T.*, neospinothalamic; *THAL*, thalamus; *PAG*, periaqueductal gray; *VPL*, ventral posterolateral nucleus; *pfCM*, parafascicularis-center median; *HYPOT*, hypothalamus; *LIMBIC*, limbic system. Descending system: *N RAPHE*, midbrain raphe nuclei. (From Charles D. Ray, Ltd. 1981. Published with permission.)

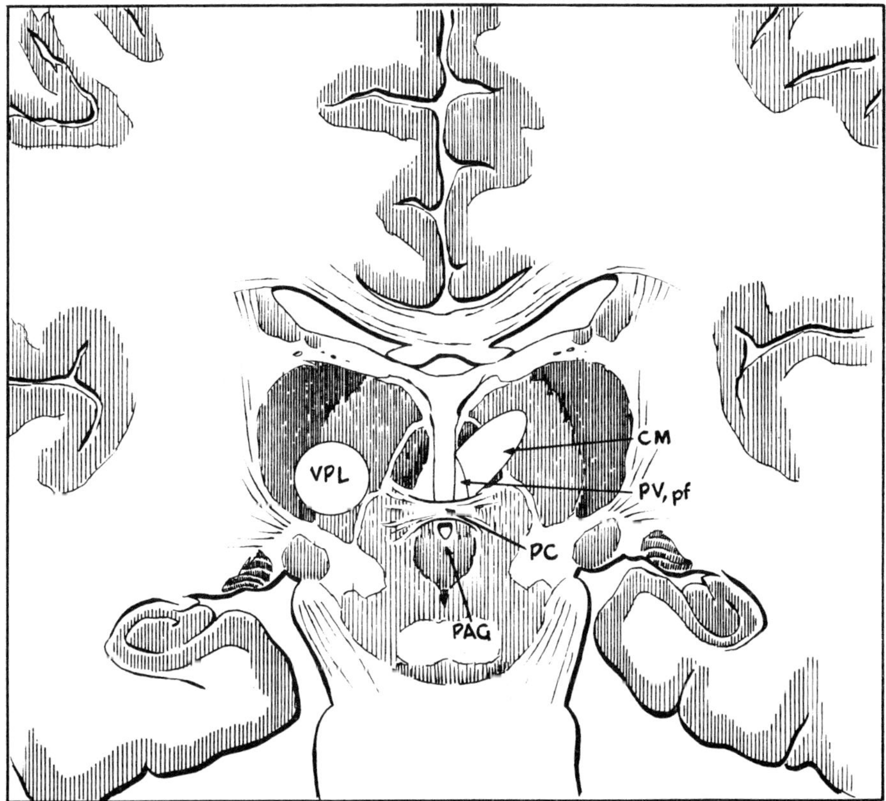

FIG. 32.2. Diagram of deep targets for DBS. Thalamic-medial (*PV*, paraventricular; *pfCM*, parafascicularis-center median) and lateral (*VPL*, ventral posterolateral). *PC*, posterior commissure. *PAG*, periaqueductal gray. (From Charles D. Ray, Ltd. 1981. Published with permission.)

thalamus produce tingling on the opposite side of the body which fortunately may inhibit the sensation or experience of pain in the same somatotopic area (25). Stimulation in the medial and intralaminar thalamus produces only some general vague feelings of warmth and restfulness and reduction in chronic, agonizing pain. The stimulation has virtually no effect on acute pain and only a little on the threshold to pinprick (1, 31). In lower animals, however, stimulation here may show true analgesia for all forms of pain. Although the systems connect upwards to cortex, the cerebral cortex seems rather unessential for pain perception. There may be some restricted regions of the cortex which are more involved but they have not been clearly identified. Cortical stimulation has had little or no effect on pain experience.

Let us point out here that there is a basic cybernetic principal that inhibition is a major function of a well-coordinated, highly complex system in order to prevent chaos and instability. Indeed there are between 100 and 1000 times more neurons and neuronal firings in the CNS that are inhibitory than are facilitatory (44). Inhibitors (regulating, controlling, limiting) abound. There is little evidence that electrical stimulation of the CNS directly produces inhibition. The current required to produce prolonged, true neuronal blockage would be destructive to the cells and the effect would cease. Inhibition must therefore come mainly from the activation of intact, normally inhibitory functions, structures, or pathways (17). In general, the activation of inhibition is apparently the principal mode of operation of neurostimulation in control of pain (and in disorders of movement).

Descending Systems

The most important site in our unfolding story is the clustered region around the PAG and the medial-intralaminar thalamus. Together called the PAG-PV (periventricular) complex. Stimulations here will not only produce important decendins impulses but will cause the release of enkephalins and endorphins. Since there is no direct connection between the PAG and the spinal cord, its main outflow, for purposes of pain control, is through the raphe nuclei (18). Fibers of the medullary raphe system descend in the dorsolateral funiculus to terminate in the substantia gelatinosa, thus completing the important closed-loop control system. Within the descending fibers of the raphe system, serotonin is pumped along, in the axons. As substance P is excitatory, and enkephalin is inhibitory, then serotonin causes the release of the latter to act on the former to produce a spinal blockage of pain transmission (Fig. 31.3). The long circuitous pathway of return of this inhibitor system allows enough of the pain to come through initially, to permit the organism to escape, but then tones down the pain later to permit the organism to go about its other business with fewer restrictions. More of this later.

Neurotransmitters of the Brain

Only 1 to 2% of the neurons in the brain are known to contain amines as transmitters. About 10% contain acetylcholine. The remaining nearly 90% contain as yet unknown neurotransmitters. There are other amino acids (such as γ-aminobutyric acid (GABA) and glycine, principally inhibitors) may be performing many of these functions. A number of other interesting hormones and a variety of other peptides have been identified as neurotransmitters (36). Several of these are located in the gastrointestinal system as well as the brain and are probably involved in a direct humoral feedback system for such things as thirst, hunger, and blood pressure, plus salt and fluid resolution. Several of the peptides that circulate in the blood may enter the brain by the choroid plexus and the

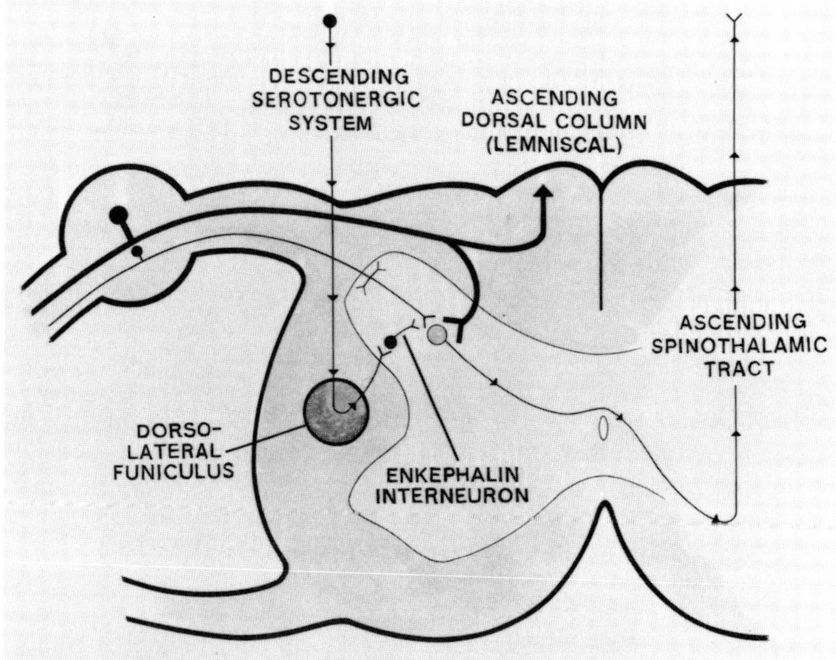

FIG. 32.3. Diagram of spinal level pain control system. Small diameter (C) fibers and larger diameter (A-δ and larger mechanoreceptor) fibers impinging on dorsal horn cells; large diameter (mechanoreceptor) fibers passing into the dorsal columns. Ascending fibers of spinothalamic tracts; ascending fibers of dorsal columns. Descending serotonergic fibers from raphe system synapsing with short enkephalinergic fibers having presynaptic terminations on C fibers (producing a blockage of substance P release at C fiber synapse), thus blocking transmission of pain signals. (From Charles D. Ray, Ltd. 1981. Published with permission.)

cerebrospinal fluid or through the pituitary and its portal system into the brain and third ventricle (26). I feel that it is important that many of the structures which are heavily loaded with exotic neurotransmitters are in close proximity to the ventricular system or cerebrospinal fluid pathway.

It has been estimated that perhaps between 1 and 5% of the brain's neurotransmitters are now known. It is unthinkable that this limited group would be the only ones involved in pain, drug actions, or mental disorders. The number of known peptide transmitters is increasing rapidly beyond the roughly 2 dozen that are now identified. Most important for our present consideration are those associated with opiate activity, endorphins, the enkephalins, serotonin, dopamine, and norepinephrine. The opiate receptors identified a few years ago in association with pain are now known to be separate from enkephalin receptor sites (14). The two may be localized very near to each other, for example, the small enkephalin interneurons in the dorsal cord that synapse on opiate receptors which in turn are localized on the endings of sensory neurons and inhibit the release of pain neurotransmitter substance P. Further, there are at least two distinct receptors for opiates: μ-receptors, which prefer morphine and probably mediate analgesia, δ-receptors, which select certain enkephalin derivatives and may preferentially regulate emotional aspects of pain behavior. It also appears that met-enkephalin and leu-enkephalin occur in distinctly separate neurons in both brain and gut. The rationale for these dual, if not competitive, locations is not yet clear.

Ribosome replication does not occur for small peptides. Instead, most biological peptides are the result of cleavage from larger precursor peptides. The difference between the two enkephalins (met- and leu-) implies that different cleaving enzymes are involved. It is also important to note that the enkephalins have a very short half-life (2 minutes) in pain regulation. β-Endorphin, which is cleaved from the β-lipotropin molecule in common with ACTH, has a much longer half-life (4 hours) (4). Under conditions of severe trauma and stress, the common precursor is split up to release both β-endorphin and ACTH to respond to the trauma.

Second to enkephalin, substance P is the most studied of the brain peptides. More pathways for substance P have been demonstrated than for any other peptide neurotransmitter (12, 16). Nonetheless, searching for them is about like looking for a pinch of salt dissolved in a swimming pool. Substance P may also be involved in axon-axonal reflexes of the skin producing local vascular effects. Neurons containing enkephalin and substance P lie close to each other in such areas as the raphe nuclei, the septum, the ventral tegmentum, and the amygdala. Substance P is also closely allied with serotonin originating in the raphe nuclei, and the two together must have an interactive regulatory role in pain suppression.

Since substance P causes a selective excitation of nociceptive neurones, a greater than normal amount of substance P or its receptor sites may account for hyperpathic sensations in response to what should be an innocuous stimulus. This would be seen in partial denervation states or certain neuralgias or perhaps causalgia. In the brain, substance P may have a dual action, in very low doses releasing endorphins and at higher doses directly exciting neuronal activity in nociceptive pathways. Endorphin release would reduce pain and excited nociceptive fibers would produce hyperalgesia (12). Morphine administration and electrical stimulation activate local and descending (serotonergic) signals that selectively inhibit the release of substance P at synapses with dorsal horn relay neurones. This action occurs through the activation of short segmental enkephalinergic interneurones that produce a presynaptic inhibition of the small diameter primary afferent nociceptive neurons (21).

Stimulus-produced Analgesia (SPA)

This term has a considerable meaning in contemporary neurophysiology but in clinical practice it is not quite correct. Many investigators have placed electrodes in several targets in the human central nervous system to produce both acute and chronic alterations of pain perception or pain awareness. However, in man true analgesia is perhaps never seen as it has been reported in lower animals. The tingling effects which come from simulation of the discriminative, direct, lateral spinothalamic or lemniscal systems produce a form of signal masking with a marked reduction in pain level (18). Pinprick sensation may also be reduced but certainly not abolished. Patients with chronic stimulators in the posterior or ventrobasal thalamus have a preservation of acute pain, such as from trauma. Similarly, chronic stimulation of the paraventricular system (PAG and intralaminar thalamus) will likewise not abolish responses to acute pain (2). We might therefore, refer to this effect as a stimulus-produced "dysalgesia" where the intensity and character of the painful process are definitely altered but not abolished. So far this difference between man and lower animals has been found regardless of the site of stimulation (cord, stem, diencephalon, or cortex).

If one simply lists the areas which will produce analgesia in animals or dysalgesia in man, it would be somewhat as follows: spinal cord, lower brain stem, midbrain, raphe nuclei, PAG, PUS (periventricular system), thalamic nuclei, internal capsule, limbic system, caudate nucleus, septal area, and cortex. There are only a few other areas which have high concentration of enkephalin or opiate receptors which do not show pain relief on stimulation (*e.g.*, subfrontal, cingulum, amygdala) (4, 36).

In the process of making stereotaxic lesions for chronic pain, as well as for movement disorders, epilepsy, and destructive behavior, anatomical targets have been found that effectively control chronic pain in humans, even if for a variable period of time. As Sweet points out, however, lesions in nearly all these targets are ineffective for acute pain and also produce no somatic sensory loss (38). They include: (*a*) inferior frontal white; (*b*) cingulum; (*c*) centrum medianum parafascicularis; (*d*) connections between medial nonspecific and lateral specific sensory relay nuclei of the thalamus; (*e*) pulvinar; (*f*) amygdala; (*g*) frontothalamic tract; (*h*) posteromedial hypothalamus; (*i*) periventricular hypothalamus; and (*j*) hypophysis. It is important to note that most of these structures are heavily endowed with opiate, enkephalin, and other receptor sites of the pain mediation system. Again, most but not all of these sites are adequate targets for pain control by neurostimulation.

This raises an important question: How can a particular anatomical structure produce pain control when it is either destroyed or it is activated by stimulation? It appears that the target structure would have to: (*a*) be an important synaptic pool; (*b*) have a facilitatory input system; and (*c*) produce a suppressor output on stimulation of the structure. In engineering terms, this very common function is performed by a phase reversing device. Destruction of the input leaves the suppressor function intact, though perhaps reduced. Stimulation would still be capable of increasing inhibitor outflow. Destroying the inhibitory output kills the function until taken over elsewhere.

Pain and More Pain

The principle interest in the use of electrical stimulation of the CNS for pain control lies in the fact that it is a nondrug, nondestructive, reversible technique with relatively few side effects. Indeed, when side effects occur they are usually eliminated or at least reduced by the simple reduction in electrical stimulation parameters.

Stimulation of the central nervous system for chronic pain is our concern here, there being little practical value for such stimulation for acute pain (except perhaps for intraoperative, obstetrical, or posttraumatic applications). We may identify three essentially elements for the development of clinically treatable chronic pain (29):

1. The injury or injurious process should persist for at least a few weeks. This should principly involve the deep, visceral, weight-bearing, paleospinothalamic system. (Hyperpathia probably represents a chronic pain involving the specific, surface, neospinothalamic system.)
2. A metabolic deficiency in antinociceptive neurotransmitters, their precursors, or associated enzymes.
3. A learned engram. There may be a behavioral predisposition or alteration in which higher functions interfere with antinociceptive functions.

In addition, there may be a psychosocial disturbance of varying degree; if this disturbance is major, the patient may not be treatable except with extensive psychotherapy. In such cases most of the established means of pain therapy (drugs, surgery, counseling, and neuroaugmentive techniques) will not work until the psychosocial problems are adequately resolved (if ever). Where psychosocial problems are not major, all three of the above elements must still be dealt with if the patient is to be cured of the chronic painful state. Clearly, wherever possible, the cause of the pain should be alleviated, *e.g.*, projecting bone spurs, ununited fractures, invasive tumors, or entrapped nerves should first be relieved.

Dealing with deficiencies in antinociceptive chemistry is at this time more difficult. Much new science is on the horizon, however. The learned element is best dealt with by behavioral modification in some form. In the presence of a learned pattern with drug-induced behavior associated with the intake of a specific drug (called state dependency), this pattern may disappear on changing or stopping the specific drug (35, 37). One sometimes sees chronic pain cases whose pain problems abates on being taken off of narcotics!

We feel that neurostimulation is helpful principally by: (*a*) stepping up the metabolic turnover of inhibitory neurotransmitter substances, (*b*) by activating ubiquitous inhibitor neurons, or by (*c*) pain signal jamming through interference with patterned neuronal firing necessary for the transmission of clear afferent signals.

Patient Selection

As yet, relatively little can actually be measured to determine the degree to which patients hurt. Acute testing with needles, tight bands, or dolorimeters poorly correlates with pain levels in chronic cases. While endorphin assays are being developed, only a few studies to date show promise in the measurement of antinociceptive neurotransmitters for distinguishing organic *vs.* psychogenic pain cases, for example. (2) Essential criteria for patient selection, beyond those obtained from a detailed history, physical, and diagnostic work-up, remain dependent upon clinical impressions and behavioral observation. Somewhat in keeping with the ancient Egyptian formula of "What I shall and what I shall not treat," we should not use neurostimulation techniques on patients who have true psychogenic pain, but they are rare. More common and more important are those patients who use their pain to manipulate their environment. The highly manipulative, chronic pain patient must be dealt with from the emotional and behavioral points of view before pain can be alleviated, regardless of its origin or the technique used for pain control (28, 39).

Just as in the real estate business it is said that the three most important elements for success are: (*a*) location, (*b*) location, and (*c*) location; since electrical stimulation can only activate existing circuits, it is clear that electrode location is by far the most significant element. Stimulus amplitude, frequency, and pulse width, although important, are no where near as much so as electrode placement. Further, the cause of the pain is of secondary significance compared to location of the pain. Of relatively lesser significance are pain duration, degree of disability caused by the pain or an intercurrent disease, and intensity of the pain or pain behavior, provided that the underlying personality structure is intact. In selecting patients for this mode of therapy, we must first ascertain that the problem is not appropriately treatable by (or has not responded to) other, standard means. This aside, in order of overall importance to good results, we must attend to the following:

A. Psychosocial Criteria
1. Adequacy of personality (nonpsychotic, nonmanipulative); there must be assurance that the pain is not a manifestation of disordered thinking
2. Motivation and cooperation by the patient
3. Freedom from habituation drugs or drug-seeking behavior.
4. Absence of impending legal actions, unsettled compensation dispute, or other major source of secondary gain
5. Absence of major marital, family, social, or occupational conflict

B. Technical Criteria
1. Location and distribution of the pain
2. Location of the stimulus site or electrode
3. Individual anatomic and physiologic variation
4. Stimulus parameters
5. Criteria by which success is judged

Less important elements for lasting results were:
1. The cause of pain (distribution is considerably more important)
2. The duration of the pain
3. Extent of disability caused by the pain or an associated intercurrent problem.

Thus, beyond the emotional and motivational aspects, it is the location (and associated with it, the type) of pain that is the primary criterion for patient selection and for electrode-target site selection.

Techniques

These things aside, decisions regarding the use of implanted neuroaugmentive devices for pain control are, in my opinion, relatively straightforward. One must not forget, as mentioned above, that neurostimulation may be selected where other methods do not work or do not work well enough. It is simply one more way of dealing with pain and is not in any way panacean.

In general, we consider that the technique is not a success if the preimplant pain is not relieved by at least 50%. Patients may be appreciative of a smaller percentage of relief and therefore refuse to have the devices taken out but this is not a truly successful result. Many clinicians require that their patients use no postimplant analgesics stronger than Tylenol or propoxyphene. We feel this is an unnecessarily strict requirement. A few tablets (up to 3 per day), of a codeine-containing pain medication is not abusive, but must be carefully monitored. Incidentally we avoid aspirin-containing medications because of the high potential for gastric irritation.

Good results from spinal stimulation have been seen in carefully selected cases of failed back surgery (especially where there is some evidence of neuronal damage but not entrapment), dysesthesias, hyperesthesias, causalgic-like syndromes, phantom limbs, partial denervation states, neuropathies, post-trauma pain, and others (6, 30). Results are better with operator experience, and also with treating the patient on a holistic basis. Reliance on stimulation alone is no more appropriate than relying entirely on a surgical procedure to rehabilitate a patient. Stimulation of the spinal cord works best for pain that is at least 60% in one limb. If the pain is bilateral, midline, deep, visceral, or involving both an arm and leg, even on the same side, it will usually not work well (32). For example, pain radiating into a leg originating from adhesive arachnoiditis may respond well whereas pain coming primarily from the central low back generally will not. If the patient has a lumbar lateral spinal stenosis causing entrapment pain plus a dysesthesia from root injury, for example, the decompression should be performed first and the stimulator implanted later. Even though the pain problem may be quite complex, spinal stimulation is sufficiently simple and safe, especially with the trial use of a percutaneously inserted spinal electrode, that it is often worthy of trial.

The percutaneously implanted spinal epidural electrical stimulator electrodes are rather easily positioned in the epidural space (30). In the typical failed back surgery case, for example, the insertion is performed under local anesthesia with image amplification x-ray control (32). Needles (17-gauge) are inserted on either side of the spinous process of L1 and the electrode are introduced, placed slightly to the side of the pain. The electrode tip can be bent about 20° and then guided through the epidural space during insertion, rather like an aortic catheter which can be guided into selected vessels. The final position of electrodes depends entirely on the patient's report of the stimulation paresthesia. Nearly all patients require that the tingling overlap the distribution of pain. Most commonly the bipolar pair of electrodes will lie at T8 and T10. A fine percutaneous extension wire is brought to the outside for a 10-day trial stimulation. The patient can even be sent back to work or put through rather rigorous exercises to determine the effectiveness of stimulation. If the trial is successful, the percutaneous extension wires are later cut off and connected to a permanent receiver implanted in a subcutaneous pocket in the anterior inferior chest wall. Patients are carefully instructed as to how to use and care for their system. They will return at regular intervals, at least once or twice yearly, and the parameters of stimulation will be optimized each time (Fig. 32.4).

The more permanent dorsal cord neurostimulator, which requires a laminectomy as did its precursor, the dorsal column stimulator, is generally reserved for those cases where a good result has been seen using

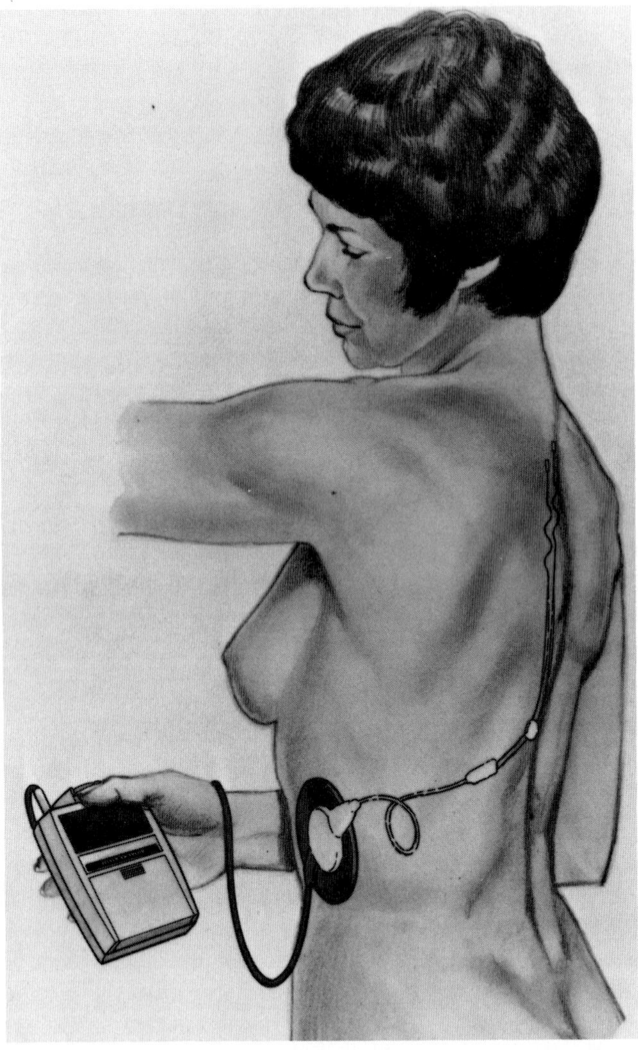

FIG. 32.4. Spinal implant system (Medtronic PISCES), showing external transmitter and antenna; implanted receiver, subcutaneous lead wire, and electrodes. (From C. D. Ray (30). Published with permission.)

the simpler percutaneously inserted spinal, stimulator but for some reason (displacement, waning of effectiveness, breakage of the wires) the system has failed after some months of success. Laminectomy dorsal cord stimulator implants involve placement of the electrodes in the endodural space (*i.e.*, between the layers of the dura) usually at T9 and slightly off the midline to the painful side. The electrodes are brought through a subcutaneous tunnel (never through muscle) over the apex of the shoulder and into a subcutaneous pocket on the subclavicular chest wall. Stimulation of the posterior spinal cord for pain control primarily works by activation of the specific (somatotopic, lemniscal, posterolateral thalamic, nonendorphinergic, neospinothalamic) pain control system. However, since it also produces stimulation of undifferentiated pain control pools in the dorsal gray, there will be an effect on pain of virtually any origin (including fibers of the paleospinothalamic system), when limited to stimulated dermatomes.

Deep brain stimulation (DBS) implants are generally reserved for cases having severe, unremitting, agonizing pain that is bilateral, deep midline, diffuse, from metastases or of central origin. Several targets are used for this technique, and they will be discussed later. In central pain states perhaps less than one-half of the cases will show good results, but it may still be worthwhile since absolutely nothing else nondestructive works well. DBS enjoys a remarkable place in the care of chronic, severe pain. In our hands, about 75% of the cases will receive good to excellent results, even when the pain has persisted, relentlessly, for years (in one case for 49 years!) (31). The technique has now been used for about 10 years, and good results continue. If there is a failure of the system, where good results have been obtained for some time, there is no question that a replacement is desirable (Fig. 32.5).

Deep brain stimulation utilizes a variety of targets, depending upon the clinician and his personal experience. The majority of the targets utilized are either those of the PAG-paraventricular complex or the specific sensory thalamus. Rich communications through the nonspecific thalamus permit good bilateral effects from a unilateral electrode.

In a brief international survey which I ran for the writing of this paper, I obtained personal communications regarding targets, clinical indications, results and numbers of cases from: J. Gybels (Louvain), Y. Hosobuchi (San Francisco), S. Larson (Milwaukee), D. Long (Baltimore), G. Mazars (Paris), B. Meyerson (Stockholm), F. Mundinser (Freiburs), J. Schvarcz (Buenos Aires), J. Siesfried (Zurich), R. Tasker (Toronto), I. Turnbull (Vancouver), and myself. Approximately 850 DBS cases were informally reported. Eleven targets were used in one or more cases. There was considerable variation among clinicians, personal experience in pain cases, targets used, and results. It is not possible to explain all of the

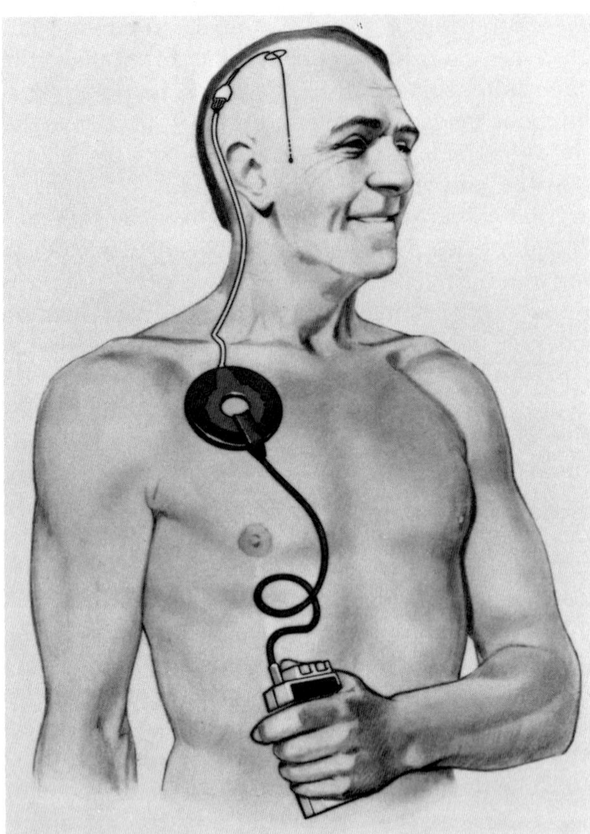

FIG. 32.5. Deep brain implant system (Medtronic DBS®), showing external transmitter and antenna; implanted receiver, substaneous lead wire, and electrodes. (From C. D. Ray (30). Published with permission.)

differences. Opinions vary from disappointment to elation. Nonetheless, the implants continue to be used since most of the cases treated have little or no alternative. The poorest results were found in patients having central or deafferentation pain; 50% or less improvement was seen, regardless of the target used (18). Nearly all the failed back surgery pain patients are from North America and show good to excellent results in about 75%. The outcome of cancer cases falls between these results. In searching for a guiding principal for electrode placement, it again appears more important to utilize a target appropriate to the location of pain (paleo-, neo-) (Table 32.1). In addition to the DBS cases, approximately 650 spinal cord implants were mentioned. In North America the majority of these are cases of failed back surgery syndrome. About 50% of spinal stimulation cases have 50% or greater relief of pain. Cancer and trauma cases were somewhat less successful. Deafferentation (phantom limb, postherpetic neuralgia) cases also enjoyed approximately 50% good results.

SUCCESSFUL RESULTS

In general, neuroaugmentive devices share a high degree of efficacy with other established means of pain control. In benign chronic pain problems, stimulation is superior to most other methods, especially destructive surgery. Behavioral intervention or modification have proven to be highly effective in a large number of cases, and this mode of therapy is often combined with one or more of the neuroaugmentive techniques. Each case requires individualization. In our practice, we utilize a multidisciplinary team approach and a comprehensive pain rehabilitation program. Further, we make a major, practical attempt to apply neuroaugmentive devices. Our reported results from the use of stimulator implants are often somewhat better than those reported elsewhere (6, 7). We feel that this is in part due to our particular concern with global management of pain and to our emphasis on nondestructive techniques.

For acute pain problems (injuries, postoperative pain) transcutaneous electrical nerve stimulation (TENS) works in about 80% of cases; for chronic pain problems, it is significantly effective in about 40%. Reported results for implanted devices range upwards from about 50% on a long-term basis. Several clinical investigators are finding that results are improved if the selection criteria (especially those relative to psychosocial factors) are strictly observed (22).

Clinical Utility

Utilizing the above concept in the clinical application of neurostimulation is rather straightforward. In short, it matters not so much what the pain is or what caused it, but where it is. Neurostimulation is a location—specific treatment mode, both in terms of pain location and electrode placement. As indicated above, the treatment must be appropriate to the particular system. That is, pain of neospinothalamic (typically surface)

TABLE 32.1
Deep Brain Stimulation Targets and Results

Location of pain	Type of Pain	Target	Reported results
Unilateral, local, surface	Protopathic, deafferented	Spec. sens. thal. int. capsule med. lemniscus	Fair to excell.
Bilateral, midline, diffuse, deep	Agonal, aversive	Paraventric. pfCM thalamus pag	Good to excel.

or somatotopic origin should be treated using electrode placements in or on that system. Pain primarily involving the deep (typically paleospinothalamic) system should utilize that system for neurostimulation therapy.

First, therefore, determine where the patient hurts (the character of pain is often typical: crawling, searing, burning sensations are usually surface-oriented; crushing, boring, sickening sensations are more likely deep). Note the anatomical distribution (unilateral, distributed, midline, one limb). Then select the neurostimulator mode and electrode location that best addresses the location of the pain. Of course, there will be cases where "crossover" treatment (from one mode to another) will suffice. Notwithstanding its simplicity, this concept serves as a practical guideline in pain management by the use of neurostimulator devices. The scheme applies to all of the available neurostimulator devices and, to a large extent as well, pain treatment by medication. Lastly, remember that the clear majority of chronic pain problems primarily involve the deep system, with its attendantly rich emotional and aversive elements. Here, as with medication, most agents used to treat acute pain do not serve well for chronic cases, and vice versa (29).

Chemical Stimulation of the CNS

Direct administration o chemical substances into the CNS has been investigated for many, many years. A considerable interest in the direct infusion, by indwelling catheters, principally utilizing catecholamines was first described about 1910 but became rather intensive in the 1950s. This is well reviewed by Myers (24). Delgado and coworkers developed a dialyzing unit for long-term intracerebral perfusion. This "dialytrode" has a semipermeable membrane on the tip of a double lumen cannula (11). Chemical materials could be washed into and through the chamber at the tip, and from there they would diffuse into the brain. A recent modification of this system permits simultaneous recording, electrical and chemical stimulation (10).

We can identify two major areas for injections: intracerebroventricular (ICV) and spinal (which may be subarachnoid or extradural). These techniques are of present or potential clinical importance because they permit the direct injection of substances that cannot otherwise easily be delivered to desired ICV or spinal targets, when we compare the administration of these compounds by indirect routes. For example, the substance may be extremely active by direct administration but is deactivated by other means (*e.g.*, by mouth, vein, or muscle). Indeed, some compounds are so fragile that they cannot be administered, except by direct means. Further, some compounds, such as morphine, exert undesirable side effects when delivered indirectly to the CNS, and these side effects are largely attenuated on direct administration. Certainly direct administration permits far greater control over the location, concentration, or dosage than is permitted by any other means. Recent discovery of the variety of neuroactive compounds that can be administered directly has increased the interest in this approach, especially substances which show antinociceptive effects when injected centrally, yet show no such effects when administered peripherally, for example, such diverse compounds as norepinephrine and baclofen (41, 42). In a real sense, an entirely new clinical pharmacology is being constructed around the concept of direct chemical stimulation of the CNS.

Direct Injection Problems

As was noted earlier, one unique thing about the use of an electrode is the fact that its effectiveness is related to a rather specific anatomical target. Whatever happens at that target may then be propagated. However, if one wants to activate a different target, one must physically move the electrode. Pharmaceuticals diffuse widely and show anatomical localization only by their site-binding specificity. By combining both a mechanical delivery system and a selective compound, one creates a new order of specificity in pharmacologic effects, but also introduces some problems, such as:

1. Selection of the delivery port location relative to the target structure.
2. Chemical characteristics of the material delivered (*e.g.*, pH, osmolarity, solubility, lipophilicity, chemical stability, and the binding to the tubing or the pump by the compounds, especially peptides).
3. Physical characteristics such as viscosity.
4. Physiological characteristics such as the direct and indirect action on cell bodies, axions, and synapses plus the distant effects as the result of axonal transport, metabolism of the material, and behavior of degradation products.

At present the chemical compounds which are being investigated include (41):

1. Neurotransmitters
2. Drugs that inhibit or facilitate (cell body metabolism, conduction, axonal transport, or synaptic behavior)
3. Precursors of neurotransmitters
4. Neuroendocrines
5. Neuronal nutrients
6. Neurotoxins

It is also quite likely that neuroimmunological agents will soon be utilized to exert a considerable effect on the selective enhancement or destruction of CNS structures.

ICV and Spinal Injection of Morphine

Intracerbroventricular (ICV) and spinal injection of morphine have been shown to exert profound control over pain, principally by inhibition of substance P release. For example, 100 μg of morphine injected intrathecally is more effective than 100 mg of morphine given intravenously (40, 42). Even though the typical, undesirable side effects of morphine are not as readily seen, dependency and respiratory depression do occur with prolonged administration of morphine in the CSF. Epidural morphine (reaching the spinal cord by diffusion) likewise requires small doses for prolonged pain relief, as compared to IM or IV administration (3). Direct injections into the ventricular system have also been done showing profound and prolonged pain relief.

The list of compounds being considered for direct injection is presently about the same as that of the neuroactive substances that have been located in the CNS. An additional interesting sidelight of this story is the fact that some antinociceptive compounds produce different effects when injected in larger than physiological quantities into the ICV spaces (*e.g.*, β-endorphin may produce a neuroleptic effect such as rigid immobility) (34). A further interesting effect is the depletion of a neuroactive material by injected compounds; for example, the intrathecal injection of capsacin (a material from hot peppers) produces a depletion of substance P and may therefore produce prolonged pain relief (43). Such effects can be both good and bad but will be the subject of much investigation. Metkephamid, an analog of methionine enkephalin, is more than 100 times as potent as morphine when injected into the ventricles and 50 times more potent on δ-receptors, yet equipotent on μ-receptors (13)! These and other effects will be the subject of much investigation.

Hardware for Chemical Delivery Systems

Techniques involving electrical or chemical stimulation of the CNS depend upon the development and use of devices. It is a general truism that the chemical, physical, and mathematical sciences are roughly about 25 years ahead of their applications in medicine. Therefore, the technology, materials science, and construction techniques exist. The principal problems that remain are the questions of targets, or, "where to go" and their effects, or "what to do when you get there." Devices for searching out targets in the human nervous system are primitive and often ill-constructed. Drug-delivery systems are also still fairly primitive but are moving along. For example, there are several types of pumps which are now available for the continuous or intermittent injection of substances into the ICV or spinal canal (Fig. 32.6.) A few external pumps are available whose rate of delivery is under direct manual or automatic control, plus the dialytrode mentioned earlier. These devices are essentially substitutes for automatic hypodermic injections. More important for the future are the totally implantable drug delivery systems, however. The ones currently available include:

1. The Ommaya reservoir (producing an intermittent delivery of the material by manual pumping)
2. Occlusive pumps (roller or peristaltic producing a constant flow output) (9)
3. The trapped propellant recoil pump (having a chamber of expanding, compressible material pressing against a second chamber containing the drug) (5)

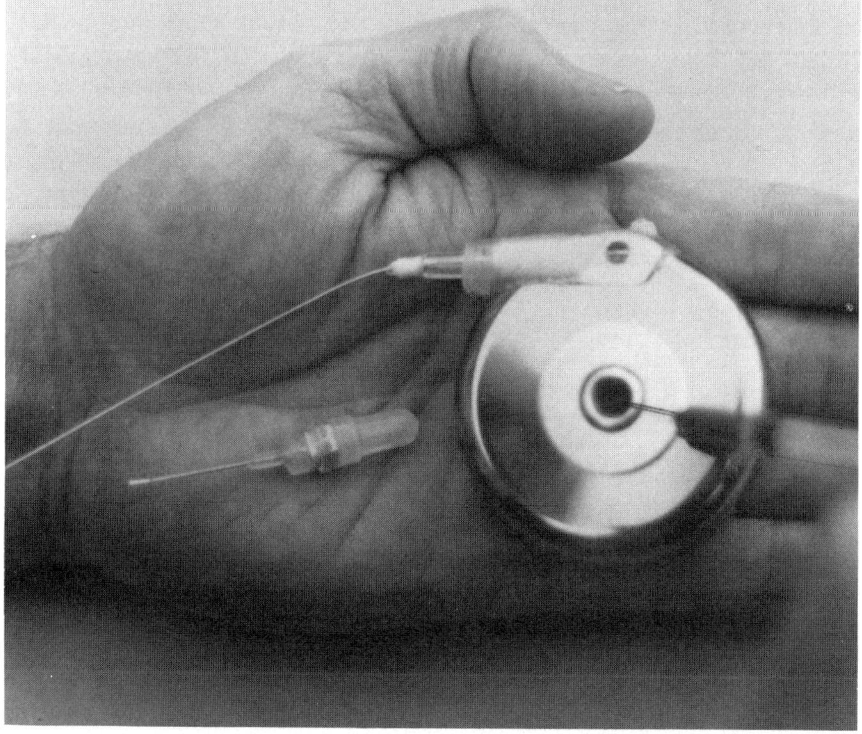

FIG. 32.6. Models of totally implantable drug delivery pump units. Larger (cardiac pacemaker appearing) unit may be roller or diaphragm operated. Long hypodermic needle penetrates rubber seal of reservoir for refilling. Delivery tube has metal coil construction to prevent collapse at bends. Smaller (osmotic minipump type) unit slowly releases drug by osmotic pressure against sealed reservoir chamber. Similar short delivery tube is attached.

4. The osmotic minipump (such as that made by Alza) (8), and
5. Implantable pellets (emitting substance by erosion or by defusion through a polymeric membrane) (20).

We should expect that the future for such devices lies in the development of specific detector transducers,, combined together with a microcomputer and the stimulator or pump, in a totally enclosed device. This system would ideally be able to detect the need for the stimulus or drug, administer it, watch the results, and then adjust subsequent output to accommodate for the effect. Such things have been anticipated by Delgado, Myers, Isaac Asimov, and myself, among many others, for several years. Indeed, at this very meeting, exactly 10 years ago, I gave a paper which in part addressed this very same topic (27). There is only a thin line which divides truth from science fiction here and that line is obviously becoming semipermeable.

Clinical applications of both electrical and chemical stimulation of the CNS for problems other than pain also appear realistic major possibilities. These would include such disorders as: addiction, malignant obesity, hormonal disturbances, memory and alertness, major psychiatric disturbances, movement disorders, and certain elements of rehabilitation of the injured or diseased CNS (15, 21, 22, 36).

REFERENCES

1. Akil, H., Richardson, D. E., Hughes, J., and Barchas, J. D. Enkephalin-like material elevated in ventricular cerebrospinal fluid of pain patients after analgetic focal stimulation. Science, *201:* 463–465, 1978.
2. Almay, B. G. L., Johansson, F., Von Knorring, L., Terenius, L., and Wahlstrom, A. Endorphins in chronic pain. I. Differences in CSF endorphin levels between organic and psychogenic pain syndromes. Pain, *5:* 153–162, 1978.
3. Behar, M., Olshwang, D., Magora, F., and Davidson, J. T. Epidural morphine in treatment of pain. Lancet, *1:* 527–529, 1979.
4. Bishop, B. Pain: Its physiology and rationale for management. Phys. Ther., *60:* 13–37, 1980.
5. Blackshear, P. J. Implantable drug-delivery systems. Sci. Am., *241:* 66–73, 1979.
6. Burton, C. V., Ray, C. D., and Nashold, B. S. (eds.). Symposium on the safety and clinical efficacy of implanted neuroaugmentive devices. Neurosurgery *1:* 185–232, 1977.
7. Burton, C. V. Safety and clinical efficacy of implanted neuroaugmentive spinal devices for the relief of pain. Appl. Neurophysiol., *40:* 175–183, 1978.
8. Capozza, R., Eckenhoff, B., and Yum, S. I. Design and performance of the implantable osmotic minipump. Med. Eng. Tech., *1:* 281–283, 1980.
9. Carlson, G. A., Love, J. T., Urenda, R. S., Spencer, W. J., and Eaton, R. P. A portable insulin infusion system with a rotary solenoid driven peristaltic pump. Med. Prog. Technol., *7:* 1–8, 1980.
10. Cornish, K. G., and Hall, R. E. A modification of the dialytrode for simultaneous CNS recording and chemical stimulation. Pharmacol. Biochem. Behav., *10:* 389–392, 1979.
11. Delgado, J. M. R., DeFeudis, F. V., Roth, R. H., Ryugo, D. K., and Mitruka, B. M. Dialytrode for long term intracerebral perfusion in awake monkeys. Arch. Int. Pharmacodyn. Ther., *198:* 9–21, 1972.

12. Ehrlich, Y. H. Volavka, J., and Brunngraber, E. G. (eds.) Modulators, mediators and specifiers in brain functions. Adv. Exp. Med. Biol., *116,* 1979.
13. Frederickson, R. C. A., Smithwick, E. L., Shuman, R., and Bemis, K. G. Metkephamid: a systemically active analog of methionine enkephalin with potent opioid d-receptor activity. Science, *211:* 603–605, 1981.
14. Goldstein, A. Opioid peptides (endorphins) in pituitary and brain. Science, *193:* 1081–1086, 1976.
15. Guillemin, R. Peptides in the brain: The new endocrinology of the neuron. Science, *202:* 390–402, 1978.
16. Henry, J. L. Substance P and pain: An updating. Trends Neurosci., *3:* 95–97, 1980.
17. Horowitz, P., Grodzins, L., Ladd, W., Ryan, J., Merriam, G., and Lechene, C. Vertebrate central nervous system: Same neurons mediate both electrical and chemical inhibitions. Science, *194:* 1166–1170, 1976.
18. Hosobuchi, Y. The current status of analgesic brain stimulation. Acta Neurochir. (Suppl.), *30:* 79–84, 1980.
19. Kerr, W. L., and Fukushima, T. New observations on the nociceptive pathways in the central nervous system. In: *Pain,* edited by J. J. Bonica. Raven Press, New York, 1980.
20. Kydonieus, A. F. (ed.). *Controlled Release Technologies: Methods, Theory and Applications.* Chemical Rubber Press, Boca Raton, Fa., 1979.
21. Langer, S. Z. Presynaptic receptors and modulation of neurotransmission: Pharmacological implications and therapeutic relevance. Trends Neurosci., *3:* 110–112, 1980.
22. Long, D. M. Current status of neuroaugmentation procedures for chronic pain. Ch 6, pp 51–69. In: *Mechanisms of Pain and Analgesic Compounds,* Chap. 6, pp. 51–69. Raven Press, New York, 1979.
23. Melzack, R., and Wall, P. Pain mechanisms: A new theory. Science, *150:* 971–979, 1965.
24. Myers, R. D. (ed.). *Handbook of Drug and Chemical Stimulation of The Brain.* Van Nostrand Reinhold, New York, 1974.
25. Ranck, J. B., Jr. Which elements are excited in electrical stimulation of mammalian central nervous system: A review. Brain Res., *98:* 417–440, 1975.
26. Rapoport, S. I., Klee, W. A., Pettigrew, K. D., and Ohno, K. Entry of opioid peptides into the central nervous system. Science, *207:* 84–86, 1980.
27. Ray, C. D. New instrumentation for *in vivo* determinations of brain function. Clin. Neurosurg., *18:* 121–154, 1971.
28. Ray, C. D. (ed.). Pain Symposium. Electrical Stimulation of the Human Nervous System for the Control of Pain (monograph). Surg. Neurol., *4:* 61–204, 1975.
29. Ray, C. D. New electrical stimulation methods for therapy and rehabilitation. Orthop. Rev., *6:* 29–39, 1977.
30. Ray, C. D. Neuroaugmentation–Neurostimulation Training Series (audio-visual): ES-2 Electrical stimulation, clinical application for therapy and rehabilitation. P-1 Pain relief through Pisces® System. IP-1 Introduction to pain relief through Pisces® system. PP-1 Relieving your pain with spinal cord stimulation. DBS-1 Pain relief through deep brain stimulation. PDBS-1 Relieving your pain with deep brain stimulation. Sister Kenny Institute, 2727 Chicago Ave., Minneapolis, Minn. 55407. Educational Materials Listing, pp. 2–3, Spring 1980.
31. Ray, C. D., and Burton, C. V. Deep brain stimulation for severe, chronic pain. Acta Neurochir. (Suppl.) *30:* 289–293, 1980.
32. Ray, C. D., Spinal epidural electrical stimulation for pain control: Practical details and results. Appl. Neurophysiol. (to be published, 1981).
33. Richardson, D. E., and Akil, H. Pain reduction by electrical brain stimulation in man (2 parts). J. Neurosurg., *47:* 178–194, 1979.
34. Segal, D. S., Bloom, F., Ling, N., and Guillemin, R. B-endorphin: Endogenous opiate or

neuroleptic? Science, *198:* 411–414, 1977.

35. Shashoua, V. E. Identification of specific changes in the pattern of brain protein synthesis after training. Science, *193:* 1264–1266, 1976.
36. Snyder, S. H. Brain peptides as neurotransmitters. Science, *209:* 976–983, 1980.
37. Swanson, J. M., and Kinsbourne, M. Stimulant-related dependent learning in hyperactive children. Science, *192:* 1354–1357, 1976.
38. Sweet, W. H. Central mechanisms of chronic pain (neuralgias and certain other neurogenic pain). pp 287–303. In: *Pain,* edited by J. J. Bonica. Raven Press, New York, 1980.
39. Vandenbergh, J. G. Behavioral biology. Science, *202:* 623–624, 1978.
40. Wei, E., and Loh, H. Chronic, intracerebral infusion of morphine and peptides with osmotic minipumps, and the development of physical dependence. Presented at the International Narcotics Research Conference, Aberdeen, Scotland, 1976.
41. Wilson, P. R., and Yaksh, T. L. Baclofen is antinociceptive in the spinal intrathecal space of animals. Eur. J. Pharmacol., *51:* 323–330, 1978.
42. Yaksh, T. L., and Rudy, T. A. Analgesia mediated by a direct spinal action of narcotics. Science, *192:* 1357–1358, 1976.
43. Yaksh, T. L., Farb, D. H., Leeman, S. E., and Jessell, T. M. Intrathecal capsaicin depletes substance P in the rat spinal cord and produces prolonged thermal analgesia. Science, *206:* 481–483, 1979.
44. Zimmermann, M. Neurophysiological models for nociception, pain and pain therapy. Adv. Neurosurg., *3:* 199–205, 1975.

CHAPTER

33

Medical and Surgical Management of Spasticity

PAUL C. SHARKEY, M.D.

Spasticity is the Dr. Jekyll and Mr. Hyde of nervous system injury. It may improve vascular flow, maintain muscle bulk and aid in maintaining upright posture; yet, it may interfere with transfer activities, make wheelchair activity almost impossible or contribute to decubitus formation, lead to breakdown of its repair, and mask or prevent retained motor activity progressing to contractures.

Spasticity is the increased muscle tone which is related to the increased rate of sensitivity of the stretch reflex (16). Its clinical presentation depends on the level and the area of the central nervous system (CNS) injury. Its most classic form, and yet most varied presentation, is seen in spinal cord injury. In brain stem injury the picture is that of decerebration whereas spasticity as a result of involvement at a hemispheric or subhemispheric level shows some dystonic features.

In spinal cord injury, flexor spasm is more frequent than extensor spasm and is seen earlier after injury. It increases in severity during the first year. Cerebral and brain stem spasticity occur earlier than spinal cord spasticity.

There was a time when spasticity was accepted as the price of nervous system injury, and physician apathy in treatment made it appear unworthy of vigorous therapy, but with the development of rehabilitation medicine and restorative neurology, the problem is being increasingly studied and more vigorously treated.

When comparing the treatment of spinal cord spasticity and its cerebral counterpart, some features are noted. As segmental hypertonia is removed and controlled on a cerebral basis, more of the extrapyramidal component, in the broadest sense, is revealed. Tone may be modified but not the postural abnormality. In general, hemiplegia is a more complex motor disorder and spinal cord injury is a less complex one.

There are a number of general principles that should be considered

Support for this work was provided by the Bob and Vivian Smith Foundation, Houston, Texas, and by Rehabilitation Services Administration, Grants 13-P-59275-6 and 16-P-56813-6, Department of Health, Education and Welfare, Washington, D.C.

and evaluated before and during treatment of spasticity. These principles are:

1. Whether the lesion is complete or incomplete
2. The age of the injury
3. The patient's age and general medical status
4. Whether the spasticity is segmental (focal) or more generalized
5. If a patient has poor volitional strength but considerable spasticity, he may use this spasticity to brace his legs so that he can walk; therefore, if an agent or technique is used that would decrease his spasticity, his ability to stand or walk may be altered
6. If the patient has good volitional strength which can't be used effectively because of spasticity, he would benefit from its modification
7. When spasm is stabilized and then becomes more severe, look for aggravating circumstances such as infections of the genitourinary (GU) system, fistula of penis or scrotum, decubitus ulcers; kidney or bladder stone and fecal impactions
8. Selective reduction or relief of spasticity is frequently needed to improve daily living activities and to treat some of the side effects of spasticity
9. When the need arises to carry out a more drastic (destructive) form of treatment, the patient and the surgeon are often reluctant to proceed. In these circumstances it is often useful to use a long-lasting local agent or weak solution of phenol or alcohol to mimic the expected result so the patient is given the opportunity to see and evaluate the effect. This often makes it easier for him to accept the procedure. In general, this is followed by a local selective treatment directed at the increased excitability of the motor cell.

Considerable assistance in selection of the best procedure is obtained by ischemic testing. This consists of a pneumatic cuff with pressure raised above systolic blood pressure for 20 minutes. It is during the later 10 minutes that hypertonia is gone and the patient is examined (16).

When we reduce the various means of treatment of spasticity to the simplest groupings, there are four basic approaches:

1. Physical therapy with its techniques and adjuncts
2. Pharmacologic treatment
3. Surgery, including the injection of chemical agents
4. Physiologic, including functional peroneal electrical stimulation (FES), spinal cord and cerebellar stimulation (SCS and CS), and biofeedback.

Treatment begins immediately after the CNS injury and precedes appearance of spasticity.

From the onset, sensitive and thoughtful nursing care is directed at prevention of bladder and bowel overdistention, prevention of pain where externally correctable, maintenance of comfortable temperatures, skin care, avoidance of rough handling, and proper positioning of extremities.

Physical therapy is important in the patient's management throughout his life, utilizing active and passive range of movements of all extremities along with indicated adjuncts such as cryotherapy, vibration and electrical stimulation of muscle to assist in obtaining maximal mobility, and supporting and maintaining any useful motor function remaining. The patient and his family are carefully trained in these techniques for continued use at home.

In association with physical therapy, as the effects of spasticity increase the various pharmacologic agents are used. They are more effective in mild to moderate spasticity and of little or no value in the severe state where toxic effects and obtundation from large doses may be seen.

Diazepam (Valium), baclofen (Lioresal), and Dantrolene sodium (Dantrium) are the main drugs in vogue at present (20–22, 27, 33–35). Drugs are somewhat limited in their useful effect because of the varied degree of impairment of different muscle groups and the fairly diffuse and equal action of these medications along with their lack of specificity. For example, in treating phasic spasticity in ambulatory patients with multiple sclerosis, these drugs are often not helpful since they do not decrease weakness, incoordination, ataxia, and fatigue (16). They are more helpful in treatment of spinal cord spasticity. All of these drugs have undesirable side effects, most of which are dose related.

Frequently these measures are inadequate for the satisfactory treatment of this problem and require other means to remedy the situation. Whether the patient is ambulatory or nonambulatory will enter into the decision as to what measures must be utilized. Usually, surgical treatment starts at the periphery with selection of the simplest and least destructive procedures. Often, satisfactory selective decrease in spasticity can be accomplished by partial block of a peripheral nerve with 6% aqueous phenol (26, 30). If a more localized block is desired, motor point blocks can be utilized (38). The motor point or nerve trunk is located first by skin stimulation with a square wave current of short duration (0.1 to 0.5 millisec) and then with an insulated needle through which injection of the blocking agent is performed.

Patients who are nonambulatory showing severe spasticity and flexor spasm with or without contracture may require chemical rhizotomy with phenol or alcohol (25, 32, 36). The use of phenol with glycerin has some advantage since the combination of drugs is hyperbaric and may be used in varying strengths ranging from 2 to 20%. This allows a more selective lesion to be made in the cauda equina that lasts from a few days or weeks up to a more permanent result, depending on the drug concentration. By this technique bowel, bladder, and penile erection, if present, can usually be spared. To use this procedure properly, each side must be done individually about 1 week apart. The use of absolute alcohol by the caudal bubble technique is very effective and is a one-stage procedure, but it should be used in the patient with severe spasms, contractures, complete absence of bowel and bladder control, and no penile erection (4). This will also control the dysreflexic syndrome. Some male patients are hesitant to proceed with chemical rhizotomy because of the loss of penile erection; this can be compensated for satisfactorily by one of the implantation procedures. This approach to spasticity control has some advantage in patients with multiple slcerosis who are apt to exacerbate following anesthesia and surgery (1).

More drastic surgical procedures have been designed to control severe spasms (41). Posterior and anterior rhizotomies were early attempts at control (18, 31). Only the anterior rhizotomy, sparing S-2,3, is still occasionally done. Anterior rhizotomy is a useful procedure for treatment of spasticity of spinal cord and brainstem origin, but not for the treatment of spasticity after stroke, cerebral palsy, and multiple sclerosis. Interest in this area continues, as evidenced by a number of reports on these modified approaches. These include selective thermal radiofrequency posterior sensory rhizotomy, partial posterior rootlet section, sectorial posterior rhizotomy, and posterior rhizotomy, in which each of the appropriate rootlets is partially sectioned under magnification (19).

A number of useful procedures were developed for controlling severe spasticity that were designed to separate the sensory from the motor output from the spinal cord. The earliest myelotomy consisted of equatorial section of the spinal cord, either a single incision from one side through 2/3 to 3/4 of the cord diameter or incisions directed from the periphery of the cord towards the central canal (2, 3, 24).

T-myelotomy and T-griseotomy were introduced and had the advantage that the motor system was preserved and the procedure was less destructive. Several modifications of this procedure have recently been offered which are better controlled, done with the microscope, and less disturbing of the remaining cord anatomy. Another approach utilized an incision between the dorsal horn of the spinal cord and the lateral corticospinal tract, preserving existing motor activity (42).

An occasional paraplegic patient who has useful extension overridden by flexor spasms precipitated by sensory stimuli can be benefited by sectioning the lateral femoral cutaneous nerve of the thigh, sensory branches of the femoral nerve, and the femoral branch of the genitofemoral nerve. Sural nerve section is also occasionally done (15).

In recent years, the physiologic approach to control of spasticity has evolved and offered nondestructive methods that utilize sensory input to further modify the nervous system responses (10, 11, 14). These methods are functional electrical stimulation of peripheral nerves (12, 28, 29), cerebellar stimulation (7, 8) and, recently, widely applied spinal cord stimulation (5, 6, 9, 17, 23, 27, 37, 40, 43).

In ambulatory patients who show an extensor thrust pattern and have ankle clonus, the use of FES will modify their spastic foot drop and their clonus (12, 13, 39). This system, which is entirely external, is based on augmentation of the physiologic mechanisms that can modify clonus. Ankle clonus or more widespread clonus and extensor spasms are also effectively controlled through spinal cord stimulation with epidural electrodes (11).

Patients who are sent to the Restorative Neurology Clinic for evaluation and treatment of spasticity are carefully screened and then the proper procedure is selected.

The protocol for the selection and study of candidates for spinal stimulation consists of the following (5):

1) Confirmation of the clinical diagnosis, including the course of the disease or injury and its recovery.
2) Evaluation of patient's general physical condition
3) Neurophysiologic evaluation of long loop reflexes, long ascending, and other sensory functions and postural and volitional brain influences on segmental reflexes. These are carried out by somatosensory visual and auditory evoked potentials, polyelectromyography, electrospinography, selective EMG studies, and EEG. These procedures are done to outline neural control mechanisms existing in the pathologic condition. It is necessary that potential candidates show an underlying neural control mechanism that can be augmented with additional input to the posterior columns of the spinal cord.
4) If these examinations qualify the patient as a potential candidate for spinal cord stimulation, temporary stimulating electrodes are placed and externalized for a 7 to 10-day test period.
5) If the effects of stimulation are beneficial as judged by the team and the patient, and the candidate is in a position to utilize improvement in motor control, then the system is implanted.
6) After the implantation the patients are started back on an

active physical therapy program, especially for the first month after implantation. They are seen at regular intervals for clinical follow-up, including functional and neurological evaluation, neurophysiological testing, and biomedical follow-up and mapping.

In the last 2 years 129 patients were referred to our program for treatment of spasticity. We have evaluated 83 patients with chronic spinal cord pathology, 23 patients with multiple sclerosis, 21 patients with head injury, and 2 patients with familial spastic paraplegia.

The spinal cord injury group consisted of 74 patients with the lesion between C-2 and T-11 level (65 males and 9 females). Their age at the time of the injury was from 5 to 64 years and they were seen 1 to 15 years after the injury. Sixty-seven of these patients had pure spinal cord injury and seven had combined spinal cord and head injuries. They are divided into 38 complete and 36 clinically incomplete lesions. Among the latter group, four additional neurological syndromes were seen: diffuse (affecting only portions of ascending, descending, and propriospinal neuronal elements) in 17 patients, and 19 circumscribed lesions, showing predominantly hemisection, anterior, and posterior syndromes.

From the 74 spinal cord-injured patients, 30 who had phasic spasticity were treated by short-term procedures such as medication, physical therapy, biofeedback training, and functional electrical stimulation. Forty-four patients had mainly tonic type spasticity interfering with their activity who required surgical procedures, including 19 who were treated with spinal cord stimulation.

Spasticity will continue to be a challenging treatment problem, but it is anticipated that increasing effort will be directed towards the neural control causing spasticity, developing treatment that will use these remaining neural mechanisms to control this problem.

This is an ongoing problem throughout the life of the patient, and its successful and useful conclusion, allowing the patient improved function, is a reward unto itself.

REFERENCES

1. Bamford, C., Sibley, W., and Laguna, J. Anesthesia in multiple sclerosis. Can. J. Neurol. Sci., *5:* 41–44, 1978.
2. Bischof, W. Die longitudinale Myelotomie. Zentralbl. Neurochir. *11:* 79–88, 1951.
3. Bischof, W. Zur dorsalen longitudinalen Myelotomie. Zentralbl. Neurochir., *28:* 123–126, 1967.
4. Bradford, K. The use of a caudal air bubble in the control of alcohol injection to relieve flexion reflexes. J. Neurosurg., *16:* 468–470, 1959.
5. Campos, R., Dimitrijevic, M., Faganel, J., and Sharkey, P. Clinical evaluation of the effect of spinal cord stimulation on motor performance in patients with upper motor neurone lesions. Appl. Neurophysiol., in press, 1980.

6. Cook, A., and Weinstein, S. Chronic dorsal column stimulation in multiple sclerosis. N. Y. State J. Med., *73:* 2868–2872, 1973.
7. Cooper, I., Amin, I., Gilman, S., and Waltz, J. The effect of chronic stimulation of cerebellar cortex on epilepsy in man. *In* The Cerebellum, Epilepsy and Behavior, edited by I. Cooper, M. Riklan, and R. Snider, pp. 119–171. Plenum Press, New York, 1974.
8. Cooper, I., Crighel, E., and Amin, I. Clinical and physiological effects of stimulation of the paleocerebellum in humans. J. Am Geriat. Soc., *21:* 40–43, 1973.
9. Davis, R., Flitter, M., and Bolton, D. Clinical efficacy and safety of chronic spinal stimulation used in multiple sclerosis and other demyelinating diseases. *In* Advances in External Control of Human Extremities, Yugoslav Committee for ETAN, pp. 557–569, 1978
10. Dimitrijevic, M. R. Use of physiological mechanisms in the electrical control of paralyzed extremities. V. External control of human extremities, pp. 27–41. Yugoslav Committee for Electronics and Automation, Belgrade, Yugoslavia, 1967.
11. Dimitrijevic, M. R., Dimitrijevic, M. M., Faganel, J., and Sharkey, P. Neurophysiological evaluation of chronic spinal cord stimulation in patients with upper motor neuron disorders. Int. Rehabil. Med., *2:* 82–85, 1980.
12. Dimitrijevic, M. R., and Gracanin, F. Control of release phenomena in hemiplegics by means of afferent electrical stimulation. Electroencephalogr. Clin. Neurophysiol., *25:* 395, 1968.
13. Dimitrijevic, M. R., Gracanin, F., and Prevec, T., *et al.* An "anticlonus" model. In Digest of the 7th International Conference on Medical and Biological Engineering, p. 196. Stockholm, Sweden, 1967.
14. Dimitrijevic, M. R., and Lenman, J. Neural control of gait in patients with upper motor neuron lesions. In: Spasticity: Disordered Motor Control, edited by R. Feldman *et al.*, pp. 110–114. Year Book Medical Publisher, Chicago, 1980.
15. Dimitrijevic, M. R., Sharkey, P., and Sherwood, A. Vibratory reflex response in spinal cord injury patients after cutaneous deafferentiation. Electroencephalogr. Clin. Neurophysiol., *43:* 622, 1977.
16. Dimitrijevic, M., and Sherwood, A. Spasticity: medical and surgical treatment. Neurology, *30*(2)*:* 19–27, 1980.
17. Dooley, D., and Sharkey, J. Electrostimulation of the nervous system for patients with demyelinating and degenerative diseases of the nervous system and vascular diseases of the extremities. Appl. Neurophysiol., *40:* 208–217, 1977/78.
18. Förster, O. Ueber eine neue operative Methode der Behandlung spastischer Lahmungen mittels Resektion hinterer Ruckenmarkswurzeln. Z. Orthop. Chir., *22:* 202, 1918.
19. Fraioli, B., and Guidetti, B. Posterior partial rootlet section in treatment of spasticity. J. Neurosurg., *46:* 618–626, 1977.
20. From, A. A doule-blind trial with baclofen (Lioresal) and diazepam in spasticity due to multiple sclerosis. Acta. Neurol. Scand., *51:* 158–166, 1975.
21. Glass, A., and Hannah, A. A comparison of dantrolene sodium and diazepam in the treatment of spasticity. Paraplegia, *12:* 170–174, 1974.
22. Haslam, R., Walcher, J., Lietman, P., Kallman, C., and Mellits, E. Dantrolene sodium in children with spasticity. Arch. Phys. Med. Rehabil., *55:* 384–392, 1974.
23. Illis, L., Sedgwick, E., and Tallis, R. Spinal cord stimulation in multiple sclerosis: clinical results. J. Neurol. Neurosurg. Psychiatry, *43:* 1–14, 1980.
24. Ivan, L., and Wiley, J. Myelotomy in the management of spasticity. Clin. Orthop., *108:* 52–56, 1975.
25. Kelly, R., and Gauthier-Smith, P. Intrathecal phenol in the treatment of reflex spasms and spasticity. Lancet, *2:* 1103–1105, 1959.

26. Khalili, A., Harmel, M., Forster, S., and Benton, J. Management of spasticity by selective peripheral nerve block in clinical rehabilitation. Arch. Phys. Med. Rehabil., *45:* 513–519, 1964.
27. Ladd, H., Oist, C., and Jonsson, B. The effect of Dantrium on spasticity in multiple sclerosis. Acta. Neurol. Scand., *50:* 397–408, 1974.
28. Levine, M., Knott, M., and Kabat, H. Relaxation of spasticity by electrical stimulation of antagonist muscles. Arch. Phys. Med. Rehabil., *33:* 668–673, 1952.
29. Liberson, W. Experiment concerning reciprocal inhibition of antagonists elicited by electrical stimulation of antagonists in a normal individual. Am. J. Phys. Med., *44:* 306–308, 1965.
30. Mooney, W., Frykam, G., and McLamb, J. Current status of intraneural phenol injections. Clin. Orthop., *63:* 122–131, 1969.
31. Munro, D. The rehabilitation of patients totally paralyzed below the waist with special reference to making them ambulatory and capable of earning their living. I. Anterior rhizotomy for spastic paraplegia. N. Engl. J. Med., *233:* 453, 1945.
32. Nathan, P. Intrathecal phenol to relieve spasticity in paraplegia. Lancet, *2:* 1099–1102, 1959.
33. Nathan, P. The action of diazepam in neurological disorders with excessive motor activity. J. Neurol. Sci., *10:* 33–50, 1970.
34. Paeslack, V. Lioresal in the treatment of spinal spasticity. Postgrad. Med. J., *48*(Suppl. 5)*:* 30–34, 1972.
35. Schlapfer, U., and Mumenthaler, M. Klinische Prüfung der muskelrelaxierenden Wirkung von Valium Roche bei Spastikern. Schweiz. Med. Wochenschr., *94:* 1425–1431, 1964.
36. Sehlden, C., and Bors, E. Subarachnoid alcohol block in paraplegia, its beneficial effect on mass reflexes and bladder dysfunction. J. Neurosurg., *5:* 385, 1948.
37. Siegfried, J., Krainick, J., Haas, H., Adorjani, C., Meyer, M., and Thoden, U. Electrical spinal cord stimulation for spastic movement disorders. Appl. Neurophysiol., *41:* 134–141, 1978.
38. Tardieu, C., Tardieu, G., Hariga, J., Gagnard, L., and Velin, J. Treatment of spasticity by injection of dilute alcohol at the motor point or by epidural route. Dev. Med. Child Neurol., *10:* 555–568, 1968.
39. Vodovnik, L., Kralj, A., and Stanic, U., *et al.* Recent applications of functional electrical stimulation to stroke patients in Ljubljana. Clin. Orthop., *131:* 64–70, 1978.
40. Waltz, J. Spinal cord stimulation for palsies? Patient Care, *13:* 118–206, 1979.
41. Yamada, S., and Mitchell, C. Control of mass spasms in paraplegia. South Med. J., *62:* 745–748, 1969.
42. Yamada, S., Perot, P., and Ducker, T., *et al.* Myelotomy for control of mass spasms in paraplegia. J. Neurosurg., *45:* 683–691, 1976.
43. Young, R., and Goodman, S. Dorsal spinal cord stimulation in the treatment of multiple sclerosis. Neurosurgery, *5:* 225–228, 1979.

Index

C

E

M